Clinical Applications of Nuclear Medicine Targeted Therapy

Emilio Bombardieri
Ettore Seregni
Laura Evangelista
Carlo Chiesa
Arturo Chiti
Editors

Clinical Applications of Nuclear Medicine Targeted Therapy

Springer

Editors
Emilio Bombardieri
Department of Nuclear Medicine
Humanitas Gavazzeni Hospital
Bergamo
Italy

Laura Evangelista
Nuclear Medicine and Molecular
Imaging Unit
Veneto Institute of Oncology IOV - IRCCS
Padova
Italy

Arturo Chiti
Nuclear Medicine
Humanitas Research Hospital
Rozzano
Milano
Italy

Ettore Seregni
Nuclear Medicine Therapy and
Endocrinology
Istituto Nazionale dei Tumori
Milano
Italy

Carlo Chiesa
Nuclear Medicine Division
Istituto Nazionale dei Tumori
Milano
Italy

ISBN 978-3-030-09684-7 ISBN 978-3-319-63067-0 (eBook)
https://doi.org/10.1007/978-3-319-63067-0

Softcover re-print of the Hardcover 1st edition 2018

Printed on acid-free paper

This Springer imprint is published by the registered company Springer International Publishing AG part of Springer Nature
The registered company address is: Gewerbestrasse 11, 6330 Cham, Switzerland

Foreword

For many decades, nuclear medicine targeted therapy or targeted systemic radiotherapy has been one of the cornerstones of Nuclear Medicine, exploiting the synergy between molecular imaging and the subsequent treatment of patients. This so called theranostic approach capitalizes the unique opportunities provided by pretreatment molecular imaging to determine the targeting of areas of interest (tumors, hyperfunctioning thyroid, etc.) and to assess the pharmacokinetics and biodistribution of radiopharmaceuticals. Thus, nuclear medicine therapy is a perfect example of individualized, precision medicine. Before exposing the patient to a therapeutic radiopharmaceutical, the disease and disease burden have been characterized, the chances for a beneficial result of treatment have been estimated and an optimal dose has been calculated

In *Clinical Applications of Nuclear Medicine Targeted Therapy*, edited by Emilio Bombardieri, Ettore Seregni, Laura Evangelista, Carlo Chiesa, Arturo Chiti, a comprehensive overview of established and novel nuclear medicine treatments is provided, mainly focusing on treatment of cancer patients. The book covers treatment of thyroid cancer with I-131, which has an unrivaled track record for patient cure for more than 75 years in an adjuvant and even in a metastatic setting. This book also provides a wealth of information and knowledge on more recent advances in nuclear medicine therapy, ranging from local treatment of hepatic metastases to systemic treatment of neuroendocrine tumors and malignant lymphoma. Of special interest is the variety of novel options for treatment of patients with metastatic prostate cancer, of which some are already widely available and used, while others are still experimental, yet highly promising to provide a significant contribution to better patient outcomes with minimal treatment-induced impact on the patients' quality of life.

Clinical Applications of Nuclear Medicine Targeted Therapy is a must-read for nuclear medicine physicians, practicing therapeutic nuclear medicine, but also highly recommended for all healthcare professionals, treating patients for whom nuclear medicine therapies are available.

Professor Wim J.G. Oyen
Professor of Nuclear Medicine and Molecular Imaging
The Institute of Cancer Research
and The Royal Marsden Hospital,
London, UK

June 2017

Preface

In spite of different experimental radiolabelled compounds for the radioisotope therapy developed and studied over the years, at present the current treatment for targeted therapies includes few clinical indications: 1-radioiodine therapy for thyroid cancer and some condition of hyperthyroidisms, 2-radionuclide microembolization with resin or glass microspheres for hepatic primary and secondary cancer, 3-radiolabelled metaiodiobenzylguanidine in neuroblastomas and pheocromocitomas, 4-radiopeptide therapy for gastrointestinal neuroendocrine tumors, 5-bone seeking radiopharmaceuticals for skeletal localizations and 6-radiolabelled antibodies in lymphomas.

The above mentioned applications have provided a very interesting improvements in patient management. However, until now, the growth of radionuclide therapies in Nuclear Medicine has been limited. The overall results, reported by many Authors in the literature, are encouraging and justify their clinical use, but different problems affect the wide diffusion of this kind of treatments.

Some conditions make difficult the diffusion and execution of radioisotope therapy, such as the request of isolated and shielded rooms for patient radiation protection, not always available; the various activities of radiopharmaceuticals given to the patients that sometimes result heterogeneous, because chosen according to an empiric experience; and the dosimetric approaches to calculate the optimal individual doses that are not always performed in the clinical practice, thus rendering the treatments not completely optimised in terms of dose distribution and efficacy.

The current clinical evidences for radioisotope therapy have been obtained worldwide in many series of patients, but mainly through retrospective studies. Perspectives controlled clinical trials able to validate the efficacy of these treatments in several indications are still missing. These objective limitations are translated into low clinical evidences reported in the current International Guidelines, thus the intrinsic clinical value of radioisotope therapy does not seem always recognized, or it is underestimated.

Nowadays, in our opinion, there are a lot of signals that radionuclide therapy is going to face a new era for growing up and being more successful. The main positive points are both the development and production of many alternative radiolabelled targeted carriers (peptides, nano and affibodies, engineered molecules) and the employment of alpha-emitters that offer many advantages of efficacy compared to beta-emitting radionuclides. The increasing introduction of dosimetric approaches is another important issue allowing to perform the internal dosimetry as a guide to optimize the calculation of the activity for the individual target in each treated patient. The advancement of technologies based on fusion imaging (such as SPECT/CT, PET/CT, PET/MRI) is able to provide better quantitative images that should be integrated in the dosimetric procedures, and new emerging theranostic radiopharmaceuticals that bring the main advantage to be applied both for diagnostic and therapeutic purpose in order to kill the tumor with minimal changes in the molecular structure. In summary, we think that radioisotope therapy will find a large space of development and is on the right way to enlarge its horizons.

This book wants to be the picture of the current situation of radioisotope therapy in the clinical practice, aiming to describe what are the established indications, the standardized procedures and the available results. Each chapter presents a general overview of the pathologies that can be treated by radioisotope therapy, and the radiopharmaceuticals that can be used by describing their biodistribution and the mechanism of action. The book provides particular attention to the operative approaches of radioisotope therapy, such as patients' preparation, pre-treatment evaluation, radionuclide administration, and the evaluation of treatment response. The dosimetric procedures are well described, taking into account the most practical aspect and the way for the calculation of optimal activity. The clinical and practical Guidelines, published by the most relevant Scientific Societies, are schematically illustrated by reporting the recommendations about radioisotope therapy based on the literature evidences. In order to enrich the content of the book, some interesting perspectives of new applications for radioisotope therapy have been added in the last part.

In conclusion, the Editors hope that the content of the book will be useful for the reader to better understand the current practical aspects and the clinical indications of radioisotope therapy. In the same time the Editors desire to leave the message that radioisotope therapy is still a "developing modality". In fact, many improvements are expected in the next future in terms of new clinical indications (novel radiopharmaceuticals), integrated procedures (by including systematic dosimetric approaches and association of radioisotopic with other non-radioisotopic treatments), and also new clinical studies (new prospective clinical trials should be encouraged).

Emilio Bombardieri
Ettore Seregni
Laura Evangelista
Carlo Chiesa
Arturo Chiti

Acknowledgments

The Editors are grateful to Ms Anna Luisa De Simone Sorrentino (Milano) for her precious collaboration in connecting Authors and assisting Authors in preparing manuscripts.

Contents

Part I Thyroid Disease

1 **Diagnosis and Treatment of Hyperthyroidism** 3
Rosa Miranda Testa, Silvia Martinelli, and Furio Pacini

2 **Radiopharmaceuticals for Therapy of Thyroid Diseases** 19
Katia Marzo

3 **Radioiodine Therapy of Hyperthyroidism** 25
Giovanna Pepe and Gennaro Cusato

4 **Dosimetry in the Radioiodine Treatment of Hyperthyroidism** 33
Cristina Canzi and Antonio Claudio Traino

5 **New Approaches in the Management of Thyroid Cancer** 45
Savvas Frangos and Ioannis Iakovou

6 **Radioiodine Therapy of Thyroid Cancer** 59
Ettore Seregni, Alice Lorenzoni, and Laura Fugazzola

7 **Radioiodine Therapy of Thyroid Cancer Dosimetry** 69
Lorenzo Bianchi

8 **Published Guidelines on Radioisotopic Treatments of Thyroid Diseases** 77
Lucia Setti, Vicinelli Riccardo, Gianluigi Ciocia, Emilio Bombardieri, and Laura Evangelista

Part II Hepatic Cancer

9 **Clinical Options for Treatment of Hepatocellular Carcinoma** 95
Matteo Virdis, Michela Monteleone, Michele Droz dit Busset, and Vincenzo Mazzaferro

10 **Medical Devices for Radioembolization** 107
Anna Bogni and Claudio Pascali

11 HCC Radioembolization with Yttrium-90 Glass Microspheres (TheraSphere) 119
Marco Maccauro, Gianluca Aliberti, Carlo Chiesa, and Carlo Spreafico

12 HCC Radioembolization with Yttrium-90 Polymer Beads (SIR-Spheres) 127
Marcello Rodari and Riccardo Muglia

13 Dosimetry in the Treatment of Liver Malignancies with Microspheres 137
Carlo Chiesa

14 The Clinical Challenge of Liver Metastasis 153
Stefano Cappato, Federica Brena, Michela Squadroni, Rosalba Barile, Davide Piccinali, Annalisa Mancin, Giorgio Quartierini, Orlando Goletti, and Giordano Beretta

15 Radioembolization of Hepatic Metastases with ^{90}Y-Microspheres: Indications and Procedure 165
Rosa Sciuto, Sandra Rea, Giuseppe Pizzi, Giulio E. Vallati, and Lidia Strigari

16 Guidelines on Radioisotope Treatment of Liver Cancer and Liver Metastases with Intra-arterial Radioactive Compounds 199
Murat Fani Bozkurt and Laura Evangelista

Part III Neuroendocrine Tumors

17 Radiopharmaceuticals for Treatment of NETs 207
Mattia Asti, Michele Iori, Pier Cesare Capponi, and Sara Rubagotti

18 Paediatric Tumours of Neuroendocrine/Peripheral Neuroectodermal Origin 235
Roberto Luksch, Carlo Chiesa, Ettore Seregni, Carlo Morosi, Marta Podda, Davide Biasoni, Gemma Gatta, Lorenza Gandola, Paola Collini, Paolo Scanagatta, Giovanna Riccipetitoni, Nadia Puma, and Maria Rita Castellani

19 Treatment with ^{131}I-mIBG (Metaiodobenzylguanidine): Indications, Procedures, and Results 253
Maria Rita Castellani, Antonio Scarale, Alice Lorenzoni, Marco Maccauro, Julia Balaguer Guill, and Roberto Luksch

20 Dosimetry for ^{131}I mIBG Therapy 273
Carlo Chiesa and Glenn Flux

21 Medical Treatment of Gastroenteropancreatic (GEP) Neuroendocrine Tumors 281
Carlo Carnaghi and Valeria Smiroldo

22 PRRT with Radiolabeled Peptides: Indications, Procedures, and Results . . . 289
Ettore Seregni and Alice Lorenzoni

23 Dosimetry in PRRT . . . 297
Marta Cremonesi, Mahila Ferrari, and Francesca Botta

24 Guidelines on Radioisotope Treatment of Neuroendocrine Tumors . . . 315
Federico Caobelli and Laura Evangelista

Part IV Prostate Cancer

25 Bone Metastases in Prostate Cancer . . . 323
Maria Bonomi, Eleonora Cerchiaro, Elisa Villa, Lucia Rebecca Setti, Letizia Gianoncelli, Emanuele Micheli, and Giovanni Luca Ceresoli

26 Radiopharmaceuticals for Bone Metastases . . . 345
Benedetta Pagano and Sergio Baldari

27 Targeted Therapy with Radium-223 of Bone Metastases . . . 365
Sergio Baldari, Alessandro Sindoni, Laura Evangelista, and Emilio Bombardieri

28 Novel Approaches of Treatment with Radium-223 Targeted Therapy . . . 379
Giovanni Luca Ceresoli, Letizia Gianoncelli, Maria Bonomi, Eleonora Cerchiaro, and Emilio Bombardieri

29 Dosimetry . . . 393
Massimiliano Pacilio, Elisabetta Verdolino, Bartolomeo Cassano, and Giuseppe De Vincentis

30 Guidelines on Radioisotope Treatment of Bone Metastases in Prostate Cancer . . . 405
Robert Murphy and Laura Evangelista

Part V Lymphomas

31 Radioimmunotherapy of Lymphomas . . . 417
Stefano Luminari, Silvia Morbelli, Lucia Garaboldi, Mahila Esmeralda Ferrari, and Alberto Biggi

32 Radioimmunotherapy in the Transplant Setting . . . 431
Liliana Devizzi

33 Guidelines on Radioisotope Treatment of Lymphomas . . . 443
Mariapaola Cucinotta and Laura Evangelista

Part VI New Approaches of Radiometabolic Therapy

34 PSMA-Based Therapy of Metastasized Castrate-Resistant Prostate Cancer . . . 451
Sarah Marie Schwarzenböck, Jens Kurth, Sascha Nitsch, and Bernd Joachim Krause

35 Locoregional Treatment of Brain Tumors . . . 465
Jolanta Kunikowska, Alfred Morgenstern, Frank Bruchertseifer, and Leszek Krolicki

36 CXCR4-Directed Endoradiotherapy as New Treatment Option in Advanced Multiple Myeloma . . . 475
Constantin Lapa, K. Martin Kortüm, and Ken Herrmann

37 Radiolabeled Somatostatin Analogues in the Treatment of Non-GEP-NET Tumors . . . 483
Annibale Versari, Angelina Filice, Massimiliano Casali, Martina Sollini, and Andrea Frasoldati

Part I

Thyroid Disease

1 Diagnosis and Treatment of Hyperthyroidism

Rosa Miranda Testa, Silvia Martinelli, and Furio Pacini

Abstract

This chapter deals with the current management of patients presenting with an excess of circulating thyroid hormones. This condition is known under two different words: hyperthyroidism and thyrotoxicosis describing two distinct pathologic conditions that should be recognized at diagnosis because they have a different natural history and may have different therapeutic approaches. The hypertiroidism indicates a condition determined by an excessive synthesis of thyroid hormones by the thyroid tissue, any cause. In the United States hyperthyroidism has a prevalence of approximately 1.2% of the population. The most common cause is Graves' disease (GD), followed by toxic nodular goiter, whose prevalence increases with age, particularly in the regions of iodine deficiency, or single hyperfunctioning thyroid adenoma (Plummer's adenoma) and, more rarely a TSH-producing pituitary adenoma. The thyrotoxicosis reflects any medical condition associated with high levels of thyroid hormones in the blood, secondary to destructive process of the thyroid or caused by improper intake of drugs or supplements containing thyroid hormones. In this manuscript the Authors report the main important condition of of hyperthyroidism and thyreotoxicosis, the current approaches for their diagnosis, and the options for the treatment of patients (medical treatments, radioisotopic treatment). The most important drugs used in the clinical practice are examined, and some clinical recommendations before particular treatments are reported.

R.M. Testa (✉) • S. Martinelli
Department of Endocrinology, Humanitas Gavazzeni, Bergamo, Italy
e-mail: rosa.testa@gavazzeni.it

F. Pacini
Department of Medical, Surgical and Neurological Sciences, University of Siena, Siena, Italy

E. Bombardieri et al. (eds.), *Clinical Applications of Nuclear Medicine Targeted Therapy*,
https://doi.org/10.1007/978-3-319-63067-0_1

1.1 Introduction

The diagnosis and treatment of patients presenting with an excess of circulating thyroid hormones will be treated in this chapter. The excess of serum thyroid hormones (defined as hyperthyroidism and thyrotoxicosis) may depend on two distinct pathologic conditions that must be immediately recognized at diagnosis because they have a different natural history and they may have a different therapeutic approach. The word hypertiroidism indicates a condition determined by an increased synthesis of thyroid hormones by the thyroid gland, any cause. In the United States hyperthyroidism has a prevalence of approximately 1.2% of the population (0.5% subclinical, 0.7% overt). The most common cause is Graves' disease (GD), followed by toxic Nodular goiter (TMNG) whose prevalence increases with age, particularly in the regions of iodine deficiency, or single hyperfunctioning thyroid adenoma (Plummer's adenoma) and, more rarely, a TSH-producing pituitary adenoma. The word thyrotoxicosis is used to indicate any medical condition associated with high levels of thyroid hormones in the blood, secondary to destructive process of the thyroid or caused by improper intake of drugs or supplements containing thyroid hormones. The common conditions of hyperthyroidism and thyreotoxicosis are described in Table 1.1.

Table 1.1 Causes of excess of thyroid hormones

Conditions of hyperthyroidism	Conditions of thyrotoxicosis
Graves' disease	Amiodarone-induced thyrotoxicosis
Toxic nodular goiter	De Quervain's thyroiditis
HCG-induced gestational hyperthyroidism	Silent or painless thyroiditis (postpartum thyroiditis, drug-induced thyroiditis, hashitoxicosis)
Thyroid-stimulating hormone (TSH)-secreting pituitary adenomas	Factitious thyrotoxicosis
	Struma ovarii
	Hydatiform moles and choriocarcinoma

1.2 Conditions of Hyperthyroidism

1.2.1 Graves' Disease

GD is the most common autoimmune disease, affecting 0.5% of the population in the US, and represents 50–80% of cases of hyperthyroidism. It occurs more commonly amongst women, smokers and patients with other autoimmune diseases or a family history of thyroid autoimmunity. Peak incidence occurs between 40 and 60 years of age but any age group may be affected [1].

It is caused by an immune defect in genetically susceptible individuals in whom the production of specific auto-antibodies against the TSH-receptor (TRAb) results in thyroid hormone excess and glandular hyperplasia. This IgG antibodies bind to and activate TSH receptor on the surface of thyroid follicular cells. This activation stimulates follicular cell growth, causing diffuse thyroid enlargement and increased production of thyroid hormones with an increase in the fraction of triiodothyronine (T3) and thyroxine (T4).

When unrecognized Graves' disease impacts negatively on quality of life and poses serious risks of tachyarrhythmia and cardiac failure. Beyond the thyroid, Graves' disease has diverse soft-tissue effects that reflect its systemic autoimmune nature. Thyroid eye disease (Graves orbitopathy) is the most common of these manifestations, affecting up to 50% of patients with Graves' disease. Characteristic features of thyroid eye disease are chemosis, eyelid oedema and retraction, swelling, exophthalmos, corneal lesions and diplopia [2].

The onset of Graves' disease is usually acute, reflecting the sudden production of stimulatory TSH-receptor antibodies, but may be indolent or subacute. Patients report the classical symptoms of hyperthyroidism that include weight loss despite increased appetite, heat intolerance, irritability, insomnia, sweatiness, diarrhoea, palpitations, muscular weakness and menstrual irregularity. Clinical signs include diffuse goitre, fine resting tremor, tachycardia, hyperreflexia, eyelid lag, warm, smooth skin and proximal myopathy.

Older patients are more likely to present with subtle symptoms such as depression and weight loss rather than overt symptoms of sympathetic overactivity. They are also more likely to present with cardiovascular features such as atrial fibrillation or congestive cardiac failure [3]. The measurement of serum anti-thyroid antibodies (anti-TPO and TRAb) are mandatory to confirm the diagnosis of Graves' disease. These antibodies, positive in 90% of patients with presumed Graves' disease, are measured as TSH-receptor binding (TBII) and stimulating antibodies (TSI), the latter reflecting the effect on thyroid function. The measurement of TSH-receptor antibodies may also have a role in assessing the risk of relapse after a course of thionamides for Graves' disease or when assessing the risk of neonatal Graves' disease in pregnant women with Graves' disease.

Technetium-labelled (^{99m}Tc—labeled) thyroid scintigraphy may aid diagnosis when the cause of hyperthyroidism remains uncertain. It effectively distinguishes Graves' disease from thyroiditis or an autonomously hyperfunctioning nodule, demonstrating diffusely increased uptake in Graves' disease, a focal area of increased uptake due to an autonomously hyperfunctioning nodule and diffusely reduced uptake in thyroiditis.

Real-time thyroid ultrasonography displaies characteristic and often striking features of Graves' disease including diffuse enlargement of the thyroid gland, marked increase in glandular vascularity and the presence of small hypoechoic patches that reflect the inflammatory process. Although the prevalence of thyroid cancer is not increased in patients with Graves' disease, a nodule that has suspicious features, such as hypoechogenicity, irregular edges or microcalcification, should be biopsied.

The three treatment modalities for Graves' hyperthyroidism include the use of thionamides (antithyroid drugs), radioactive iodine (RAI) therapy or surgery. Patients in Australia, the UK and Europe are more likely than their North American counterparts to receive an initial course of thionamide therapy prior to the consideration of RAI [4]. Surgery has the highest long-term remission rate (95%) but is not without risks.

The two thionamides that have been in use since the 1940s are propylthiouracil (PTU) and methimazole (MMI). These drugs work by blocking the synthesis of thyroid hormone. PTU has the additional action of inhibiting peripheral conversion of T4 to the more active T3. These drugs may also possess immunosuppressive and anti-inflammatory properties, but this is controversial [5, 6].

Patients should be informed of potential side effects including rash, arthralgia, ANCA-positive vasculitis, hepatitis and agranulocytosis and should be advised to stop antithyroid drugs if any potential symptoms of agranulocytosis develop, such as fever, oral ulceration or painful throat. This rare idiosyncratic reaction affects 0.1–0.3% of patients on antithyroid drugs, occurs acutely without prior warning and is not dose related. MMI is the treatment of choice, particularly in children, because of less side effects compared to PTU. The last is the treatment of choice when dealing with pregnant women because it is associated with less frequent congenital anomalies in the offspring.

Whenever anti-thyroid drugs are not able to induce stable remission after a complete course or when a definitive cure is required, the other treatment options are RAI therapy or surgery, the so called "definitive treatments".

RAI may be given following an unsuccessful course of thionamides. Before RAI therapy, the patient must be rendered perfectly euthyroid with Thionamides, which are discontinued a few days before the administration of RAI. In patients with severe hyperthyroidism or those in whom persistent hyperthyroidism poses serious risks (such as the elderly or cardiac patients), beta blockers therapy is useful after RAI in order to control the transient (usually 2 weeks) thyrotoxicosis observed after RAI therapy. The dose of radioactive iodine to be administered should be sufficient to completely destroy the thyroid gland, rendering the patient permanently hypothyroid. The recommended dose is usually the maximum (15 mCi) that can be administered on an outpatient basis. Tretament should be associated with a 2–3 months therapy with low dose corticosteroids aimed to prevent the development of Graves orbitopathy induced by RAI therapy.

Surgery is indicated in the presence of big goiters, or when rapid ablation of the thyroid gland is required, such as in case of severe

Graves' ophthalmopathy or suspicious nodules. It is also considered when the patient refuse RAI administration. Surgery consists of total thyroidectomy and should be performed when the patient is perfectly euthyroid. There is some suggestion that thyroidectomy may prevent the later development of thyroid eye disease but this is anecdotal and should not be an indication for surgery in most patients.

Rituximab, a monoclonal CD20 antibody, has been advocated for the treratment of thyroid eye disease. However, its utility is limited by both cost and toxicity and, most of all, by the fact that its effect has not been reproduced in some prospective studies [7, 8].

1.2.2 Toxic Nodular Goiter

Thyroid nodules are frequent in clinical practice, occurring with a prevalence of 4% by palpation, 33 to 68% by ultrasound examination, and 50% on autopsy series.

As the initial step for evaluation of a thyroid nodule is measurement of serum thyroid stimulating hormone (TSH), it is not uncommon that the patient has low-suppressed TSh (subclinical hyperthyroidism) ort overt hyperthyroidism. In this setting, the thyroid nodule may represent a solitary hyperfunctioning thyroid nodule in an otherwise normal thyroid gland or within a multinodular goiter. Thyroid scintigraphy employs radioiodine (^{123}I, ^{131}I) or technetium-99m-(^{99m}Tc) pertechnetate in order to differentiate these diagnostic possibilities.

The distinction is important, because hyperfunctioning nodules—also referred to as "autonomous," "autonomously-functioning," or "hot" nodules—are thought to only rarely harbor malignancy, such that fine needle aspiration (FNA) is not ususally indicated in this circumstance but need a treatment.

Total thyroidectomy or radioiodine therapy represent the treatments of choice for autonomous functioning solitary nodules but also in case of multinodular goiter. RAI is indicated provided that there are no compressive symptoms. Long-term anti-thyroid drugs are not recommended. RAI may also be preferred in elderly patients with significant comorbidities, previous surgery to the neck or with a small goiter. In multinodular goiter, non-functioning nodules should be submitted to FNAC, before surgery or RAI, to rule out malignancy.

1.2.3 HCG-Induced Gestational Hyperthyroidism

Gestational transient thyrotoxicosis of non-autoimmune origin is a rare condition caused by stimulation of the TSH receptor by placental hCG. May occurs in about 1.4% of pregnant women, mostly when hCG levels are above 70–80,000 IU/l.

hCG and TSH share the common glycoprotein alpha subunit and the beta subunit is highly homologous. At high doses, hCG cross-reacts with the TSH receptor, and this stimulation can lead to an increase in secretion of T4 and T3, with subsequent suppression of TSH secretion [9]. The thyroid gland of normal pregnant women may be stimulated by hCG to secrete slightly excessive quantities of T4 and induce a slight suppression of TSH, but it only induces overt hyperthyroidism in a subset of pregnant women. The increased secretion of hCG result in the physiological decrease in TSH levels that are characteristic of the first trimester of pregnancy, or in overt hyperthyroidism [10].

When hyperthyroidism is mild, the signs and symptoms of hyperthyroidism are not specific and overlap with those of normal pregnancy. Because of the decrease in the levels and bioactivity of hCG later in pregnancy, hCG-induced gestational hyperthyroidism is usually transient and limited to the first 3–4 months of gestation. In a subset of women, the manifestations of hCG-induced hyperthyroidism are more severe and they are often associated with hyperemesis. Hyperemesis patients had significantly greater mean serum levels of hCG, free T4, total T3, and estradiol, and lesser serum TSH concentrations compared to controls. The degree of biochemical hyperthyroidism and hCG concentration correlated directly with the severity of vomiting. The hyperemesis may be caused by a marked hCG-induced increase in estradiol levels. However, the relation between hyperemesis and gestational hyperthyroidism varies among patients, and unidentified mechanisms may be involved.

The diagnosis is established by measuring TSH, free or total T4, and T3. The physiological decrease in TSH levels and the increase in total thyroid hormone concentrations associated with the increase in thyroxine-binding globulin (TBG) have to be considered when interpreting the results. TBG levels increase in response to elevated estradiol levels and plateau by about 20 weeks of gestation [11]. Treatment with antithyroid medications is often not necessary. Women with hyperemesis need therapy with antiemetics. In patients in whom total T4 levels are higher than 1.5 times the upper reference range, therapy with antithyroid drugs may be indicated. Propylthiouracil (PTU) is the preferred medication during the first trimester of pregnancy. Overtreatment with antithyroid drugs can result in hypothyroidism in the fetus. Therefore, free T4 should be kept close or slightly above the normal range with the lowest possible dose of antithyroid drugs.

1.2.4 Thyroid-Stimulating Hormone (TSH)-Secreting Pituitary Adenomas

(TSH)-secreting pituitary adenomas are a rare cause of hyperthyroidism. They account for 0.5–3% of all functioning pituitary tumors and much less than 1% of all cases of hyperthyroidism [12].

The diagnosis should be considered in all hyperthyroid patients with detectable TSH, especially those with a diffuse goiter and no typical manifestations of Graves' disease.

TSH-secreting adenomas secrete biologically active TSH in a more or less autonomous fashion, and its biological activity varies considerably; as a result, serum immunoreactive TSH concentrations range from normal (albeit inappropriately high in the presence of hyperthyroidism) to markedly elevated.

TSH-secreting pituitary adenomas must be differentiated from the syndrome of resistence to thyroid hormone, a rare genetic condition, in which thyroid hormone levels are increased and TSH is inappropriately detectable due to mutation in the TSH receptor. Since the TSH-receptors are different in different tissue, the sign and symptoms may be very individual in different patients. Some patients may not be hyperthyroid, while others may have cardiac symptoms only.

The differential diagnosis is based on clinical presentation, a-subunit protein levels, imaging, and occasionally, the T3 suppression test and the TRH stimulation test.

Approximately 20–25% of the adenomas secrete one or more other pituitary hormones, predominantly growth hormone or prolactin co-secretion of TSH and prolactin is approximately five times more common in women than in men.

As well as typical symptoms and signs of hyperthyroidism patients with TSH pituitary adenoma may have symptoms related to the expanding tumor mass or to the other hormonal co-secretion: visual field defects, menstrual disturbances, headache, galactorrhea, symptoms of acromegaly.

When discovered, management of these tumors has traditionally been through transsphenoidal resection as first-line therapy. Treatment is often difficult because of its large size and common cavernous sinus involvement at presentation, the resection is often incomplete or the tumor recurs. Despite debulking, the remaining small component of the tumor continues to produce enough TSH to cause persistent hyperthyroidism.

Adjuvant therapy with somatostatin analogs and radiosurgery has been used to treat patients not in remission after surgery. Cosecretion of GH does not predict tumor response to somatostatin analogs. TSH-secreting adenoma treatment by somatostatin analogs can be reduced TSH and a-subunit levels with the restoration of a euthyroid state in the majority of patients with an intact thyroid. Three-quarters of patients also can improved visual field findings and nearly half had decreased tumor size [13].

Dopamine agonists have failed to control TSH-secreting adenomas, except those cosecreting PRL in which case a decreased tumor mass has been noted.

1.3 Conditions of Thyrotoxicosis

1.3.1 Amiodarone-Induced Thyrotoxicosis

Amiodarone is an anti-arrhythmic drug that commonly affects the thyroid, causing hypothyroidism or thyrotoxicosis. Amiodarone inhibits both thyroid hormone uptake into peripheral tissues such as the liver and the activity of the 50-monodeiodinase, which is responsible for the conversion of T4 to T3 in these tissues. The primary result is that serum levels of T4 rise and T3 fall. Changes in serum thyrotropin (TSH) are not uncommon and often occur within days of amiodarone administration, these alterations don't need treatment [14, 15].

Amiodarone-induced thyrotoxicosis (AIT) may develop early during amiodarone treatment, but it has been reported that AIT may develop even several month after amiodarone withdrawal, since amiodarone and its metabolites have a long half-life due to accumulation in several tissues, especially fat. This is the reason that in the case of amiodarone-induced adverse effects stopping the therapy usually has little short-term benefit.

AIT is more frequent in males than in females (M/F = 3/1) and occurs in 3% of patients treated with amiodarone in North America, but is much more frequent (up to 10%) in countries with a low iodine dietary intake. The signs and symptoms of AIT usually begin as a reappearance of the underlying cardiac disease state, such as arrhythmias or angina.

AIT is caused by excessive thyroid hormone biosynthesis in response to iodine load in autonomously functioning thyroid glands, in patients with a preexisting nodular goiter or Graves' disease (type 1 or AIT 1), or by a destructive thyroiditis typically occurring in normal glands (type 2 or AIT 2) [16].

Color flow Doppler ultrasonography is useful to differentiate between type 1 and type 2 AIT. Intra-thyroidal vascular flow is increased in type 1 AIT and reduced or absent in type 2, determination of anti-thyroid antibodies (TgAb, TPOAb, TRAb) are often useful to distinguish AIT type 1, but high levels of Tg and TPOAb have also been reported in 8% of type 2 AIT.

Differential diagnosis AIT, between the two forms is critical, since treatments are different.

Type 1 AIT should be treated with high doses of thioamides (20–40 mg/day of methimazole; or 400–600 mg/day of propylthiouracil) to block the synthesis of thyroid hormones. Potassium perchlorate can also be used to increase sensitivity of the gland to thyonamides by blocking iodine uptake in the thyroid. KClO4 should be used for no more than 30 days at a daily dose <1 g/day, since this drug, especially in higher doses, is associated with aplastic anemia. Once thyroid hormones are back to normal, definitive treatment of the hyperthyroidism should be considered. If thyroid uptake is sufficient (>10%) radioactive iodine can be used. Thyroid surgery is a good alternative. If thyrotoxicosis worsens after initial control, a mixed form type1-type 2 should be considered, and treatment for type 2 AIT should be started.

Type 2 AIT can be treated with prednisone, starting with an initial dose of 0.5–0.7 mg/kg body weight per day, and the treatment is generally continued for 3 months. If a worsening of the thyrotoxicosis occurs during the taper, doses should be increased again. Thioamides are generally not useful in type 2 AIT, but to consider in mixed form or in non responder. For patients with persisting hyperthyroidism surgery is the optimal choice. Beta blockers will be helpful in preparation for surgery.

1.3.2 De Quervain's Thyroiditis

Inflammatory disorders of the thyroid gland are divided into three groups according to their duration: acute, subacute and chronic. De Quervain's thyroiditis (also termed giant cell or granulomatous thyroiditis) is a subacute inflammation of the thyroid, which accounts for 5% of thyroid disorders. The etiology is unknown, but it is presumed to be due to viral infection and it usually appears 2 weeks after an upper viral respiratory infection.

Clinically, the condition is associated with severe pain that is aggravated during swallowing, usually localized to the anterior aspect of the neck and may radiate up to the jawor ear. In addition, tenderness of the thyroid gland upon palpation and small diffuse goiter are frequently present. Common initial clinical features and laboratory investigation results include fever, fatigue, mild thyrotoxic manifestations, suppressed thyroid stimulating hormone (TSH), and elevated erythrocyte sedimentation rate, the leukocyte count, C-reactive protein are normal or slightly elevated.

The natural history of granulomatous thyroiditis involves four phases: the destructive inflammation results temporarily in thyrotoxicosis followed by euthyroidism. After a transient hypothyroidism the disease becomes inactive and the thyroid function is normalized, rarely patients developed permanent hypothyroidism and need thyroxine replacement therapy (less than 1%). Ultrasonographic findings are diffuse or pseudonodular hypoechogenic structures with typical reduction of vascular flow [17, 18]. Clinical picture and laboratory results are the bases for the diagnosis, while radioiodine uptake and cytological diagnosis are often not required.

There is no special treatment, but high dose steroid should be given immediately to relieve the pain. Salicylates and nonsteroidal antiinflammatory drugs can be used in patients with mild or moderate forms of the disorder. In more severe forms of the condition, corticosteroids in suitable pharmacological dosage will generally cause a rapid relief of symptoms within 24–48 h. Prednisone may be initiated in dosages of 50 mg daily, with a gradual reduction in dosage thereafter over several weeks. Recurrences do appear in a small percentage of patients, necessitating restoration of a higher dose once again [19].

1.3.3 Silent or Painless Thyroiditis

Silent thyroiditis is characterized by lymphocytic infiltration and can lead to transient thyrotoxicosis and hypothyroidism. Although the disease was earlier considered to be a mild form of subacute (De Quervain's) thyroiditis, there is now convincing evidence that it is a lymphocytic thyroiditis. Many patients with silent thyroiditis have a personal or a family history of other autoimmune diseases, thereby indirectly supporting the concept that it is an autoimmune thyroiditis. There is no significant association with viral infections. There is a significant association with HLA genotype DR3. Postpartum thyroiditis is considered to be a form of silent thyroiditis occurring after delivery [20].

The duration of the thyrotoxic phase is variable, but for the most part, it lasted less than 1 year. The mean duration was 3.6 months (range 1–12.5). Symptoms began about 2 months preceding the initial evaluation. Exophthalmos and pretibial myxedema were absent. The thyroid gland is typically firm in consistency. Forty three percent of patients had a mild enlarged thyroid. The clinical course of the disease consists usually of an initial hyperthyroid phase, followed by a hypothyroid phase, and sometimes subsequent restoration of a euthyroid metabolic state.

Development of Graves' disease, after painless thyroiditis has been documented and TSH receptor antibodies have been found in these patients.

During the first phase of the disease, discharge of hormone from the inflamed thyroid results in increases in serum T4, T3 and a decrease in serum TSH. During this phase, there is no uptake of radioactive iodine in the thyroid. In patients with silent thyroiditis, antithyroglobulin antibodies and antimicrosomal antibodies are positive [21]. The echogenicity is decreased and a correlation between the decrease in the echo signal at the onset and nadir of the T3 level has been suggested [22].

As thyrotoxicosis is usually mild in silent thyroiditis, there is often no need for any treatment. In some patients, therapy with a beta-blocker can be considered during the thyrotoxic phase. In patients with more severe thyrotoxicosis, administration of NSAIDs and prednisone may be of benefit [23]. After the thyrotoxic phase, many patients become temporarily hypothyroid and therapy with levothyroxine should be initiated in symptomatic patients. After a few months, levothyroxine therapy should be gradually withdrawn in order to assess whether the hypothyroidism is transient or permanent. Only a small proportion of patients remain permanently hypothyroid. Some patients, who initially recovered, may ultimately develop permanent thyroid failure. In a series of 54 patients, Nikolai et al. reported that about half of the patients developed permanent hypothyroidism [24]. This is in contrast with subacute thyroiditis where permanent hypothyroidism is less common.

In this group of thyroiditis, we can consider some forms of drug-induced thyroiditis (cytokines, lithium, tyrosine kinase inhibitors) which may give destructive thyrotoxicosis, followed by hypothyroidism.

1.3.4 Factitious Thyrotoxicosis

Is due to the voluntary or involuntary intake of supraphysiological amounts of exogenous thyroid hormone. Most commonly, it is iatrogenic, either intentionally in order to suppress TSH in thyroid cancer patients or unintentionally in patients treated for primary hypothyroidism. In both instances, subclinical thyrotoxicosis is more common. The risk of atrial fibrilliation is increased in patients with long-standing suppression of TSH. Several cardiac parameters can be affected, but the severity of these effects is somewhat controversial. Suppressive doses of thyroid hormones can also affect bone mineral density, but this has not been confirmed in all studies. Non-iatrogenic thyrotoxicosis factitia can occur in patients of all ages with psychiatric illnesses. In addition, some patients may take excessive amounts of thyroid hormones, sometimes prescribed by physicians, for weight loss, treatment of depression, or infertility. These patients often deny the intake of thyroid hormones or an excessive intake. In these instances, a heightened suspicion is needed in order to readily diagnose the disorder. Thyrotoxicosis induced by excessive thyroid hormone intake due to consumption of meat containing bovine thyroid tissue has been reported repeatedly. Patients are clinically thyrotoxic, without signs of endocrine ophthalmopathy. The thyroid may be small because of long-standing suppression of TSH.

Serum TSH is suppressed, (free) T4 and T3 levels are variably elevated. The T4 and T3 levels depend on the type of ingested thyroid hormone preparation. Poisoning with T3 may be particularly severe, but even very high doses are often well tolerated, especially by children. When the diagnosis of thyrotoxicosis factitia is suspected, measurement of serum thyroglobulin levels is useful. During ingestion of levothyroxine, little or no thyroglobulin is present is necessary to exclude the presence of thyroglobulin antibodies that can potentially interfere with the assay. The thyroidal uptake of radioiodine or technetium are decreased like in silent thyroiditis but, in this, the serum thyroglobulin is elevated.

In most patients, adjustment or discontinuation of the thyroid hormone preparation is sufficient to normalize thyroid function tests. Patients with surreptitious intake of thyroid hormones for eating disorders or psychiatric illnesses can be difficult to treat and may need psychiatric consultation and assistance. In patients with severe intoxication, beta-blockers can be useful.

1.3.5 Struma Ovarii

Is a rare tumor consisting primarily of thyroid components occurring in a teratoma or dermoid in the ovary (1% of all ovarian tumors and 2–4% of all ovarian teratomas) 5–10% are malignant [25]. Thyrotoxicosis occurs in about 8% of affected patients. Thyroglobulin is secreted by benign and malignant ovarian strumae. Radioiodine uptake will reveal uptake in the pelvis, while the uptake in the thyroid is diminished or absen. Imaging with computed tomography or magnetic resonance imaging will demonstrate of unilateral or bilateral ovarian masses [26]. CA125 may be elevated. Malignant thyroid tissue shows the characteristic patterns of papillary or follicular thyroid cancer and can be positive for mutations in BRAF [27]. Metastasis is uncommon but has been reported. Unilateral or bilateral open or laparoscopic oophorectomy is the primary therapy. Thyrotoxic women should be treated with antithyroid drugs and, if needed, with beta-blockers prior to surgery. In the case of malignant lesions, the patient should undergo thyroidectomy followed by treatment with 131 iodine. The subsequent surveillance for residual or recurrent cancer does not differ from primary thyroid carcinomas.

1.3.6 Hydatiform Moles and Choriocarcinoma

Hydatiform moles and choriocarcinomas are gestational trophoblastic diseases that secrete high amounts of hCG and can cause hyperthyroidism. In men, choriocarcinomas can arise in the testis and cause hyperthyroidism by secreting hCG.

A correlation between serum hCG levels and thyroid stimulating activity in both serum and urine was found in women and men who had widely metastatic choriocarcinoma and marked hyperthyroidism.

Most women with hydatiform moles present with uterine bleeding in the first half of pregnancy. The size of the uterus is large for the duration of gestation, molar pregnancies can cause nausea and vomiting, pregnancy-induced hypertension or pre-eclampsia. The signs and symptoms of thyrotoxicosis are present in some women, but they may be obscured by toxemic signs. Women with choriocarcinomas present within 1 year after conception. The tumor may be confined to the uterus, more frequently it is metastatic to multiple organs such as the liver and lungs, among others. In men, choriocarcinomas of the testes is often widely metastatic at initial presentation. Gynecomastia is a common finding. Measurement of serum hCG concentrations is needed for the diagnosis of moles and choriocarcinomas, and hCG serves as a sensitive and specific tumor marker during therapy and surveillance. In women, hCG concentrations are significantly higher than those found during normal pregnancies. Ultrasonography of the uterus shows a characteristic “snowstorm” pattern.

Hydatiform moles are treated by suction rather than curettage. Serum T4, T3, TSH, and hCG levels normalize rapidly after removal of the mole [28].

Choriocarcinomas can be divided into two groups: a low risk group treated by monotherapy, most often with methotrexate or actinomycine D and a success rate close to 100% and an high risk group treated with polychemotherapy (etoposide, methotrexate, actinomycine D, cyclophosphamide, vincristine) with a response of about 86%. In patients that are not responding to chemotherapy, the 5-year survival rate is about 43%. Longitudinal measurement of hCG as specific and sensitive tumor marker is key for long-term surveillance.

1.4 The Differential Diagnosis of Hyperthyroidism and Thyrotoxicosis

Blood sampling for TSH has the highest sensitivity and specificity to reveal thyroid disease and it can be used as a screening test, but is not sufficient to define the entity of hyperthyroidism, for this is also required the determination of both FT4 and FT3, taking into account that there are forms of hyperthyroidism with prevailing T3 secretion.

The patient’s clinical examination is main to identify patients with increased cardio-vascular risks, complications, or more debilitated and symptomatic, which requiring a faster resolution of hormonal imbalance [29, 30].

1.4.1 Search the Etiology of Thyrotoxicosis

The determination of both TSH and thyroid hormones allows to detect rare forms of TSH-mediated hyperthyroidism, once has been excluded interference to the assay (Table 1.1). The relationship between T3 and T4 can be useful in understanding the causes of thyrotoxicosis:

(a) A gland overactive tends to produce more T3 than T4.

(b) T4 is usually higher than T3 in thyrotoxicosis factitia (by exogenous L-thyroxine), iatrogenic, or attributable to autoimmune thyroiditis.

The distinction of subacute thyroiditis is usually not difficult, thanks to painful swelling of the neck, intensely accentuated by palpation, and low-grade fever with elevated inflammatory indices.

When the etiologic diagnosis is not sufficiently clear with the aid of clinical presentation and biochemical tests, further examinations are recommended:

TSH receptor antibody (TRAb) sampling: If they exceeding normal limits, are diagnostic of GD, with lower costs and faster results than the determination of the radioiodine uptake. Indeed TBII (TSH-binding inhibition immunoglobulin) third generation dosages have very high sensitivity and specificity and are positive in 96% of patients with GD.

Thyroid ultrasound examination with vascular signal (ecodoppler): the presence of increased blood flow could distinguish GD from the destructive thyroiditis and, if we exclude thyroiditis, ultrasound examination will highlight the presence of thyroid nodules and their characteristics.

Thyroid scintigraphy (with 123I or 99Tc pertechnetate) is useful if the clinical presentation and ultrasound examination suggests a toxic adenoma (TA) or TMNG.

Determination of radioiodine uptake (RAIU) provides further information: absent in the case of subacute, silent or postpartum thyroiditis, improper ingestion of thyroid hormones, excess iodine, increased in all cases of glandular hyperfunction.

Thyroglobulin (Tg) sampling is useful only for detecting unaware or psychotic intake of exogenous thyroid hormones, in which case it is suppressed (consider that positivity of anti-thyroglobulin antibodies interfere with serum Tg) [31].

Determination of urine iodine when we suspect an excess of iodine.

1.5 Antithyroid Drugs

The antithyroid drugs are the first choice in GD. They are thioamides (propylthiouracil, thiamazole, and carbimazole) and the mechanism of action is the inhibition of thyroid peroxidase [32].

Thiamazole is the preferred drug in Graves' disease, especially with a good chance of complete disease remission. In some conditions, such as hyperthyroidism during pregnancy (except for the first trimester), elderly patients with multiple comorbidities, cardiological patients requiring prompt correction of hyperthyroidism, this is the only therapeutical option.

In hyperthyroidism related to multi nodular goiter or Plummer toxic adenoma, drug therapy may be considered before surgery or RAI therapy for the improvement of clinical signs of hyperthyroidism (Table 1.2).

Thiamazole is considered the first line therapy; it has several advantages over propylthiouracil, such as better efficacy; longer half-life and duration of action, and less severe side-effects.

The use of propylthioracil is preferred during the first trimester of pregnancy and in patients with minor adverse reactions to thiamazole, who refuse surgery or RAI therapy [6].

The goal of the therapy is to reach the normal thyroid function as quickly and safely as possible. These medications in adequate doses are very effective in controlling the hyperthyroidism and they might also have anti-inflammatory and immunosuppressive effects [33, 34].

Patients should be informed about possible side effects of these drugs and the necessity of

Table 1.2 Indications of RAI vs thyroidectomy in hyperthyroidism

RAI	Total thyrodectomy
High surgical risk	Goiter with compressive symptoms
Previous surgery or RT neck	Moderate to severe Graves' ophthalmopathy
Planned pregnancy beyond 6 months	Planned pregnancy before 6 months
Diffused struma or little nodules (low ATA risk)	Multiple nodules or suspected malignancy

informing the referring physician promptly. Minor side-effects such as pruritic rash, arthralgia, and gastrointestinal distress occur in about 5% of patients. In minor skin reactions, an antihistamine can be added to the therapy or in some cases the antithyroid drug could be replaced with another one. Major side-effects of ATDs are rare and they usually develops within the first 3 months of therapy.

Agranulocytosis is the most frequent major side-effect (annual incidence 0.1–0.3%); it requires the immediate withdrawal of the medication if the granulocyte count is less than 1000 cells/mm^3. When patients receiving ATDs present with fever or sore throat, chills, diarrhea, or myalgia, a white blood cell count should be obtained. Trial of another ATD is contraindicated in this circumstance because of the documented cross-reactivity. Other very rare haematological side-effects of ATDs include aplastic anaemia, thrombocytopenia, and hypoprothrombinaemia.

Another major side-effect is hepatotoxicity (0.1–0.2%); it can rarely present as acute liver failure, which is associated with propylthiouracil more frequently than with thiamazole (0.25 vs 0.08%), and might require liver transplant.

It is recommended to obtain a baseline complete blood count and a serum liver profile before the initiation of therapy [35].

The starting dose of thiamazole depends on the severity of the hyperthyroidism and the size of the thyroid gland and could vary from 10–15 to 20–40 mg daily. The equivalent dose of carbimazole is approximately 140% of that of thiamazole. Thyroid function should be checked 4–6 weeks after initiation of therapy and then every 2–3 months once the patient is euthyroid.

TSH might remain suppressed for several months, which is why serum T4 and T3 should be monitored to assess efficacy of therapy.

Once euthyroidism is achieved, a maintenance dose (thiamazole 5–10 mg daily, or propylthiouracil 50–100 mg daily) should be continued for at least 12–18 months.

In presence of fever or symptoms suggestive for side effects, blood count and a serum liver profile should be checked, especially in the first 3 months of therapy.

Therapy can be gradually reduced and then suspended when a stable euthyroidism is reached and maintained.

1.5.1 Therapy During Pregnancy

Hyperthyroidism during pregnancy should be adequately treated to prevent maternal and fetal complications.

The treatment of choice for overt hyperthyroidism in pregnant women is ATD; radioiodine treatment is not recommended. If ATDs are not tolerated, the alternative treatment is thyroidectomy, preferably in the second trimester of pregnancy. Hyperthyroidism should be treated with the lowest possible dose to keep mother's level of T4 and T3 at or slightly above the normal range and the TSH below the normal range for pregnancy. Current guidelines recommend the use of PTU in the first trimester of pregnancy, and to switch to MMI in the second trimester considering the possible higher risk of hepatotoxicity associated with the use of PTU [36].

The drugs are equally effective in the treatment of hyperthyroidism, and they all pass the placenta, which may lead to fetal hypothyroidism in late pregnancy. The major concern to the use of these drugs in early pregnancy is, however, the potential risk of birth defects, including aplasia cutis, choanal atresia, oesophageal atresia, and omphalocele, described with thiamazole administration; although less common, propylthiouracil has also been shown to be associated with birth defects in the face and neck, and urinary systems [37].

1.5.2 The Use of Beta-Blockers

Beta-adrenergic blockade is recommended in patients with symptomatic hyperthyroidism to control the peripheral effects of excess thyroid hormones, especially in elderly patients with heart disease or tachycardia. The β blocker therapy in addiction can slightly decrease T4 to T3 conversion. These drugs are contraindicated in patients with asthma or history of bronchospasm;

in these patients could be used calcium channel blockers as verapamil or diltiazem to reduce the heart rate [38].

1.6 Radioactive Iodine (^{131}I)

As reported above radioactive iodine (^{131}I) can be used as treatment of patients with of hyperthyroidism. The indcations of radioactive iodine therapy (RAI) are discussed in details in a dedicated session of this textbook (see Chap. 3). However in the following paragraphs are summarized some recommendations and patient's preparation for patients with hyperthyroidism candidate to radioisotopic therapy.

1.7 Clinical Recommendation and Preparation Before Radioactive Iodine Therapy in Hyperthyroidism

Radioactive iodine therapy is safe and cost-effective and can be the first-line treatment for hyperthyroidism due to Graves' disease, toxic adenoma, and toxic multinodular goiter [39–41].

RAI should be preferred in women planning a pregnancy in the future (more than 6 months following the therapy), patients with high surgical risk, previously neck surgery or neck external irradiation or failure to obtain a normal thyroid function with pharmacological therapy. The indications and contraincications of RAI therapy versus surgery are summarized in Tables 1.2 and 1.3.

Absolute contraindications to RAI therapy are: pregnancy, breastfeeding, planning pregnancy (within 6 months), inability to comply with radiation safety recommendations, thyroid cancer or suspicion of thyroid cancer.

Table 1.3 Contraindication of RAI vs thyroidectomy in hyperthyroidism

RAI	Total thyrodesctomy
Pregnancy or lactation	Pregnancy (in the second quarter)
Thyroid cancer	High surgical risk
Severe Graves' ophthalmopathy	No experienced surgeons
Inability to follow the safety recommendations	Thyroid storm

In GD RAI therapy is contraindicated in patients with active moderate-to-severe Graves' orbitopathy, while in mild active Graves' orbitopathy, radioactive iodine treatment should be followed by prophylactic steroid treatment [34]. Patients with inactive Graves' orbitopathy, but no risk factors, can be given radioactive iodine therapy without corticosteroids.

In patients with thyroid nonfunctioning nodules or with suspicious ultrasound characteristics, fine needle aspiration with cytological examination should be performed before RAI treatment and, if they are suspicious or diagnostic of thyroid cancer, radioactive iodine is contraindicated and surgery is recommended.

Medical therapy for hyperthyroidism should be optimized prior RAI therapy and b-adrenergic blockade should be considered even in asymptomatic patients who are at increased risk for complications due to possible transient worsening of hyperthyroidism. Pharmacological therapy should be discontinued 3–5 days before radioactive iodine therapy, then restarted 3–7 days later, especially in high risk patients, and withdrawn as soon as thyroid function normalizes.

Before treatment patient should be informed about avoid nutritional supplements or radiologic contrasts containing iodine and seaweeds for at least 1 week.

In women should be obtained a pregnancy test within 48 h prior the treatment and patients must be informed about the need to delay the conception for at least 6 months and until normalization of the thyroid hormones is established. No adverse effects were reported on the health of offspring of patients given radioactive iodine for hyperthyroidism before pregnancy.

During breastfeeding RAI should not be administered for at least 6 weeks after lactation stop to avoid active concentration of radioactivity in breast tissues; breastfeeding should not be resumed after treatment.

Thyroid function should be monitored at least every 6–8 weeks after treatment and levothyroxine replacement should be started as soon as hypothyroidism occurs. The timing for the thyroid hormone replacement therapy should be determined by results of thyroid function tests, clinical symptoms, and physical examination.

In the 40% of patients with GD hypothyroidism occur within 8 weeks and more than the 80% within 16 weeks. In multinodular goiter and toxic adenoma the resolution of hyperthyroidism occurs in approximately 55 and 75% of cases respectively within 3 months and the average size reduction is about 45% in 2 years. In patients with a persistent hyperthyroidism after 6 months following RAI therapy, a retreatment sholud be considered.

With the development of hypothyroidism, TSH levels may remain suppressed for some months after the resolution of hypothyroidism and consequently they should not be used initially to determine the need for levothyroxine.

Until TSH level is suppressed the levothyroxine dose should be adjusted based on an assessment of free T4. The required dose may be less than the typical full replacement, expecially in the first period of therapy, due to the possibility of an underlying persistent thyroid function.

Overt hypothyroidism should be avoided, especially in patients with active Graves' orbitopathy and in patients with cardiac disease.

Once euthyroidism is achieved, lifelong annual thyroid function testing is recommended.

1.8 Clinical Recommendation and Preparation for Surgery in Hyperthyroidism

Surgery should be taken into account in GD not responding to drug therapy, with large nodules or large goiter, when radioiodine (RAI) therapy it is not useable (Table 1.3). In these cases the chosen procedure is total thyroidectomy. When thyroid nodules are present, cytological examination must be performed before surgery if they have suspicious ultrasonographic characteristics or if they are cold or not avid at scintigraphic examination.

In toxic multinodular goiter or toxic adenoma the most appropriate therapies are RAI or surgery, while the long-term drug therapy is chosen only in selected situations.

RAI may be preferred in elderly patients with significant comorbidities, previous neck surgery, a small goiter or the unavailability of an experienced surgeon. If there are cold nodules these have to be subjected to cytological examination before treatment. In the presence of large goiters with compressive symptoms, in the suspicion of thyroid tumor coexistence or when hyperthyroidism rapid correction is necessary, surgical therapy should be preferred. The chosen procedure should be total thyroidectomy in multinodular goiter, while in uninodular toxic adenoma, can be performed hemithyroidectomy.

Appropriate medical preparation before surgery is necessary to reach the euthyroidism condition; this therapy must be stopped immediately before the intervention.

In patients with GD is recommended preoperative treatment with a potassium iodide solution (Lugol's solution) for about 7–10 days before the operation at a dose of 5–7 drops three times a day. Preoperative Lugol solution treatment decreases the rate of blood flow, and intraoperative blood loss during thyroidectomy [42].

It is recommended to control calcium and vitamin D before surgery; several studies demonstrated that the pre-existing vitamin D deficiency is an additional risk factor for postoperative hypocalcemia; moreover the GD itself is a risk factor for post surgical hypocalcemia. In these patients a vitamin D supplementation before surgery can be considered for a demonstrated role in the reduction of the risk of postoperative transient hypocalcemia.

Levothyroxine therapy for hypothyroidism should be undertaken immediately after total thyroidectomy at replacement dose (approximately 1.5 mcg/kg). After 6–8 weeks TSH and FT4 must be checked to verify the adequacy of the LT4 dose.

After lobectomy replacement therapy should not be necessary but periodical checks of thyroid function are needed and therapy should be considered only in case of evolution in hypothyroidism (about 20% of cases).

After total thyroidectomy it is recommended to check the levels of serum calcium and PTH after 6 and 12 h after surgery, administering calcium and calcitriol if necessary. If the PTH is normal when the patient reaches the normocalcaemia, calcium and calcitriol may be gradually reduced up to the suspension.

References

1. Manji N, Carr-Smith JD, Boelaert K, Allahabadia A, Armitage M, Chatterjee VK, et al. Influences of age, gender, smoking and family history on autoimmune thyroid disease phenotype. J Clin Endocrinol Metab. 2006;91:4873–80.
2. Brent GA. Clinical practice: Graves' disease. N Engl J Med. 2008;358:2544–54.
3. Shapiro LE, Sievert R, Ong L, Ocampo EL, Chance RA, Lee M, Nanna M, Ferrick K, Surks MI. Minimal cardiac effects in asymptomatic athyreotic patients chronically treated with thyrotropin-suppressive doses of L-thyroxine. J Clin Endocrinol Metab. 1997;82(8):2592–5.
4. Wartofsky L, Glinoer D, Solomon B, Nagataki S, Lagasse R, Nagayama Y, Izumi M. Differences and similarities in the diagnosis and treatment of Graves' disease in Europe, Japan, and the United States. Thyroid. 1991;1(2):129–35.
5. Cooper DS, Rivkees SA. Putting propylthiouracil in perspective. J Clin Endocrinol Metab. 2009;94:1881–2.
6. Bahn RS, Burch HS, Cooper DS, et al. The role of propylthiouracil in the management of Graves' disease in adults: report of a meeting jointly sponsored by the American Thyroid Association and the Food and Drug Administration. Thyroid. 2009;19:673–4.
7. Neumann S, Eliseeva E, McCoy JG, Napolitano G, Giuliani C, Monaco F, et al. A new smallmolecule antagonist inhibits Graves' disease antibody activation of the TSH receptor. J Clin Endocrinol Metab. 2011;96:548–54.
8. Neumann S, Huang W, Eliseeva E, Titus S, Thomas CJ, Gershengorn MC. A small molecule inverse agonist for the human thyroid- stimulating hormone receptor. Endocrinology. 2010;151:3454–9.
9. Glinoer D. The regulation of thyroid function in pregnancy: pathways of endocrine adaptation from physiology to pathology. Endocr Rev. 1997;18:404–33.
10. Goodwin TM, Montoro M, Mestman JH, Perkary AE, Hershman JM. The role of chorionic gonadotropin in transient hyperthyroidism of hyperemesis gravidarum. Trans Assoc Am Phys. 1991;104:233–7.
11. Glinoer D. The regulation of thyroid function during normal pregnancy: importance of the iodine nutrition status. Best Pract Res Clin Endocrinol Metab. 2004 Jun;18(2):133–52.
12. Beck-Peccoz P, Brucker-Davis F, Persani L, Smallridge RC, Weintraub BD. Thyrotropin-secreting pituitary tumors. Endocr Rev. 1996;17:610–38.
13. Beck-Peccoz P, Persani L. Medical management of thyrotropinsecreting pituitary adenomas. Pituitary. 2002;5:83–8.
14. Cohen-Lehman J, Dahl P, Danzi S, Klein I. Effects of amiodarone therapy on thyroid function. Nat Rev Endocrinol. 2010;6:34–41.
15. Bogazzi F, Tomisti L, Bartalena L, Aghini-Lombardi F, Martino E. Amiodarone and the thyroid: a 2012 update. J Endocrinol Investig. 2012;35:340–8. https://doi.org/10.3275/8298.
16. Tanda ML, Piantanida E, Lai A, Liparulo G, Sassi L, Bogazzi F, Wiersinga WM, Braverman LE, Martino E, Bartalena L. Diagnosis and management of amiodarone-induced thyrotoxicosis: similarities and differences between North American and European thyroidologists. Clin Endocrinol. 2008; 69(5):812–8.
17. Cappelli C, Pirola I, Gandossi E, Formenti A, Agosti B, Castellano M. Ultrasound findings of subacute thyroiditis: a single institution retrospective review. Acta Radiol. 2014;55(4):429–33.
18. Tokuda Y, Kasagi K, Iida Y, Yamamoto K, Hatabu H, Hidaka A, Konishi J, Ishii Y. Sonography of subacute thyroiditis: changes in the findings during the course of the disease. J Clin Ultrasound. 1990;18(1):21–6.
19. Fatourechi V, Aniszewski JP, Fatourechi GZE, Atkinson EJ, Jacobsen SJ. Clinical features and outcome of subacute thyroiditis in an incidence cohort: Olmsted County, Minnesota, study. J Clin Endocrinol Metab. 2003;88(5):2100–5.
20. Muller AF, Drexhage HA, Berghout A. Postpartum thyroiditis and autoimmune thyroiditis in women of childbearing age: recent insights and consequences for antenatal and postnatal care. Endocr Rev. 2001;22: 605–30.
21. Iitaka M, Morgenthaler NG, Momotani N, Nagata A, Ishikawa N, Ito K, Katayama S, Ito K. Stimulation of thyroid-stimulating hormone (TSH) receptor antibody production following painless thyroiditis. Clin Endocrinol. 2004;60(1):49–53.
22. Miyakawa M, Tsushima T, Onoda N, Etoh M, Isozaki O, Arai M, Shizume K, Demura H. Thyroid ultrasonography related to clinical and laboratory findings in patients with silent thyroiditis. J Endocrinol Investig. 1992;15(4):289–95.
23. Nikolai TF, Coombs GJ, McKenzie AK, Miller RW, Weir GJ Jr. Treatment of lymphocytic thyroiditis with spontaneously resolving hyperthyroidism (silent thyroiditis). Arch Intern Med. 1982;142(13): 2281–3.
24. Nikolai TF, Coombs GJ, McKenzie AK. Lymphocytic thyroiditis with spontaneously resolving hyperthyroidism and subacute thyroiditis. Long-term follow-up. Arch Intern Med. 1981;141:1455–8.
25. Roth LM, Talerman A. The enigma of struma ovarii. Pathology. 2007;39:139–46.

26. Yassa L, Sadow P, Marqusee E. Malignant struma ovarii. Nat Clin Pract Endocrinol Metab. 2008;4:469–72.
27. Dardik RB, Dardik M, Westra W, et al. Malignant struma ovarii: two case reports and a review of the literature. Gynecol Oncol. 1999;73:447–51.
28. Noal S, Joly F, Leblanc E. Management of gestational trophoblastic disease. Gynecol Obstet Fertil. 2010;38(3):193–8.
29. Ross DS, Burch HB, Cooper DS, Greenlee MC, Laurberg P, Maia AL, Rivkees SA, Samuels M, Sosa JA, Stan MN, Walter MA. 2016 American Thyroid Association guidelines for diagnosis and management of hyperthyroidism and other causes of thyrotoxicosis. Thyroid. 2016;26(10):1343–421.
30. De Leo S, Lee SY, Braverman LE. Hyperthyroidism. Lancet. 2016;388(10047):906–18.
31. Pacini F, Pinchera A. Serum and tissue thyroglobulin measurement: clinical applications in thyroid disease. Biochimie. 1999;81(5):463–7. Review.
32. Cooper DS. Antithyroid drugs. N Engl J Med. 2005;352(9):905–17.
33. Baskin HJ, Cobin RH, Duick DS, Gharib H, Guttler RB, Kaplan MM. American Association of Clinical Endocrinologists medical guidelines for the evaluation and treatment of hyperthyroidism and hypothyroidism. Endocr Pract. 2002;8:457–69.
34. Bartalena L, Marcocci C, Bogazzi F, Manetti L, Tanda ML, Dell'Unto E, et al. Relation between therapy for hyperthyroidism and the course of Graves' ophthalmopathy. N Engl J Med. 1998;338:73–8.
35. Otsuka F, Noh JY, Chino T, Shimizu T, Mukasa K, Ito K, Ito K. Taniyama M Hepatotoxicity and cutaneous reactions after antithyroid drug administration. Clin Endocrinol. 2012;77(2):310–5.
36. Mandel SJ, Cooper DS. The use of antithyroid drugs in pregnancy and lactation. J Clin Endocrinol Metab. 2001;86:2354–9.
37. Andersen SL, Olsen J, Wu CS, Laurberg P. Severity of birth defects after propylthiouracil exposure in early pregnancy. Thyroid. 2014;24:1533–40.
38. Ventrella S, Klein I. Beta-adrenergic receptor blocking drugs in the management of hyperthyroidism. Endocrinologist. 1994;4:391–9.
39. Tarantini B, Ciuoli C, Di Cairano G, Guarino E, Mazzucato P, Montanaro A, Burroni L, Vattimo AG, Pacini F. Effectiveness of radioiodine (131-I) as definitive therapy in patients with autoimmune and non-autoimmune hyperthyroidism. J Endocrinol Investig. 2006;29(7):594–8.
40. Acharya SH, Avenell A, Philip S, Burr J, Bevan JS, Abraham P. Radioiodine therapy (RAI) for Graves' disease (GD) and the effect on ophthalmopathy: a systematic review. Clin Endocrinol. 2008;69(6):943–50.
41. Ross DS. Radioiodine therapy for hyperthyroidism. N Engl J Med. 2011;364(6):542–50.
42. Erbil Y, Ozluk Y, Giriş M, Salmaslioglu A, Issever H, Barbaros U, Kapran Y, Ozarmağan S, Tezelman S. Effect of lugol solution on thyroid gland blood flow and microvessel density in the patients with Graves' disease. J Clin Endocrinol Metab. 2007;92(6):2182–9.

2 Radiopharmaceuticals for Therapy of Thyroid Diseases

Katia Marzo

Abstract

Since the discovery of radium, the medical community has been interested in the application of unsealed radioactive isotopes to target and treat cancer and benign proliferative conditions. Radioactive iodine-131, as non radioactive Iodine, is taken up by thyroid cells, either normal or pathological, therefore thanks to its gamma and beta emissions, represents a radiopharmaceutical of choice for thyroid diseases. We give here a summary of the chemistry, mechanism of uptake and biodistribution of 131-Iodine with regard of its applications in thyroid benign and malignant diseases. The medical community has been interested in the application of unsealed radioactive isotopes to target and treat cancer and benign systemic and locoregional proliferative conditions. Lack of effective system agents coupled with the intention to use targeted therapy for treating cancer made radioisotopes an option for use in cancer.

Radioactive iodine-131 given the abundant beta and gamma emissions and thanks to the normal physiological uptake of elemental iodine in the thyroid gland, was the most logical choice for treating a number of thyroid disorders.

K. Marzo
Humanitas Research Hospital, Rozzano, MI, Italy
e-mail: katia.marzo@cancercenter.humanitas.it

E. Bombardieri et al. (eds.), *Clinical Applications of Nuclear Medicine Targeted Therapy*,
https://doi.org/10.1007/978-3-319-63067-0_2

Iodine-131 has a convenient half-life and energy characteristics ($t_{1/2}$ = 8.1 days; E_{max} beta = 600 keV). Normal physiological uptake of iodine in functioning thyroid tissue is the primary reason for its role in treating several thyroid disorders and malignancies.

This fact, coupled with the energetic beta emission, has made it a standard treatment. Sodium iodide has the convenience of easy oral administration.

Its high-energy gamma radiation (364 keV), which requires additional radiation safety measures, can be considered advantageous for biodistribution studies and radiation-absorbed dose evaluation.

Sodium iodide in liquid form is highly volatile and needs special handling in a fume hood with exhaust system to avoid inhalation of the iodine vapor during labeling.

It also means that personnel handling the radiopharmaceutical should be subjected to periodic assay to exclude uptake in their thyroid glands. However, I-131 remains the most commonly used radionuclide in nuclear medicine for therapy purposes.

2.1 Chemistry

Sodium iodide I-131 radioisotopic in its various forms is one of the most precociously introduced radionuclides in nuclear medicine practice.

The most common way to mark with radioiodine complex molecules is achievable, thanks to the possibility of replacing, by means of a radical redox reaction with the hydroxyl-OH-I-ion, which has the same valence and spatially occupies a similar volume to that of -OH-radical.

Iodine-131 is used both for therapeutic (beta emission) and diagnostic (gamma emission) purposes [1].

131_iodine is used for therapeutic purposes in the treatment of hyperthyroidism and thyroid carcinomas that take up iodide. Palliative effects may be observed in patients with advanced thyroid malignancy with metastatic lesions [2].

2.2 Pharmaceutical Form

Sodium Iodide I 131 (Na I-131) Capsules Therapeutic is supplied for oral administration in opaque white gelatin capsules.

The capsules are available in different activities ranging from 28 to 3700 MBq (0.75–100 mCi) at the time of calibration. Sodium iodide I-131 capsules are packaged in shielded cylinders.

Sodium Iodide I 131 (Na I-131) Solution Therapeutic is supplied for oral administration as a stabilized aqueous solution.

The solution is available in vials that contain 185 to 5550 MBq (5–150 mCi) iodine-131 at the time of calibration.

The solution contains 0.1% sodium bisulfite and 0.2% edetate disodium as stabilizers, 0.5% sodium phosphate anhydrous as a buffer, and sodium iodide I-131 at concentrations of 185 or 925 MBq (5 or 25 mCi) per milliliter. The pH has been adjusted to between 7.5 and 9. The iodine-131 utilized in the preparation of the solution contains not less than 99% iodine-131 at the time of calibration. The expiration date is not later than 1 month after the calibration date. The calibration date and the expiration date are stated on the label.

2.3 Action Mechanism

Taken orally, sodium iodide I-131 is rapidly absorbed and distributed within the extracellular fluid of the body. The iodide is concentrated in the thyroid via the sodium/iodide symporter and subsequently oxidized to iodine. The destruction of thyroidal tissue is achieved by the beta emission of sodium iodide I-131 [3].

2.4 Pharmacodynamics

The therapeutic effects of sodium iodide I-131 are due to absorbed dose by the thyroidal tissue.

Tissue damage is the result of direct insult to molecules by ionization and excitation and the consequent dissociation of those molecules. About 90% of local irradiation from sodium iodide I-131 is the result of beta radiation, and 10% is the result of gamma radiation.

2.5 Pharmacokinetics

After oral administration, sodium iodide I-131 is absorbed rapidly from the upper gastrointestinal tract (90% in 60 min). The pharmacokinetics follow the same of the non radioactive iodide. After entering the bloodstream, the iodide is distributed into the extrathyroidal compartment. From here, it is predominantly taken up by the thyroid or excreted renally. In the thyroid, the trapped iodide is oxidized to iodine and organified. The sodium/iodide symporter (NIS) is responsible for the concentration of iodide in the thyroid. This active transport process is capable of concentrating iodide 20–40 times the plasma concentration under normal circumstances, and this may increase tenfold in the hyperthyroid state. NIS also mediates active iodide transport in other tissues, including salivary glands, nasolacrimal duct, lacrimal sac, gastric mucosa, lactating mammary gland, and the choroid plexus. The non-thyroidal iodide transporting tissues do not have the ability to organify accumulated iodide.

Depending on renal and thyroid gland function, urinary excretion is 37–75% of the administered dose, fecal excretion is about 10%, and excretion in sweat is almost negligible.

2.6 Biodistribution

The pharmacokinetics is identical to that of unlabeled iodide.

After entering the bloodstream, the drug is distributed in the radio sector extrathyroidal. From this seat, it is picked up mainly by the thyroid or eliminated through the kidneys.

The uptake of iodide in the thyroid reaches its maximum after 24–48 h, with 50% of the maximum peak reached after 5 h.

The uptake is influenced by several factors: patient age, thyroid volume, renal clearance, and level of circulating iodide. The clearance of iodide by the thyroid is about 5–50 ml/min.

In the case of iodine deficiency, the value is obviously increased up to 100 ml/min and hyperthyroidism up to 1000 ml/min. In the case of iodine overload, the value may be reduced up to 2–5 ml/min. The iodide also accumulates in the kidneys [4].

The iodide which is absorbed by the thyroid follows the metabolism of thyroid hormones and is incorporated in organic compounds from which thyroid hormones are synthesized (Fig. 1) [5].

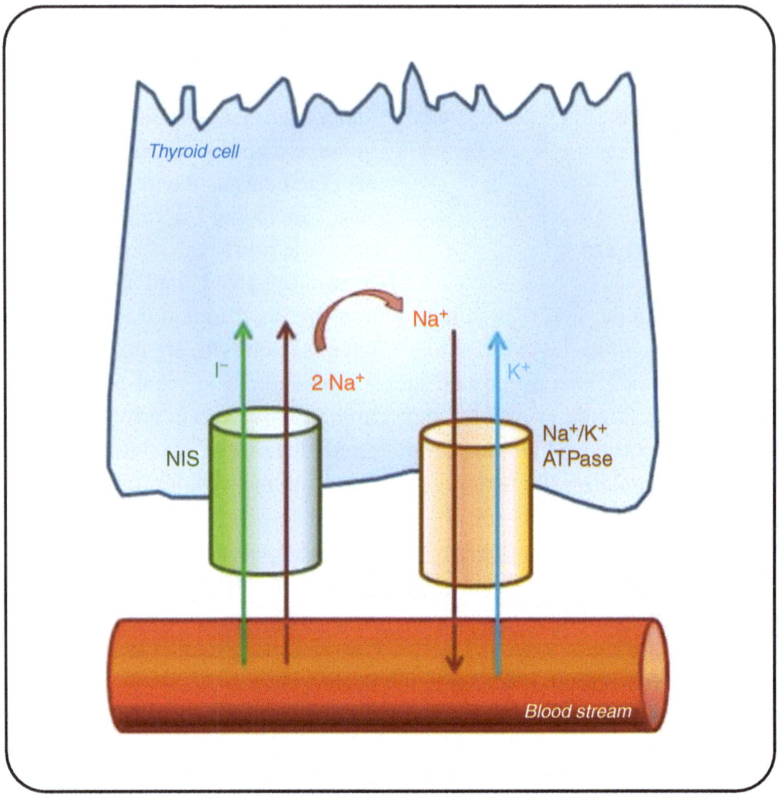

Fig. 2.1 Mechanism of uptake of Iodine in thyroid cells

2.7 Excretion

Elimination occurs mainly via the urine. Urinary excretion accounts for 37–75%, foecal excretion accounts for roughly 10%. Elimination with sweat is negligible.

Urinary excretion is characterized by renal clearance, which constitutes approximately 35% in renal blood flow and is relatively constant from one person to another. Renal excretion can be reduced in hypothyroidism and impaired renal function. coversely, hyperthyroidism can cause an increased renal excretion.

2.8 Activity

2.8.1 Hyperthyroidism

For hyperthyroidism, the usual sodium iodide I-131 dose range is 148–370 MBq (4–10 mCi). Higher activities may be necessary for the treatment of toxic nodular goiter and other special situations. Consider discontinuation of antithyroid therapy in a severely hyperthyroid patient 3–4 days before administration of sodium iodide I-131. Evaluate patients for risk of thyroid enlargement and obstruction of structures in the neck.

2.8.2 Thyroid Carcinoma

For thyroid carcinoma, the usual sodium iodide I-131 therapeutic administered activity is 3700–5550 MBq (100–150 mCi). For ablation of postoperative residual thyroid tissue, the usual activity is 1850 MBq (50 mCi).

2.8.3 Individualization of Therapy

Personalized sodium iodide I-131 therapy, including activity selection, is based on patient-specific factors such as the nature of the underlying condition, comorbidities, age, estimated thyroid tissue iodine uptake, thyroid size, as well as ability of the patient to comply with the therapeutic regimen and radiation safety procedures. Perform a clinical assessment, including history, physical examination, and laboratory testing, when preparing patients for sodium iodide I-131 therapy in order to detect conditions which may alter thyroid iodine uptake and increase the risks of the therapy or diminish its effectiveness. For example, intake of iodine in radiographic contrast may diminish thyroid iodine uptake, while low serum chloride or nephrosis may increase thyroid iodine uptake. Obtain a drug history, and ascertain whether any medications need to be discontinued before the administration of the radioiodine therapy [3].

References

1. Eary JF, Bennet W. Nuclear medicine therapy. Boca Raton, FL: CRC Press; 2007.
2. Sodium Iodide I-131. https://www.drugs.com/pro/sodium-iodide-i-131.html.
3. Volterrani D, Erba PA, Mariani G. Fondamenti di Medicina Nucleare. Milano: Springer; 2010.
4. AIFA. https://farmaci.agenziafarmaco.gov.it/aifa/servlet/PdfDownloadServlet?pdfFileName=footer_000908_039083_RCP.pdf&retry=0&sys=m0b1l3.
5. Courtesy of G. Pepe. Re-designed from: Ahn BC. Sodium iodide symporter for nuclear molecular imaging and gene therapy: from bedside to bench and back. Theranostics. 2012;2(4):392–402.

3 Radioiodine Therapy of Hyperthyroidism

Giovanna Pepe and Gennaro Cusato

Abstract

Thyroid benign disorders have been successfully treated by means of administration of 131iodine since the 1940s. The efficacy and safety of this treatment and the advantages over thyroid surgery made its success worldwide. In this chapter we outline indication, Patients preparation and precautions regarding radioiodine. We also discuss the procedures and the safety and side effects of this treatment.

3.1 Brief Introduction

Thyroid benign disorders have been successfully treated by means of administration of 131iodine since the 1940s [1]. The efficacy and safety of this treatment and the advantages over thyroid surgery made its success worldwide, and recommendations have been released by several scientific societies including the European Association of Nuclear Medicine and Molecular Imaging and the American Society of Nuclear Medicine, whose procedural guidelines we also refer to, in this chapter [2, 3].

G. Pepe (✉) • G. Cusato
Nuclear Medicine Unit, Humanitas Research Hospital, Rozzano, MI, Italy
e-mail: giovanna.pepe@cancercenter.humanitas.it

3.2 Indications

Indications for 131iodine treatment of thyroid benign diseases include:

- Hyperfunctioning conditions (hyperthyroidism)
- Subclinical hyperthyroidism
- Non-hyperfunctioning conditions (euthyroid goitre)

Clinically evident hyperthyroidism may be caused by:

- Multiple or single hyperfunctioning nodules (toxic goitre and thyroid adenoma)
- Autoimmune toxic diffuse goitre (also known as Graves or Basedow disease)

E. Bombardieri et al. (eds.), *Clinical Applications of Nuclear Medicine Targeted Therapy*,
https://doi.org/10.1007/978-3-319-63067-0_3

For persistent hyperthyroidism due to toxic nodular goitre, radioiodine represents the treatment of choice since antithyroid drugs (ATD) are not curative in this condition and the administration of 131iodine is aiming to a reduction in either function or size of the gland.

For patients affected by solitary toxic adenoma, since the radiopharmaceutical is concentrated by the toxic nodule, there is also a partial sparing of the surrounding normal tissue from radiation-induced changes.

In Graves patients radioiodine may represent a first-line treatment or it could be administered after a treatment with ATDs has failed to result in long-term remission. In fact treatment with antithyroid medications may result not only difficult with regard to the patient management, but it is also burdened by serious side effects (including minor rashes and, in rare cases, agranulocytosis and hepatitis), possible drug resistance as well as relapse of disease after drug discontinuation (Table 3.1).

A large number of patients affected by Graves disease (GD) are younger than 40 years old, and GD is the most common cause of hyperthyroidism in childhood affecting 1 in 10,000 children.

In this group of patients, iodine can be prescribed as a first-choice treatment in view of the long-term morbidity associated with poorly controlled thyrotoxicosis and in consideration of the difficult management of long-term therapy with ATDs. Controversies in the administration of 131iodine in the paediatric age do exist; nonetheless interesting results are available in literature, and iodine administration in younger Patients has become more frequent in the routine clinical practice [4].

131iodine is also indicated when hyperthyroidism is not controlled or recurs after partial thyroid surgery: in these cases radioiodine should be administered before the patient becomes symptomatic [5, 6].

Even if there are few studies assessing the potential benefit of TSH (thyroid-stimulating hormone) normalization, treatment of *subclinical hyperthyroidism* has gained importance in recent years [7].

Radioiodine is recommended when solitary/multiple functioning nodules or GD are the underlying disease in subclinical hyperthyroidism and when the biochemical abnormality is persistent, being this condition associated with increased risk of coronary disease, atrial fibrillation, heart failure and fractures in patients with serum TSH levels <0.1 mIU/l [8] (Table 3.2).

For different causes of subclinical hyperthyroidism, other treatments should be contemplated (see Table 3.3).

Non-hyperfunctioning thyroid diseases (*euthyroid goitre*) could benefit from a reduction in size (to relieve compressive symptoms), thanks to the application of radioactive iodine.

For significantly sized goitres causing symptoms or signs of obstruction of the oesophagus or the trachea, surgery is still considered the treatment of choice; however radioiodine can be discussed as options especially when surgery is not indicated for co-morbidity or it is refused by the patient [10] (Table 3.4).

We can then summarize the clinical settings for this treatment into three categories as in Table 3.5.

Table 3.1 Factors that influence the decision-making in hyperfunctioning disease (hyperthyroidism)

• Diagnosis (toxic goitre, toxic adenoma, Graves disease)
• Thyroid tracer uptake
• Patient age
• Gender
• Severity of hyperthyroidism
• Other co-existing medical conditions
• Access to radioiodine
• Patient preference

Table 3.2 Factors that influence the decision-making process in subclinical hyperthyroidism

• Diagnosis (underlying disease)
• TSH serum levels over the time
• Thyroid tracer uptake
• Patient age
• Co-morbidity

Contraindications for radioiodine treatment are as in EANM guidelines [2]:

Table 3.3 Treatment options for subclinical hyperthyrodism of different origin

Causes of subclinical hyperthyroidism	Treatment suggested
Autonomous thyroid hormone secretion	
• Multinodular autonomous goitre	Radioactive iodine
• Solitary hyperfunctioning adenoma	Radioactive iodine
Excessive TSH-receptor stimulation	
• Graves disease	Antithyroid medication/radioiodine
• Gestational transient thyrotoxicosis	'Wait and see'
• hCG-producing molar or choriocarcinoma	Surgery
• TSH-producing pituitary adenoma	Surgery
Thyroiditis	Steroids
Iatrogenic thyrotoxicosis	Adjust dosage
External sources	Stop self-administration of medication/stop intake of food supplements
Other diseases	
• Struma ovarii	Surgery

Modified from Carle et al. [9]

Table 3.4 Factors that influence the decision-making process in non-hyperfunctioning disease (euthyroid goitre)

• Goitre size
• Tracer uptake
• Patient age
• Likelihood of surgical complications

- Relative
  - Uncontrolled hyperthyroidism
  - Active thyroid orbitopathy (particularly in smokers)
- Absolute
  - Pregnancy
  - Breastfeeding

When prescribing radioiodine treatment in women planning a pregnancy, it is mandatory to either postpone the treatment or to inform the patient that it is advisable not to get pregnant within 6 months after taking iodine.

There is neither reported reduction in fertility after radioiodine treatment nor evidence of any foetal or maternal risk for women previously treated.

Breast-feeding must be discontinued permanently when radioiodine is administered as iodine is concentrated in milk, but is safe in subsequent pregnancies.

3.3 Patient Preparation

Thyroid disease always needs close cooperation between the endocrinologist and the nuclear medicine physician. The first one refers to the treatment and usually follows the patient up; the latter takes the overall responsibility for the radioiodine treatment being in charge of assessing the indication, prescribing and administering radioiodine as well as giving all the information about radiation safety.

A pre-evaluation in the outpatient clinic can be organized, during which the nuclear medicine physician will have to collect the following information:

Table 3.5 Clinical indications for 131iodine treatment in thyroid benign disease

Hyperfunctioning	Intermediate	Non-hyperfunctioning
Multiple toxic nodules	Subclinical hyperthyroidism • Solitary/multiple functioning nodules • GD	Large non-toxic goitre
Solitary toxic nodule		
Autoimmune toxic goitre (Graves/Basedow)		

Table 3.6 Drugs interactions

Medication	Suggested withdrawal
Methimazole	3–4 days
Propylthiouracil	2–3 weeks
Thyroid hormones	10 days for T3[a]
	4 weeks for T4[a]
Lugol solution	2–3 weeks
Topical iodine (surgical disinfection)	2–3 weeks
Potassium iodide	2–3 weeks
Radiological contrast media	2–3 months according to the type
Amiodarone	6 months

Modified from SNM guidelines [3]
[a]T3 or T4 treatment discontinuation should rather be discussed in conjunction with the endocrinologist

- Patient history with regard to duration of disease, previous treatment including antithyroid drugs and/or previous radioiodine, medical treatment for co-morbidity as some drugs may interfere with tracer uptake (see Table 3.6)
- Laboratory test: free T4, free T3, TSH, anti-TSH rec, TPO
- Recent (less than 3 months) neck ultrasound with/without FNA of larger suspicious nodules to exclude malignancy and volumetric evaluation of the gland (or at least goitre extension)
- Recent (less than 6 months) thyroid scintigraphy performed either with 99mTc-pertechnetate or 123iodine and thyroid tracer uptake
- Previous administration of contrast media for radiological imaging (it may cause reduction in tracer uptake)
- GD evaluation of ophthalmopathy, possibly assessed by a dedicated ophthalmologist

Clear communication between the nuclear medicine physician and the patient is the core point to ensure the treatment is prescribed and performed according to good clinical practice and to guarantee correct application of the radiation safety measures.

A written informed consent for the treatment must be obtained during the patient's interview or upon the administration of treatment.

With regard to medical preparation to the radioiodine therapy, ATDs must be discontinued for a sufficient time before 131iodine to avoid reduction in tracer uptake. It is important to bear in mind that among ATD, methimazole needs to be stopped for 3 days before planned radioiodine administration; propylthiouracil needs discontinuation for at least 2 weeks because of its radioprotective action [11, 12].

However in patients affected by GD, a certain period of 'premedication' with such drugs may be required to deplete thyroid hormone stores.

There are also other medications containing iodine that need to be stopped before nuclear medicine treatment (as summarized in Table 3.6) to avoid interferences.

Fasting is needed for at least 4 h prior to the administration of iodine and in the following two, to improve the gastrointestinal absorption.

Debate exists regarding the optimal treatment strategy in paediatric patients; despite a prolonged use of ATDs is considered a valid approach, it does not increase the chances of remission. Moreover risks and side effects from antithyroid drugs are known as well as in the adult population [13].

It is possible to plan radioiodine treatment for young patients after antithyroid drug failure in remission or in known side effects caused by these medications.

The use of radioactivity even in these patients is safe even though it may require some additional precautions. A stratification of risk is mandatory to choose the best therapy options (Fig. 3.1).

As seen for adults, antithyroid medications need withdrawal for very similar time lapse; however in young patients, the discontinuation of thyroid/antithyroid medication can be more problematic than in the adults, thus requiring a close look by the paediatric endocrinologist.

Thyroid scintigraphy and tracer uptake measurement are mandatory before treatment and together with a volumetric evaluation of the gland may contribute to the definition of a personalized therapy by means of the dosimetric analysis.

131Iodine has proven to show less efficacy in thyroid glands larger than 80 g in children; therefore it is not recommended in these cases (Fig. 3.1).

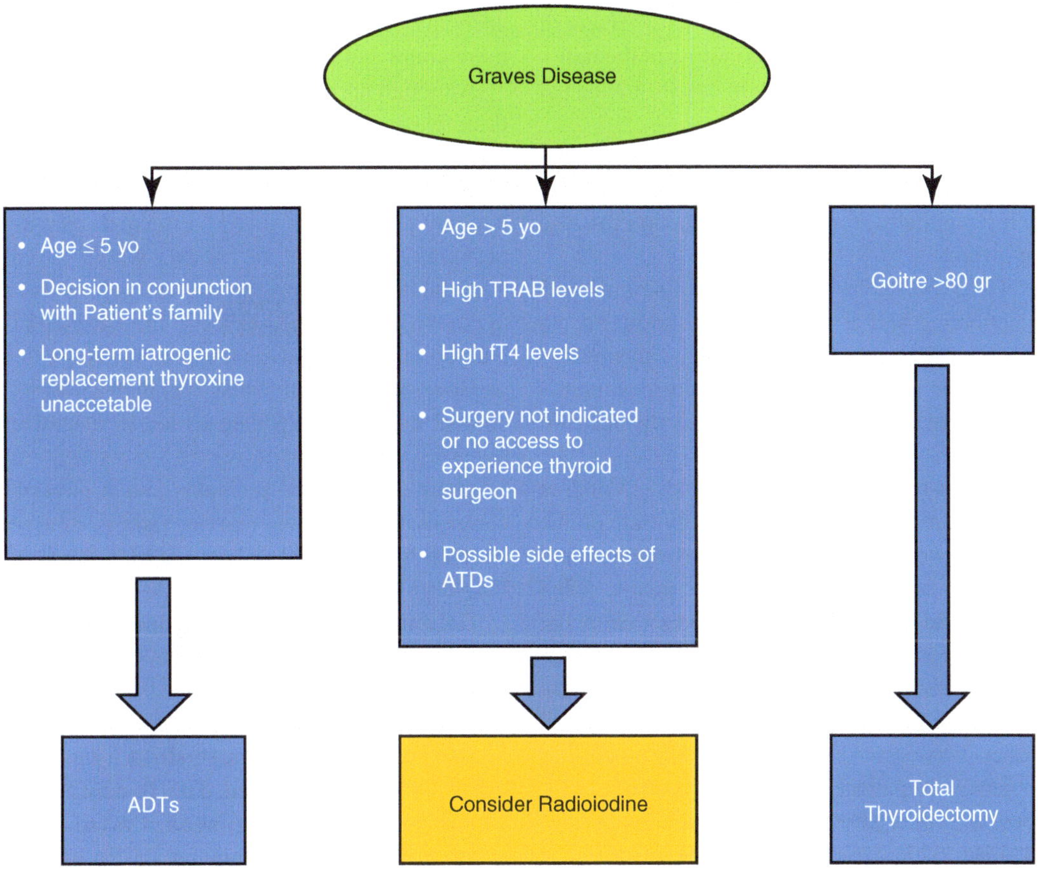

Fig. 3.1 Risk stratification and therapeutic approach flow-chart in Graves disease

3.3.1 Precautions

Radioiodine administration is very unlikely to elicit an allergic reaction, even in known iodine sensitivity, as the elemental iodine content of radioiodine preparations is 0.05–0.18 μg (very significantly lower than average daily iodine intake). There is no need for hyposensitizing premedication in these patients.

Lithium is known to be able to block the radioiodine release but not the uptake, so it is possible in selected cases to plan premedication with lithium to enhance the iodine uptake [14].

Additional care is needed with patients incontinent of urine (bladder catheterization before radioiodine therapy or even admission to the hospital for in-patient treatment should be considered).

Any peculiar case ought to be discussed within a multidisciplinary team meeting.

3.4 Procedures and Results

The administration of 131iodine is allowed only in premises that have registration and authorisation from the appropriate regulatory body according to the national laws.

It is carried out by a nuclear medicine physician after written informed consent is obtained by the patient or her/his legal representative (parents in case of paediatric patients). In case of women in fertile age, a pregnancy test must be checked prior to iodine administration.

This therapy does not usually need hospital admission, a part from specific cases and unless the local authorities impose hospitalization, so it is usually performed within the out-patient clinic activity.

The presence of specialized non-medical staff such as nurses or technologists and of a medical physicist is advisable for the safe management of the patient and for a correct handling of the radiopharmaceutical, particularly in case of incidental contamination and spread.

Iodine is commonly administered orally, but in patients affected by severe dysphagia or unable to be compliant, an intravenous injection can also be given.

The expected results of radioiodine in hyperfunctioning and/or subclinical disease are to achieve a non-hyperthyroid status—either euthyroidism or iatrogenic hypothyroidism (which is going to be compensated afterwards by means of levothyroxine).

In non-toxic goitre, the aim of 131iodine administration is the reduction of thyroid volume and consequent relief of compressive symptoms.

There are two approaches in adults, fixed activity and personalized activity, decided on the basis of the dosimetric analysis (that will be further discussed in the next section of this book).

The range of activities currently prescribed varies between 300 and 800 MBq, with the majority of patients receiving 400–600 MBq; these activities have been empirically established [15]. In Table 3.7 there is a range of activities commonly used in clinical practice.

In selected cases, especially in non-functioning goitre, higher activities may be required needing a switch from out-patient to in-patient setting. In these patients, iodine uptake evaluation test or even dosimetry may be advisable to ensure an adequate irradiation of the gland is achieved.

When treating *hyperthyroidism*, success following 131iodine administration has been defined the elimination of hyperthyroidism, which is expected to rate an average of 80%, whether the underlying disease is GD, toxic goitre or toxic adenoma with even higher rates up to 90% in toxic goitre and hyperfunctioning adenoma [16].

Table 3.7 Range of 131-iodine activities commonly used in clinical practice

Clinical scenario	131Iodine prescribed activity
GD	400–600 MBq
Toxic multinodular goitre	500–800 MBq
Toxic adenoma	500 MBq
Non-toxic goitre	600–800 MBq[a]
Retreatment in hyperthyroidism relapse	Individual risk assessment

[a]Higher activities may be required, thus implying hospitalization

Although normalization of thyroid function is desirable and can be accomplished after radioiodine, the majority of patients will become hypothyroid eventually. The incidence of hypothyroidism has been estimated ranging between 20 and 40% of patients within 1 year after radioiodine treatment, and the probability of hypothyroidism increases over the years, thus making regular follow-up necessary [17].

However it is notable that hypothyroidism is a clinical condition exposing to lower risks than hyperthyroidism with regard especially to cardiovascular-related problems and it is easily compensated by levothyroxine administration, which is not burdened by heavy side effects from long-term therapy as opposed to ATDs.

Patients affected by autoimmune thyroid disease should also be monitored for complications, such as Graves' opthalmopathy.

When treating *non-hyperfunctioning* thyroid disease, in patients with a small to a medium-sized goitre, an approximate reduction by 50% of volume has been estimated as an effect of radioiodine therapy with evidence already in the first months after the 131iodine.

Radioiodine has been shown to be effective also in retrosternal goitre even if this treatment is relatively contraindicated in those with very large goitre because of the need for higher activities or repeated treatments [18].

When treating *children* affected by GD, the reluctance to use radioiodine derives mainly from concerns about short- and long-term complications, but a 95% remission rate is expected as seen in literature in more than 1200 cases, and radioiodine seems to show superior efficacy as compared to ATDs, in several studies [19, 20].

There is experience of excellent results for iodine treatment even in children as young as 1 year old, even though the administration of radioiodine in such young patients is not common and not routinely recommended. As seen for adults, the response rate is partially related to the gland size and to the administered activity, but there are data supporting that thyroid tissue of children is more sensitive to 131iodine-induced ablative effects than adults [21].

3.5 Side Effects and Safety

Most patients notice no side effects from the treatment; however in either adults or children, nausea can occur soon after iodine as well as pain in the neck region mimicking sore throat, both symptoms when not self-limiting can be treated with anti-inflammatory drugs.

Graves' ophthalmopathy that is at risk of exacerbation in adults does not seem to worsen in children following iodine treatment, but it is possible to prevent it by means of steroid therapy upon administration of 131iodine. The administration of steroids in children should be discussed with the paediatric endocrinologist [22].

Soon after radioiodine treatment, especially in those patients already affected by hyperfunctioning goitre, a transient thyrotoxicosis may show up, and therefore treatment with antithyroid drugs could be prescribed from 4 days after radioiodine for 10 up to 20 days in order to control the symptoms. β-Blockers may also be used to relieve the cardiac symptoms in the first 2 weeks after iodine.

Iodine treatment is safe as there is no evidence of increased incidence of leukaemia or solid tumours in patients that had been treated with radioiodine [23, 24].

The small increased risk of thyroid cancer after radioiodine reported in some epidemiological studies seems associated more to the underlying thyroid disease rather than treatment itself [25].

In a retrospective analysis of patients younger than 20 years old treated and followed for three decades did not show excess of adverse effects, providing evidence of safety in children and adolescents [26].

3.6 Radiation Safety Information

Before releasing the patient, the nuclear medicine physician should provide her/him with written instructions and recommended precautions to lower unnecessary irradiation to the public and to family members. Children and pregnant women should be kept away from the patients for around 1 week (this period may vary according to the administered activity); there are no significant restrictions for all other adults (Table 3.8) [27].

Table 3.8 Behaviour restriction and radiation safety instructions after treatment

	Activity of administered iodine		
Behaviour restriction	300–400 MBq	600 MBq	800 MBq or superior
Stay at least 1 m away from children <10 years old and pregnant women	5 days	7–10 days	14 days
Sleep separately from comforters and acrers	–	2 days	7 days
Avoid prolonged close contact (more than 3 h, less than 1 m) with other adults	–	–	1 day

Modified from 'Royal College of Physicians. Radioiodine in the management of benign thyroid disease: clinical guidelines. Report of a Working Party. London: RCP, 2007' [27]

No hazard derives for any of the family member from what the patient has touched, including food. Disposable plates can be used for the first days after treatment but are not strictly necessary.

Due to the urinary excretion of the radiopharmaceutical, it is advisable that men urinate sitting down and that all patients should flush the toilet twice after any use. There is no need for separate wash of patients' clothes. Prolonged use of public transport is discouraged at least in the first days after radioiodine as well as attendance to theatre and cinema.

3.7 Follow-Up

Follow-up is usually carried by the endocrinologist, albeit there is tradition in some countries for the nuclear medicine physician to do so.

Patients should be instructed to promptly report to the referring physician major side effects such as worsening of the Graves' ophthalmopathy or transient thyrotoxicosis and cardiac symptoms.

Significant reduction of the thyroid activity is rarely seen before 6–8 weeks after treatment;

hence it is useful to check blood levels of thyroid hormones not prior to 45 days after treatment.

Subsequent laboratory test could be asked with a time interval of 2 months to monitor the ensuing of the hypothyroidism in order to correct it with levothyroxine.

Relapse of hyperthyroidism can also occur especially in severe GD, and a second treatment may be required, but an interval of 6 months before another cycle of radioiodine therapy is recommended.

References

1. Chapman EM. History of the discovery and early use of radioactive iodine. JAMA. 1983;250(15):2042–4.
2. Stokkel MPM, Handkiewicz DJ, Lassmann M, et al. EANM procedure guidelines for therapy of benign thyroid disease. Eur J Nucl Med Mol Imaging. 2010;37:2218–28.
3. Silberstein EB, Abass A, Balon HR, et al. The SNM practice guideline for therapy of thyroid disease with 131I 3.0. JNM. 2012;53(10):1633–51.
4. Rivkees SA. Controversies in the management of Graves' disease in children. J Endocrinol Investig. 2016;39:1247–57.
5. Cooper DS. Hyperthyroidism. Lancet. 2003;362:459–68.
6. Franklyn JA. The management of hyperthyroidism. N Engl J Med. 1994;330:1731–8.
7. McDermott MT, Woodmansee WW, Haugen BR, et al. The management of subclinical hyperthyroidism by thyroid specialists. Thyroid. 2003;13:1133–9.
8. Biondi B, Bartalena L, Cooper DS, et al. The 2015 European Thyroid Association guidelines on diagnosis and treatment of endogenous subclinical hyperthyroidism. Eur Thyroid J. 2015;4:149–63.
9. Carle A, Andersen SL, Boelaert K, et al. Management of endocrine disease: subclinical thyrotoxicosis: prevalence, causes and choice of therapy. Eur J Endocrinol. 2017;176(6):R325–37. https://doi.org/10.1530/EJE-16-0276.
10. Wesche MF, Tiel-V Buul MM, Lips P, et al. A randomized trial comparing levothyroxine with radioactive iodine in the treatment of sporadic nontoxic goiter. J Clin Endocrinol Metab. 2001;86: 998–1005.
11. Braga M, Walpert N, Burch HB, et al. The effect of methimazole on cure rates after radioiodine treatment for Graves' hyperthyroidism: a randomized clinical trial. Thyroid. 2002;12:135–9.
12. Santos RB, Romaldini JH, Ward LS. Propylthiouracil reduces the effectiveness of radioiodine treatment in hyperthyroid patients with Graves' disease. Thyroid. 2004;14:525–30.
13. West JD, Cheetham TD, Dane C, et al. Should radioiodine be the first-line treatment for paediatric Graves' disease? – review article. J Pediatr Endocrinol Metab. 2015;28(7-8):797–804.
14. Bal CS, Kumar A, Pandey RM. A randomized controlled trial to evaluate the adjuvant effect of lithium on radioiodine treatment of hyperthyroidism. Thyroid. 2002;12:399–405.
15. Lazarus JH. Guidelines for the use of radioiodine in the management of hyperthyroidism: a summary. The Radioiodine Audit Subcommittee of the Royal College of Physicians Committee on Diabetes and Endocrinology, and the Research Unit of the Royal College of Physicians. J R Coll Physicians Lond. 1995;29:464–9.
16. Collier A, Gosh S, Hair M, et al. Comparison of two fixed activities of radioiodine therapy (370 vs. 555 MBq) in patients with Graves' disease. Hormones (Athens). 2009;8:273–8.
17. Hagen GA, Ouellette RP, Chapman EM. Comparison of high and low dosage levels of 131-I in the treatment of thyrotoxicosis. N Engl J Med. 1967;277(11):559–62.
18. Bachmann J, Kobe C, Bor S, et al. Radioiodine therapy for thyroid volume reduction of large goitres. Nucl Med Commun. 2009;30:466–71.
19. Rivkees SA, Sklar C, Freemark M. Clinical review 99: the management of Graves' disease in children, with special emphasis on radioiodine treatment. J Clin Endocrinol Metab. 1998;83:3767–76.
20. Ma C, Kuang A, Xie J, et al. Radioiodine treatment for pediatric Graves' disease. Cochrane Database Syst Rev. 2008;3:CD006294.
21. Rivkees SA, Cornelius EA. Influence of iodine-131 dose on the outcome of hyperthyroidism in children. Pediatrics. 2003;111(4 Pt 1):745–9.
22. Bartalena L, Baldeschi L, Dickinson A, et al. Consensus statement of the European Group on Graves' orbitopathy (EUGOGO) on management of GO. Eur J Endocrinol. 2008;158:273–85.
23. Hall P, Berg G, Bjelkengren G, et al. Cancer mortality after iodine-131 therapy for hyperthyroidism. Int J Cancer. 1992;50:886–90.
24. Hall P, Boice JD, Berg G, et al. Leukaemia incidence after iodine-131 exposure. Lancet. 1992;340:1–4.
25. Dobyns BM, Sheline GE, Workman JB, et al. Malignant and benign neoplasms of the thyroid in patients treated for hyperthyroidism: a report of the cooperative thyrotoxicosis therapy follow-up study. J Clin Endocrinol Metab. 1974;38:976–98.
26. Read CH, Tansey MJ, Menda Y. A 36-year retrospective analysis of the efficacy and safety of radioactive iodine in treating young Graves' patients. J Clin Endocrinol Metab. 2004;89:4229–33.
27. Royal College of Physicians. Radioiodine in the management of benign thyroid disease: clinical guidelines. Report of a Working Party. London: RCP; 2007.

Dosimetry in the Radioiodine Treatment of Hyperthyroidism

4

Cristina Canzi and Antonio Claudio Traino

Abstract

Radioiodine therapy has largely replaced surgery and is nowadays commonly used because it is easy to perform and has proved to be effective in the definitive treatment of hyperthyroidism.

Hundreds of thousands of patients have been treated all over the world, but still there isn't a clear evidence about the optimal method to determine the activity to administer to reach the therapeutic objective. The discussion is still open on when to use fixed activities or to perform a pre-therapeutic dosimetric study to personalize the administered activity to the single patient's morphological and metabolic characteristics. The rationale behind pretreatment personalized dosimetry is to determine the ^{131}I activity that is most likely to lead to the therapeutic success but that limits the radiation exposure to the strictly necessary amount as also required by the recent European Directives about protection against the dangers due to ionizing radiation. Hyperthyroidism is a benign condition, so the aim of the treatment is to heal it in a short time with the minimum activity and, if possible, with a unique administration. Personalized dosimetry aims to tailor the therapeutic activity to be administered to the morphological and metabolic characteristics of each patient's thyroid because there is quite a wide interpatient variability. Some indications about how to perform a personalized dosimetry are reported with a short review of literature data about the clinical results of different methods.

C. Canzi
Health Physics and Nuclear Medicine Units, Fondazione IRCCS Ca' Granda Ospedale Maggiore Policlinico, Milan, Italy
e-mail: ccanzi@policlinico.mi.it

A.C. Traino (✉)
Health Physics Unit, Azienda Ospedaliero-Universitaria Pisana, Pisa, Italy
e-mail: c.traino@ao-pisa.toscana.it

4.1 Goal of Dosimetry in Hyperthyroidism

The first administration of ^{131}I to a patient for the treatment of hyperthyroidism was on January 1, 1941 [1]. Radioiodine therapy has largely replaced surgery and is nowadays commonly

E. Bombardieri et al. (eds.), *Clinical Applications of Nuclear Medicine Targeted Therapy*,
https://doi.org/10.1007/978-3-319-63067-0_4

used because it is easy to perform and has proved to be effective in the definitive treatment of hyperthyroidism.

Hundreds of thousands of patients have been treated all over the world, but still there isn't a clear evidence about the optimal method to determine the activity to administer to reach the therapeutic objective. The discussion is still open on when to use fixed activities or to perform a pretherapeutic dosimetric study to personalize the administered activity to the single patient's morphological and metabolic characteristics.

Although the administration of fixed activities is still admitted by the EANM procedure guidelines for therapy of benign thyroid disease [2], mainly for patients >45 of age, there is an increasing evidence that personalized treatments could improve the quality and outcome of radionuclide therapy [3]. The rationale behind pretreatment personalized dosimetry is to determine the ^{131}I activity that is most likely to lead to the therapeutic success but that limits the radiation exposure to the strictly necessary amount. Such an approach was introduced in 1997 by the "European Council Directive 97/43/Euratom on health protection of individuals against the dangers of ionizing radiation in relation to medical exposure" [4] that at article 4 stated that "…for all medical exposure of individuals for radiotherapeutic purposes…, exposures of target volumes shall be *individually planned*; taking into account that doses of non-target volumes and tissues shall be as low as reasonably achievable and consistent with the intended radiotherapeutic purpose of the exposure."

In 2013 the new Council Directive 2013/59/EURATOM "Laying down basic safety standards for protection against the dangers arising from exposure to ionising radiation" [5] (that repeals the previous one and must be adopted by member states by February 2018) again underlines this concept and, moreover, at article 56 adds that not only exposures of target volumes shall be *individually planned* but also "their delivery appropriately verified."

Even in the USA, on January 2015, the ex-president Barack Obama in his State of the Union Address announced the Personalized Medicine Initiative calling for hundreds of million dollars to support it. The concept of Personalized Medicine is prevention and treatment strategies that take into account individual variability [6].

Implementation of dosimetry prior to therapy varies among the different European nations: in some countries it is mandatory, such as in Germany [7], while in others it remains exceptional, such as in Italy [8].

Individual patient dosimetry is essential not only for optimizing the administered activity through the establishment of the minimum effective dose but also for determining a dose-response relationship as a basis for predicting clinical outcome.

In nuclear medicine, the most easy quantity to measure is the activity (intended as number of decay per second (Bq, becquerel) of a radioactive source) because all laboratories are equipped with a dose calibrator. However, the same activity given to different patients can distribute in the body in a different way depending on many factors such as their physiopathological conditions (e.g., because of some organ impairment or different kinds of disease), organ dimensions, organ uptake, and retention, and so the energy released by the radioactivity can vary from each other. The energy released in a mass is called absorbed dose and is expressed in Gray (Gy; 1 Gy = 1 J/Kg). The clinical effect of radionuclide administration should be correlated to the absorbed dose and not to the bare activity, and this concept is the pillar of the individualized dosimetry when radioactivity is administered for therapeutic aims. In fact, personalized dosimetry aims to tailor the therapeutic activity such that the absorbed dose to the thyroid or diseased parts of the thyroid amount to the prescribed dose value.

Hyperthyroidism is a benign condition, so the aim of the treatment is to heal it in a short time with the minimum activity and, if possible, with a unique administration.

4.2 The Practical Implementation of Dosimetry in Hyperthyroidism

Iodine kinetics in thyroid is characterized by an intake phase reaching a maximum of about 24–48 h after the administration, followed by a washout one (see Fig. 4.1).

This behavior can be described by the following mathematical function (derived from a two-compartmental model):

$$U(t) = \frac{U_{\max}\lambda_{in}}{\lambda_{out} - \lambda_{in}}\left(e^{-\lambda_{in}t} - e^{-\lambda_{out}t}\right) \quad (4.1)$$

where $U_{\max}$ = maximum uptake

λ_{in} = rate of iodine intake in thyroid
λ_{out} = rate of iodine washout from thyroid including physical decay and biologic dismission. This parameter can be converted in a more intuitive quantity, the effective half-life:

$$T_{\frac{1}{2}\text{eff}} = \frac{In(2)}{\lambda_{out}} \quad (4.2)$$

These three parameters are specific for each thyroid or even for each substructure present in the same gland, and they can be determined by fitting experimental data (circles in Fig. 4.1) with Eq. (4.1).

It is therefore evident that a patient-specific dosimetric study implies the measurements of uptake values at different times to describe the radioiodine kinetics in the therapy target. If the uptake assessments are at least 3 including measurements at about 2–4 h, 1–2 days, and 5–8 days, according to the MIRD formalism and Eq. (4.1), the therapeutic activity can be calculated as:

$$A(MBq) = 24.7\frac{D(Gy)m(g)}{U_{\max}T_{\frac{1}{2}eff}(d)} \quad (4.3)$$

If less than three uptake measurements are performed, how to determine the therapeutic activity is well described in the EANM guidelines for dosimetry prior to radioiodine therapy of benign thyroid diseases [9].

Uptake at time t is defined as the ratio between the activity present at that time in a biological structure and the administered activity; its measurement can be performed with a dedicated probe or by means of planar scintigraphy acquired with a gamma camera. Activity can be administered orally both in liquid form and as capsules: this second way is preferable to limit the possibility of contaminations. An intravenous administration is also possible.

The tracer activity to be used for the pre-therapy dosimetry must be measured before the administration using a phantom mimicking the neck. It must be made of a material that has radiation absorption and scatter characteristics similar to those of human soft tissue and the same geometrical structures and sizes of real necks. The one proposed by the International Atomic Energy Agency (IAEA) and the American National Standards Institute is made of Lucite and is represented in Fig. 4.2.

If a probe is used to measure the activity in the thyroid, the distance between the detector and the patient's neck must be at least 25 cm from the detector to assure that the field of view covers the entire thyroid. If measurements are performed at different times, it is very important that this distance is always kept exactly the same because the count rate varies according to the inverse square

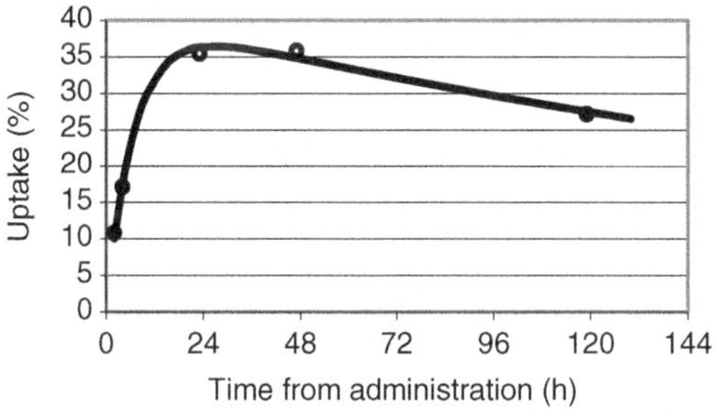

Fig. 4.1 Iodine kinetics in thyroid

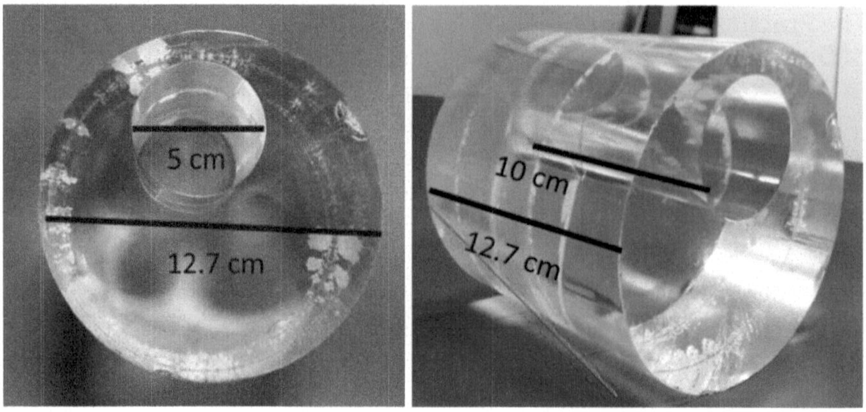

Fig. 4.2 Neck phantom

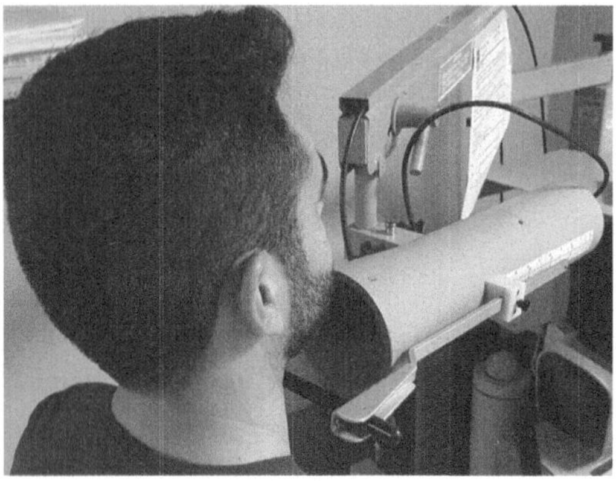

Fig. 4.3 Measurements of thyroid uptake with a probe

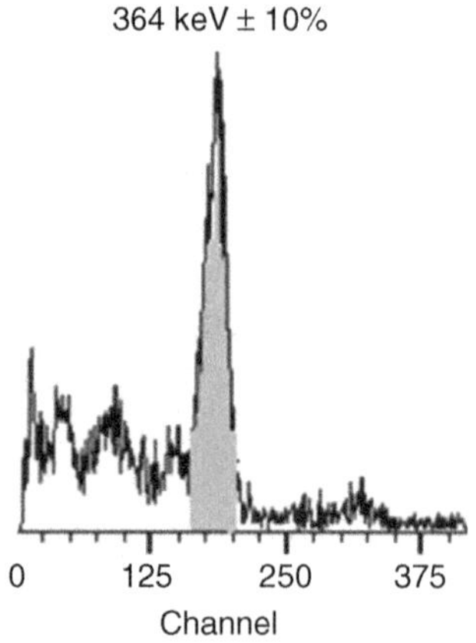

Fig. 4.4 ^{131}I spectrum

law. A spacer between detector and neck can help in reproducing the same geometrical conditions as shown in Fig. 4.3.

If a gamma camera is used, geometrical conditions are not a critical aspect because the count rate doesn't follow the inverse square law but depends on the collimator characteristics.

If a probe is used, a spectrum is obtained with a peak centered at 364 keV (main ^{131}I gamma emission), and an energy window of ±10% must be set to register the counts as reported in Fig. 4.4. The tracer activity of ^{131}I should be about 2 MBq and the acquisition time about 1 min.

The use of the probe to measure uptake is good when the activity is uniformly distributed inside the therapeutic target such as in Graves' disease and in solitary adenoma without uptake in extranodular healthy tissue as reported in Fig. 4.5.

If the activity is not uniformly distributed inside the gland due to the presence of multi-substructures, the use of images acquired with a gamma camera is suggested to estimate the dose to each different area. Iodine kinetics of substructures in the same gland usually are different from each other, and proportions are not conserved along time as shown in Fig. 4.6, so it is discouraged to perform uptake measurements with a probe acquiring just one image with a gamma camera to calculate the proportions among the different areas and keep them fixed.

If a gamma camera is used, the tracer ^{131}I activity should be increased to about 10 MBq.

With the gamma camera, the employment of ^{123}I can be suggested because the image quality is quite better than with ^{131}I due the lower emitted energy (159 keV) as can be seen in Fig. 4.7.

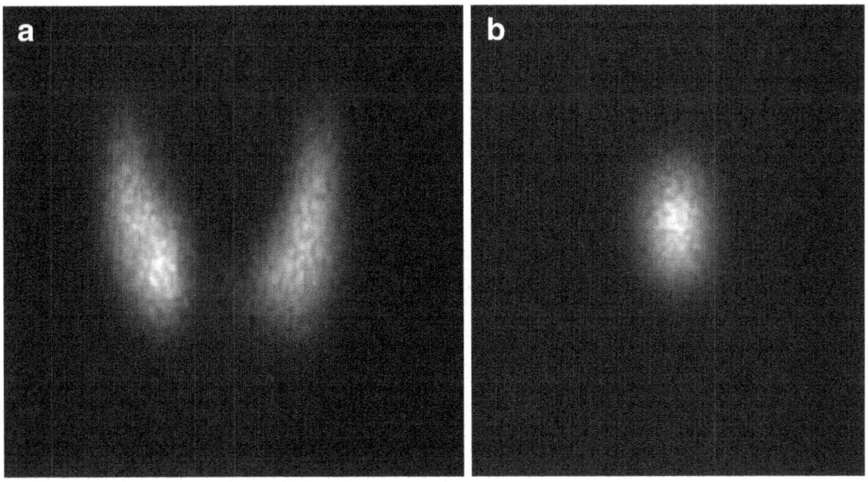

Fig. 4.5 Iodine distribution in Graves' disease and in a solitary adenoma

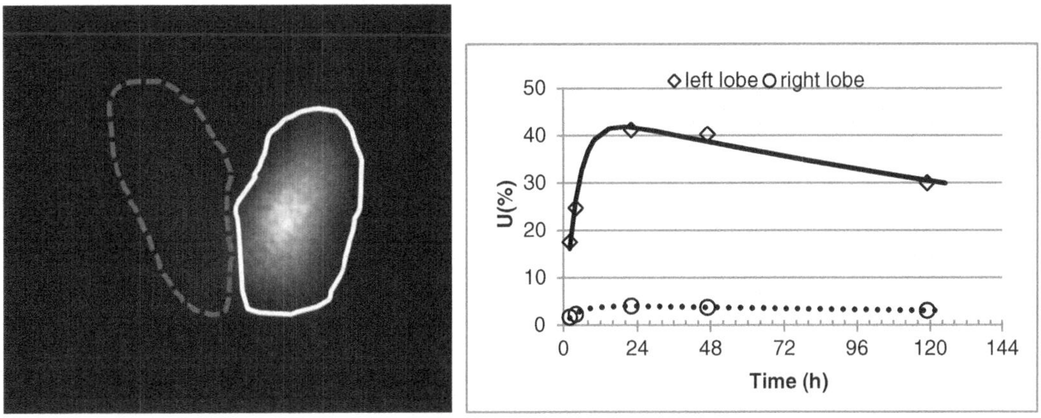

Fig. 4.6 Iodine kinetics in two different subthyroidal structures

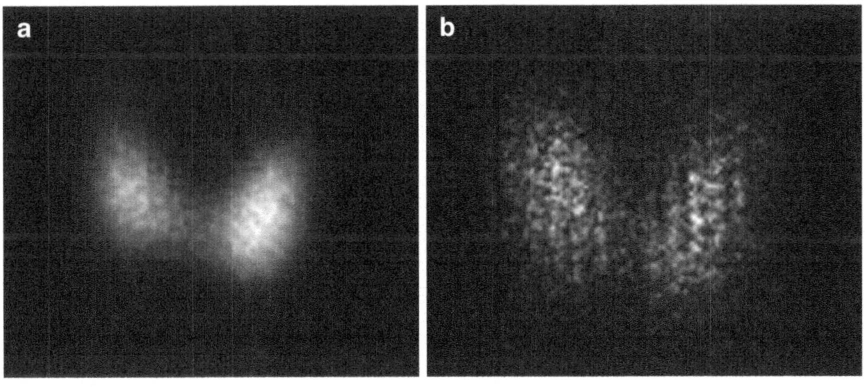

Fig. 4.7 Graves' disease. (**a**) 4-h image of dosimetry with 74 MBq of ^{123}I and (**b**) 4-h image of dosimetry with 5 MBq of ^{131}I

If ^{123}I is used for dosimetry, uptake data must be corrected for the radioactive decay to take into consideration that dosimetry and therapy are performed with different radionuclides. The biologic uptake data obtained must be then corrected for the ^{131}I halftime when therapeutic activity is calculated (^{131}I $T_{1/2}$ = 192 h, ^{123}I $T_{1/2}$ = 13.2 h).

The mass value to insert in Eq. (4.3) usually is obtained by ultrasonography; it should always be compared to a ^{99m}Tc scintigraphy to verify that the measured volume corresponds to the accumulating target volume. Mass is calculated with the ellipsoid formula

$$m(g) = \rho\frac{\pi}{6}*\text{height}(\text{cm})*\text{width}(\text{cm})*\text{depth}(\text{cm}) \quad (4.4)$$

where ρ is the density set equal to 1 g/cm^3.

Axes measurements can also be done on scintigraphic images, but in this case the depth is missed and is set equal to width (rotational ellipsoid).

There is a great interpatient variability of the three parameters necessary to calculate the administered activity according to Eq. (4.3) as indicated in Fig. 4.8. This is the evidence of the necessity of a personalized approach to radiometabolic therapy as reported in the example of Table 4.1: to give the same dose to two thyroidal structures with different morphological and kinetics characteristics, you need quite different (tenfold) therapeutic activities.

From these considerations, it results that the approach based on a fixed activity administration is only an empirical, very inaccurate way to choose the ^{131}I therapeutic activity. It doesn't take into account the differences in radioiodine kinetics and in basal mass between the patients.

The aim of treatment is to quickly achieve a non-hyperthyroid status trying to restore a long-lasting euthyroid status in the case of nodularities and to obtain a complete ablation of thyroid functions (hypothyroidism) in the case of Graves' disease; the therapeutic dose recommended to reach these clinical results is 300–400 Gy and 200–300 Gy, respectively [2], even if it must be noted that the Italian Guidelines for nuclear medicine therapy [8] suggest lower doses for the treatments of nodularities (200 Gy for single nodules and 300 Gy for multinodular goiters).

Starting from these dose values and knowing the characteristics of the therapy target, it is possible to calculate the therapeutic ^{131}I activity to administer using Eq. (4.3).

It is very important to underline the importance of the verification of the agreement between any pretreatment dosimetric study and what really happens after the therapeutic administration: what was measured during the dosimetry should be the same after the therapeutic administration, or, if there is a systematic variation, it

Table 4.1 Example of therapeutic activity calculations in two different cases

Dose (Gy)		Mass (g)	U (%)	$T_{1/2}$eff (d)	A (MBq)
200	Case 1	5.5	48.4	6.7	63
	Case 2	13.3	26.5	3.0	599

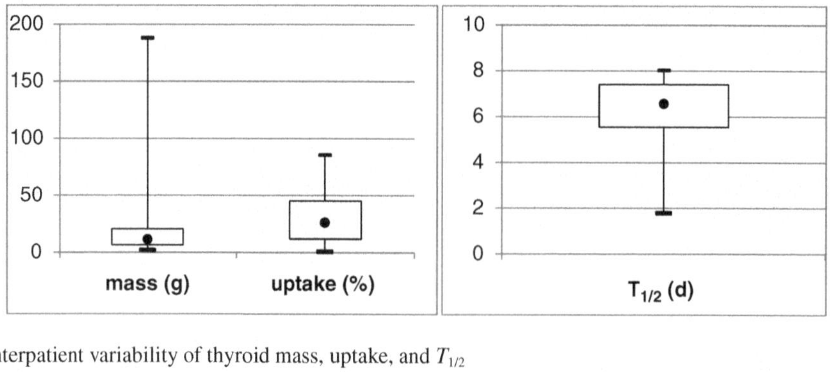

Fig. 4.8 Interpatient variability of thyroid mass, uptake, and $T_{1/2}$

should be considered during the therapy planning. Dosimetry and therapy conditions are quite similar but not identical, just only for the fact that in the first case a tracer activity is given and in the second one a therapeutic amount is administered that can produce some immediate effects. Some authors have already reported the presence of systematic disagreements mainly in the maximum uptake [10–12].

In the case of Graves' disease, another method to calculate the therapeutic activity is suggested by the group of Traino [13–17]. They considered the results published by other groups trying to decide an "optimal" absorbed dose value [18–22]. According to these papers, you can obtain different rates of cure with the same dose values, and conversely with different dose values, you can have the same cure rate.

More recently, relationships between post-therapeutic thyroid volume (mass) and therapy outcome in Graves' disease patients have been reported in literature [23, 24]. These works conclude that an adjustment of the target doses based on thyroid basal volumes will lead to an appropriate reduction of thyroid volumes. This means that the "optimal" absorbed dose value is individual, i.e., it depends on the characteristics of the patient and on the "appropriate" reduction of his thyroid volume. Note that all those results are based only on statistical considerations, without any theoretical model, and for this reason the debate on the optimization of ^{131}I therapy of Graves' disease has a very weak grounding. The hypothesis of an optimum value of thyroid absorbed dose seems to disagree also with the radiobiological linear-quadratic (LQ) model which predicts that the dose needed to reduce a target organ depends on its basal mass. According to it, it seems possible to decide the optimal activity based on the desired reduction of thyroid mass: knowing the optimal value of the final thyroid mass for each patient, the LQ model allows to decide predictively, i.e., after a diagnostic activity (0.37–1.85 MBq) administration, the optimal therapeutic activity A_0, based on the thyroid absorbed dose needed to reduce the basal mass to the optimum mass value [13]. Note that this new modality of optimal activity calculation allows an individualized treatment of the pathology.

The possibility to treat Graves' disease based on the desired reduction of the thyroid mass follows from two main hypotheses:

1. In Graves' disease, the ^{131}I activity is uniformly distributed throughout the gland, i.e., the uptake can be considered almost uniform. This means that thyroid iodine trapping, organification, and function are uniform throughout the gland.
2. There is a linear correlation between the uptake concentration U_0/m_0 before therapy and the uptake concentration U_1/m_1 at the end of therapy (the reduction of the thyroid uptake depends linearly on the reduction of the thyroid mass).

From hypothesis no. 1, it follows that the thyroid functional tissue can be described as a set of identical traps uniformly distributed throughout the gland. These traps are able to concentrate iodine from the blood. Each of them is assumed to take up the same fraction of radioiodine from the blood; thus, the radioiodine uptake depends on the number of the traps in the gland. For each patient, the number of the traps is linearly related to the mass (volume) of his thyroid, i.e., the mass (volume) of the gland is individually linearly related to the uptake. This doesn't mean that patients with the same thyroid mass (volume) have the same number of traps (it depends on thyroid uptake) but that reducing of a fraction f the mass (volume) of the gland one reduces the thyroid uptake of a fraction related to f.

For lovers of mathematics, hypothesis no. 2 can be expressed by equation:

$$\frac{U_1}{m_1} = \phi \frac{U_0}{m_0} \tag{4.5}$$

where m_0 is the basal mass of the gland, U_0 is the basal maximum thyroid uptake, m_1 is the mass of the gland 6 months to 1 year after therapy administration, and U_1 is the maximum thyroid uptake 6 months to 1 year after therapy administration, i.e., at the end of ^{131}I therapy; Φ is a coefficient which takes into account the adjustment of uptake per unit mass due to radioiodine therapy.

Note that $U_1 = U_G$ and $m_1 = m_G$ can be the maximum uptake, and the mass of the gland at the moment of Graves' disease "cure" correspondent to TSH = 0.3 mUI/ml (in the absence of antithyroid drug therapy).

Based on previously published studies, Eq. (4.5) can be rewritten:

$$m_G = 0.24\frac{m_0}{U_0} \qquad (4.6)$$

The final mass of the thyroid due to ^{131}I therapy can be evaluated using the equation:

$$m_{\text{fin}} = m_0 \exp\left(-\alpha D_T\right) \qquad (4.7)$$

where α = 0.0038 Gy^{-1} is a constant typical of thyroid tissue. From Eqs. (4.6) and (4.7), it follows:

$$D_T = D_{TG} = -\frac{1}{\alpha}\ln\left(\frac{0.24}{U_0}\right) \qquad (4.8)$$

D_{TG} is the thyroid dose needed to obtain a final thyroid mass m_G, i.e., the "optimal" thyroid final mass value (see Eq. (4.8)). Note that Eq. (4.7) can be considered a "macroscopic" representation of the LQ model without the quadratic term (that can be neglected if the dose rate is negligible).

Equation (4.8) can be used to evaluate the thyroid absorbed dose which "cures" Graves' disease. Remembering that (MIRD formalism) the absorbed dose in a target is related to the administered activity (among other parameters), also this last value can be calculated based on Eq. (4.8).

It has been demonstrated [14] that the "volume-reduction"-based method reduces the activity and the thyroid absorbed dose compared to the "empirical"-based method, allowing to optimize the therapy administration.

4.3 Feasibility in the Routine

The implementation of dosimetric studies requires availability of personnel and equipment like any other nuclear medicine practice. If a probe is used for uptake measurements, this device is usually dedicated only to these studies, and so the other department activities are not hindered. If a gamma camera is used, the acquisition time is short, of the order of some minutes, so these patients can be set in the agenda early in the morning or at the end of the working day.

Patients usually don't complain about their time engagements if they are properly informed about the reasons of any step. It is suggested to have a talk with the patient where, in addition to all the clinical considerations required to make the decisions about the opportunity to perform the radiometabolic therapy, a clear description about how all the process is organized should be given.

In this practice different professional figures are involved such as physicians, physicists, technologists, and nurses, so a multidisciplinary team must be created and educated to work in synergy to optimize any action.

4.4 Short Review

A lot of papers have been published about the radioiodine treatment of hyperthyroidism, but comparisons are difficult because often it is not clear:

- How the therapeutic activity is determined or, if the dose is considered, what relationship between dose and activity is used
- What the real follow-up of the patients is

Hereafter a short review of some recent works is reported. In most of the papers, activity is calculated as a fixed iodine concentration (4–13 MBq/g) multiplied by the gland mass and divided by the follow-up.

In Table 4.2 data about treatment of single nodules are reported in decreasing order of cure rate intended as a quick resolution of hyperthyroidism; a second therapy aim is to try to reach a euthyroid status stable on time avoiding the incidence of hypothyroidism.

It is evident that the best clinical results with the lowest administered activity are for the series in which a personalized pretreatment dosimetric

Table 4.2 Literature data about treatment of single nodules

Author	Method	A (MBq)	Resolution (%)	Euthyroidism (%)	Hypo (%)	Hyper (%)
Huysmans [25]	Fixed activity	740	100	88	12	0
Walter [26]	Eq. (4.3) *with* $D = 400$ Gy	*592*	*100*	*90*	*10*	*0*
Schiavo [27]	*Traino's method with* $D = 300$ Gy	*304*	*99*	*91*	*8*	*1*
Regalbuto [28]	Eq. (4.3) *with* $D = 300$ Gy *and a fixed* $T_{1/2}$eff = 5.6 d	*374*	*97*	*79*	*17*	*3*
Zingrillo [29]	12.6 MB/g	488	96	78	18	4
Tarantini [30]	Not declared	444	94	75	19	6
Mariotti [31]	6.7 MB/g	466	91	88	4	9
Erdogan [32]	3.7 MB/g	740	87	77	10	13
Ratcliff [33]	Fixed activity	555	87	87	0	13
Nygaard [34]	3.7 MB/g	310	86	78	8	14
Jarlov [35]	3.7 MB/g	259	56	56	0	44
Ustun [36]	4.4 MB/g	370	45	45	0	55

Table 4.3 Literature data about treatment of multinodularity

Author	Method	A (MBq)	Resolution (%)	Euthyroidism (%)	Hypo (%)	Hyper (%)
Kok [37]	Activity intervals based on mass intervals	766	93	74	19	7
Kok [37]	7.5 MB/g	317	90	78	12	10
Schiavo [38]	*Traino's method with* D = 300 Gy	*526*	*82*	*69*	*13*	*18*
Tarantini [30]	Not declared	481	81	62	19	19
Walter [26]	Eq. (4.3) *with* D = 150 Gy	*444*	*78*	*68*	*10*	*23*
Jarlov [35]	Activity intervals based on mass intervals	324	71	67	4	29
Jarlov [35]	5.6 MB/g	316	68	63	5	32

study was performed (indicated in italics). The same activities administered to patients with a nonpersonalized method can lead to high failure levels. Good clinical results are obtained also by Huysmans, but he administered a fixed high activity that is over the maximum limit allowed for outpatient treatments in some countries such as Italy (600 MBq) and Switzerland (200 MBq).

As far as multinodularity is concerned, less paper has been published with respect to single nodule therapy; some results are reported in Table 4.3.

Clinical results are worse than in the case of single nodules because the situation is more complex to deal with: more than one target inside the same gland with different morphological and functional characteristics. Globally, the probability of hyperthyroidism persistency is higher, and the best result is with a very high activity.

The same author, Kok, reports almost the same clinical results with quite different therapeutic activities, and two papers with the same administered activity (Kok and Jarlov) have given quite different results: this means that the therapeutic methods must be improved. Even the two personalized methods (Schiavo and Walter) have not reached very good results maybe because they both measured the uptakes with a probe without considering separately the different subthyroidal structures.

As far as the Graves' disease is concerned, a lot of studies have been made and many papers published trying to decide an "optimal" absorbed dose value. In their paper, Peters et al. [18] report a success rate of about 40–50% in patients who received a target dose of 100 Gy (with considerable differences due to the basal mass of the thyroid) and a success rate of 80% in patients who received a target dose of 200 Gy. In another paper from the same group [19], they demonstrate a strong correlation between the outcome of therapy and the radiation dose absorbed by the thyroid. The rate is 11% for 50 Gy, 50% for 100 Gy, 67% for 150 Gy, 80% for 200 Gy, 84% for 250 Gy, 90% for 300 Gy, and 93% for 400 Gy. Reinhardt et al. [20] report a success rate of 73% for 150 Gy, increasing to 92% for 300 Gy. Bajnok et al. [21] report a success rate of 72% 6 months after therapy administration for a thyroid absorbed dose ranging from 70 to 100 Gy. They relate the success of the therapy to the size of the gland. In their study Howarth et al. [22] randomly divide the patients into two groups, one receiving 60 Gy and the other receiving 90 Gy. They report a positive response of 41% of patients of the second group (90 Gy) and of 39% of patients of the first group (60 Gy) 6 months after ^{131}I administration. They conclude that no significant advantage in response rate is gained by using a dose of 90 Gy instead of 60 Gy.

More recently, an empirical relationship between post-therapeutic thyroid volume (mass) and therapy outcome in Graves' disease patients has been reported in literature. Gomez-Arnaiz et al. [23] report a relation between the thyroid volume 3 and 6 months after therapy and final thyroid function outcome. Haase et al. [24] divide the patients into three groups depending on the basal thyroid volume (mass) and adjust the dose calculation to the patient's thyroid volume. They report a therapeutic success associated with different target doses in each of the three groups (150 Gy for thyroid volumes <15 ml; 220 Gy for thyroid volumes in the range 15–25 ml; 260 Gy for thyroid volumes >25 ml), and they find a significant correlation between post-therapeutic thyroid volume (mass) and clinical outcome. They conclude that an adjustment of the target doses based on thyroid basal volumes will lead to an appropriate reduction of thyroid volumes. This means that the "optimal" absorbed dose value is individual, i.e., it depends on the characteristics of the patient and on the "appropriate" reduction of his thyroid volume.

The theoretical possibility of curing Graves' disease based on the reduction of the thyroid volume has been demonstrated, based on a two-compartmental model [15]. In this work a new approach to ^{131}I iodide administration in Graves' disease is presented. This new approach was confirmed in references [16, 17]. In this paper the possibility to administer the radioiodine activity based on the desired thyroid mass reduction instead of a constant value of optimal thyroid absorbed dose was presented. The optimum final mass of the gland depends on the maximum thyroid uptake $\underline{U}_0$ end on the thyroid basal mass m_0. The results of the studies on the effectiveness of this method are reported in references [13, 14].

4.5 Future Perspectives

Hyperthyroidism treatments with radioiodine planned with a personalized dosimetric study can reach the double objectives of optimal clinical results with the lowest necessary activity decreasing the radiation protection impact of the treatment itself as required by the most recent European Directives.

It is desirable that the concept of tailoring the therapy to any single patient could spread out and put its roots into the mentality of physicians, of physicists, and also of hospital managers that should recognize the effort to optimize the use of radioactive agents with high clinical standards being guaranteed. In Italy there is a slow but continuous increasing interest in the application of dosimetric strategies limiting the use of empirical solutions [13–17, 27, 38–41].

References

1. McCready VR. Radioiodine – the success story of nuclear medicine. Eur J Nucl Med Mol Imaging. 2017;44:179–82.
2. Stokkel MPM, Handkiewicz Junak D, Lassmann M, Dietlin M, Luster M. EANM procedure guidelines for therapy of benign thyroid disease. Eur J Nucl Med Mol Imaging. 2010;37:2218–28.
3. Salvatori M, Luster M. Radioiodine therapy dosimetry in benign thyroid disease and differentiated

thyroid carcinoma. Eur J Nucl Med Mol Imaging. 2010;37:821–8.
4. Council Directive 97/43/Euratom of 30 June 1997 on health protection of individuals against the dangers of ionizing radiation in relation to medical exposure, and repealing Directive 84/466/Euratom. Off J Eur Communities. 1997;180:07.
5. Council Directive 2013/59/Euratom of 5 December 2013 laying down basic safety standards for protection against the dangers arising from exposure to ionising radiation, and repealing Directives 89/618/Euratom, 90/641/Euratom, 96/29/Euratom, 97/43/Euratom and 2003/122/Euratom. Off J Eur Communities. 2014.
6. Collins FS, Varmus H. A new initiative on precision medicine. N Engl J Med. 2015;372:793–5.
7. Dietlin M, Grunwald F, Schmidt M, Schneider P, Verburg FA, Luster M. Radioiodtherapie bei benignen Schilddrüsenerkrankungen (Version 5). Nuklearmedizin. 2016;55:213–20.
8. Giovannella L, Salvatori M,Testori O, Brianzoni E, Pace L, Perotti G, Dottorini M, Traino C, Bodei L, Chiesa, C, Rufini, V, Castellani R. Raccomandazioni procedurali per la terapia medico-nucleare. 2012.
9. Hanscheid H, Canzi C, Eschner W, Flux G, Luster M, Strigari L, Lassmann M. EANM Dosimetry Committee series on standard operational procedures for pre-therapeutic dosimetry II. Dosimetry prior to radioiodine therapy of benign thyroid disease. Eur J Nucl Med Mol Imaging. 2013;40:1126–34.
10. Bockish A, Jamitzky T, Derwanz R, Biersack HJ. Optimized dose planning of radioiodine therapy of benign thyroidal diseases. J Nucl Med. 1993;34:1632–8.
11. Hilditch TE, Dempsey MF, Bolster AA, McMenemin RM, Reed NS. Self-stunning in thyroid ablation: evidence from comparative studies of diagnostic 131I and 123I. Eur J Nucl Med. 2002;29:783–8.
12. Canzi C, Zito F, Voltini F, Reschini E, Gerundini P. Verification of the agreement of two dosimetric methods with radioiodine therapy in hyperthyroid patients. Med Phys. 2006;33:2860–7.
13. Traino AC, Grosso M, Mariani G. Possibility of limiting the unjustified irradiation in ^{131}I therapy of Graves' disease: a thyroid mass-reduction based method for the optimum activity calculation. Phys Med. 2010;26:71–9.
14. Orsini F, Traino AC, Grosso M, Guidoccio F, Boni G, Volterrani D, Mariani G. Personalization of radioiodine treatment for Graves' disease: a prospective, randomized study with a novel method for calculating the optimal 131I-iodide activity based on target reduction of thyroid mass. Q J Nucl Med Mol Imaging. 2012;56:496–502.
15. Di Martino F, Traino AC, Brill AB, Stabin MG, Lazzeri M. A theoretical model for prescription of the patient-specific therapeutic activity for radioiodine therapy of Graves' disease. Phys Med Biol. 2002;47:1493–9.
16. Traino AC, Di Martino F, Grosso M, Monzani F, Dardano A, Caraccio N, Mariani G, Lazzeri M. A predictive mathematical model for the calculation of the final mass of Graves' disease thyroids treated with ^{131}I. Phys Med Biol. 2005;50:2181–91.
17. Traino AC, Di Martino F, Grosso M, Monzani F, Dardano A, Caraccio N, Mariani G, Lazzeri M. A study of the possibility of curing Graves' disease based on the desired reduction of thyroid mass (volume) as a consequence of 131I therapy: a speculative paper. Nucl Med Commun. 2006;27:439–46.
18. Peters H, Fischer C, Bogner U, Reiners C, Schleusener H. Radioiodine therapy of Graves' hyperthyroidism: standard vs. calculated 131-iodine activity. Results from a prospective, randomized, multicentre study. Eur J Clin Investig. 1995;25:186–93.
19. Peters H, Fischer C, Bogner U, Reiners C, Schleusener H. Treatment of Graves' hyperthyroidism with radioiodine: results of a prospective randomized study. Thyroid. 1997;7(2):247–51.
20. Reinhardt MJ, Brink I, Joe AY, von Mallek D, Ezziddin S, Palmedo H, Krause TM. Radioiodine therapy in Graves' disease based on tissue-absorbed dose calculations: effect of pre-treatment thyroid volume on clinical outcome. Eur J Nucl Med. 2002;29(9):1118–24.
21. Bajnok L, Mezosi E, Nagy E, Szabo J, Sztojka I, Varga J, Galuska L, Leovey A. Calculation of the radioiodine dose for the treatment of Graves' hyperthyroidism: is more than seven-thousand rad target dose necessary? Thyroid. 1999;9(9):865–9.
22. Howarth D, Epstein M, Lan L, Tan P, Booker J. Determination of the optimal minimum radioiodine dose in patients with Graves' disease: a clinical outcome study. Eur J Nucl Med. 2001;28(10):1489–95.
23. Gomez-Arnaiz N, Andia E, Guma A, Abos R, Soler J, Gomez JM. Ultrasonographic thyroid volume as a reliable prognostic index of radioiodine-131 treatment outcome in Graves' disease hyperthyroidism. Horm Metab Res. 2003;35:492–7.
24. Haase A, Bahre M, Lauer I, Meller B, Richter E. Radioiodine therapy in Graves' hyperthyroidism: determination of individual optimum target dose. Exp Clin Endocrinol Diabetes. 2000;108:133–7.
25. Huysmans DA, Corstens FH, Kloppenborg PW. Long-term follow-up in toxic solitary nodules treated with radioactive iodine. J Nucl Med. 1991;32:27–30.
26. Walter MA, Christ-Crain M, Eckard B, Schindler C, Nitzsche EU, Muller-Brand J, Muller B. Radioiodine therapy in hyperthyroidism: inverse correlation of pre-therapeutic iodine uptake level and post-therapeutic outcome. Eur J Clin Investig. 2004;34:365–70.
27. Schiavo M, Bagnara MC, Camerieri L, Pomposelli E, Giusti M, Pesce G, Reitano C, Caputo M, Bagnasco M. Clinical efficacy of radioiodine therapy in multinodular toxic goiter, applying an implemented dose calculation algorithm. Endocrine. 2015;48:902–8.
28. Regalbuto C, Marturano I, Condorelli A, Latina A, Pezzino V. Radiometabolic treatment of hyper-

thyroidism with a calculated dose of 131-iodine: results of one-year follow-up. J Endocrinol Investig. 2009;32:134–8.
29. Zingrillo M, Urbano N, Suriano V, Modoni S. Radioiodine treatment of Plummer and multinodular toxic and nontoxic goiter disease by the first approximation dosimetry method. Cancer Biother Radiopharm. 2007;22:256–60.
30. Tarantini B, Ciuoli C, Di Cairano G, Guarino E, Mazzucato P, Montanaro A, Burroni L, Vattimo AG, Pacini F. Effectiveness of radioiodine (131-I) as definitive therapy in patients with autoimmune and non-autoimmune hyperthyroidism. J Endocrinol Investig. 2006;29:594–8.
31. Mariotti S, Martino E, Francesconi M, Ceccarelli C, Grasso L, Lippi F, Baschieri L, Pinchera A. Serum thyroid autoantibodies as a risk factor for development of hypothyroidism after radioactive iodine therapy for single thyroid "hot" nodule. Acta Endocrinol. 1986;113:500–7.
32. Erdogan MF, Kucuk NO, Anil C, Aras S, Ozer D, Aras G, Kamel N. Effect of radioiodine therapy on thyroid nodule size and function in patients with toxic adenomas. Nucl Med Commun. 2004;25:1083–7.
33. Ratcliffe G, Cooke S, Fogelman I, Maisey M. Radioiodine treatment of solitary functioning thyroid nodules. Br J Radiol. 1986;59:385–7.
34. Nygaard B, Hegedus L, Gerhard Nielsen K, Ulriksen P, Hansen JM. Long-term effect of radioactive iodine on thyroid function and size in patients with solitary autonomously functioning toxic thyroid nodules. Clin Endocrinol. 1999;50:197–202.
35. Jarlov AE, Hegedus L, Kristensen LO, Nygaard B, Hansen JM. Is calculation of the dose in radioiodine therapy of hyperthyroidism worthwhile? Clin Endocrinol. 1995;43:325–9.
36. Ustun F, Yuksel M, Durmus-Altun G, Kaya M, Cermik TF, Sarikaya A, Berkarda S. The incidence of recurrence and hypothyroidism after radioiodine treatment in patients with hyperthyroidism in Trakya, a mild iodine deficiency area, during the period 1991–2003. Ann Nucl Med. 2005;19:737–42.
37. Kok SW, Smit JW, De Craen AJM, Goslings BM, Van Eck-Smit BLF, Romijin JA. Clinical outcome after standardized versus dosimetric radioiodine treatment of hyperthyroidism: an equivalence study. Nucl Med Commun. 2000;21:1071–8.
38. Schiavo M, Bagnara MC, Pomposelli E, Altrinetti V, Calamaia I, Camerieri L, Giusti M, Pesce G, Reitano C, Bagnasco M, Caputo M. Radioiodine therapy of hyperfunctioning thyroid nodules: usefulness of an implemented dose calculation algorithm allowing reduction of radioiodine amount. Q J Nucl Med Mol Imaging. 2013;57(3):301–7.
39. Matheoud R, Canzi C, Reschini E, Zito F, Voltini F, Gerundini P. Tissue-specific dosimetry for radioiodine therapy of the autonomous thyroid nodule. Med Phys. 2003;30:791–8.
40. Amato E, Campennì A, Leotta S, Ruggeri RM, Baldari S. Treatment of hyperthyroidism with radioiodine targeted activity: a comparison between two dosimetric method. Phys Med. 2016;32:847–53.
41. Skanjeti A, Miranti A, Delgado Yabar GM, Bianciotto D, Tevisiol E, Stasi M, Podio V. A simple and accurate dosimetry protocol to estimate activity for hyperthyroidism treatment. Nucl Med Rev. 2015;18:13–8.

5 New Approaches in the Management of Thyroid Cancer

Savvas Frangos and Ioannis Iakovou

Abstract

With 98.1% 5-year survival rate, differentiated thyroid carcinoma is one of the best in prognosis among all cancers. The primary treatment of thyroid cancer is the surgical removal of thyroid, in most of the cases total thyroidectomy, which is followed by iodine-131 ablation therapy. Last years' new trends apply in small thyroid carcinomas: Hemithyroidectomy is suggested, and even in cases of total thyroidectomy iodine-131 therapy should not be used. In localized thyroid carcinoma, the 5-year survival rate is more than 99% This is the main reason of choosing lobectomy and for not using the iodine-131 therapy for thyroid cancers less than 1 cm. Nevertheless, the 5-year relative survival rate in patient with distant metastasis is 55.3%. Approximately 1.2% of men and women in the USA will be diagnosed with thyroid cancer at some point during their lifetime, based on 2011–2013 data. The estimated new cases in the USA for 2017 are 56,870 individuals. Out of them about 2275 (4%) will have distant metastasis. From them about 1150 will not survive until 2022. Even though we do not have exact numbers, the same situation should be in Europe. In other parts of the world, given the situation that the diagnosis comes later, the numbers of metastatic patients should be in a higher percent. These numbers are a challenge in the management of thyroid cancer, and the progress is not impressive. The scope of the chapter is to show how these difficult cases should be managed starting on the possibility to recognize the people who will develop thyroid cancer, the initial surgical treatment of the disease, and if any progress in diagnosis and therapy has been made in the last years. The questions that we will try to answer in the next paragraphs are the following: Is there any possibility to find out the patients that will develop thyroid cancer? Can the details of the histopathology reports add information about

S. Frangos (✉)
Department of Nuclear Medicine, Bank of Cyprus Oncology Centre, Nicosia, Cyprus
e-mail: savvas.frangos@gmail.com

I. Iakovou
Department of Nuclear Medicine, Aristotle University, Papageorgiou Hospital, Thessaloniki, Greece
e-mail: iiakovou@icloud.com; iiakovou@auth.gr

E. Bombardieri et al. (eds.), *Clinical Applications of Nuclear Medicine Targeted Therapy*,
https://doi.org/10.1007/978-3-319-63067-0_5

the patient at risk to improve their management? Is the initial surgery a predictive factor in the prognosis of each patient and how this could be improved? Are the new methods of surgery adding in value regarding the managements of thyroid cancer patient? How and when surgery should be used in relapses of thyroid cancer? Localization of distant metastasis is very important. What is the role of PET/CT? What is the role of systemic therapy in treating metastatic thyroid cancer? Is there any role of external beam radiation in the management of thyroid cancer?

5.1 Background

With 98.1% 5-year survival rate, differentiated thyroid carcinoma is one of the best in prognosis among all cancers [1].

The primary treatment of thyroid cancer is the surgical removal of thyroid, in most of the cases total thyroidectomy, which is followed by iodine-131 ablation therapy. Last years' new trends apply in small thyroid carcinomas: Hemithyroidectomy is suggested, and even in cases of total thyroidectomy iodine-131 therapy should not be used.

In localized thyroid carcinoma, the 5-year survival rate is more than 99% [1]. This is the main reason of choosing lobectomy and for not using the iodine-131 therapy for thyroid cancers less than 1 cm.

How and when iodine-131 should be used will be covered in other chapters of this book.

Nevertheless, the 5-year relative survival rate in patient with distant metastasis is 55.3% [1].

Approximately 1.2% of men and women in the USA will be diagnosed with thyroid cancer at some point during their lifetime, based on 2011–2013 data [2].

The estimated new cases in the USA for 2017 are 56,870 individuals [2]. Out of them about 2275 (4%) will have distant metastasis. From them about 1150 will not survive until 2022. Even though we do not have exact numbers, the same situation should be in Europe. In other parts of the world, given the situation that the diagnosis comes later, the numbers of metastatic patients should be in a higher percent. These numbers are a challenge in the management of thyroid cancer, and the progress is not impressive.

The scope of the chapter is to show how these difficult cases should be managed starting on the possibility to recognize the people who will develop thyroid cancer, the initial surgical treatment of the disease, and if any progress in diagnosis and therapy has been made in the last years.

The questions that we will try to answer in the next paragraphs are the following:

- Is there any possibility to find out the patients that will develop thyroid cancer?
- Can the details of the histopathology reports add information about the patient at risk to improve their management?
- Is the initial surgery a predictive factor in the prognosis of each patient and how this could be improved?
- Are the new methods of surgery adding in value regarding the managements of thyroid cancer patient?
- How and when surgery should be used in relapses of thyroid cancer?
- Localization of distant metastasis is very important. What is the role of PET/CT?
- What is the role of systemic therapy in treating metastatic thyroid cancer?
- Is there any role of external beam radiation in the management of thyroid cancer?

5.2 Is There Any Possibility to Find Out the Patients that Will Develop Thyroid Cancer?

Thyroid cancer is the most common endocrine malignancy and the fifth most common malignant neoplasm of the female sex [3]. During the past several decades, an increasing incidence of thyroid cancer has been reported. The mortality from thyroid cancer is comparatively low and remains almost stable showing a slight increase [4]. It is currently unclear whether the observed increases in thyroid cancer are real or are due to increased diagnosis, as clinical and pathological findings recognize the real increase in the incidence and mortality of thyroid cancer of all sizes and all stages, with different distributions depending on gender, race, age, and environmental conditions [5]. Therefore, the question arises: Is there any possibility to find out the patients that will develop thyroid cancer?

Despite considerable progress in the understanding of the biology and molecular pathways of carcinogenesis in the thyroid gland, much less achievements have been made in terms of defining a risk profile for thyroid cancer. The only risk factor which is systematically documented as carcinogenic for thyroid is exposure to ionizing radiation during childhood [6]. Recently several studies are examining risk factors such as diet and exercise, benign thyroid diseases, as well as genetic factors that influence the incidence and mortality of the disease [7]. To the best of our knowledge, there are only few epidemiological studies examining the effects of exposure to chemical agents on thyroid cancer's "behavior" [8].

The most well-documented risk factor for the onset of thyroid malignant neoplasms, in current literature, is ionizing radiation, which makes it more likely for exposed populations to develop TC [9]. The anatomical position and the radiosensitivity of the thyroid tissue make it particularly vulnerable to the carcinogenic effects of ionizing radiation [10, 11]. The use of nuclear technology leads to the formation of long-lived radionuclides, of which the 137Cs is the most abundant. Artificial radionuclides found in the environment are mostly a result of nuclear weapon tests, nuclear power accidents, and geological storage of nuclear waste [12–14]. Moreover, an increase in the global annual per caput effective radiation dose has been described (from 3 mSv/year in 1980 to 6 mSv/year in 2006), partly as a result of medical exposure. External beam radiation therapy of the head and neck region has attributed to this trend [15]. The effects of exposure to ionizing radiation may be apparent either directly or within decades. The development of malignant neoplasms in the thyroid gland is the most common stochastic effect of exposure to ionizing radiation, and it is still possible to occur after the absorption dose of less than 1 Gy [9]. Thus, the possibility of developing thyroid cancer is higher among people who have been exposed to ionizing radiation rather than the general population.

Our current understanding of the molecular pathogenesis of thyroid cancer resulted from identification of genetic and epigenetic alterations in various signaling pathways, including the mitogen-activated protein kinase (MAPK), the phosphatidylinositol-3 kinase (PI3K), protein kinase (AKT), the nuclear factor-kB (NF-kB), the Ras association domain-containing protein 1 (RASSF1)-mammalian sterile (STE20)-like protein kinase 1 (MST1), the forkhead box O3 (FOXO3), the WNT-b-catenin, the hypoxia-inducible factor 1a (HIFIa), and the TSH receptor pathways. Among the various pathways, the MAPK and PI3K/AKT are the pathways best characterized to indicate the patients that are most likely to develop thyroid cancer and show promise in thyroid cancer treatment. Activation of the MAPK pathway mainly drives the development of papillary thyroid cancer (PTC). By contrast, activation of the PI3K/AKT pathway is involved in the formation of follicular adenoma and carcinoma. Upon simultaneous activation of both pathways with an accumulation of genetic alterations, PTC or follicular carcinoma may progress to poorly differentiated carcinoma or anaplastic carcinoma [16].

Medullary thyroid carcinoma constitutes 5–10% of all thyroid malignancies. About 25% of the cases of MTC are familial, and the disease is inherited in an autosomal dominant manner. The inherited forms present as multiple endocrine neoplasia syndromes, MEN2A and MEN2B. Those without further tumors are characterized as familial medullary thyroid carcinoma (FMTC) only. The molecular pathology of inherited MTC is constitutive activation of the RET proto-oncogene. The human RET gene comprises 21 exons and its size is 53.3 kb. It encodes a tyrosine kinase receptor with a cysteine-rich extracellular 44 domain, a transmembrane domain, and an intracellular tyrosine kinase domain. Mutations in the gene lead to abnormalities in cell proliferation and differentiation of tissues derived from neural crest cells, such as the C-cells of the thyroid and the adrenal medulla. The number and type of recognized RET mutations have increased over the last years due to the wider application of genetic screening [17]. The RET mutation testing for inherited MTC is a unique paradigm of the value of genetic screening in the early diagnosis, prevention, and treatment of cancer which has been of great importance for the management of patients with MTC. The indications for screening and intervention follow a mutation-based risk classification for MTC patients and carriers according to the guidelines of the American Thyroid Association (ATA) [18] and the European Thyroid Association (ETA) [19].

Although oncogenes and other growth factors are involved in thyroid cancer growth and development, it seems probable that TSH can act as a cancer stimulus. This hypothesis is supported by improved survival in thyroid cancer patients treated with suppressive doses of levothyroxine and by cases of tumor growth post-T4 withdrawal or recombinant TSH [20]. Autoimmune thyroiditis, of which Hashimoto's thyroiditis represents the most frequent form, is an inflammatory state of the thyroid gland. The incidence of Hashimoto's thyroiditis has increased substantially over the past decades. Meanwhile, the incidence of thyroid cancer has more than doubled. These findings lead to the conclusions, after intensive research, that autoimmune thyroiditis predisposes patients to the development of thyroid cancer. Moreover, several other malignant thyroid diseases including goiters, adenomas, and nodules in the gland's parenchyma have been also associated with an increased incidence of TC, which makes it more possible for those patients to develop thyroid cancer [21]. Therefore, higher surveillance is imperative for this patients' group.

Nutritional factors such as iodine deficiency may induce an increasing incidence of benign thyroid conditions, but very high iodine intake also affects thyroid function and, possibly, thyroid cancer risk [22]. Furthermore, the relationship between obesity and lack of exercise and risk of thyroid cancer has been studied for more than 10 years. Although, the results remained uncertain, according to Mas' meta-analysis, obesity is definitely associated with an increased thyroid cancer risk, except medullary thyroid cancer [23]. Finally, other risk factors including the age (with increasing incidence among young population), the gender (female), and the reproductive and menstrual history have been also associated with the development of papillary thyroid cancer [24]. To the best of our knowledge, there are only few epidemiological studies examining the effects of exposure to chemical agents on thyroid cancer's "behavior." There is substantial evidence that polychlorinated biphenyls, dioxins, and furans cause hypothyroidism in exposed animals and that environmentally occurring doses affect human thyroid homeostasis. Similarly, flame retardants reduce peripheral thyroid hormone (TH) levels in rodents, but human studies are scarce. Studies also indicate thyroid-disruptive properties of phthalates, but the effect of certain phthalates seems to be stimulative on TH production, contrary to most other groups of chemicals. Thyroid disruption may be caused by a variety of mechanisms, as different chemicals interfere with the hypothalamic-pituitary-thyroid axis at different levels. Mechanisms of action may involve the sodium-iodide symporter, thyroid peroxidase enzyme, receptors for THs or TSH, transport proteins, or cellular uptake mechanisms. The peripheral metabolism of the THs can be affected through effects on iodothyronine deiodinases or hepatic enzymes [25, 26]. It is therefore urgent to clarify the populations exposed to these factors in order to predict those with a higher possibility of developing thyroid cancer.

5.3 Can the Details of the Histopathology Reports Add Information About the Patient at Risk to Improve Their Management?

It is well accepted that the important information regarding cancer are extracted from the histopathology report of each cancer [27]. With very few exceptions, definitive therapy for cancer should not be undertaken in the absence of a tissue diagnosis.

Thyroid cancer could not make an exception on this. According to the British Thyroid Association [28], "A careful, accurate and thorough histopathology report is essential because many of the histological features affect staging and prognosis and may therefore influence clinical management decisions." The importance of histopathology is also emphasized in ATA 2015 [29].

The College of American Pathologists [30] descripts in details how the histopathology should be created and reported.

The essential parts of the report are summarized as follows:

In addition to the basic tumor features required for thyroid cancer staging including status of resection margins, pathology reports should contain additional information helpful for risk assessment, such as the presence of vascular invasion and the number of invaded vessels, number of lymph nodes examined and involved with tumor, size of the largest metastatic focus to the lymph node, and the presence or absence of extra-nodal extension of the metastatic tumor.

Histopathologic variants of thyroid carcinoma associated with more unfavorable outcomes (e.g., tall cell, columnar cell, and hobnail variants of PTC; widely invasive FTC; poorly differentiated carcinoma) or more favorable outcomes (e.g., encapsulated follicular variant of PTC without invasion, minimally invasive FTC) should be identified during histopathologic examination and reported.

The pathologist should also comment on the presence or absence of extra-nodal extension since the latter was shown to increase the risk for distant metastases and death (reference Update to the College of American Pathologists Reporting on Thyroid Carcinomas).

The standard histopathology diagnosis depends on examination of routine hematoxylin- and eosin-stained slides, but interobserver or intraobserver disagreements in the diagnosis of papillary and follicular thyroid lesions are well known and documented in the literature [31].

Immunohistochemistry can add in the certainty of diagnosis. Various newer immunohistochemistry markers are being described and validated for differentiating benign nodules from malignant ones and follicular variant of papillary carcinoma from follicular carcinoma or follicular adenoma. Further assessment with molecular markers can also add in the diagnosis and future prognosis of the thyroid cancer patient. Details regarding immunohistochemistry or molecular markers are beyond the scope of this chapter.

To answer the question: The details on the histopathology report are essential in the management of thyroid cancer patients. The report should be made for experienced pathologists, and the reporting should be done according to pregiven templates in order to have constancy.

5.4 Is the Initial Surgery a Predictive Factor in the Prognosis of Each Patient and How Could This Be Improved?

The treatment of thyroid cancer is primarily surgical.

Surgical options for thyroid cancer are hemithyroidectomy, with or without the removal of isthmus, near-total thyroidectomy (leaving less than 1 g of thyroid tissue), and total thyroidectomy (removing all visible thyroid tissue).

According to the American Thyroid Association [29], the primary goal for thyroid cancer treatment is to improve overall and disease-specific survival, reduce the risk of persistent/recurrent disease and associated morbidity, and permit accurate disease staging and risk stratification while minimizing treatment-related morbidity and unnecessary therapy. The specific goals of initial therapy are to remove the primary tumor including lymph node metastasis. Completeness of the surgery is the most important factor influencing the prognosis of each patient. Radioiodine treatment and TSH suppression play in most of the cases an adjuvant role.

Without the appropriate surgical removal of the thyroid, the radioiodine therapy is not a clinically feasible option due to possible complications resulting from large amounts of remnant thyroid tissue and limited prospects for successful treatment by stricter criteria [32]. The accurate diagnosis could not be done without surgery including the removal of lymph nodes to allow the exact histopathology reporting and staging of the tumor.

The extent of surgery and the experience of the surgeon both play important roles in determining the risk of surgical complications.

Both surgeon experience and completeness of surgery are well-documented as critical to patient outcome.

The 2008 EANM guidelines [33] state: “When thyroid surgery is performed in highly expert hands at selected tertiary referral centres, though, the positive influence of radioiodine ablation may not be Apparent.” In other words if the ablation is already done from the surgeon, there is no further need of the radioiodine ablation. This statement of course applies only in selected cases.

In our study [34] it has been shown that only experienced surgeons can perform truly total thyroidectomy, and a surgeon score based on the number of patients referred for postoperative 131I ablation of thyroid cancer independently predicted the size of the thyroid remnant.

Many of the surgical quality measures currently in use are not disease specific. For thyroid cancer, mortality and even recurrence are difficult to measure since mortality is rare and recurrence can take decades to occur. Therefore, there is a critical need for quality indicators in thyroid cancer surgery that are easily measured and disease specific [35]. There are two potential quality indicators in thyroid cancer surgery. The uptake percentage on postoperative radioactive iodine scans indicates the completeness of resection. Another measure, the lymph node ratio, is the proportion of metastatic nodes to the total number of nodes dissected. This serves as a more global measure of quality since it indicates not only the completeness of lymph node dissection but also the preoperative lymph node evaluation and decision-making. Together, these two quality measures offer a more accurate, disease-specific oncologic indicator of quality that can help guide quality assurance and improvement. Another very important indicator is the level of the postoperative thyroglobulin level [34]. It is easy to perform and repeatable. According to the NCCN guidelines [36], the level of postoperative thyroglobulin not only evaluates the completeness of surgery but also guides the decision for radioiodine ablation.

Surgeon volume is a significant predictor of thyroid surgery outcomes [37, 38]. High-volume surgeons were more likely to perform more extensive surgery for thyroid disease, including neck dissection, and had lower incidences of recurrent laryngeal nerve injury and postoperative hypocalcemia. The risk of complication diminishes when a high-volume or experienced surgeon performs the thyroidectomy. The British Thyroid Association guidelines [28] suggest that surgeons who operate on patients with thyroid cancer should perform a minimum of 20 thyroidectomies per year. Taking into consideration that the precise total thyroidectomy and the extent of surgery predict the outcome of the patient, the differences in relapse rates and even the 5- or 10-year survival rates depend on the accurate diagnosis. It is obvious with the above that only experienced surgeons should operate on thyroid cancer patient. Identifying the surgeon is not an easy task, but it is possible.

The important next step is to answer the question: “How much is enough?” In most of the cases in medicine, there are controversies: Hemithyroidectomy? Total thyroidectomy? Central lymph node dissection? Lateral lymph node dissection?

According to the ATA 2015 guidelines [29], hemithyroidectomy is indicated for small tumors less than 1 cm without evidences of extrathyroidal extension or lymph node involvement and in the absence of prior head and neck radiation, familial thyroid carcinoma, or clinically detectable cervical nodal metastases. Similar criteria are mentioned in the NCCN guidelines [36]. Regarding patients with thyroid cancer >1 and <4 cm without evidences of extrathyroidal extension or lymph node involvement, hemithyroidectomy is controversial. The American Thyroid Association [29] supports it as one reasonable method, but EANM [32] saw in this particular recommendation a reason to decline the endorsement of ATA 2015 guidelines. The rationale behind this decision is that in patients who have undergone hemithyroidectomy only, administering a postoperative course of 131I is not a clinically feasible option, and this could affect the prognosis of the patient especially regarding possible relapse.

Another important issue regarding surgery is the central lymph node dissection. If we have positive nodes, there is no discussion about the necessity of the dissection. The questions arise about prophylactic central lymph node dissection. The importance of surgeon experience leads to insert the following paragraph in ATA 2015 guidelines [29]: "The preceding recommendations should be interpreted in light of available surgical expertise." If surgical expertise is not available, then central neck dissection should be avoided even though this could increase future relapses. The majority of the patient will avoid surgical complications, which are increased in not so experienced hands. The best example of surgeon experiences is the famous surgeon Albert Kocher. By 1882, Kocher's mortality rate was 2.4%, and by the end of the nineteenth century, this rate was as low as 0.18%. Kocher had over 5000 cases by the time of his death in 1917 (https://www.nobelprize.org/nobel_prizes/medicine/laureates/1909/kocher-article.html).

To answer the question: The initial surgery and the surgeon play an essential role in the prognosis of thyroid cancer patient. To improve the outcome of the surgery, the preoperative evaluation is important but also the creation of specialist surgical clinics to operate on thyroid cancer patients.

5.5 Are the New Methods of Surgery Adding in Value Regarding the Managements of Thyroid Cancer Patient?

5.5.1 Transaxillary Thyroidectomy

During his presentation in 1912, Dr. Albert Kocher describes the incision used by his father Theodor Kocher as follows: "This is done with Kocher's symmetrical' collar incision across the middle of both lobes" [39]. It is still the most used method in thyroid operations. This method is used in thousands of patients around the world.

The last decades and especially in Asia, a new method was used under the pressure to find a way for better cosmetic effect, the transaxillary thyroidectomy. The main benefit of this method is the avoidance of scarring in the neck. In one study it is shown that people are willing to travel long distances and to pay more money to have a better cosmetic outcome [40].

There are multiple studies, which compare the endoscopic technique with open thyroidectomies. The transaxillary approach was originally described in Korea, but modifications should be done if the method should be applied to other population. The height and weight of the patient and also the size of the thyroid play an important role in the success of the transaxillary thyroidectomy. Similar to the conventional thyroidectomy, experienced hands are needed to achieve the necessary high standard of total thyroidectomy.

5.5.2 Outpatient Thyroid Surgery

Outpatient management of surgical procedure is increasing over the last years. The definition of outpatient surgery is the same-day discharge, not requiring an overnight hospital stay [41]. The benefits of outpatient thyroidectomy are the cost and patient satisfaction. Additionally, the short stay in the hospital can minimize the exposure to potential nosocomial infection [42]. The main risk is hematoma that could lead to airway compromise and life-threatening situation. Other complications could be hypoparathyroidism and recurrent laryngeal nerve injury. For those reasons the main requirement for performing outpatient thyroid surgery is the expertise of the surgeon. In the hands of high-volume thyroid surgeons, the possibility of complication is diminished. Therefore, only those surgeons should operate in outpatient basis. Another important issue is the patient selection. For the latest the following conditions should be met according to the position paper of ATA [41]: no major comorbidities, to be able to understand preoperative education, team approach to education and clinical care, primary caregiver willing and available, social setting conducive to safe postoperative management, and proximity to skilled facility. The important issue for outpatient thyroid surgery is the criteria for discharge. According to the position paper of ATA, the patient should have all of the following abilities: ability to take liquids and postoperative medications; adequate pain control on oral medications; ability to void satisfactorily; ability to ambulate as preoperatively and perform essential activities of daily living; satisfactory postoperative assessment with attention to the surgical wound, neck swelling/hematoma, dysphonia, dyspnea, and dysphagia; adequate social support and understanding of instructions; and adequate oxygenation, vital signs, and blood pressure control.

Both outpatient and robotic thyroid surgery can add in the comfort of the patient, reduce the cost, and also offer a better cosmetic result, but it is still not clear if and how these influence the prognosis and the risk of relapse for thyroid cancer patients.

5.6 Locoregional Recurrence

Lymph node metastasis occurs in up to 50% of patients with papillary thyroid cancer [43]. If micrometastasis in lymph nodes is considered, this percentage reaches up to 90% [44]. Both ATA 2015 [29] and NCCN [36] guidelines suggest surgery (if resectable) for locoregional recurrence in thyroid carcinoma. Essential according to NCCN is the preoperative vocal cord assessment, if central neck recurrence occurred.

There are three forms of relapse in thyroid cancer [45]: distant metastasis, "true" local recurrence, and, the most usual appearance, disease within lymph nodes. The latest is most probably due to persistence of microscopic disease in lymph nodes that was not detected at the initial operation. Proof of this is the fact that half of the recurrences were detected within the first 3 years of follow-up [46].

An important issue is to put the indication for surgery. We need to take into consideration that suspicious cervical lymph nodes in the lateral neck usually remain stable for long periods of time and can be safely followed with serial ultrasounds [47]. An important aspect is the involvement of vital structures. In those cases, surgery should be performed regardless of the size of the nodules. For all other cases for central compartment, the lymph nodes should be >8 mm and for lateral neck >10 mm. The positive lymph nodes should be proven by biopsy and/or thyroglobulin washout [48].

Also in those cases, the experience of the surgeon plays a vital role to achieve the cure of the patient.

5.7 Localization of Distant Metastasis Is Very Important. What Is the Role of PET/CT?

The primary imaging for thyroid cancer is the iodine-131 scintigraphy. This method can show all foci of thyroid cancer in a simple examination, and it was well known in the first administration of iodine-131 to the human [49]. Sodium-iodide symporter [50, 51] is expressed at the highest level in the thyroid [52]. Since NIS confers highly efficient iodide accumulation in cells, its expression in cancer cells allows for the diagnostic use of radioactive iodide (^{123}I, ^{124}I, and ^{131}I). A majority (68–86%) of thyroid cancer retains functional NIS expression [53, 54]. Unfortunately, in the rest of the cases, thyroid cancer cells are losing the ability to concentrate iodine. Positron emission tomography in combination with computer tomography (PET/CT) is used in the localization of relapses and distant metastasis. In case that the thyroid cancer cells preserve the ability to concentrate iodine, then the use of I-124 as positron emitter could add value to identify foci of the disease [55]. The first use of I-124 was in the 1960s [56]. With the introduction of hybrid PET/CT devices to the clinic, ^{124}I-PET/CT is becoming a powerful tool in the management of patients with thyroid cancer [57, 58]. Serial ^{124}I-PET can be used for lesion dosimetry [59].^{124}I-PET provides higher spatial resolution and imaging sensitivity than gamma camera.

In case that the thyroid cancer cell loses their ability to concentrate iodine, then other methods should be used with the scope to identify local relapse or metastasis. Fluorine-18 fluorodeoxyglucose (FDG) is known to be retained in malignant tissue, depending on the grade of malignancy [60]. Usually, carcinomas of a high malignancy grade show a more intensive tracer uptake than low-grade tumors. 18FDG-PET/CT is primarily considered in high-risk thyroid cancer patients with elevated serum Tg (generally >10 ng/mL) with negative iodine-131 imaging [29].

The expression of somatostatin receptors (SSTR) in thyroid cells [61] may offer the possibility to identify metastatic lesions and to select patients for peptide receptor radionuclide therapy (PRRT). The use of [62] ^{68}Ga-DOTATOC or ^{68}Ga-DOTATATE positron emission tomography/computed tomography (PET/CT) can show uptake of the radiopharmaceutical in select patients with progressive differentiated thyroid cancer [63]. Disease localization by ^{68}Ga-DOTANOC PET-CT can give the possibility for treatment of differentiated thyroid cancer with peptide receptor radionuclide therapy (PRRT) using ^{177}Lu/^{90}Y-DOTA-peptides.

5.8 What Is the Role of Systemic Therapy in Treating Metastatic Thyroid Cancer?

What is the role of systemic therapy (kinase inhibitors, other selective therapies, conventional chemotherapy, bisphosphonates, denosumab) in treating metastatic DTC?

Over recent decades, the trend of an increasing incidence of thyroid cancer has inevitably given rise to a number of patients who present with aggressive disease and eventually succumb to it. The survival rate in patients with RAI-refractory metastatic DTC has been estimated to be 10% at 10 years. Until recently, the therapeutic options available for patients with progressive, metastatic, RAI-refractory DTC have been limited. C-cell-derived medullary thyroid carcinoma (MTC), although uncommon, has a much worse prognosis than iodine-positive DTC, which is approximately the same with RAI-refractory DTC. In most cases, MTC is already metastatic at initial presentation, with no available effective therapeutic options other than surgery, when possible. Novel tyrosine kinase inhibitors (TKIs), such as vandetanib, sorafenib, axitinib, pazopanib, sunitinib, and cabozantinib, have been used recently for the treatment of refractory cases of thyroid cancer, where all conventional treatment options (surgery, RAI, chemotherapy) have been proven ineffective. These molecules inhibit cellular signaling by targeting multiple tyrosine kinase receptors as well as platelet-derived growth factor receptors and vascular endothelial growth factor receptors, which play a role in both tumor angiogenesis and proliferation of tumor cells. Simultaneous inhibition of these targets leads to reduced tumor vascularization, apoptosis of cancer cells, and ultimately tumor shrinkage. Some phase II and III trials have reported promising results regarding favorable response rates in metastatic thyroid cancer that has been nonresponsive to conventional treatment. Recently, vandetanib and cabozantinib were approved for patients with MTC, and sorafenib was approved for those with DTC. However, because both agents target many different receptors, they have numerous side effects, including hematological, skin, and cardiac toxicities that may have a negative impact on patients' quality of life [64].

Leboulleux et al. attempted to assess efficacy and safety of vandetanib, a tyrosine kinase inhibitor of RET, VEGFR, and EGFR signaling, finding that it is the first targeted drug to show evidence of efficacy in a randomized phase II trial in patients with locally advanced or metastatic differentiated thyroid carcinoma [65]. Brose et al. investigated the efficacy and safety of orally administered sorafenib in the treatment of patients with this type of cancer, concluding that it can significantly improve progression-free survival compared with placebo in patients with progressive radioactive iodine-refractory differentiated thyroid cancer [66]. In their multi-institutional study, Cohen et al. assessed the activity and safety of axitinib, an oral, potent, and selective inhibitor of vascular endothelial growth factor receptors (VEGFR) 1, 2, and 3 in patients with advanced thyroid cancer. They found responses were noted in all histologic subtypes, indicating that axitinib is a selective inhibitor of VEGFR with compelling antitumor activity in all histologic subtypes of advanced thyroid cancer [62]. Similarly, pazopanib, sunitinib, and cabozantinib proved to represent a promising therapeutic option for patients with progressive, radioiodine-refractory, metastatic differentiated, and medullary thyroid cancers, pointing that the correlation of the patient's response and pazopanib concentration during the first cycle might indicate that treatment can be individualized to achieve optimum outcomes [67–69].

Despite the different receptors targeted, the vast majority of TKI-related adverse events (AEs) are common to different drugs. The most frequent AEs are diarrhea, anorexia, weight loss, fatigue, hypertension, hypothyroidism, hand-and-foot syndrome, and skin rash. The most frequent drug-related AEs for the different drugs investigated in the largest clinical trials are summarized in the table above. The majority of these AEs are generally mild or moderate (G1–G2), and only in less than 5–10% of cases are they severe or life-threatening (G3–G4), based on the common terminology criteria for adverse events. Death related to AEs (G5) is, fortunately, a very rare event.

The majority of AEs are easily prevented or managed with drug treatment, but in a nonnegligible percentage of cases, dose reduction (up to 79% for cabozantinib), interruption (up to 66.2% for sorafenib), or withdrawal (up to 26% for lenvatinib) was needed in clinical trials. Because of this, after drug approval, a number of phase IV studies were designed to evaluate the efficacy/tolerability of the drugs at lower doses, which can be better tolerated, and to determine if the same results on the disease progression are observed (vandetanib, NCT01496313; cabozantinib, NCT01896479; lenvatinib, NCT02211222). From a practical point of view, side effects should be known and prevented by both patients and doctors to avoid the need for and the risk of unnecessarily stopping the drug treatment. Some practical suggestions are given in the "Management of thyroid cancer patients undergoing TKI treatment: practical suggestions" section. In particular, patients should be instructed to report any types of side effects as soon as they appear to allow doctors to immediately start a therapeutic strategy. According to some observations, TKI toxicities could also be used as a surrogate marker of the efficacy of the drug. TKI toxicities have recently been classified as being an "on-target" toxicity (On-TT) and an "off-target" toxicity (Off-TT). An On-TT is a primary effect of the drug that occurs because of a common pathway/target among neoplastic and normal cells, whereas an Off-TT is a secondary effect of the drug that is due to the inhibition of the kinases that are not the intended target of the drug. A paradigmatic example is the association between TKI-induced hypertension and drug efficacy in terms of OR, PFS, and OS outcomes in patients treated with sunitinib and sorafenib for renal cell carcinoma and hepatocellular carcinoma. In cases of thyroid cancer, this phenomenon has been recently reported for hypertension in patients treated with lenvatinib [70].

It should be highlighted also that broadly construed, systemic therapy encompasses not only more recently emerging "targeted" approaches but also historical "mainstay" therapies including TSH suppression and RAI. Although more "novel" approaches have attracted attention recently, it is important to optimally apply fundamental approaches. In this regard, therapeutic RAI should also be used to optimal effect prior to the initiation of more recent/novel therapies. To accomplish this requires attention to detail, including assurance of adequate TSH stimulation, patient adherence to low-iodine pre-RAI therapy dietary restrictions, and avoidance of proximal preceding iodine contamination from intravenous contrast agents—with verification by urinary iodine concentration measurements in selected cases. In this context, occasional patients previously declared "RAI-refractory" can be found instead to have RAI-responsive disease when such details are attended to if previously neglected [29]. However, nowadays another promising pathway seems to enhance iodine avidity in previously declared "RAI-refractory" cases.

Experiments in cell line and animal models provided proof-of-principle data that pharmacologic manipulation of the MAPK pathway with small molecule inhibitors may be a novel approach for enhancing iodide avidity. In a mouse model of poorly differentiated thyroid cancer driven by inducible thyroid-specific expression of BRAFV600E, treatment with downstream MAPK pathway inhibitors targeting either BRAF or MEK partially restored expression of NIS and iodine avidity [71]. These preclinical data led to a pilot clinical trial evaluating the impact of the MEK inhibitor selumetinib upon iodide uptake in patients with RAI-refractory thyroid cancers. In this study, recombinant human TSH (rh-TSH) I-124 PET/CT lesional dosimetry was utilized to quantify drug-induced changes in iodide incorporation within specific lesions. This pilot study provided a critical proof of concept that selumetinib produces clinically meaningful increases in iodine uptake and retention in a subgroup of patients with thyroid cancer that is refractory to radioiodine; the effectiveness may be greater in patients with RAS-mutant disease [72].

In summary, although some of the data discussed in this section appear promising, optimizing and defining the efficacy and safety of various novel drugs will only be accomplished through larger prospective clinical trials. Imaging, including PET/CT with I-124 and FDG, as well as SPECT/CT with I-123 and I-131, will be a critical part of clinical trials and will be essential to guide and monitor novel targeted therapies. We expect these therapies will ultimately translate into improved outcomes for patients with advanced thyroid cancer over the next decade [73].

Cytotoxic chemotherapies provided low response rates in patients with advanced and progressive refractory thyroid cancer, and toxicity was high. The more frequently tested agent in thyroid cancer patients is doxorubicin, used either alone or in combination with cisplatin. Tumor response rates range from 0 to 22%, with all responses being partial and only lasting a few months. Newer cytotoxic drugs, such as taxanes, gemcitabine, or irinotecan, have not been reported in a significant number of DTC patients [74].

Metastatic bone disease represents a particularly challenging clinical problem in patients with RAI-refractory DTC, especially given the high rate of multiple skeletal-related events in patients following detection of an initial bone lesion. Bisphosphonate or denosumab therapy should be considered in patients with diffuse and/or symptomatic bone metastases from RAI-refractory DTC, either alone or concomitantly with other systemic therapies. Adequate renal function (bisphosphonates) and calcium and vitamin D25 level (bisphosphonates and denosumab) should be documented prior to each dose, and dental evaluation should take place before initial use. Unfortunately, kinase inhibitors appear to be less effective in controlling bone metastatic disease in comparison to disease at other soft tissue sites such as lungs and lymph nodes. Progression of bone metastases while on kinase inhibitor therapy commonly occurs despite maintained benefit with respect to disease at other metastatic sites. Hence, kinase inhibitor therapy cannot be relied upon to control diffuse bone metastases in many patients with RAI-refractory DTC [29].

5.9 Is There Any Role of External Beam Radiation in the Management of Thyroid Cancer?

Both NCCN [36] and ATA 2015 [29] see a limited role for external beam radiation regarding thyroid cancer.

ATA emphasized that there is *no* role for routine adjuvant external beam radiation, and NCCN guidelines mention that it could be considered in non-iodine-avid thyroid cancer with gross residual disease in the neck. ATA guidelines could recommend external beam radiation in patient with serial operation when the risk of reoperation is high. Another indication for external beam radiation could be the management of aerodigestive invasive disease in combination with radioiodine therapy.

References

1. Howlader N, Noone AM, Krapcho M, Miller D, Bishop K, Altekruse SF, Kosary CL, Yu M, Ruhl J, Tatalovich Z, Mariotto A, Lewis DR, Chen HS, Feuer EJ, Cronin KA, editors. SEER cancer statistics review, 1975–2013. [Online]; 2015 [cited 2017 March 31]. Available from: http://seer.cancer.gov/csr/1975_2013/.
2. www.cancer.org. [Online]; 2017 [cited 2017 March 31]. Available from: www.cancer.org/cancer/thyroidcancer/detailedguide/thyroid-cancer-key-statistics.
3. Kilfoy BA, Zheng T, Holford TR, et al. International patterns and trends in thyroid cancer incidence, 1973–2002. Cancer Causes Control. 2009;20(5):525–31.
4. World Health Organization. International Agency for Research on Cancer. Globocan 2012: estimated can-

cer incidence, mortality and prevalence worldwide in 2012. Available at: http://globocan.iarc.fr/Pages/fact_sheets_cancer.aspx. Accessed 7 Feb 2016.
5. Hall SF, Irish J, Groome P, Griffiths R. Access, excess, and overdiagnosis: the case for thyroid cancer. Cancer Med. 2014;3(1):154–61.
6. Ermak G, Figge JJ, Kartel NA, Davies KJ. Genetic aberrations in Chernobyl-related thyroid cancers: implications for possible future nuclear accidents or nuclear attacks. IUBMB Life. 2003;55(12):637–41.
7. Giannoula E, Iakovou I, Chatzipavlidou V. Risk factors and the progression of thyroid malignancies. Hell J Nucl Med. 2015;18(3):275–84.
8. Leux C, Guénel P. Risk factors of thyroid tumors: role of environmental and occupational exposures to chemical pollutants. Rev Epidemiol Sante Publique. 2010;58(5):359–67.
9. Shah DJ, Sachs RK, Wilson DJ. Radiation-induced cancer: a modern view. Br J Radiol. 2012;85:e166–e73.
10. Gaussen A, Legal JD, Beron-Gaillard N, et al. Radiosensitivity of human normal and tumoral thyroid cells using fluorescence in situ hybridization and clonogenic survival assay. Int J Radiat Oncol Biol Phys. 1999;44(3):683–91.
11. Ivanov VK, Kashcheev VV, Chekin SY, et al. Radiation-epidemiological studies of thyroid cancer incidence in Russia after the Chernobyl accident (estimation of radiation risks, 1991–2008 follow-up period). Radiat Prot Dosim. 2012;151(3):489–99.
12. Moysich KB, Menezes RJ, Michalek AM. Chernobyl-related ionising radiation exposure and cancer risk: an epidemiological review. Lancet Oncol. 2002;3(5):269–79.
13. Rashed-Nizam QM, Rahman MM, Kamal M, Chowdhury MI. Assessment of radionuclides in the soil of residential areas of the Chittagong metropolitan city, Bangladesh and evaluation of associated radiological risk. J Radiat Res. 2015;56(1):22–9.
14. Taylor DM, Taylor SK. Environmental uranium and human health. Rev Environ Health. 1997;12(3):147–57.
15. Mettler FA Jr, Bhargavan M, Thomadsen BR, et al. Nuclear medicine exposure in the United States, 2005–2007: preliminary results. Semin Nucl Med. 2008;38(5):384–91.
16. Huang CJ, Jap TS. A systematic review of genetic studies of thyroid disorders in Taiwan. J Chin Med Assoc. 2015;78(3):145–53.
17. Sarika L, Papathoma A, Garofalaki M, et al. Genetic screening of patients with medullary thyroid cancer (MTC) in a referral center in Greece during the past two decades. Eur J Endocrinol. 2015;172(4):501–9.
18. American Thyroid Association Guidelines Task Force, Kloos RT, Eng C, Evans DB, Francis GL, Gagel RF, Gharib H, et al. Medullary thyroid cancer: management guidelines of the American Thyroid Association. Thyroid. 2009;19:565–612.
19. Elisei R, Alevizaki M, Conte-Devolx B, Frank-Raue K, Leite V, Williams GR. European Thyroid Association guidelines for genetic testing and its clinical consequences in medullary thyroid cancer. Eur Thyroid J. 2012;1:216–31.
20. Haymart MR, Repplinger DJ, Leverson GE, et al. Higher serum thyroid stimulating hormone level in thyroid nodule patients is associated with greater risks of differentiated thyroid cancer and advanced tumor stage. J Clin Endocrinol Metab. 2008;93(3):809–1.
21. Liu CL, Cheng SP, Lin HW, Lai YL. Risk of thyroid cancer in patients with thyroiditis: a population-based cohort study. Ann Surg Oncol. 2014;21(3):843–9.
22. Dal Maso L, Bosetti C, La Vecchia C, Franceschi S. Risk factors for thyroid cancer: an epidemiological review focused on nutritional factors. Cancer Causes Control. 2009;20(1):75–86.
23. Ma J, Huang M, Wang L, Ye W, et al. Obesity and risk of thyroid cancer: evidence from a meta-analysis of 21 observational studies. Med Sci Monit. 2015;21:283–91.
24. Sakoda LC, Horn-Ross PL. Reproductive and menstrual history and papillary thyroid cancer risk: the San Francisco Bay Area thyroid cancer study. Cancer Epidemiol Biomark Prev. 2002;11(1):51–7.
25. Boas M, Main KM, Feldt-Rasmussen U. Environmental chemicals and thyroid function: an update. Curr Opin Endocrinol Diabetes Obes. 2009;16(5):385–91.
26. Capen CC. Mechanistic data and risk assessment of selected toxic end points of the thyroid gland. Toxicol Pathol. 1997;25(1):39–48.
27. Kufe DW, Pollock RE, Weichselbaum RR, et al. Holland-Frei cancer medicine. 6th ed. Hamilton: BC Decker; 2003.
28. Perros P, Boelaert K, Colley S, Evans C, Evans RM, Gerrard Ba G, Gilbert J, Harrison B, Johnson SJ, Giles TE, Moss L, Lewington V, Newbold K, Taylor J, Thakker RV, Watkinson J, Williams GR, British Thyroid Association. Guidelines for the management of thyroid cancer. Clin Endocrinol. 2014;81(Suppl 1):1–122.
29. Haugen BR, Alexander EK, Bible KC, Doherty GM, Mandel SJ, Nikiforov YE, et al. 2015 American Thyroid Association management guidelines for adult patients with thyroid nodules and differentiated thyroid cancer: the American Thyroid Association guidelines task force on thyroid nodules and differentiated thyroid cancer. Thyroid. 2016;26:1–133.
30. Seethala RR, Asa SL, Cart SE, Hodak SP, McHugh JB, Shah J, Thompson LDR, Nikiforov YE. Protocol for the examination of specimens from patients with carcinomas of the thyroid gland. Version Thyroid 3.1.0.0 College of American Pathologists. Available from: www.cap.org/apps/docs/committees/cancer/cancer_protocols/2014/Thyroid_ 14Protocol_3100.pdf. Accessed 31 Mar 2017.
31. Elsheikh TM, Asa SL, Chan JKC, DeLellis RA, Heffess CS, Livolsi VA, et al. Interobserver and intraobserver variation among experts in the diagnosis of thyroid follicular lesions with borderline nuclear features of papillary carcinoma. Am J Clin Pathol. 2008;130:736–44.

32. Verburg FA, Aktolun C, Chiti A, et al. Why the European Association of Nuclear Medicine has declined to endorse the 2015 American Thyroid Association management guidelines for adult patients with thyroid nodules and differentiated thyroid cancer. Eur J Nucl Med Mol Imaging. 2016;43:1001–5. https://doi.org/10.1007/s00259-016-3327-3.
33. Luster M, Clarke SE, Dietlein M, Lassmann M, Lind P, Oyen WJ, et al. Guidelines for radioiodine therapy of differentiated thyroid cancer. Eur J Nucl Med Mol Imaging. 2008;35:1941–59.
34. Frangos S, Iakovou IP, Marlowe RJ, Eftychiou N, Patsali L, Vanezi A, et al. Difficulties in deciding whether to ablate patients with putatively "low-intermediate-risk" differentiated thyroid carcinoma: do guidelines mainly apply in the centres that produce them? Results of a retrospective, two-centre quality assurance study. Eur J Nucl Med Mol Imaging. 2015;42:2045–55.
35. Schneider DF, Sippel RS. Measuring quality in thyroid cancer surgery. Adv Endocrinol. 2014;2014:1–6.https://doi.org/10.1155/2014/714291. Article ID 714291.
36. NCCN Clinical Practice Guidelines in Oncology. www.nccn.org. [Online]; 2017 [cited 2017 April 8]. Available from: https://www.nccn.org/professionals/physician_gls/PDF/thyroid.pdf.
37. Lifante JC, Duclos A, Couray-Targe S, Colin C, Peix JL, Schott AM. Hospital volume influences the choice of operation for thyroid cancer. Br J Surg. 2009;96(11):1284–8.
38. Pieracci FM, Fahey TJ III. Effect of hospital volume of thyroidectomies on outcomes following substernal thyroidectomy. World J Surg. 2008;32(5):740–6.
39. Kocher A. Discussion on partial thyroidectomy under local anaesthesia, with special reference to exophthalmic goitre. Proc R Soc Med. 1912;5:89–96.
40. Coorough NE, Schneider DF, Rosen MW, et al. A survey of preferences regarding surgical approach to thyroid surgery. World J Surg. 2014;38:696–703.
41. Terris DJ, Snyder S, Carneiro-Pla D, et al. American Thyroid Association statement on outpatient thyroidectomy. Thyroid. 2013;23(10):1193–202.
42. Balentine CJ, Sippel RS. Outpatient thyroidectomy: is it safe?. In: Surgical oncology clinics of North America, vol. 25, Number 1. Philadelphia: Elsevier; 2015. p. 61–76.
43. Grubbs EG, Evans DB. Role of lymph node dissection in primary surgery for thyroid cancer. J Natl Compr Cancer Netw. 2007;5:623–30.
44. Qubain SW, Nakano S, Baba M, et al. Distribution of lymph node micrometastasis in pN0 well-differentiated thyroid carcinoma. Surgery. 2002;131:249–56.
45. Grant CS. Recurrence of papillary thyroid cancer after optimized surgery. Gland Surg. 2015;4:52–62.
46. Durante C, Montesano T, Torlontano M, et al. Papillary thyroid cancer: time course of recurrences during postsurgery surveillance. J Clin Endocrinol Metab. 2013;98:636–42.
47. Robenshtok E, Fish S, Bach A, Domínguez JM, Shaha A, Tuttle RM. Suspicious cervical lymph nodes detected after thyroidectomy for papillary thyroid cancer usually remain stable over years in properly selected patients. J Clin Endocrinol Metab. 2012;97(8):2706–13.
48. Giovanella L, Bongiovanni M, Trimboli P. Diagnostic value of thyroglobulin assay in cervical lymph node fine-needle aspirations for metastatic differentiated thyroid cancer. Curr Opin Oncol. 2013;25:6–13.
49. Smithers DW. Some varied applications of radioactive isotopes to the localization and treatment of tumors. Acta Radiol. 1951;35(1):49–61.
50. Dai G, Levy O, Carrasco N. Cloning and characterization of the thyroid iodide transporter. Nature. 1996;379:458–60.
51. Smanik PA, Ryu KY, Theil KS, Mazzaferri EL, Jhiang SM. Expression, exon-intron organization, and chromosome mapping of the human sodium iodide symporter. Endocrinology. 1997;138:3555–8.
52. Dohan O, De la Vieja A, Paroder V, Riedel C, Artani M, Reed M, et al. The sodium/iodide Symporter (NIS): characterization, regulation, and medical significance. Endocr Rev. 2003;24:48–77.
53. Castro MR, Bergert ER, Goellner JR, Hay ID, Morris JC. Immunohistochemical analysis of sodium iodide symporter expression in metastatic differentiated thyroid cancer: correlation with radioiodine uptake. J Clin Endocrinol Metab. 2001;86:5627–32.
54. Wapnir IL, van de Rijn M, Nowels K, Amenta PS, Walton K, Montgomery K, et al. Immunohistochemical profile of the sodium/iodide symporter in thyroid, breast, and other carcinomas using high density tissue microarrays and conventional sections. J Clin Endocrinol Metab. 2003;88:1880–8.
55. Freudenberg LS, Jentzen W, Stahl A, et al. Clinical applications of 124I-PET/CT in patients with differentiated thyroid cancer. Eur J Nucl Med Mol Imaging. 2011;38(Suppl 1):48–56. https://doi.org/10.1007/s00259-011-1773-5.
56. Phillips AF, Haybittle JL, Newberry GR. Use of iodine-124 for the treatment of carcinoma of the thyroid. Acta Unio Int Contra Cancrum. 1960;16:1434–8.
57. Lassmann M, Reiners C, Luster M. Dosimetry and thyroid cancer: the individual dosage of radioiodine. Endocr Relat Cancer. 2010;17(3):R161–72.
58. Freudenberg LS, Antoch G, Knust J, Görges R, Müller SP, Bockisch A, et al. Value of 124I-PET/CT in staging of patients with differentiated thyroid cancer. Eur Radiol. 2004;14:2092–8.
59. Freudenberg LS, Jentzen W, Petrich T, Frömke C, Marlowe RJ, Heusner T, et al. Lesion dose in differentiated thyroid carcinoma metastases after rhTSH or thyroid hormone withdrawal: 124I PET/CT dosimetric comparisons. Eur J Nucl Med Mol Imaging. 2010;37:2267–76.
60. Strauss LG, Conti PS. The application of PET in clinical oncology. J Nucl Med. 1991;32:623–48.
61. Ain KB, Taylor KD, Tofiq S, Venkataraman G. Somatostatin receptor subtype expression in human thyroid and thyroid carcinoma cell lines. J Clin Endocrinol Metab. 1997;82:1857–62.

62. Cohen EE, Rosen LS, Vokes EE, et al. Axitinib is an active treatment for all histologic subtypes of advanced thyroid cancer: results from a phase II study. J Clin Oncol. 2008;26(29):4708–13.
63. Kundu P, Lata S, Sharma P, et al. Eur J Nucl Med Mol Imaging. 2014;41:1354. https://doi.org/10.1007/s00259-014-2723-9.
64. Chrisoulidou A, Mandanas S, Margaritidou E, et al. Treatment compliance and severe adverse events limit the use of tyrosine kinase inhibitors in refractory thyroid cancer. Onco Targets Ther. 2015;8:2435–42.
65. Leboulleux S, Bastholt L, Krause T, et al. Vandetanib in locally advanced or metastatic differentiated thyroid cancer: a randomised, double-blind, phase 2 trial. Lancet Oncol. 2012;13(9):897–905.
66. Brose MS, Nutting CM, Jarzab B, et al. Sorafenib in radioactive iodine-refractory, locally advanced or metastatic differentiated thyroid cancer: a randomised, double-blind, phase 3 trial. Lancet. 2014;384(9940):319–28.
67. Bible KC, Suman VJ, Molina JR, et al. Efficacy of pazopanib in progressive, radioiodine-refractory, metastatic differentiated thyroid cancers: results of a phase 2 consortium study. Lancet Oncol. 2010;11(10):962–72.
68. Carr LL, Mankoff DA, Goulart BH, et al. Phase II study of daily sunitinib in FDG-PET-positive, iodine-refractory differentiated thyroid cancer and metastatic medullary carcinoma of the thyroid with functional imaging correlation. Clin Cancer Res. 2010;16(21):5260–8.
69. Sherman SI, Clary DO, Elisei R, et al. Correlative analyses of RET and RAS mutations in a phase 3 trial of cabozantinib in patients with progressive, metastatic medullary thyroid cancer. Cancer. 2016;122(24):3856–64.
70. Viola D, Valerio L, Molinaro E, et al. Treatment of advanced thyroid cancer with targeted therapies: ten years of experience. Endocr Relat Cancer. 2016;23(4):R185–205.
71. Chakravarty D, Santos E, Ryder M, et al. Small-molecule MAPK inhibitors restore radioiodine incorporation in mouse thyroid cancers with conditional BRAF activation. J Clin Invest. 2011;121(12):4700–11.
72. Ho AL, Grewal RK, Leboeuf R, et al. Selumetinib-enhanced radioiodine uptake in advanced thyroid cancer. N Engl J Med. 2013;368(7):623–32.
73. Grewal RK, Ho A, Schöder H, et al. Novel approaches to thyroid cancer treatment and response assessment. Semin Nucl Med. 2016;46(2):109–18.
74. Schlumberger M, Sherman SI. Approach to the patient with advanced differentiated thyroid cancer. Eur J Endocrinol. 2012;166(1):5–11.

Radioiodine Therapy of Thyroid Cancer

6

Ettore Seregni, Alice Lorenzoni, and Laura Fugazzola

Abstract

Differentiated thyroid cancers are typically iodine-avid and can be effectively treated with radioiodine. In most patients, radioactive iodine therapy (RAI) is done for ablation of residual tissue or with adjuvant intent in case of suspected persistent disease after surgery. Patient with advanced or metastatic disease may also benefit from RAI. In this chapter, we will discuss the current role of 131I-iodide therapy, including patient's selection and preparation, and the importance of individual response to therapy to guide subsequent patient management.

6.1 Differentiated Thyroid Cancer

Thyroid cancer is the most common endocrine malignancy, accounting approximately for 1% of all new cancers diagnosed each year in the United States and Europe [1]. The thyroid cancer incidence rate has tripled in the United States since the 1980s, especially among women, and the increase is mostly due to small-sized tumors. This trend has been attributed to increased detection due to the wider availability of ultrasound and fine-needle aspiration [2]. Thyroid cancer comprises different histologic subtypes arising from follicular epithelial cell and less frequently from the neural crest-derived parafollicular C cells. Other rare primary thyroid malignancies include non-epithelial tumors (sarcomas and malignant hemangioendothelioma), thyroid lymphoma, and an extremely rare group of carcinomas characterized by the presence of mucin-producing cells, keratin, or both.

Differentiated thyroid cancer (DTC), arising from thyroid follicular epithelial cells, accounts for the vast majority of all thyroid malignancies (>90%). They are characterized by the maintenance of the specific features of the follicular normal cells, such as the ability to accumulate iodine and to produce thyroglobulin and the TSH dependence. Among DTCs, papillary thyroid

E. Seregni (✉) • A. Lorenzoni
Nuclear Medicine, Fondazione IRCCS Istituto Nazionale Tumori, Milan, Italy
e-mail: ettore.seregni@istitutotumori.mi.it

L. Fugazzola
Division of Endocrine and Metabolic Diseases, IRCCS Istituto Auxologico Italiano, Milan, Italy

Department of Pathophysiology and Transplantation, University of Milan, Milan, Italy

E. Bombardieri et al. (eds.), *Clinical Applications of Nuclear Medicine Targeted Therapy*,
https://doi.org/10.1007/978-3-319-63067-0_6

cancer (PTC) accounts for about 80% of cases, while 10–20% have a follicular histology (FTC), which includes conventional and oncocytic (Hurthle cell) carcinomas [3].

Papillary carcinoma (PTC) demonstrates characteristic microscopic nuclear features: nuclear overlapping, large-sized nuclei, ground-glass appearance, longitudinal nuclear grooves, and invaginations of the cytoplasm into the nucleus. Although a papillary growth pattern is frequently seen, it is not required for the diagnosis. About 50% of PTCs are also characterized by the presence of calcium deposits called "psammoma bodies". About 50–60% of PTCs are multifocal, affecting both thyroid lobes in more than 30% of the cases. More than ten microscopic variants of papillary carcinoma have been documented [4]. Some of them are associated with more aggressive or conversely more indolent tumor behavior. The variants with more unfavorable outcomes are the tall cell, columnar cell, and hobnail variants. The tall cell variant is characterized by predominance (>50%) of tall columnar tumor cells whose height is at least three times their width. These tumors present at an older age and more advanced stage than classic papillary carcinoma and demonstrate a higher recurrence rate and decreased disease-specific survival. The columnar cell variant of PTC is characterized by predominance of columnar cells with pronounced nuclear stratification. These tumors have a higher risk of distant metastases and tumor-related mortality, the latter seen mostly in patients with an advanced disease stage at presentation. Other variants of PTC, such as the solid variant and the diffuse sclerosing variant, may be associated with a less favorable outcome, although the data remain conflicting. The encapsulated follicular variant of papillary carcinoma is characterized by a follicular growth pattern with no papillae formation and total tumor encapsulation and associated with a low risk of recurrence, particularly in the absence of capsular or vascular invasion. The diagnosis is performed upon the finding of characteristic nuclear features of PTC.

Follicular thyroid cancer shows follicular cell differentiation and the lack of the diagnostic nuclear features of papillary thyroid carcinoma. It displays variable morphology ranging from small-/medium-sized follicles containing colloid to trabecular or solid growth pattern. Follicular tumors that exhibit vascular and/or capsular invasion should be regarded as follicular carcinomas. Depending on the degree of their invasiveness, follicular carcinomas have been divided into two major categories: minimally invasive or encapsulated (the most common) and widely invasive [5].

6.2 Radioiodine Therapy in Differentiated Thyroid Cancer After Surgical Intervention

Radioactive iodine therapy (RAI) is administered in patients with differentiated thyroid cancer (DTC) for eradication of thyroid remnant after total thyroidectomy or, in patients with metastatic disease, for curative or palliative treatment.

Depending on the postoperative risk stratification of the individual patient, the primary goal of postoperative administration of RAI after surgery includes:

1. RAI remnant ablation to eliminate any normal thyroid tissue left after total or near-total thyroidectomy, thereby simplifying disease surveillance by examinations such as thyroglobulin (Tg) measurements or whole-body RAI scans.
2. RAI adjuvant therapy to theoretically destroy suspected, but unproven residual disease with the aim to improve disease-free survival.
3. RAI therapy to treat persistent disease in higher-risk patients to improve disease-specific and disease-free survival.

In the past years, thyroid remnant ablation was indicated in almost every patient with a diagnosis of DTC. Nowadays, careful revision of patients' outcome has introduced the concept of risk-based selection of patients candidate to thyroid remnant ablation. In recent years, and especially upon the publication of the 2015 American Thyroid Association (ATA) Differentiated Thyroid Cancer

(DTC) guidelines [6], the systematic use of RAI has declined or at least has been called into question. The decision on whether to give RAI, and if so what 131I activity to administer, increasingly relies upon risk stratification systems (RSS) such as the ATA risk of recurrence system or the DTC-specific survival oriented UICC/AJCC TNM staging system. Each system takes into account the extent of disease at surgery and additional characteristics such as age, histology, and possibly other patient- or treatment-related factors.

6.3 Risk Stratification in Differentiated Thyroid Cancer

Thyroid cancer is usually a well-differentiated, slowly growing disease with a very low disease-specific mortality rate for local-regional disease after complete initial therapy (5-year survival 99.9% for localized disease and 97.8% for regional metastatic disease); however, some patients are at high risk of developing distant metastatic disease associated with significantly worse prognosis (5-year survival 55.3%) [7]. These patients should be identified at the time of diagnosis to individualize the treatment to their specific risk. Postoperative staging for thyroid cancer, as for other cancer types, is useful to provide prognostic information, which is of value when considering disease surveillance and therapeutic strategies. Accurate initial staging requires a detailed understanding of all pertinent risk stratification data, whether they were obtained as part of preoperative testing, during the operation(s), or as part of postoperative follow-up.

Over the years, multiple staging systems have been developed to predict the risk of mortality in patients with DTC [8]. Each of the systems uses some combination of age at diagnosis, size of the primary tumor, specific tumor histology, and extrathyroidal spread of the tumor (direct extension of the tumor outside the thyroid gland, locoregional metastases, and/or distant metastases) to stratify patients into one of several categories with different risks of death from thyroid cancer. Because the AJCC/TNM risk of mortality staging system does not adequately predict the risk of recurrence in DTC [9–12], the 2009 version of the ATA thyroid cancer guidelines proposed a three-tiered clinicopathologic risk stratification system that classified patients as having low, intermediate, or high risk of recurrence [13]. Low-risk patients are defined as having intrathyroidal DTC with no evidence of extrathyroidal extension, vascular invasion, or metastases. Intermediate-risk patients harbor either microscopic extrathyroidal extension, cervical lymph node metastases, RAI-avid disease in the neck outside the thyroid vascular invasion, or aggressive tumor histology. High-risk patients display gross extrathyroidal extension, incomplete tumor resection, distant metastases, or inappropriate postoperative serum Tg values.

6.4 Radioiodine Therapy Indications

Guidelines of the American Thyroid Association (ATA) [6] and the European Thyroid Association (ETA) [14] define the population of patients who do not require radioiodine remnant ablation, mainly those with small (<1 cm uni-multifocal), intrathyroidal tumors without nodal or vascular invasion or aggressive histology or in case of known distant metastases. Otherwise radioiodine remnant ablation is recommended after total thyroidectomy for patients with large (>4 cm) primary tumors or with gross extrathyroidal extension. In patients at intermediate risk, radioiodine remnant ablation should be considered, but the decision must be individualized.

In the remaining cases, the evidence is inadequate or conflicting, so that clear recommendations cannot be made and RAI should be considered after total thyroidectomy in intermediate-risk level (Table 6.1).

Radioiodine adjuvant therapy is performed in patient with no clinical evidence of residual cancer after resection but at increased risk for recurrence (i.e., they are suspected to have microscopic residual cancer after surgery). This scenario is considered in patients who have undergone comprehensive

Table 6.1 RAI indications

ATA category (2015)	Description	RAI
Low risk	Tumor size <1 cm (uni- or multifocal) Tumor size >1–4 cm	No indication Not routine—May be considered for patients with aggressive histology or vascular invasion
Low to intermediate risk	Tumor size >4 cm Microscopic extra-thyroid extension, any tumor size Central compartment neck lymph node metastases Lateral neck or mediastinal lymph node metastases	Should be considered
High risk	Any size, gross extra-thyroid extension Distant metastases	Recommended
ETA category (2006)	*Description*	*RAI*
Very low risk	Unifocal microcarcinoma (<1 cm) with no extension beyond the thyroid capsule and without lymph node metastases	No indication
High risk	Documented persistent disease or at high risk of persistent or recurrent disease	Recommended
Low-risk group	Includes all other patients	No consensus

resection of extensive locoregional disease without known gross residual cancer. Successful adjuvant treatment will prevent or delay the development of clinically detectable disease.

6.5 Patient Preparation

1. RAI must be performed under adequate TSH stimulation (>30 mU/l), which is needed in order to increase the uptake of radioiodine by thyroid cells [15]. It can be obtained after thyroid hormone withdrawal to increase endogenous thyroid-stimulating hormone or with exogenous TSH stimulation by the administration of recombinant human TSH (rhTSH) [16, 17]. In the first case, sufficient levels of TSH are most commonly achieved with levothyroxine (LT4) withdrawn for 3–4 weeks. Upon LT4 withdrawal, liothyronine (LT3) may be administered in the initial 2 weeks, but it should be withdrawn for at least 2 weeks. In the second case, the administration of rhTSH which induces high TSH levels without clinical hypothyroidism is an alternative way of preparation for RAI (Table 6.2). Recombinant TSH (0.9 mg) is injected i.m. for 2 consecutive days (days 1 and 2) and 131I is administered on day 3.

Table 6.2 Indications of use of rTSH

Category	rTSH stimulation
• ATA low risk • ATA intermediate risk without extensive lymph node involvement (i.e.,T1–T3, N0/Nx/N1a, M0)	• Acceptable alternative
• ATA intermediate risk with extensive lymph node disease (multiple clinically involved LN) without distant metastases	• May be considered
• Any risk level with significant comorbidity that may preclude thyroid hormone withdrawal	• Should be considered
• ATA high risk with attendant higher risks of disease-related mortality and morbidity	• No recommendation

In low-risk thyroid cancer patients, the rate of ablation and the outcome were found not to differ in patients prepared with LT4 withdrawal or with rhTSH [18].

2. A low-iodine diet should be advised for a period of 2–3 weeks before 131I administration. All patients must discontinue use of iodide-containing drugs and preparation that could potentially affect the ability of thyroid tissue to accumulate iodide for a sufficient time before therapy (Table 6.3).

Table 6.3 Iodide-containing preparations

Products/drugs	Length of withdrawal
High-iodine content foods/products (i.e., seafood, eggs, soy products, red hair coloring)	At least 2 weeks
Topical iodine (e.g., surgical skin preparation)	3 weeks
Iodinated radiographic contrast agents:	
Intravenous (water soluble)	4 weeks
Lipophilic	>4 weeks
Amiodarone	>3 moths

3. Female patients who have the potential to be pregnant should routinely be tested for pregnancy.
4. Breastfeeding must be stopped, and therapy must be delayed until lactation ceases in order to minimize the radiation dose to the breast.
5. Serum thyroglobulin (Tg) should be measured immediately before 131I administration in the case of withdrawal or on the third day after the second injection in the case of preparation with rhTSH. Low Tg levels in this setting are associated with a favorable outcome [19].

6.6 Administered Activities

Administration of 131I-iodide in activities pre-fixed irrespective of pretreatment dosimetric estimates is the most widely employed approach.

For ablation purposes, a single administration of either 1.11 or 3.7 GBq (30 or 100 mCi) of 131I-iodide ensues complete destruction of the remnants in 90% of the cases when uptake of a tracer amount of radioiodide in the residue is <2%, while ablation is successful in only one third of the cases when uptake is >2% [20]. In low-risk patients in whom remnant ablation is planned, recent data support the use of reducing activity of 131I-iodide (1.1 GBq rather than 3.7 GBq) to maintain a reasonable ablation rate. Indeed, two large randomized studies published in 2012 showed essentially equivalent ablation success rates whether patients were treated with 1.1 or 3.7 GBq (and whether thyroid hormone withdrawal or recombinant human thyroid-stimulating hormone was used for stimulation). These two studies included not only low-risk patients but also patients at intermediate risk of recurrence, including those showing minimal extrathyroidal extension of the primary tumor or lymph node metastases. A prospective, randomized study comparing the rate of recurrent disease in low-risk patients ablated with 30 or 100 mCi showed that in 10 years of follow-up, the rate of persistent disease was similar in both groups [21]. Also in intermediate-risk DTC patients, the final outcome was similar between patients treated with low and high activities of 131I at ablation in a study by Castagna and colleagues [22]. The rates of disease remission (76.5 vs. 72.1%), persistent (biochemical or metastatic) disease (18.8 vs. 23.6%), recurrent disease (2.4 vs. 2.1%), and death (2.4 vs. 2.1%) were not statistically different in patients treated with 1.11 GBq (30 mCi) versus 3.7 GBq (100 mCi). On the contrary, a higher DTC-related mortality in low- and high-risk patients treated with low activities of 131I at ablation (≤2 GBq) when patients were at least 45 years of age at diagnosis and a higher recurrence rate in older high-risk patients without distant metastases have recently been reported [23]. In this study, performed by Verburg and colleagues, 1298 patients with low-risk (698 pts), high-risk M0 (434 pts), and M1 (136 pts) DTC were grouped according to ablation activity administered (I, ≤2000 MBq); II, 2000–3000 MBq; and III, >3000 MBq), subdivided by age (<45 and ≥45 years at diagnosis). In low-risk patients at least 45 years of age, DTC-specific mortality was significantly higher in group I than in groups II and III; in high-risk M0 patients at least 45 years of age, the recurrence rate and DTC-specific mortality were significantly higher in group I than in groups II and III.

In most cases, ablative treatments are limited to the range of 1.1–5.6 GBq.

Table 6.4 Administered activity of 131I-iodide

ATA risk group	Activity of 131I
Low risk	1.1 GBq (30 mCi)
Intermediate risk	1.1 GBq (30 mCi) in case of low-volume central neck nodal metastases with no other known residual disease 1.1–5.5 GBq (30–150 mCi) in case of extensive lymph node disease, multiple clinically involved LN, or suspected or documented microscopic residual disease
High risk	3.7–5.5 GBq (100–150 mCi)

Among adjuvant therapy, there is a wide range of potentially recommended administered activities and the data less strong to help guide choice. When RAI is used to treat suspected or documented residual disease in ATA high-risk patients, administered activities of 3.7–5.5 GBq are generally recommended (Table 6.4).

The 131I-iodine activity administered with therapeutic purpose frequently ranges from 3.7 to 7.4 GBq.

A post-therapeutic whole-body scan (WBS) is recommended 3–5 days after the administration of 131I to confirm the presence and the extent of the thyroid remnant and to reveal the presence of unsuspected metastatic foci in 10–26% of the cases [24], thus allowing the reclassification of disease stage [25]. Whenever possible, a SPECT-CT can be useful to better define the neck uptake and distinguish the remnant from local lymph node or paratracheal tumor.

6.7 Clinical Implications of Response to Radioiodine Therapy

Initial recurrence risk estimates should be continually modified during follow-up (ongoing risk stratification), because the risk of recurrence and disease-specific mortality can change over time as a function of the clinical course of the disease and the response to therapy. Many patients initially classified as intermediate or high risk of recurrence using initial staging systems can be reclassified as having a subsequent low risk of recurrence based on having an excellent response to initial therapy [11, 12].

All clinical, biochemical, imaging (structural and functional), and cytopathologic findings obtained during follow-up should be used to redefine the clinical status of the patient and to assess their individual response to therapy.

Response to initial therapy may be categorized as follows:

- *Excellent response*: no clinical, biochemical, or structural evidence of disease. It is defined as a TSH-stimulated Tg of <1 ng/mL in the absence of structural or functional evidence of disease (and in the absence of anti-Tg antibodies).
- *Biochemical incomplete response*: abnormal suppressed and/or stimulated Tg values (Tg values of >1 ng/mL or TSH-stimulated Tg values of >10 ng/mL) or rising anti-Tg antibodies without structural evidence of disease.
- *Structural incomplete response*: structural or functional evidence of persistent or newly identified locoregional or distant metastases.
- *Indeterminate response*: nonspecific biochemical or structural findings that cannot be confidently classified as either excellent response or persistent disease. This includes patients with stable or declining anti-Tg antibody levels without definitive structural evidence of disease, faint uptake in the thyroid bed with undetectable stimulated Tg on follow-up imaging, nonstimulated Tg values detectable but <1 ng/mL, and TSH-stimulated Tg values between 1 and 10 ng/mL.

An excellent response to initial therapy is achieved in 86–91% of ATA low-risk patients, 57–63% of ATA intermediate-risk patients, and 14–16% of ATA high-risk patients. The risk of recurrence over 5–10 years of follow-up ranged from 1% to 4%.

A biochemical incomplete response is seen in 11–19% of ATA low-risk patients, 21–22% of ATA intermediate-risk patients, and 16–18% of ATA high-risk patients. Only 8–17% of patients develop structurally identifiable disease over 5–10 years of follow-up.

A structural incomplete response to initial therapy is seen in 2–6% of ATA low-risk patients, 19–28% of ATA intermediate-risk patients, and 67–75% of ATA high-risk patients.

Despite additional treatments, the majority of patients will have persistent structural and/or biochemical evidence of persistent disease. Death from disease is seen in 11% of patients with a locoregional incomplete response and in 57% of patients with structurally identifiable distant metastases.

An indeterminate response to initial therapy is seen in 12–29% of ATA low-risk patients, 8–23%of ATA intermediate-risk patients, and 0–4% of ATA high-risk patients. The clinical outcomes in patients with an indeterminate response to therapy are intermediate between patients with an excellent response and those with incomplete responses. Only 13–20% of patients with an indeterminate response to therapy are reclassified as persistent/recurrent disease over approximately 10 years of follow-up, and the majority of patients remain disease-free during prolonged follow-up.

This ongoing risk stratification is useful to guide early surveillance and therapeutic management decisions (Table 6.5).

6.8 Radioiodine Therapy of Locoregional Recurrences and Metastatic Disease

6.8.1 Locoregional Disease

Surgery is the main treatment of local and regional recurrences whenever feasible. A complete work-up is mandatory to detect the extent of locoregional recurrence and to identify the presence of potential distant metastases. For regional nodal metastases, RAI may be employed in patients with low-volume disease or in combination with surgery. In patients with local or locoregional recurrence, treatment with 131I-iodide is often effective, leading to a reduction of further subsequent recurrences in 50% of the cases and decreasing disease-specific mortality [26].

The optimal therapeutic activity remains uncertain and controversial. There are three approaches to 131I therapy: empiric fixed amounts, therapy determined by the upper limit of blood and body dosimetry, and quantitative tumor or lesional dosimetry. Empirical activities are generally safe, but caution is mandatory in administering empiric activities higher than 3.7–5.5 GBq in certain populations such as elderly patients and patients with renal insufficiency. An activity of 7.4 GBq would exceed the maximum tolerated radiation-absorbed dose, defined as

Table 6.5 Response to therapy and correlation with clinical outcome and implications

Category	Clinical outcome	Clinical implication
Excellence response	1–4% recurrence <1% disease-specific death	Decrease in intensity and frequency of follow-up degree of TSH suppression
Biochemical incomplete response	At least 30% evolve to NED 20% achieve NED after additional therapy 20% develop structural disease <1% disease-specific death	Additional investigations and therapies in case of rising Tg or anti-Tg antibody TSH suppression
Structural incomplete response	50–85% persistent disease despite additional therapy 11% disease-specific death with locoregional disease and 50% with distant metastases	Additional treatments or ongoing observation
Indeterminate response	15–20% structural disease during follow-up <1% disease-specific death	Continued observation with appropriate serial imaging and serum Tg monitoring

200 cGy to blood, in 8–15% of patients younger than 70 years and in 22–38% of patients aged 70 years and older [27].

The patient preparation with recombinant TSH may be indicated in selected patients with underlying comorbidities making iatrogenic hypothyroidism potentially risky, in patients with pituitary disease whose serum TSH cannot be raised, or in patients in whom a delay in therapy might be deleterious.

6.8.2 Metastatic Disease

Distant metastatic disease represents the most common cause of thyroid cancer-related deaths occurring in 10–15% of the cases [28]. Only 1–4% of patients with DTC present with distant metastatic disease at the time of diagnosis (50% lungs, 25% bones, 20% lungs and bones, and 5% other sites); in the remaining cases, metastases can be discovered from 2 to 3 up to more than 10 years after initial treatment [29].

Individual prognosis depends upon factors including histology of the primary tumor, distribution and number of sites of metastasis (e.g., brain, bone, lung), tumor burden, age at diagnosis of metastases, and RAI avidity.

In the management of the patient with pulmonary metastases, the size of metastatic lesions (macronodular typically detected by chest radiography, micronodular typically detected by CT) and iodine avidity play a pivotal role. Lung macronodules may benefit from radioiodine therapy but the definitive cure rate is very low; otherwise, highest rates of complete remission after treatment with RAI may be obtained in case of pulmonary micrometastases. The selection of RAI activity to administer can be made empirically (3.7–7.4 GBq) or by lesional dosimetry or whole-body dosimetry if available in order to limit whole-body retention to 80 mCi at 48 h and 200 cGy to the bone marrow. Pulmonary pneumonitis and fibrosis are rare complications of high-dose RAI treatment and may limit the possibility of further RAI treatments.

Bone metastases should be treated by a combination of surgery whenever possible, RAI if uptake is present, and external beam radiotherapy either as curative or palliative treatment. Radioiodine therapy of iodine-avid bone metastases, though rarely curative, is associated with improved survival. The activity administered can be given empirically (100–200 mCi) or determined by dosimetry.

Brain metastases are relatively rare and usually associated with a poor prognosis. Whenever possible they should be resected; if not resectable and non-iodine-avid, external beam radiation may provide palliation.

6.9 Complication of Radioiodine Therapy

A minority of patients may have early- and late-onset complications from 131I-iodine treatment.

Early effects may include:

- Radiation thyroiditis with swelling and discomfort; it is more frequent in patients with large thyroid remnants and can be limited by the use of corticosteroids.
- Abnormalities of taste and smell are frequent but transient.
- Nausea and vomiting can be minimized by antiemetic drugs.
- Sialadenitis can be limited by hydration and by lemon juice given 24 h after radioiodine.
- Dry eye.
- Hypospermia is usually transient. Pretreatment sperm banking should be offered if multiple treatments are planned.
- Amenorrhea. An earlier onset of menopause has been reported after repeated courses of radioiodine.

Radiation exposure of the bladder and gonads may be limited by hydration and colon exposure by laxative treatment.

Women of childbearing age should avoid pregnancy for 6–12 months after radioiodine therapy. Male patients should avoid conception for a minimum of 4 months.

Late effects may include:

- Xerostomia and xerophthalmia.
- Radiation fibrosis in patients with pulmonary metastases.
- Bone marrow (BM) depression; low activities (<7.4 GBq) are not usually associated with clinically relevant BM depression; highest activities may induce transient BM depression.
- Increased risk of leukemia and secondary cancers has been reported in patients treated with high cumulative activities of radioiodine (>22 GBq) [30].

Conclusion

Radioiodine therapy of differentiated thyroid cancer is an effective and low-risk treatment for eradication of thyroid remnant after total thyroidectomy, to theoretically destroy suspected but unproven residual disease after surgery (adjuvant therapy) or in patients with metastatic disease with curative or palliative intent. In the past years, thyroid remnant ablation was indicated in almost every patient with a diagnosis of DTC. Recently, revision of patients' outcome has introduced the concept of risk-based selection of patients candidate to thyroid remnant ablation. However, to date, dilemmas exist in indication for postoperative 131I therapy, pretreatment TSH stimulation, and activity to be administered. The major goal of posttreatment surveillance of patients with DTC is still the timely detection and effective management of persistent or recurrent cancer; however, increasing emphasis has been put on the use of the ongoing risk stratification after initial treatment to guide surveillance and therapeutic management decisions.

References

1. Curado MP, Edwards B, Shin HR, et al. Cancer incidence in five continents. vol 9. IARC Scientific Publications No. 160. Lyon: IARC; 2007.
2. Pellegriti G, Frasca F, Regalbuto C, et al. Worldwide increasing incidence of thyroid cancer: update on epidemiology and risk factors. J Cancer Epidemiol. 2013;2013:965212.
3. Aschebrook-Kilfoy B, Ward MH, Sabra MM, Devesa SS. Thyroid cancer incidence patterns in the United States by histologic type, 1992–2006. Thyroid. 2011;21(2):125–34.
4. LiVolsi VA. Papillary neoplasms of the thyroid. Pathologic and prognostic features. Am J Clin Pathol. 1992;97:426–34.
5. Ghossein R. Encapsulated malignant follicular cell-derived thyroid tumors. Endocr Pathol. 2010;21:212–8.
6. Haugen BR, Alexander EK, Bible KC, et al. 2015 American thyroid association management guidelines for adult patients with thyroid nodules and differentiated thyroid cancer: the American Thyroid Association guidelines task force on thyroid nodules and differentiated thyroid cancer. Thyroid. 2016;26(1):1–133.
7. SEER Stat Fact Sheets: Thyroid Cancer. Surveillance, Epidemiology, and End Results Program. http://seer.cancer.gov/statfacts/html/thyro.html. Accessed 12 Mar 2017.
8. Jukkola A, Bloigu R, Ebeling T, et al. Prognostic factors in differentiated thyroid carcinomas and their implications for current staging classifications. Endocr Relat Cancer. 2004;11:571–9.
9. Orlov S, Orlov D, Shaytzag M, et al. Influence of age and primary tumor size on the risk for residual/recurrent well-differentiated thyroid carcinoma. Head Neck. 2009;31:782–8.
10. Baek SK, Jung KY, Kang SM, et al. Clinical risk factors associated with cervical lymph node recurrence in papillary thyroid carcinoma. Thyroid. 2010;20:147–52.
11. Tuttle RM, Tala H, Shah J, et al. Estimating risk of recurrence in differentiated thyroid cancer after total thyroidectomy and radioactive iodine remnant ablation: using response to therapy variables to modify the initial risk estimates predicted by the new American Thyroid Association staging system. Thyroid. 2010;20:1341–9.
12. Vaisman F, Momesso D, Bulzico DA, et al. Spontaneous remission in thyroid cancer patients after biochemical incomplete response to initial therapy. Clin Endocrinol. 2012;77:132–8.
13. American Thyroid Association (ATA) Guidelines Taskforce on Thyroid Nodules and Differentiated Thyroid Cancer, Cooper DS, Doherty GM, Haugen BR, Kloos RT, Lee SL, Mandel SJ, Mazzaferri EL, McIver B, Pacini F, Schlumberger M, Sherman SI, Steward DL, Tuttle RM. Revised American Thyroid Association management guidelines for patients with thyroid nodules and differentiated thyroid cancer. Thyroid. 2009;19(11):1167–214.
14. Pacini F, Schlumberger M, Dralle H, Elisei R, Smit JW, Wiersinga W. European thyroid cancer taskforce. European consensus for the management of patients with differentiated thyroid carcinoma of the follicular epithelium. Eur J Endocrinol. 2006;154(6):787–803.

15. Edmonds CJ, Hayes S, Kermode JC, et al. Measurement of serum TSH and thyroid hormones in the management and treatment of thyroid carcinoma with radioiodine. Br J Radiol. 1977;50:799–807.
16. Pacini F, Schlumberger M, Harmer C, et al. Post-surgical use of radioiodine (131I) in patients with papillary and follicular thyroid cancer and the issue of remnant ablation: a consensus report. Eur J Endocrinol. 2005;153:651–9.
17. Pacini F, Ladenson PW, Schlumberger M, et al. Radioiodine ablation of thyroid remnants after preparation with recombinant human thyrotropin in differentiated thyroid carcinoma: results of an international, randomized, controlled study. J Clin Endocrinol Metab. 2006;91:926–32.
18. Elisei R, Schlumberger M, Driedger A, et al. Follow-up of low-risk differentiated thyroid cancer patients who underwent radioiodine ablation of post-surgical thyroid remnants after either recombinant human thyrotropin or thyroid hormone withdrawal. J Clin Endocrinol Metab. 2009;94(11):4171–9.
19. Piccardo A, Arecco F, Puntoni M, et al. Focus on high-risk DTC patients: high postoperative serum thyroglobulin level is a strong predictor of disease persistence and is associated to progression-free survival and overall survival. Clin Nucl Med. 2013;38:18–2.
20. Maxon HR 3rd, Englaro EE, Thomas SR, et al. Radioiodine-131 therapy for well-differentiated thyroid cancer-a quantitative radiation dosimetric approach: outcome and validation in 85 patients. J Nucl Med. 1992;33:1132–6.
21. Maenpaa HO, Heikkonen J, Vaalavirta L, et al. Low vs. high radioiodine activity to ablate the thyroid after thyroidectomy for cancer: a randomized study. PLoS One. 2008;2(3):e1885.
22. Castagna MG, Cevenini G, Theodoropoulou A, et al. Postsurgical thyroid ablation with low or high radioiodine activities results in similar outcomes in intermediate risk differentiated thyroid cancer patients. Eur J Endocrinol. 2013;169:23–9.
23. Verburg FA, Mader U, Reiners C, et al. Long term survival in DTC is worse after low-activity initial post-surgical I-131 therapy in both high and low risk patients. J Clin Endocrinol Metab. 2014;99:4487–96.
24. Fatourechi V, Hay ID, Mullan BP, et al. Are post-therapy radioiodine scans informative and do they influence subsequent therapy of patients with differentiated thyroid cancer? Thyroid. 2009;10:573–7.
25. Souza Rosario PW, Barroso AL, Rezende LL, et al. Post I-131 therapy scanning in patients with thyroid carcinoma metastases: an unnecessary cost or a relevant contribution? Clin Nucl Med. 2004;29:795–8.
26. Van Nostrand D. The benefits and risks of I-131 therapy in patients with well-differentiated thyroid cancer. Thyroid. 2009;19:1381–91.
27. Klubo-Gwiezdzinska J, Van Nostrand D, Atkins F, et al. Efficacy of 131 dosimetric versus empiric prescribed activity of I for therapy of differentiated thyroid cancer. J Clin Endocrinol Metab. 2011;96(10):3217–25.
28. Baudin E, Schlumberger M. Metastasis of differentiated cancers of the thyroid. Ann Endocrinol (Paris). 1997;58:326–9.
29. Nixon IJ, Whitcher MM, Palmer FL, et al. The impact of distant metastases at presentation on prognosis in patients with differentiated carcinoma of the thyroid gland. Thyroid. 2012;22:884–9.
30. Sawka AM, Thabane L, Parlea L, Ibrahim-Zada I, Tsang RW, Brierley JD, Straus S, Ezzat S, Goldstein DP. Second primary malignancy risk after radioactive iodine treatment for thyroid cancer: a systematic review and meta-analysis. Thyroid. 2009;19:451–7.

Radioiodine Therapy of Thyroid Cancer Dosimetry

7

Lorenzo Bianchi

Abstract

Radioactive iodine therapy has been established in the management of patients with metastatic thyroid cancer therapy. The optimal activity to be administered has been under discussion since its first use. The activity can be determined using two approaches, empiric and dosimetry based. Administering an empirical activity is low cost and easy, and the rate and severity of side effects are well known and accepted. However, it can lead to undertreat or overtreat patients, due to the different specific characteristics of the iodine kinetics in each patient.

Therefore, an individual dosimetry-based approach is advisable to determine the correct activity to be administered in order to be effective and, at the same time, to limit severe side effects.

Here a simple method to perform individual dosimetry is proposed, based on the Committee on Medical Internal Radiation Dose schema. It can be applied both to perspective and peri-therapy dosimetry, depending on the goal and the available resources; since it improves awareness in taking a decision in patient's management, it represents a powerful instrument to support clinical strategies aimed at improving safety and efficacy of treatments.

7.1 Introduction

Patients affected by metastatic differentiated thyroid cancer (MDTC) undergo radioactive iodine therapy (RAIT) since the 1940s [1]. RAIT has proved to be effective to ablate thyroid remnant and to treat lymph node metastases (LMTS) and distant metastases which the most commonly are pulmonary (PMTS) and bone (BMTS).

Since its first use [2], there has been a discussion about the optimal activity to be administered in order to be effective and safe, i.e., to maximize the tumor dose and to avoid severe myelotoxicity at the same time.

Red marrow (RM) is historically considered the main organ at risk (OAR), and the absorbed dose constraint suggested in 1962 by Benua et al. [3] of

L. Bianchi
Struttura Complessa di Fisica Sanitaria, ASST della Valle Olona, Busto Arsizio, VA, Italy
e-mail: lorenzo.bianchi@asst-valleolona.it

E. Bombardieri et al. (eds.), *Clinical Applications of Nuclear Medicine Targeted Therapy*,
https://doi.org/10.1007/978-3-319-63067-0_7

2 Gy absorbed dose to RM is generally accepted. Moreover, in presence of pulmonary metastases, an activity less than 4.44 GBq (120 mCi) in the total body at 48 h after administration is advisable [4]; in case of miliary pulmonary metastases, the limit is lowered to 2.96 GBq (80 mCi).

Concerning the efficacy, an activity of 1.11–3.7 GBq (30–100 mCi) is considered sufficient to ablate the remnant; in presence of lymph node metastases, the suggested activity is 3.7–7.4 GBq (100–200 mCi), while in the presence of distant metastases, an activity of 7.4 GBq (200 mCi) is advisable.

However, already in 1983 Hurley and Becker [5] showed that administering a fixed activity of 7.4 GBq leads to undertreat 53% of patients and to overtreat 3% of them. So, the administration of a "maximum safe fixed activity" seems not to be an optimal strategy, and an individual dosimetry-based approach is advisable.

7.2 Goal of Dosimetry in the Treatment of MDTC

Further to the above considerations, an integral approach to individualized dosimetry should lead to administer an activity considered both *safe* and *effective*. A *safe* activity should result in an *equivalent dose* to OARs lower than the appropriate constraint (for example, 2 Gy for RM). An activity can be considered *effective* when delivering an equivalent dose not less than 300 Gy to the remnant and/or not less than 80 Gy to the metastases [6]. Recently Jentzen et al. [7] suggested that 80 Gy seems to be effective in case of LMTS, while to treat effectively BMTS, at least 650 Gy is needed.

Therefore, an individual estimate of the activity to be administered to be safe and effective requires a perspective dosimetry to singularly evaluate the dose delivered per unit of administered activity both to OARs and to tumor. In case of pulmonary metastases, perspective dosimetry allows also the estimate of the maximum activity to be administered to comply with the further exposed constraints (total body activity at 48 h after administration).

Since that metastases dosimetry requires considerable efforts in terms of time and equipment employed, one can choose to perform only RM and lungs perspective dosimetry, in order to calculate the maximum tolerable activity (MTA); so, the administered activity of ^{131}I that will comply the dose constraints for RM and lungs. The rationale is that safety has to be considered first; under this point of view, optimizing a treatment means to administer an activity *as high as safely achievable* (AHASA). Moreover, there is some evidence [8] that *one big shot* is more effective than repeated treatments with lower administered activities.

If perspective dosimetry isn't carried out for some reason, anyway peri-therapy dosimetry is advisable in order to correlate absorbed dose and effects, both for RM and metastases.

The calculation methods set out below, based on Committee on Medical Internal Radiation Dose (MIRD) schema, apply both to perspective and peri-therapy dosimetry.

Owing to the difficulties in obtaining reliable data for an accurate remnant dosimetry, the topic is not discussed here. The discussion will therefore be limited to RM, lungs and metastases dosimetry.

7.3 Red Marrow Dosimetry: The Calculation Model

To estimate the absorbed dose to RM, two sources have to be considered: RM and remainder of the body (RB). Under such hypotheses, according to the MIRD schema, the equation describing RM absorbed dose is

$$D_{\mathrm{RM}} = S_{\mathrm{RM}\leftarrow\mathrm{RM}}\tilde{A}_{\mathrm{RM}} + S_{\mathrm{RM}\leftarrow\mathrm{RB}}\tilde{A}_{\mathrm{RB}} \quad (7.1)$$

where $\tilde{A}_{\mathrm{RM}}$ and $\tilde{A}_{\mathrm{RB}}$ are, respectively, RM and RB cumulated activity to be assessed for each patient, and $S_{i\leftarrow j}$ are the *S factors* tabulated in the MIRD schema, representing the dose to the target *i* per unit of activity cumulated in the source organ *j*; in particular, $S_{RM\leftarrow RM}$ is the absorbed dose to RM per unit of cumulated activity in RM itself, while $S_{RM\leftarrow RB}$ is the absorbed dose to RM per unit of cumulated activity in RB.

Under the hypothesis of mono-exponential kinetics, absorbed dose to RM of adult male and female patients are, respectively:

$$\text{Male } D_{RM}(Gy/MBq) = \frac{1.06\times10^{-4}}{m_p(\text{kg})\lambda_{TB}(\text{h}^{-1})} + 6.1\times10^{-5}\frac{[U_{Bl}]_{max}(\text{kg}^{-1})}{\lambda_{Bl}(\text{h}^{-1})} \quad (7.2)$$

$$\text{Female } D_{RM}(Gy/MBq) = \frac{9.43\times10^{-5}}{m_p(\text{kg})\lambda_{TB}(\text{h}^{-1})} + 6.5\times10^{-5}\frac{[U_{Bl}]_{max}(\text{kg}^{-1})}{\lambda_{Bl}(\text{h}^{-1})} \quad (7.3)$$

where m_p is the patient mass; λ_{TB} and $\lambda_{Bl}$are the effective decay constants of radioiodine in total body and blood, respectively; and $[U_{Bl}]_{max}$ is the maximum fraction of administered activity per unit of mass of patient's blood.

When decay curves of activity show long-term components, a multi-exponential kinetic has to be considered; usually, a bi-exponential model is enough to describe with a sufficient degree of accuracy both short- and long-term components. Under such conditions Eqs. (7.2) and (7.3) become:

$$\text{Male } D_{RM}(Gy/GBq) = \frac{0.106}{m_p(\text{kg})}\tau_{TB}(h) + 61\,\tau_{BL}^{1\text{mL}}(\text{h}/\text{mL}) \quad (7.4)$$

$$\text{Female } D_{RM}(Gy/GBq) = \frac{0.0943}{m_p(\text{kg})}\tau_{TB} + 65\tau_{BL}^{1\text{ mL}}(\text{h}/\text{mL}) \quad (7.5)$$

where m_p is the patient mass, $\tau_{TB}$is the residence times of radioiodine in total body, and τ_{BL}^{1mL} is the residence time of radioiodine in 1 ml of blood.

7.4 Red Marrow Dosimetry: Data Acquisition

The parameters mentioned above (uptake, residence times, decay times) are acquired with serial total body and blood sample measurements.

Total body measurements. Total body measurements are performed with an external probe after the activity administration. Geiger counters, ionization chambers, proportional counters, and NaI probes can be used for this purpose.

The measurements have to be performed always under the same geometrical conditions. An example is proposed in Fig. 7.1.

The distance d can be 3 m or, in case of high administered activities, 4 m, in order to avoid significant levels of dead time.

AP and PA measurements have to be performed, and total body counts at time t, $N_{TB}(t)$, are obtained as geometric mean of them:

$$N_{TB}(t) = \sqrt{[N_{AP}(t) - N_B]\cdot[N_{PA}(t) - N_B]} \quad (7.6)$$

where N_B are the background counts.

The reference value of $N_{TB}(0)$ has to be measured after 2 h in the case of oral administration or immediately in the case of iv administration; patients have to avoid urinating before the first measurement. The counts N_{TB} obtained correspond to the administered activity A_0.

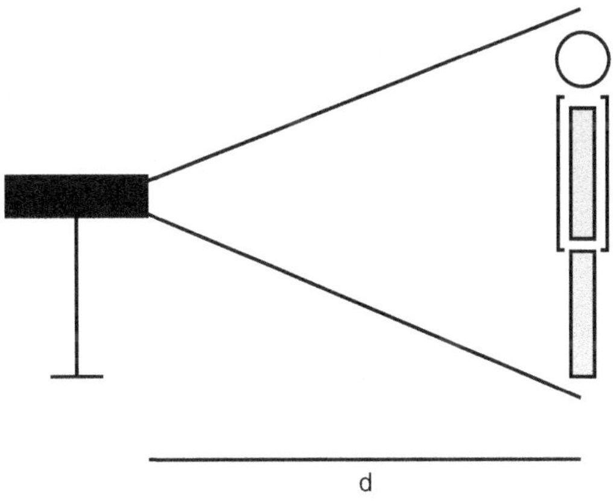

Fig. 7.1 Total body measurement conditions

Afterward, counts have to be acquired at least at 6, 24, 48, and 96 h after administration, after the patient has urinated. Measurements after 120 h or more are advisable, especially in the case of long-term components. Although time-consuming, a more frequent sampling is advisable to obtain more accurate statistics.

After construction of time-count curve, a fitting has to be performed using the corresponding equations above exposed in order to evaluate λ_{TB} or τ_{TB}.

Software OLINDA-EXM [9] or other reliable software can be used to fit data.

Blood samples collection. Blood samples are collected immediately before or after total body measurements. It's suggested to collect about 2 ml samples. Measurements of samples are performed using calibrated gamma counters, well counters, or similar.

Blood concentrations in 1 ml are determined by fitting time-count curves obtained with the corresponding equations above exposed.

Other simpler methods have been proposed to assess absorbed dose to RM [10] in which blood activity concentration is expressed as a function of total body retention, avoiding blood samples collection.

7.5 Tumor Dosimetry: The Calculation Model

Imaging isn't required to calculate absorbed dose to RM, but it becomes mandatory when calculating absorbed dose to tumor.

MIRD Pamphlet No. 16 [11] is a good reference to approach the problem of quantifying radiopharmaceutical biodistribution in the absorbed dose assessment. Here the simplest approach will be considered, based on planar images acquisition. Further extensions are well discussed in the pamphlet. Commercial codes have been developed too, all of them based on MIRD schema.

According to MIRD schema, assuming that the major lesion dose contribution is given by the activity cumulated in the lesion itself, the basic equation to calculate lesion absorbed dose is

$$D = \tilde{A}S \tag{7.7}$$

where $\tilde{A}$ is the cumulated activity in the lesion and S is the Snyder S factor. $\tilde{A}$ is estimated performing serial scans after administration, and S is calculated from the lesion mass.

7.6 Tumor Dosimetry: Data Acquisition

S factors calculation. S factors expressed in mGy/MBqh depend on the lesion mass m according to the equations below:

$$S = 110.02 / m^{-0.9734} \quad (m < 10\text{g}) \tag{7.8}$$

$$S = 107.80 / m^{-0.9673} \quad (10\text{g} < m < 100\text{g}) \tag{7.9}$$

$$S = 97.10 / m^{-0.9673} \quad (100\text{g} < m < 1000\text{g}) \tag{7.10}$$

$$S = 74.53 / m^{-0.9052} \quad (1000\text{g} < m < 6000\text{g}) \tag{7.11}$$

So, tumor dosimetry requires, first of all, an accurate determination of the lesion mass. Regions of interest (ROIs) on CT or MR images need to be contoured slice by slice to determine lesion volumes V; the volumes are converted into masses multiplying by the corresponding density values, usually 1 g/cm^3.

In case of bone metastases or diffuse lung micro-metastases, density may differ significantly from 1 g/cm^3. In such cases, ICRP Publication No. 70 [12] is a good reference for bone density values. Otherwise, density ρ can be estimated basing on CT numbers of the lesion (CT_L) according to the following equation:

$$\rho = CT_L / 1000 + 1 \tag{7.12}$$

and mass m calculated as

$$m = \rho V \tag{7.13}$$

where V is the lesion volume.

CT or RM scans must be performed not more than 2 months before dosimetry, and iodinated contrast agents must be avoided to prevent competition with radioactive iodine.

Small lesion volumes are particularly difficult to be determined. When a lesion is visible only on 2 or 3 slices, the determination of volume's value is affected by partial volume effect. The error so introduced can propagate, and the application of this protocol is discouraged.

$\tilde{A}$ *calculation*. A time-activity curve has to be constructed in order to calculate $\tilde{A}$.

Scans have to be performed at 24, 48, 72, and 96 h after administration of radioactive iodine. Further, a tardive scan (at least 120 h after administration) is necessary to take into account long-term components.

For each scan, the activity A in the lesion has to be determined. The conjugate views method [11] is the simplest way to determine it. It's based on the acquisition of two opposite images with a gamma camera in a planar scan. For each scan, the activity is calculated according to the expression below:

$$A = \sqrt{\frac{I_A^{'} I_P^{'}}{\exp\left(-\mu\left({}^{131}I\right)^{*} T\right)}}^{*} f / C \quad (7.14)$$

where $\mu(^{131}I)$ is the linear attenuation correction coefficient for ^{131}I, to be evaluated in water on the gamma camera with the same collimators employed with the patient; I_A and I_P are the anterior and posterior counts, respectively, in the ROI defined around the object of study, after background subtraction; T is the patient effective thickness in the region of the lesion; f = *z*/*hip sin (z)* (usually 1, except in case of very big lesions); $z = \mu(^{131}I)$ *t/2*; t is the mean lesion thickness, estimated as volume to area ratio of the ROI; and C is the system calibration factor, i.e., count rate per unit activity.

Patient thickness T in the ROI can be determined with a double scan with a planar source of ^{57}Co, the first one in the absence of patient (*blank*), the second one in the presence of patient; thickness is then obtained by simple calculation described in MIRD pamphlet No. 16.

Other corrections are needed:

- Dead time correction, when the high activity in the patient may cause very high dead time
- Scatter correction
- Partial volume effect correction

For every correction mentioned above, various methods are proposed in MIRD pamphlet No. 16.

System calibration factor C is needed in order to convert count rate into activity. According to MIRD 16, it is obtained by counting for a fixed time, a point source of known activity placed in air at a distance from the collimator similar to that used for patient protocol. Alternatively, it is possible to obtain it by measuring an extended source at different depths in water; extended source is advisable rather than point source to take into account both partial volume effects and clinical acquisition conditions.

Once time-activity curve is made, the cumulated activity $\tilde{A}$ is calculated as area under the curve. It's also possible to fit the curve using the same software, described above, employed to fit time-count curves for absorbed dose to RM assessment.

7.7 Practical Considerations

When choosing whether subjecting a patient to RAIT or not, Table 14 in 2015 American Thyroid Association Guidelines [13] should be considered. According to the risk stratification here proposed, RAIT is mandatory in the case of high-risk patients, not indicated in low-risk patients, and has to be considered for low/intermediated risk and intermediate risk. Furthermore, in the case of advanced thyroid cancer and elevated thyroglobulin levels, the *New Theranostic Paradigm* proposed by Pattinson et al. [14] for patient management should be considered, in order to choose the optimal diagnostic and therapeutic path.

When a patient is framed in intermediate or high risk, according to ATA guidelines, perspective dosimetry should be performed before subjecting a patient to RAIT: RM dosimetry and lung dosimetry can lead to determine MTA, but the real goal should be to understand if this activity can be effective in order to obtain therapeutic efficacy also for the lesions.

Perspective dosimetry has to be performed administering an activity sufficiently high to see the lesions and to evaluate the uptake with a satisfactory statistical accuracy. At the same time, activity should be not too high in order to avoid stunning effects [15–17]. Considering these constraints, an activity ranging from 37 to 111 MBq (1–3 mCi) could be suitable. If only absorbed dose to RM is required, also lower activities can be administered, such as 15–30 MBq.

Acquisitions and evaluations according to the scheme proposed above provide the estimate of the absorbed dose to lesion per unit of administered activity *D/A* (mGy/MBq or Gy/GBq). The activity A_E to be administered considered *effective* can be easily derived by dividing the dose D_E, considered effective, by *D/A*. For example, in the case of a lymph node lesion for which A/D calculated corresponds to 6 Gy/GBq, according to Maxon [6], the activity *A* to be administered to give an absorbed dose to the lesion of 80 Gy at least should be

$$A = 80Gy / 6Gy / Gbq \cong 13.3GBq \quad (7.15)$$

Then, in order to check for the *safety* of treatment, this activity A has to be multiplied by the absorbed dose per unit of administered activity *D/A* estimated for RM. For example, in the case of A/D calculated for RM corresponding to 0.1 Gy/GBq, the corresponding RM absorbed dose will be

$$D = 13.3Gbq * 0.1Gy / GBq \cong 1.33Gy \quad (7.16)$$

Since the estimated RM absorbed dose is less than 2 Gy, the treatment could be considered safe, according to the traditional constraint proposed by Benua.

In the case of A/D calculated for RM corresponding to 0.2 Gy/GBq, the corresponding RM absorbed dose will be about 2.7 Gy; so, according to Benua constraint, the RM dose could cause serious hematological toxicity.

In case of pulmonary metastases, further considerations concerning the activity *A* to be administered must be taken into account. As exposed above, basing on total body retention curve determined with perspective dosimetry measurements, the maximum activity to be administered *A* for a safe treatment can be easily derived from the total body retention at 48 h after the administration $U_{TB}(48)$. For example, in case of focal pulmonary metastases, if $U_{TB}(48)$ is 0.32 (i.e., 32%), the maximum activity *A* to be administered should be

$$A = 4.44GBq / 0.32 \cong 13.88GBq \quad (7.17)$$

where 4.44 GBq is the permitted constrain.

In case of diffused pulmonary metastases, the total body at 48 h activity constraint lowers to 2.96 and, accordingly, the maximum activity to be administered *A* lowers to 9.25 GBq.

If the workload for a complete dosimetry (both RM and metastases) is deemed excessive, at least RM perspective dosimetry should be performed, for the purpose of estimating the maximum tolerable activity and to ensure a safe treatment. Of course, in case of pulmonary metastases, specific constraints recalled above have to be taken into account too.

Especially when high activities are administered, important differences between estimated RM dose in perspective dosimetry and calculated RM dose during therapy could be noticed, owing to the different kinetics [18].

Perspective dosimetry when administering Rh-TSH to treat patients under euthyroidism regimen doesn't provide reliable data, because the kinetic can change significantly when administering the therapeutic activity [19].

Under the clinical point of view, some considerations must be done. Brans et al. in 2007 [20] cite Dorn's paper [21], where administered activity is maximized to an absorbed dose to the bone marrow of 3 Gy or 30 Gy to the lungs, resulting in mean of 22.1 GBq administered activity (range 7.4–38.5 GBq); many institutions will find difficult to administer these amounts, notwithstanding that rarely bone marrow depression has been reported, the rate of leukemia has been estimated to be approximately 1% in 5–10 years, and lung fibrosis as consequence of micronodular iodine avid metastases has been reported in 1% of patients suffering from pulmonary metastases. Bianchi et al. [22], in their experience of RAIT both and peri-therapy dosimetry, refer about five cases of RM absorbed dose above 2 Gy (range 2.03–6.67 Gy); all the cases showed severe toxicity, but in all of them it was transient, with a complete recovery of platelets and WBC within 3–6 months.

Dorn's experience and the above exposed data may suggest that further considerations could be made about the possibility of exceeding the 2 Gy constraint, paying attention to other side effects, such as radioiodine sialadenitis [23], which may seriously compromise patient's quality of life. In any case, perspective dosimetry has to be considered a powerful tool to improve the consciousness of what we can reach out when performing RAIT, both in terms of safety and efficacy.

7.8 Further Developments

The schema proposed is easily implemented and can be considered a good basis to be improved, depending on the availability of personnel and instrumentation, both hardware and software. A first limitation is that mean dose to the lesions is considered, regardless of not-uniform distributions of the activity that should be taken into account, especially in the case of extended lesions. Voxel dosimetry [24], requiring a better quantitative imaging, takes into account the microdistribution of the activity and offers S values estimated at the voxel level.

Under the diagnostic point of view, ^{124}I PET imaging proved to be a superior diagnostic tool compared to low-dose diagnostic ^{131}I scans [25, 26]. ^{124}I scans showed to be a better predicting tool of findings in scans subsequent to high-dose RAIT, owing to the high resolution and the possibility to combine with CT scans, and could lead to improved clinical decision-making.

Conclusions

Dosimetry in RAIT is a powerful instrument to support clinical strategies in order to improve the safety and the efficacy of a treatment. Depending on the available resources, various levels of implementation are available, and every center where RAIT is performed can make the best choice.

Key Points

- RAIT is traditionally based on empirical ^{131}I activity administered to patients, basing on their clinical conditions.
- Administering fixed empirically determined activities may cause both overtreatment and undertreatment.
- Treatment optimization requires to administer an activity sufficiently high to ablate residuals and/or kill metastases and, at the same time, to avoid side effects.
- Perspective dosimetry allows, in principle, to assess the optimal activity both to administer a curative dose to metastases and doses to organs at risk (such as red marrow) lower than the appropriate constraints.
- Peri-therapy dosimetry is useful to assess red marrow and lesion absorbed dose.

References

1. Luster M, Clarke SE, Dietlein M, et al. Guidelines for radioiodine therapy of differentiated thyroid cancer. Eur J Nucl Med Mol Imaging. 2008;35:1941–59.
2. Seidlin SM, Marinelli LD, Oshry E. Radioactive iodine therapy: effect on functioning metastases of adenocarcinoma of thyroid. JAMA. 1946;132:838–47.
3. Benua RS, Cicale NR, Sonemberg M, Rawson RW. The relation of radioiodine dosimetry to results and complications in the treatment of metastatic thyroid cancer. Am J Roentgenol Radium Therapy, Nucl Med. 1962;87:171–82.
4. Benua RS, Leeper RD. A method and rationale for treating metastatic thyroid carcinoma with the largest safe dose of I-131. In: Medeiros-Neto G, Gaitan E, editors. Frontiers in thyroidology, vol. 2. New York: Plenum Medical Book; 1986. p. 1317–21.
5. Hurley JR, Becker DV. The use of radioiodine in the management of thyroid cancer. In: Freeman LM, Weissmann HS, editors. Nuclear medicine annual. New York: Raven Press; 1983. p. 329.

6. Maxon HR, Thomas SR, Hertzberg VS, Kerejakes JG, Chen IW, Sperling MI, Saenger EI. Relation between effective radiation dose and outcome of radioiodine therapy for thyroid cancer. N Engl J Med. 1983;309:937–41.
7. Jentzen W, Verschure V, van Zon A, van de Kolk R, Wierts R, Schmitz J, Bockisch A, Binse I. ^{124}I PET Assessment of response of bone metastases to initial radioiodine treatment of differentiated thyroid cancer. J Nucl Med. 2016;57:1499–504.
8. Klubo-Gwiezdzinska J, Van Nostrand D, Atkins F, Burman K, Jonklaas J, Mete M, Wartofsky L. Efficacy of dosimetric versus empiric prescribed activity of ^{131}I for therapy of differentiated thyroid cancer. J Clin Endocrinol Metab. 2011;96:3217–25.
9. Stabin MG, Sparks RB, Crowe E. OLINDA/EXM: the second-generation personal computer software for internal dose assessment in nuclear medicine. J Nucl Med. 2005;46:1023–7.
10. Heinscheid H, Lassmann M, Luster M, Kloos RT, Reiners C. Blood dosimetry from a single measurement of the whole body radioiodine retention in patients with differentiated thyroid carcinoma. Endocr Relat Cancer. 2009;16:1283–9.
11. Siegel JA, et al. MIRD pamphlet no. 16: techniques for quantitative radiopharmaceutical biodistribution data acquisition and analysis for use in human radiation dose estimates. J Nucl Med. 1999;40:37S–61S.
12. International Commission on Radiological Protection Publication 70. Basic anatomical & physiological data for use in radiological protection – the skeleton. In: Ann. Annals of the ICRP, vol 25(2). Oxford:Pergamon Press; 1995.
13. Haugen BR, et al. 2015 American Thyroid Association management guidelines for adult patients with thyroid nodules and differentiated thyroid cancer. Thyroid. 2016;26:1–160.
14. Pattison DA, Solomon B, Hicks RJ. A new theranostic paradigm for advanced thyroid cancer. J Nucl Med. 2016;57:1493–4.
15. Pacini F, Lippi F, Formica N, Elisei R, Anelli S, Ceccarelli C, et al. Therapeutic doses of iodine-131 reveal undiagnosed metastases in thyroid cancer patients with detectable serum thyroglobulin levels. J Nucl Med. 1987;28:1888–91.
16. Cholewinski SP, Yoo KS, Klieger PS, O'Mara RE. Absence of thyroid stunning after diagnostic whole-body scanning with 185 MBq ^{131}I. J Nucl Med. 2000;41:1198–202.
17. Park HM, Perkins OW, Edmondson JW, Schnute RB, Manatunga A. Influence of diagnostic radioiodines on the uptake of ablative dose of iodine-131. Thyroid. 1994;4:49–54.
18. Miranti A, Giostra A, Richetta E, Gino E, Pellerito RE, Stasi M. Comparison of mathematical models for red marrow and blood absorbed dose estimation in the radioiodine treatment of advanced thyroid carcinoma. Phys Med Biol. 2015;60:1141–57.
19. Heinsched H, et al. Iodine biokinetics and dosimetry in radioiodine therapy of thyroid cancer: procedures and results of a prospective international controlled study of ablation after rhTSH or hormone withdrawal. J Nucl Med. 2006;47:648–54.
20. Brans B, Bodei L, Giammarile F, Linden O, Luster M, Oyen WJG, Tennvall J. Clinical radionuclide therapy dosimetry: the quest for the "Holy Gray". Eur J Nucl Med Mol Imaging. 2007;34:772–86.
21. Dorn R, Kopp J, Vogt H, Heidenreich P, Carroll RG, Gulec SA. Dosimetry-guided radioactive iodine treatment in patients with metastatic differentiated thyroid cancer: largest safe dose using a risk-adapted approach. J Nucl Med. 2003;44:451–6.
22. Bianchi L, Baroli A, Lomuscio G, Pedrazzini L, Pepe A, Pozzi L, Chiesa C. Dosimetry in the therapy of metastatic differentiated thyroid cancer administering high ^{131}I activity: the experience of Busto Arsizio Hospital (Italy). Q J Nucl Med Mol Imaging. 2012;56:515–21.
23. Fard-Esfahani A, Emami-Ardekani A, Fallahi B, Fard-Esfahani P, Beikia D, Hassanzadeh-Rada A, Eftekharia M. Adverse effects of radioactive iodine-131 treatment for differentiated thyroid carcinoma. Nucl Med Commun. 2014;35:811–7.
24. Bolch WE, Bouchet LG, Robertson JS, Wessels BW, Siegel JA, Howell RW, Erdi AK, Aydogan B, Costes S, Watson EE. MIRD pamphlet no. 17: the dosimetry of nonuniform activity distributions—radionuclide S values at the voxel level. J Nucl Med. 1999;40:118–368.
25. Phan HTT, Jager PL, Paans MJ, Plukker JTM, Sturkenboom MGG, Sluiter WJ, Wolffenbuttel BHR, Dierckx RAJO, Links TP. The diagnostic value of ^{124}I-PET in patients with differentiated thyroid cancer. Eur J Nucl Med Mol Imaging. 2008;35:958–65.
26. Pettinato C, Monari F, Nanni C, Allegri V, Marcatili S, Civollani S, Cima S, Spezi E, Mazzarotto R, Fanti S. Usefulness of ^{124}I PET/CT imaging to predict absorbed doses in patients affected by metastatic thyroid cancer and treated with ^{131}I. Q J Nucl Med Mol Imaging. 2012;56:509–14.

Check for updates

Published Guidelines on Radioisotopic Treatments of Thyroid Diseases

8

Lucia Setti, Vicinelli Riccardo, Gianluigi Ciocia, Emilio Bombardieri, and Laura Evangelista

8.1 Introduction

The present chapter has the aim to provide the current position of nuclear medicine for the treatment of benign and malignant thyroid disease with 131-Iodine (131-I), in the main international guidelines.

A general comment should be added in order to introduce the current position of radioiodine therapy as reported by the most important guidelines dealing with the treatment of thyroid diseases. Over the last 60 years, radioiodine therapy has always been considered one of the first options for treating both benign and malignant pathologies of the thyroid gland. As awaited, clinical indications, procedures, and treatment modalities should be already well-defined and established, but, on the contrary, many differences still result among the published guidelines, both in terms of level of evidences, recommended activities, and the best standard of diagnosis and care. These discrepancies, clearly reported in the present chapter, can be explained by summarizing the critical points that have been reported in the preface of this book. Being a huge quantity of clinical data about the radioiodine therapy of benign and malignant thyroid diseases published over the last years by many authors, we can say that the overall results now can justify the clinical adoption of this therapy. However, the majority of these results were obtained worldwide in very large series of patients but mainly through retrospective studies. Perspective controlled clinical trials, able to validate the efficacy of the nuclear medicine therapy, are still missing. Therefore the intrinsic value of radioisotope therapy is not always recognized, or it is even underestimated. In fact, the prescribed radioiodine activities to the patients, results often heterogeneous, being chosen according to an empiric experience. The correct dosimetric approaches to calculate the individual doses for the patients were not always carried out in the clinical practice; thus rendering the target irradiation is not completely optimized in terms of dose distribution and efficacy. The advancement of technology and the progressive application of dosimetry are going to improve the efficacy of this targeted therapy. The reader can find in the mentioned guidelines some contradictory statements. However, we decided to report in this text the complete state of the art based on the literature evidences.

L. Setti • G. Ciocia • E. Bombardieri
Department of Nuclear Medicine, Humanitas Gavazzeni Hospital, Bergamo, Italy

V. Riccardo
School Specialization of Nuclear Medicine, University Milano Bicocca, Milan, Italy

L. Evangelista (✉)
Nuclear Medicine and Molecular Imaging Unit, Veneto Institute of Oncology IOV, IRCCS, Padua, Italy
e-mail: laura.evangelista@iov.veneto.it

E. Bombardieri et al. (eds.), *Clinical Applications of Nuclear Medicine Targeted Therapy*,
https://doi.org/10.1007/978-3-319-63067-0_8

8.2 Comments and Suggestions About Benign Thyroid Disease

In Table 8.1 a summary of clinical indications is reported for benign thyroid disease. In the context of benign thyroid disease are present two guidelines about the procedural information provided by EANM and SNMMI. Moreover, clinical recommendation is mainly driven by ATA guidelines. The directions recommended by the ACR proposed the use of different activities of 131-I to be administered for the treatment of hyperthyroidism in toxic diffuse goiter/Graves' disease and for the hyper functioning multinodular goiter or toxic adenoma. The ATA guideline for the treatment of hyperthyroidism indicates the 131-I therapy in patients with Graves' disease, particularly in patients with contraindications to surgical treatment or poor hyperfunction control on antithyroid drugs (ATDs). Table 8.2 illustrates the recommended 131-I activities for the treatment of benign thyroid disease.

8.3 Comments and Suggestions About Malignant Thyroid Disease

In Table 8.3 a summary of clinical indications is reported for malignant thyroid disease. Similarly, in the treatment of malignant thyroid disease, we can distinguish between procedural and clinical guidelines. However, a large discrepancy between ATA and the other clinical/procedural guidelines emerges.

The ATA 2015 guideline indicates in a clear way the different purposes (therapy, adjuvant therapy, or ablation of the residual thyroid tissue) for which the radioiodine treatment may be indicated. These guidelines allow the clinicians to have a certain degree of decision-making autonomy, indicating the postsurgical treatment in patients with low-differentiated thyroid carcinoma (DTC) and medium risk only as "to consider" in case of particular features of greater aggressiveness of the disease, even in the presence of primary lesions greater than 4 cm.

The wide freedom of choice left to the clinicians that the application of these guidelines allow is one of the reasons leading the EANM to deny the endorsement required by the ATA for this document. The objection promoted by the EANM is based on the fear that the reduction in the number of patients with indication for radioiodine treatment may result in an increase of recurrent disease and, subsequently, of deaths related to thyroid disease. A further reason to disagree is about the possible to use of rTSH, which is proposed as an alternative is the second choice, instead of the hormone therapy withdrawal, despite what is reported in the literature. The ATA guidelines also introduce the concept of dynamic risk assessment, calculated on the basis of the response to primary therapy (including surgery and radioiodine therapy) and allow you to modulate the follow-up and possible further treatment on the basis of serum Tg on OT therapy or stimulated and clinical or instrumental evidence of persistent disease. Contrary to what is indicated by the ATA, the EANM considers 131-I therapy as a standard treatment procedure for patients with DTC, with one exception for the unifocal papillary carcinoma sizes of <1 cm, with no other risk factors. There is no consensus instead of 131-I activity to be administered, between 1 and 5 GBq in single administration for the ablation of thyroid remnant, and between 3.7 and 7.4 GBq or even increased activity, for repeated administration over time in case of evident disease at a distance iodo-sensitive and not operable.

NCCN and BTA guidelines are completely in line with the ATA guidelines, by indicating the treatment with 131-I mainly in patients with a large size thyroid cancer (> 4 cm), with extensive extranodal extension, and with the presence of known or suspected distant metastases.

Table 8.4 illustrates the recommended 131-I activities for the treatment of malignant thyroid disease, according to the main international guidelines.

Table 8.1 Treatment with 131-I in benign thyroid disease

Name of guidelines [ref]	Year pub.	Link	Clinical indication	Level of recommendation, grade of evidence
EANM procedure guidelines [1]	2010	http://eanm.org/publications/guidelines/gl_EJNMMI_therapy_of_benign_thyroid_disease.pdf	Graves' disease, toxic multinodular goiter, solitary hyperfunctioning nodule, nontoxic multinodular goiter, goiter recurrence, ablation of residual thyroid tissue in case of malignant ophthalmopathy after surgery, but during an active state of the orbitopathy	NA
SNMMI practice guidelines [2]	2012	http://interactive.snm.org/docs/Therapy%20of%20Thyroid%20Disease%20with%20Iodine-131%20v2.0.pdf	Graves' disease, toxic uni-multinodular goiter, and nontoxic nodular goiter	NA
ACR (https://www.acr.org/~/media/99393BE60E964AF6830B57C3E52E2339.pdf)	2014	https://www.acr.org/~/media/99393BE60E964AF6830B57C3E52E2339.pdf	Treatment of hyperthyroidism	NA
ATA guidelines [3]	2016	http://online.liebertpub.com/doi/pdf/10.1089/thy.2015.0020	*Recommendation 3*. RAI is an alternative treatment in patients with GD. RAI is the treatment of choice in women planning a pregnancy in the future (in more than 6 months following RAI administration, provided thyroid hormone levels are normal),individuals with comorbidities increasing surgical risk, and patients with previously operated or externally irradiated necks, or lack of access to a high-volume thyroid surgeon, and patients with contraindications to ATD use or failure to achieve euthyroidism during treatment with ATDs. Patients with periodic thyrotoxic hypokalemic paralysis, right heart failure pulmonary hypertension, or congestive heart failure should also be considered good candidates for RAI therapy. Definite contraindications include pregnancy, lactation, coexisting thyroid cancer, or suspicion of thyroid cancer, individuals unable to complywith radiation safety guidelines and used with informed caution in women planning a pregnancy within 4–6 months	Strong recommendation, moderate-quality evidence

(continued)

Table 8.1 (continued)

Name of guidelines [ref]	Year pub.	Link	Clinical indication	Level of recommendation, grade of evidence
			Recommendation 4. (preparation of the patients): because RAI treatment of GD can cause a transient exacerbation of hyperthyroidism, b-adrenergic blockade should be considered even in asymptomatic patients who are at increased risk for complications due to worsening of hyperthyroidism (i.e., elderly patients and patients with comorbidities)	Weak recommendation, low-quality evidence
			Recommendation 5. In addition to b-adrenergic blockade (see Recommendations 2 and 4), pretreatment with MMI prior to RAI therapy for GD should be considered in patients who are at increased risk for complications due to worsening of hyperthyroidism. MMI should be discontinued 2–3 days prior to RAI	Weak recommendation, moderate-quality evidence
			Recommendation 6. In patients who are at increased risk for complications due to worsening of hyperthyroidism, resuming MMI 3–7 days after RAI administration should be considered	Weak recommendation, low-quality evidence
			Recommendation 7. Medical therapy of any comorbid conditions should be optimized prior to RAI therapy	Strong recommendation, low-quality evidence
			Recommendation 8. Sufficient activity of RAI should be administered in a single application, typically a mean dose of 10–15 mCi (370–555 MBq), to render the patient with GD hypothyroid	Strong recommendation, moderate-quality evidence
			Recommendation 9. A pregnancy test should be obtained within 48 h prior to treatment in any woman with childbearing potential who is to be treated with RAI. The treating physician should obtain this test and verify a negative result prior to administering RAI	Strong recommendation, low-quality evidence

Table 8.1 (continued)

Name of guidelines [ref]	Year pub.	Link	Clinical indication	Level of recommendation, grade of evidence
			Recommendation 10. The physician administering RAI should provide written advice concerning radiation safety precautions following treatment. If the educations cannot be followed, alternative therapy should be selected	Strong recommendation, low-quality evidence
			Recommendation 11. Follow-up within the first 1–2 months after RAI therapy for GD should include an assessment of free T4, total T3, and TSH. Biochemical monitoring should be continued at 4- to 6-week intervals for 6 months, or until the patient becomes hypothyroid and is stable on thyroid hormone replacement	Strong recommendation, low-quality evidence
			Recommendation 12. When hyperthyroidism due to GD persists after 6 months following RAI therapy, retreatment with RAI is suggested. In selected patients with minimal response 3 months after therapy, additional RAI may be considered	Weak recommendation, low-quality evidence
			Recommendation 37. We suggest that patients with overtly TMNG or TA be treated with RAI therapy or thyroidectomy. On occasion, long-term, low-dose treatment with MMI may be appropriate	Weak recommendation, moderate-quality evidence
			Recommendation 38. Because RAI treatment of MNG or TA can cause a transient exacerbation of hyperthyroidism, b-adrenergic blockade should be considered even in asymptomatic patients who are at increased risk for complications due to worsening of hyperthyroidism (i.e., elderly patients and patients with comorbidities)	Weak recommendation, low-quality evidence

(continued)

Table 8.1 (continued)

Name of guidelines [ref]	Year pub.	Link	Clinical indication	Level of recommendation, grade of evidence
			Recommendation 39. In addition to b-adrenergic blockade (see Recommendations 2 and 38), pretreatment with MMI prior to RAI therapy for TMNG or TA should be considered in patients who are at increased risk for complications due to worsening of hyperthyroidism, including the elderly and those with cardiovascular disease or severe hyperthyroidism	Weak recommendation, low-quality evidence
			Recommendation 40. In patients who are at increased risk for complications due to worsening of hyperthyroidism, resuming ATDs 3–7 days after RAI administration should be considered	Weak recommendation, low-quality evidence
			Recommendation 42. Sufficient activity of RAI should be administered in a single application to alleviate hyperthyroidism in patients with TMNG	Strong recommendation, moderate-quality evidence
			Recommendation 43. Sufficient activity of RAI should be administered in a single application to alleviate hyperthyroidism in patients with TA	Strong recommendation, moderate-quality evidence
			Recommendation 44. Follow-up within the first 1–2 months after RAI therapy for TMNG or TA should include an assessment of free T4, total T3, and TSH. Biochemical monitoring should be continued at 4- to 6-week intervals for 6 months, or until the patient becomes hypothyroid and is stable on thyroid hormone replacement	Strong recommendation, low-quality evidence

Table 8.1 (continued)

Name of guidelines [ref]	Year pub.	Link	Clinical indication	Level of recommendation, grade of evidence
			Recommendation 45. If hyperthyroidism persists beyond 6 months following RAI therapy for TMNG or TA, retreatment with RAI is suggested. In selected patients with minimal response 3 months after therapy, additional RAI may be considered	Weak recommendation, low-quality evidence

ATA American thyroid association, *RAI* radioimmunotherapy, *GD* Graves' disease, *ATD* antithyroid drug, *MMI* methimazole, *TSH* thyrotropin, *TMNG* toxic multinodular goiter, *TA* toxic adenoma, *NMG* nontoxic multinodular goiter, *EANM* European Association of Nuclear Medicine, *NA* not available, *SNMMI* Society of Nuclear Medicine and Molecular Imaging, *ACR* American College of Radiology

Table 8.2 Recommended activities in accordance with the main international guidelines

Guidelines [ref]	Disease	Recommended activity
EANM [1]	Hyperthyroidism in toxic diffuse goiter/Graves' disease	The dose with the aim of restoring a euthyroid status is approximately 150 Gy, whereas the dose to achieve complete ablation is in the range 200–300 Gy
	Hyperfunctioning multinodular goiter or toxic adenoma	An absorbed radiation dose of 100–150 Gy is recommended, requiring about 3.7–5.5 MBq per gram of thyroid tissue corrected for the 24-h 131-I uptake
SNMMI [2]	Hyperthyroidism in toxic diffuse goiter/Graves' disease. Hyperfunctioning multinodular goiter or toxic adenoma	Delivered activity of 2.96–7.4 MBq (80–200 μCi) per gram of thyroid tissue is generally appropriate
ACR (https://www.acr.org/~/media/99393BE60E964AF6830B57C3E52E2339.pdf)	Hyperthyroidism in toxic diffuse goiter/Graves' disease. Hyperfunctioning multinodular goiter or toxic adenoma	1.85–7.4 MBq/500–200 μCi for gram of thyroid up to 1.22 GBq/33 mCi
ATA [3]	Hyperthyroidism in toxic diffuse goiter/Graves' disease. Hyperfunctioning multinodular goiter or toxic adenoma	370 and 555 MBq (10–15 mCi)

Table 8.3 Treatment with 131-I for malignant thyroid disease

Guidelines [ref]	Year pub	Link	Clinical indication	Level of recommendation, grade of evidence
EANM practical guidelines [4]	2008	http://eanm.org/publications/guidelines/gl_radio_ther_259_883.pdf	Selective irradiation of thyroid remnants, microscopic DTC or other nonresectable or incompletely resectable DTC, or both purposes	NA
ESMO clinical guidelines [5]	2012	http://www.esmo.org/Guidelines/Endocrine-Cancers/Thyroid-cancer	All patients with: 1-known distant metastases; 2-documented lymph node metastases; 3-gross extra thyroidal extension of the tumor regardless of tumor size; 4-primary tumor size >2 cm even in the absence of other higher-risk features (tall cell, columnar, insular and solid variant as well as poorly DTC and follicular and Hurthle cell cancer, intrathyroidal vascular invasion, gross or microscopic multifocal disease)	NA
SNMMI procedural guidelines [2]	2012	http://snmmi.files.cms-plus.com/docs/I-131_V3.0_JNM_pub_version.pdf	Differentiated papillary and follicular thyroid cancer, residual or recurrent thyroid cancer, and metastatic disease after near-total thyroidectomy	NA
ACR (https://www.acr.org/~/media/99393BE60E964AF6830B57C3E52E2339.pdf)	2014	https://www.ncbi.nlm.nih.gov/pubmed/24824115	Indications for postoperative adjuvant RAI are (1) tumor >1–1.5 cm; (2) patient age > 45 years; (3) capsular, vascular, or soft tissue invasion; (4) multifocal, residual, or recurrent disease; (5) lymph node metastasis; (6) distant metastasis; and (7) intermediate or high-risk disease based on a prognostic system	NA
ATA management guidelines for adult patients with thyroid nodules and differentiated thyroid cancer [3]	2015	http://online.liebertpub.com/doi/pdf/10.1089/thy.2015.0020	*Recommendation 32(B)*. RAI ablation may be used to ablate the remnant lobe in selected cases	Weak recommendation, low-quality evidence
			Recommendation 50(A). Postoperative disease status (i.e., the presence or absence of persistent disease) should be considered in deciding whether additional treatment (e.g., RAI, surgery, or other treatment) may be needed	Strong recommendation, low-quality evidence
			Recommendation 50(C). The optimal cutoff value for postoperative serum Tg or state in which it is measured to guide decision-making regarding RAI administration is not known	No recommendation, insufficient evidence

Table 8.3 (continued)

Guidelines [ref]	Year pub	Link	Clinical indication	Level of recommendation, grade of evidence
			Recommendation 51. ATA low-risk T1a N0, Nx, M0, Mx, tumor size <1 cm (uni-or multifocal) not indicated postsurgical RAI	Strong recommendation, moderate-quality evidence
			ATA low-risk T1b,T2, N0, Nx, M0, Mx tumor size >1–4 cm, indication to RAI is not routine: considered for patients with aggressive histology or vascular invasion	Weak recommendation, low-quality evidence
			ATA low- to intermediate-risk T3 N0, Nx, M0, Mx tumor size >4 cm, indication to RAI is to consider the need to consider the presence of other adverse features. Advancing age may favor RAI use in some cases, but specific age and tumor size cutoffs subject to some uncertainty	Weak recommendation, low-quality evidence Weak recommendation, low-quality evidence
			ATA low- to intermediate-risk T3 N0, Nx, M0, Mx with microscopic ETE, any tumor size. Indication: consider, generally favored based on risk of recurrent disease. Smaller tumors with microscopic ETE may not require RAI	Weak recommendation, low-quality evidence Weak recommendation, low-quality evidence
			ATA low- to intermediate-risk T1-3 N1a M0, Mx with central compartment neck lymph node metastases, indication: consider, generally favored, due to somewhat higher risk of persistent or recurrent disease, especially with increasing number of large (>2–3 cm) or clinically evident lymph nodes or presence of extranodal extension and advanced age. No sufficient data in RAI use in patients with few (<5) microscopic nodal metastases in central compartment in absence of other adverse features	Strong recommendation, moderate-quality evidence Strong recommendation, moderate-quality evidence
			ATA low- to intermediate-risk T1-3 N1b M0, Mx with lateral neck or mediastinal lymph node metastases considered—generally favored—due to higher risk of persistent or recurrent disease, especially with increasing number of macroscopic or clinically evident lymph nodes or presence of extranodal extension. Advancing age may also favor RAI use	
			ATA high-risk T4 any N any M any size, gross ETE. Clinical indication to RAI: YES	
			ATA high-risk M1 any T any N distant metastases. Clinical indication to RAI: YES	

(continued)

Table 8.3 (continued)

Guidelines [ref]	Year pub	Link	Clinical indication	Level of recommendation, grade of evidence
			Recommendation 52. The role of molecular testing in guiding postoperative RAI use has yet to be established; therefore, no molecular testing to guide postoperative RAI use can be recommended at this time	(No recommendation, insufficient evidence)
			Recommendation 53(A). If thyroid hormone withdrawal is planned prior to RAI therapy or diagnostic testing, LT4 should be withdrawn for 3–4 weeks. Liothyronine (LT3) may be instituted for LT4 in the initial weeks if LT4 is withdrawn for 4 or more weeks, and in such circumstances, LT3 should be withdrawn for at least 2 weeks. Serum TSH should be measured prior to radioisotope administration to evaluate the degree of TSH elevation	Strong recommendation, moderate-quality evidence
			Recommendation 53(B). A goal TSH of >30 mIU/L has been generally adopted in preparation for RAI therapy or diagnostic testing, but there is uncertainty relating to the optimum TSH level associated with improvement in long-term outcomes	Weak recommendation, low-quality evidence
			Recommendation 55(A). If RAI remnant ablation is performed after total thyroidectomy for ATA low-risk thyroid cancer or intermediate-risk disease with lower-risk features, a low administered activity of approximately of 30 mCi is generally favored over higher administered activities	Strong recommendation, high-quality evidence
			Recommendation 55(B). Higher administered activities may need to be considered for patients receiving less than a total or near-total thyroidectomy in which a larger remnant is suspected or in which adjuvant therapy is intended	Weak recommendation, low-quality evidence

Table 8.3 (continued)

Guidelines [ref]	Year pub	Link	Clinical indication	Level of recommendation, grade of evidence
			Recommendation 56. When RAI is intended for initial adjuvant therapy to treat suspected microscopic residual disease, administered activities above those used for remnant ablation up to 150 mCi are generally recommended (in absence of known distant metastases). It is uncertain whether routine use of higher administered activities (>150 mCi) in this setting will reduce structural disease recurrence for T3 and N1 disease	Weak recommendation, low-quality evidence
			Recommendation 57. A low iodine diet (LID) for approximately 1–2 weeks should be considered for patients undergoing RAI remnant ablation or treatment	Weak recommendation, low-quality evidence
			Recommendation 58. A post-therapy WBS (with or without SPECT/CT) is recommended after RAI remnant ablation or treatment, to inform disease staging and document the RAI avidity of any structural disease	Strong recommendation, low-quality evidence
			Recommendation 61. There is no role for routine systemic adjuvant therapy in patients with DTC (beyond RAI and/or TSH D40 suppressive therapy using LT4)	Strong recommendation, low-quality evidence
			Recommendation 66. After the first posttreatment WBS performed following RAI remnant ablation or adjuvant therapy, low-risk and intermediate-risk patients (lower-risk features) with an undetectable Tg on thyroid hormone with negative anti-Tg antibodies and a negative US (excellent response to therapy) do not require routine diagnostic WBS during follow-up	Strong recommendation, moderate-quality evidence
			Recommendation 67(A). Diagnostic WBS, either following thyroid hormone withdrawal or rhTSH, 6–12 months after adjuvant RAI therapy, can be useful in the follow-up of patients with high- or intermediate-risk (higher-risk features) of persistent disease and should be done with 123-I or low activity 131-I	Strong recommendation, low-quality evidence

(continued)

Table 8.3 (continued)

Guidelines [ref]	Year pub	Link	Clinical indication	Level of recommendation, grade of evidence
			Recommendation 67(B). SPECT/CT RAI imaging is preferred over planar imaging in patients with uptake on planar imaging to better anatomically localize the RAI uptake and distinguish between likely tumors and nonspecific uptake	Weak recommendation, moderate-quality evidence
			Recommendation 72. When technically feasible, surgery for aerodigestive invasive disease is recommended in combination with RAI and/or EBRT	Strong recommendation, moderate-quality evidence
			Recommendation 73(A). Although there are theoretical advantages to dosimetric approaches to the treatment of locoregional or metastatic disease, no recommendation can be made about the superiority of one method of RAI administration over another	No recommendation, insufficient evidence
			Recommendation 73(B). Empirically administered amounts of 131-I exceeding 150 mCi that often potentially exceed the maximum tolerable tissue dose should be avoided in patients over age 70 years	Strong recommendation, moderate-quality evidence
			Recommendation 74.There are currently insufficient outcome data to recommend rhTSH-mediated therapy for all patients with distant metastatic disease being treated with 131-I	No recommendation, insufficient evidence
			Recommendation 75. Recombinant human TSH-mediated therapy may be indicated in selected patients with underlying comorbidities making iatrogenic hypothyroidism potentially risky, in patients with pituitary disease whose serum TSH cannot be raised, or in patients in whom a delay in therapy might be deleterious. Such patients should be given the same or higher activity that would have been given had they been prepared with hypothyroidism or a dosimetrically determined activity	Strong recommendation, low-quality evidence

Table 8.3 (continued)

Guidelines [ref]	Year pub	Link	Clinical indication	Level of recommendation, grade of evidence
			Recommendation 76. Since there are no outcome data that demonstrate a better outcome of patients treated with lithium as an adjunct to 131-I therapy, the data are insufficient to recommend lithium therapy	No recommendation, insufficient evidence
			Recommendation 77. Pulmonary micrometastases should be treated with RAI therapy, and RAI therapy should be repeated every 6–12 months as long as disease continues to concentrate RAI and respond clinically because the highest rates of complete remission are reported in these subgroups. RAI activity to administer can be empiric (100–200 mCi or 100–150 mCi for patients ‡70 years old) or estimated by dosimetry to limit whole-body retention to 80 mCi at 48 h and 200 cGy to the bone marrow	Strong recommendation, moderate-quality evidence
			Recommendation 78. Radioiodine-avid macronodular metastases may be treated with RAI, and treatment may be repeated when objective benefit is demonstrated (decrease in the size of the lesions, decreasing Tg), but complete remission is not common, and survival remains poor. The selection of RAI activity is reported in recommendation 77	Weak recommendation, low-quality evidence
			Recommendation 79(A). RAI therapy of iodine-avid bone metastases has been associated with improved survival and should be employed, although RAI is rarely curative, with activity described in recommendation 77	Strong recommendation, moderate-quality evidence
			Recommendation 80. In the absence of structurally evident disease, patients with stimulated serum Tg < 10 ng/mL with thyroid hormone withdrawal or <5 ng/mL with rhTSH (indeterminate response) can be followed without empiric RAI therapy on continued thyroid hormone therapy alone, reserving additional therapies for those with rising serum Tg levels over time or other evidence of structural disease progression	Weak recommendation, low-quality evidence

(continued)

Table 8.3 (continued)

Guidelines [ref]	Year pub	Link	Clinical indication	Level of recommendation, grade of evidence
			Recommendation 81. Empiric (100–200 mCi) or dosimetrically determined RAI therapy may be considered in patients with more significantly elevated serum Tg levels, rapidly rising serum Tg levels, or rising anti-Tg antibody levels, in whom imaging has failed to reveal a tumor source that is amenable to directed therapy	Weak recommendation, low-quality evidence
			Recommendation 82. If persistent nonresectable disease is localized after an empiric dose of RAI, and there is objective evidence of significant tumor reduction, then consideration can be made for RAI therapy to be repeated until the tumor has been eradicated or the tumor no longer responds to treatment. The risk of repeated therapeutic doses of RAI must be balanced against uncertain long-term benefits	Weak recommendation, low-quality evidence
			Recommendation 83. The evidence is insufficient to recommend for or against the routine use of measures to prevent salivary gland damage after RAI therapy	Weak recommendation low-quality evidence
			Recommendation 87. Patients receiving therapeutic doses of RAI should have baseline complete blood count and assessment of renal function	Weak recommendation, low-quality evidence
			Recommendation 88. Women of childbearing age receiving RAI therapy should have a negative screening evaluation for pregnancy prior to RAI administration and avoid pregnancy for 6–12 months after receiving RAI	Strong recommendation, low-quality evidence
			Recommendation 89. Radioactive iodine should not be given to nursing women. Depending on the clinical situation, RAI therapy could be deferred until lactating women have stopped breastfeeding or pumping for at least 3 months	Strong recommendation, moderate-quality evidence

Table 8.3 (continued)

Guidelines [ref]	Year pub	Link	Clinical indication	Level of recommendation, grade of evidence
			Recommendation 90. Men receiving cumulative RAI activities >400 mCi should be counseled on potential risks of infertility	Weak recommendation, low-quality evidence
BTA [6]	2014	http://onlinelibrary.wiley.com/doi/10.1111/cen.12515/pdf	*Definitive indication*: (1) tumor >4 cm; (2) any tumor size with gross extra thyroidal extension; and (3) distant metastases present *No indications*: (1) tumor ≤1 cm unifocal or multifocal; (2) histology classical papillary or follicular variant of papillary carcinoma or follicular carcinoma; (3) minimally invasive without angioinvasion; (4) no invasion of thyroid capsule (extrathyroidal extension)	2+; C
NCCN thyroid cancer (www.nccn.org)	2017	https://www.nccn.org/store/login/login.aspx?ReturnURL=https://www.nccn.org/professionals/physician_gls/pdf/thyroid.pdf	*Not typically recommended (if all present)*: (1) primary tumor < 2 cm; (2) intrathyroidal; (3) no vascular invasion; (4) clinical N0; (5) no detectable anti-Tg antibodies; (6) postoperative unstimulated Tg < 1 ng/mL *Selectively recommended (if present)*: (1) primary tumor 2–4 cm; (2) minor vascular invasion; (3) cervical lymph node metastases; (4) postoperative unstimulated Tg < 5–10 ng/mL *Recommended (if any present)*: (1) gross extrathyroidal extension; (2) primary tumor >4 cm; (3) extensive vascular invasion; (4) postoperative unstimulated Tg > 5–10 ng/L; (5) known or suspected distant metastases at presentation	NA

EANM European Association of Nuclear Medicine, *DTC* differentiated thyroid cancer, *ESMO* European Society of Medical Oncology, *SNMMI* Society of Nuclear Medicine and Molecular Imaging, *ACR* American College of Radiology, *ATA* American Thyroid Association, *RAI* radioablation therapy, *ETE* extrathyroidal extension, *WBS* whole-body scan, *SPECT* single-photon emission computed tomography, *CT* computed tomography, *Tg* thyroglobulin, *rhTSH* recombinant TSH, *BTA* British Thyroid Association, *NCCN* National Cancer Comprehensive Network

Table 8.4 Recommended activities in accordance with the main international guidelines

Guidelines [ref]	Stage disease	Recommended activity
EANM [4]	– Remnant ablation – Non-operable iodine-avid distant metastases	(1) A single administration of 1–5 GBq (2) Multiple administrations, each 3.7–7.4 GBq or more
ESMO [5]	Remnant ablation	1110–1850 MBq
SNMMI [2]	– Remnant ablation – Lymph node involvement – Known or suspected distant metastases – Residual or recurrent thyroid cancer	(1) 11–3.7 GBq (30–100 mCi) (2) 5.55–7.4 GBq (150–200 mCi) (3) 7.4 GBq (200 mCi) or more (4) 5.55–7.40 GBq (150–200 mCi)
ACR (https://www.acr.org/~/media/99393BE60E964AF6830B57C3E52E2339.pdf)	– Remnant ablation – Suspected or obvious residual disease or lymph node involvement – Known or suspected distant metastases – High-risk patients with negative diagnostic WBS and stimulated Tg values > 10 ng/ml	(1) 1.11 to 3.7 GBq (30–100 mCi) (2) 5.55 and 3.7 GBq (100–150 mCi) (3) Equal to or greater at 5.55 GBq (150 mCi) (4) 3.7–5.55 GBq/100–150 mCi
ATA [3]	– Remnant ablation Low-risk thyroid cancer or intermediate-risk disease – Lymph node involvement (patients with low- to intermediate-risk disease, N1a-N1b) – Lung metastases – Recurrent disease	(1) Up at 5.55 GBq (150 mCi)[a] (2) 30 mCi (3) 1.1 GBq (30 mCi) (4) 100–200 mCi, or 100–150 mCi for patients ‡70 years old (5) 100–200 mCi
BTA [6]	– Remnant ablation pT1-T2, N0, M0, R0 T3 and/or N1 – Known residual local disease	(1) 1.1GBq (2) Decided by MDT (3) 3.7–5.5 GBq
NCCN (www.nccn.org)	– Lymph node involvement – Cancer growing through the thyroid capsule – Distant metastases – Diffuse pulmonary metastases	(1) 100–175 mCi (3700–6475 MBq) (2) 150–200 mCi (5550–7400 MBq) (3) 200 mCi (7400 MBq) (4) 150 mCi (5550 MBq)

MDT multidisciplinary team
[a]No distant metastases

References

1. Stokkel MPM, Junak DH, Lassman M, Dietlein M, Luster M. EANM procedure guidelines for therapy of benign thyroid disease. Eur J Nucl Med Mol Imaging. 2010;37:2218–28.
2. Silberstein EB, Alavi A, Balon HR, Becker DV, Brill DR, Clarke SEM, et al. Society of nuclear medicine procedure guideline for therapy of thyroid disease with iodine-131 (Sodium Iodide). www.snmmi.com.
3. Hauger BR, Alexander EK, Bible KC, Doherty GM, Mandel SJ, et al. 2015 American Thyroid Association management guidelines for adult patients with thyroid nodules and differentiated thyroid cancer. Thyroid. 2016;26:1–133.
4. Luster M, Clarke SE, Dietlein M, Lassman M, Lind P, Oyen WJG, et al. Guidelines for radioiodine therapy of differentiated thyroid cancer. Eur J Nucl Med Mol Imaging. 2008;35(10):1941. https://doi.org/10.1007/s00259-008-0883-1.
5. Pacini F, Castagna MG, Brilli L, Pentheroudakis G, ESMO Guidelines Working Group. Ann Oncol. 2012;23(S7):vii110–9.
6. Perros P, Colley S, Boelaert K, Evans C, Gerrard GE, Gilbert JA, et al. Guidelines for the management of thyroid cancer. Yorkshire: British Thyroid Association; 2014.

Part II

Hepatic Cancer

9 Clinical Options for Treatment of Hepatocellular Carcinoma

Matteo Virdis, Michela Monteleone, Michele Droz dit Busset, and Vincenzo Mazzaferro

Abstract

Management of HCC depends on tumor stage, liver function, and patient performance status (BCLC stage) and requires a multidisciplinary approach for optimal treatment. Hepatic resection, liver transplantation, and local ablation of HCC up to 3 cm are curative options in the early stage of disease. There have been significant advances in transarterial embolotherapies (TACE and TARE) in intermediate/advanced stages. Drug-eluting beads have improved the efficacy and safety of conventional TACE, and radioembolization has set a new standard of treatment that delivers the radiation effect to tumor location without compromising the surrounding fragile liver tissue. Molecular studies on HCC have identified aberrant activation of several signaling pathways, which may represent key targets for novel molecular therapies. Immunotherapy is emerging as an additional option in properly selected patients.

Abbreviations

AFP	Alpha-fetoprotein
BCLC	Barcelona Clinic Liver Cancer
CT	Computed tomography
DAA	Direct-acting antiviral
DEB	Drug-eluting beads
DFS	Disease-free survival
HBV	Hepatitis B virus
HCC	Hepatocellular carcinoma
HCV	Hepatitis C virus
HDV	Hepatitis D virus
LA	Laser ablation
LDLT	Living donor liver transplantation
LR	Liver resection

M. Virdis • M. Monteleone • M.D.d. Busset
Hepato-Oncology Group, Surgical Oncology, HPB and Liver Transplantation, Istituto Nazionale Tumori (National Cancer Institute) IRCCS Foundation, Milan, Italy

V. Mazzaferro (✉)
Hepato-Oncology Group, Surgical Oncology, HPB and Liver Transplantation, Istituto Nazionale Tumori (National Cancer Institute) IRCCS Foundation, Milan, Italy

University of Milan, Milan, Italy
e-mail: vincenzo.mazzaferro@istitutotumori.mi.it

E. Bombardieri et al. (eds.), *Clinical Applications of Nuclear Medicine Targeted Therapy*,
https://doi.org/10.1007/978-3-319-63067-0_9

LT	Liver transplantation
MDCT	Multiple detector computed tomography
MELD	Model for end-stage liver disease
MRI	Magnetic resonance imaging
MW	Microwave
NAFLD	Non-alcoholic fatty liver disease
OS	Overall survival
PEI	Percutaneous ethanol injection
PS	Performance status
PVT	Portal vein thrombosis
RFA	Radiofrequency ablation
TACE	Transarterial chemoembolization
TARE	Transarterial radioembolization
UCSF	University of California at San Francisco

9.1 Introduction

Hepatocellular carcinoma (HCC) is one of the leading causes of cancer-related death worldwide. According to recent data, incidence continues to rise despite screening and prevention programs. Cirrhosis is the major condition for development of HCC. Independent risk factors are represented by hepatitis B (HBV) and hepatitis C (HCV) chronic infection. Continuous alcohol consumption and metabolic syndrome play a relevant role in liver inflammation, thus promoting carcinogenesis.

In the setting of cirrhosis, diagnosis of HCC doesn't usually require histopathology confirmation but is mainly based on imaging. Ultrasound is the most widely used imaging modality for screening. For lesions less than 1 cm, a close follow-up with 3-month repeated imaging is usually undertaken. For lesions >1 cm, typical findings in one imaging modality (either triple-phase MDCT or MRI with hepatospecific contrast agent) are sufficient for diagnosis. In the case of atypical features, two imaging modalities are required for diagnosis. Alpha-fetoprotein (aFP), if elevated, can be useful for screening and follow-up of patients with previously treated HCC.

In the Western world, treatment is mainly tailored according to Barcelona Clinic Liver Cancer (BCLC) staging system, where number and size of HCC nodules, presence of portal vein invasion or extrahepatic spread, performance status, and Child-Pugh score define the best approach for each patient (Fig. 9.1).

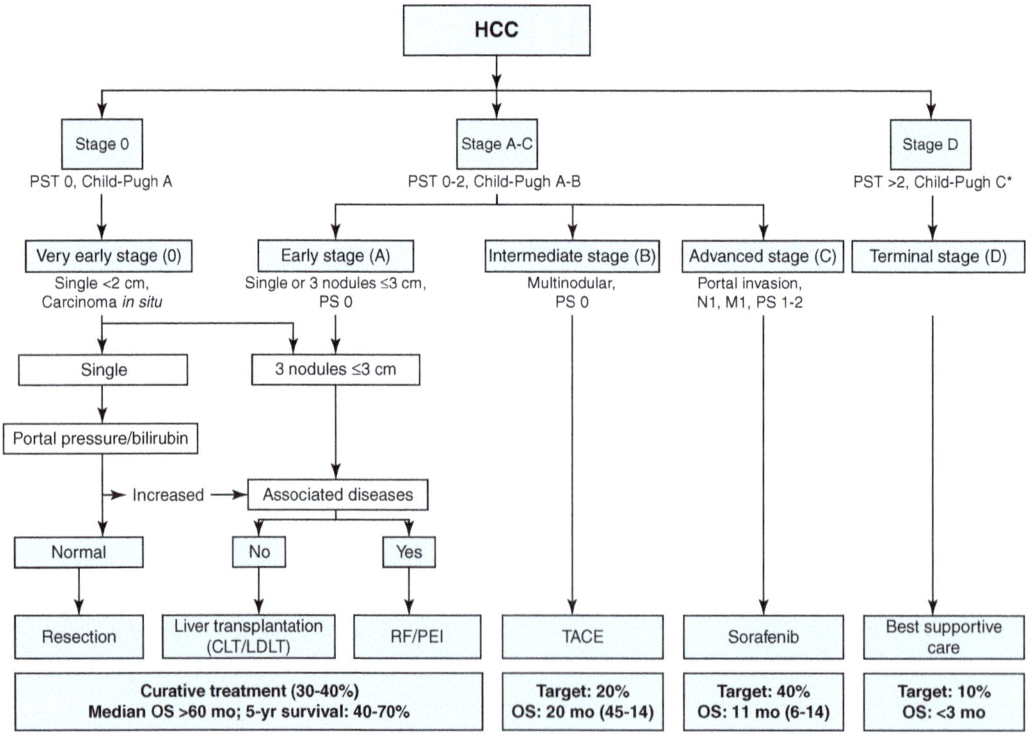

Fig. 9.1 BCLC staging and treatment algorithm

Patients in early stage can benefit from curative treatments including orthotopic liver transplantation (LT), hepatic resection (LR), and thermal ablation. In the palliative setting, locoregional embolotherapies are mainly used. Advanced HCC with preserved liver function requires systemic treatment with molecular targeted agents, such as sorafenib or regorafenib. Best supportive care is reserved to advanced patients with impaired performance status (PS) or compromised liver function.

In the present article, we will review the current epidemiology of HCC, the main risk factors, and the available treatment options depending on the stage of disease.

9.2 Epidemiology

HCC is the fifth most frequently diagnosed cancer in the world, and currently the second leading cause of cancer-related death worldwide, with an estimated 15.3 per 100,000 newly diagnosed cases that almost equates the registered 14.3 deaths per 100,000 persons every year.

Chronic liver disease and cirrhosis are the most important risk factors for the development of HCC, of which viral hepatitis and excessive alcohol intake are the leading risk factors worldwide. According to large data set (i.e., GLOBOCAN report), the highest incidence of HCC is in China, Japan, Southeast Asia, and sub-Saharan Western and Eastern Africa (ranging from 11 to 25 per 100,000/year inhabitants). Countries with low incidence include most of Europe and North America (5 per 100,000/year population) [1].

Currently, 80% of HCCs are related to chronic viral hepatitis, and incidence varies widely according to geographic locations and ethnic groups, due to regional variations in exposure to hepatitis viruses and environmental pathogens. Chronic HBV infection is the predominant risk factor for HCC in Southeast Asia and Africa, whereas chronic infection with HCV is the main risk factor for HCC in Western countries and Japan, accounting for up to 70% of HCC patients. Currently, there is a rising trend of HCC in the West, such as in the USA and Canada where the incidence used to be low. This is partly due to the HCV epidemic in the 1960s and 1970s and the prevalence of metabolic syndrome (obesity and diabetes mellitus) and non-alcoholic fatty liver disease (NAFLD) in the Western population. A decreasing incidence of HCC in intermediate- to high-incidence areas has been recently registered, partly as a result of the implementation of HBV vaccination programs in many areas of Asia. However, due to changes in diet and sedentary lifestyle, the prevalence of NAFLD in some parts of East Asia has increased to almost as that of Europe and the USA. It is expected that HCC related to obesity, diabetes mellitus, and metabolic syndrome will rise globally and finally overcome the trend of decreasing HCC rates related to other causes [2].

HBV transmission occurs via contaminated venous injections and blood transfusions and sexual contact. Vertical transmission from mother to fetus is common and is the main cause of HBV infection. Chronic HBV presence is related to significant carcinogenicity, even in the absence of cirrhosis. Suppression of the viremia can result in a significant 5-year reduction of the incidence of HCC, mainly in cirrhotic patients, from 14 to 4%. The implementation of HBV vaccination has resulted in significant declines in the incidence of related HCC. Coinfection with hepatitis D virus (HDV) appears to increase threefold the risk of HCC among patients with HBV.

With respect to HCV infection, 80% of patients progress to chronic hepatitis, with 20% eventually developing cirrhosis in a mean period of 10–20 years. Development of HCC related to HCV mainly occurs in established cirrhosis. Dual infection with HBV and HCV in a cirrhotic patient increases the risk of HCC, and a synergistic effect with alcohol has been described too, with an increased risk of developing HCC between 1.7- and 2.9-fold as compared to HCV alone. The cumulative lifetime incidence of HCC for patients with HCV alone is around 17–24%.

HCV-induced HCC is related to the degree of inflammation and necrosis and seems to be caused by inflammation rather than specific oncogene activation. By contrast, HBV-related

HCC appears to arise after induction of specific oncogenes by the virus. The risk of HCC is reduced significantly in patients who obtain a sustained viral response after antiviral treatment, with a 50% reduction in all-cause mortality.

In all countries, men are more likely than women to develop HCC (mean 3.5:1). Such difference in sex distribution is thought to be secondary to variations in exposure to environmental toxins, effects of androgens, and potentially protective effects of estrogens in modulation of inflammatory response.

The relationship between alcohol and chronic liver disease is proportional with the lifetime alcohol intake. Alcohol abuse accounts for about 40% of all HCC cases in Europe. The risk of alcohol-induced HCC after the onset of cirrhosis can be amplified by the concomitant presence of viral hepatitis.

Chronic conditions such as diabetes mellitus and obesity increase the risk of HCC.

Diabetes mellitus directly affects the liver because of the essential role the liver plays in glucose metabolism and due to the dysregulation of insulin that normally controls the anti-inflammatory cascade, inducing cellular proliferation. Diabetes is considered an independent risk factor leading to chronic hepatitis, steatosis, and cirrhosis and increases by 2- to 4-fold the risk of tumorigenesis.

Obesity too is associated with non-alcoholic fatty liver disease (NAFLD), steatosis, and cryptogenic cirrhosis that can all lead to the development of HCC with a 1.5–4-fold increased risk. The mean age of presentation is 70 years. Up to 50% of cases of NAFLD-related HCC occur in the absence of cirrhosis.

Progressive iron deposition in the liver in hemochromatosis is also associated with primary liver cancer: HCC is responsible for approximately 45% of all deaths in patients with hemochromatosis, which increases liver cancer risk from 20- to 200-fold.

Finally, cigarette smoking seems to be associated with a significant increase in the development of HCC. Studies have confirmed the association between smoking and liver cancer with a hazard ratio of 1.6 for current smokers and 1.5 for former smokers [3].

9.3 Diagnosis

The main goal of surveillance in high-risk patients (patients with cirrhosis, HBV infection, and HCV hepatitis with liver fibrosis) is to identify small HCC (<2 cm) that carries lower risk of satellite nodules and microvascular invasion. Surveillance is usually based on periodic liver ultrasound. CT scan and MRI are supplementary imaging techniques in the presence of conditions that limit the accuracy of liver ultrasound examination.

When a new nodule is identified on ultrasound in patients at risk of HCC occurrence, strategy varies according to the size of the lesion. The recall strategy for lesions ≥1 cm is based on contrast-enhanced imaging techniques with use of vascular contrast media. The lesion should be assessed prior to contrast injection and after contrast injection in multiphasic protocol (i.e., arterial, portal, venous, and late venous phases) by CT scan or MRI. Hallmark of HCC diagnosis is the intense contrast uptake in the arterial phase ("wash-in") followed by rapid contrast discharge ("wash-out") in the portal phase. If radiologic features of a liver lesion are not typical for HCC, alternative imaging technique (CT or MRI) or percutaneous biopsy may be necessary.

Lesions <1 cm usually enter a close follow-up protocol based on ultrasound assessments at 3–6 months interval considering the limited specificity of digital imaging and biopsy in very small lesions in cirrhosis. If the size of such lesions does not increase over a 2-year period, a 6-month interval surveillance can be restored.

Alpha-fetoprotein (AFP) should not be used as a diagnostic test due to the possibility of elevated levels in various diseases and of non-AFP-producing HCC. However, if elevated in previously treated HCC patients, it can be a useful tool to complement screening and follow-up [4].

9.4 Treatment Options

Treatment of HCC predominantly depends on cancer stage, liver function, and performance status. The most widely adopted staging system in

Western nations is the Barcelona Clinic Liver Cancer (BCLC) algorithm, which incorporates prognostic factors and stratifies patients in different disease stages based on patients' life expectancy. As summarized in Fig. 9.1, the BCLC stage system considers very-early-stage (stage 0), early-stage (stage A), intermediate-stage (stage B), advanced-stage (stage C), and terminal-stage (stage D) HCC [5].

Herein, the treatment alternatives summarized in Table 9.1 will be discussed according to the tumor stage described in the BCLC algorithm.

9.4.1 Very Early and Early HCC

Asymptomatic patients with a single nodule or up to 3 nodules of maximum diameter of 3 cm, Child-Pugh status A or B, and performance status 0 (fully functional), without vascular invasion or extrahepatic spread, are classified as "early-stage HCC" (BCLC A). Among these patients, those with a single nodule ≤2 cm are defined as "very early-stage HCC" (BCLC 0) [6].

The standard of care for patients with "very early HCC" and "early HCC" with a single nod-

Table 9.1 Summary of alternatives, advantages and disadvantages for each technique in the treatment of HCC

Treatment	Pros	Cons	Observations
Liver resection (LR)	– High curability rate with wide margins (anatomical resection) – Optimal HCC local control	– High recurrence rate – Lack of accepted universal selection criteria	– Feasible only if liver function and adequate volume preservation are respected
Liver transplantation (LT)	– Best curability potentials of both HCC and carcinogenic cirrhosis if restrictive criteria are applied	– Limitations in graft availability and priority with respect to non-HCC patients – Permanent immunosuppression	– New perspectives with effective HCV treatment – Access to living donation – Post-LT survival may relate to pre-LT response to locoregional therapies
Radiofrequency ablation (RFA)	– High curability rate up to 3 cm, especially in borderline liver function and in case of comorbidities – Repeatability and low complication rate	– High recurrence rate (as for surgery) – Suboptimal results in difficult locations	– Feasible in almost all patients, alone or associated with surgery or combined treatments (multiple RFA) – Frequent change in technology and cost
Embolotherapies: transarterial chemoembolization (TACE) and radioembolization (TARE)	– Treatment of multifocal HCC repeatability and low complication rate – TARE is applicable to tumoral portal vein thrombosis	– Risk of liver decompensation – Decreased effect as the number of treatment increase	– Can be used as downstaging treatment to transplantation criteria
Systemic treatments (sorafenib and regorafenib)	– Indicated once HCC progression is detected after surgery and/or locoregional treatments – Proven efficacy in prolonging survival in advanced HCC	– Systemic toxicity up to 30% of patients – Liver function must be preserved – Not proven effect in the adjuvant setting	– In randomized trials more selective compounds failed to improve results of multikinase inhibitor as sorafenib – Immuno-checkpoint inhibitors are likely to be competitive with sorafenib and regorafenib

ule, compensated cirrhosis (Child-Pugh A), and no portal hypertension is liver resection (LR), with an expected 5-year OS around 70%.

Thanks to advances in surgical technique and postoperative care, perioperative mortality has been drastically reduced and in referral centers does not exceed 1%, with a blood transfusion requirement below 10%. In cirrhotic patients, a liver remnant of at least 40% after resection is recommended. Whenever possible, an anatomical resection should be performed, given the lower risk of local recurrence shown by some authors in case of removal of the tumor together with the entire segmental territory in which is located [7].

According to American and European guidelines, LR is contraindicated in the presence of clinically relevant portal hypertension and abnormal bilirubin, as these factors are predictive of early mortality from postoperative decompensation [6]. Portal hypertension is defined as a hepatic vein-portal vein pressure gradient ≥10 mmHg. Presence of esophageal varices at gastroscopy, splenomegaly, and a platelet count <100,000/μL are indirect signs of portal hypertension. The risk of post-hepatectomy liver failure can be predicted combining the grade of portal hypertension, the extent of hepatectomy, and the model for end-stage liver disease (MELD) score [8, 9]. In clinical practice, the presence of portal hypertension, hyperbilirubinemia, and multinodularity are not considered absolute contraindications to LR, but the associated increased risks of postoperative decompensation have been shown in meta-analyses.

The main oncology issue related with LR for HCC is the high rate of tumor recurrence, around 70–80% at 5 years [10]. Recurrent HCC mainly affects the liver itself and is classified as "early recurrence," when occurring within 2 years after LR—as a consequence of residual microscopic tumor foci left at the time of primary resection—or "late recurrences," occurring more than 2 years after LR and more commonly related to development of new tumor sites within the carcinogenetic cirrhotic liver [11].

An alternative treatment option for patients with up to 3 nodules ≤3 cm is local ablation by means of radiofrequency (RFA), microwave (MW) application, or ethanol injection [11]. RFA is more effective than percutaneous alcohol injection (PEI), especially for HCCs >2 cm. Ablation techniques become suboptimal and less cost-effective for the treatment of tumors between 3 and 5 cm and are definitely suboptimal above 5 cm. RFA and MW achieve complete responses in more than 70% of nodules <3 cm, with reported 5-year patient survival ranging in the 55–65% interval [12]. Results of ablation are now similar to those ones achieved after LR, with the potential advantages of reduced invasiveness, complication rate, hospital stay, and costs [13]. Consequently, RFA has become the standard of care for patients with very early HCC not amenable to surgical treatment.

The debate on superiority of LR or ablation in treating small HCC remains open, as randomized clinical trials have been impeded by too many biases in patients selection and tumor presentation. According to current guidelines, resectable HCC especially above 2–3 cm and carrying a low risk of complication should be resected in experienced centers. Conversely, nonsurgical patients with tumors <3 cm associated with borderline liver function should be offered ablation.

Modern techniques of minimally invasive LR (laparoscopic resections)—when feasible—may increase the safety of LR and reduce the current limitations of surgical intervention for early-stage HCC.

In patients with portal hypertension or increased bilirubin, in the absence of significant comorbidities, liver transplantation (LT) is the best treatment option for HCC. As a matter of fact, LT can achieve cure for both the tumor and the underlying oncogenic liver disease. Milan criteria (single nodule <5 cm or up to 3 nodules ≤3 cm) are the benchmark guiding patients' selection for LT. HCC patients transplanted under such restrictive criteria are expected to survive more than 75% at 5 years [14]. In patients with >2 cm tumors, bridge treatment by means of RFA or transarterial chemoembolization (TACE) is usually undertaken while on the wait list. Although this approach is not supported by data, there is some evidence that bridge therapies may prevent tumor progression and reduce wait list dropout. It is unclear whether tumor recurrence following LT can be reduced as well.

Although the widespread application of Milan criteria to select patients for LT greatly improved the survival outcomes of transplanted patients, extended criteria may be applied under different circumstances. The group of the University of California at San Francisco (UCSF) was the first to attempt an expansion of Milan criteria, including a single nodule ≤6.5 cm or 2–3 nodules each ≤4.5 cm, up to a total sum of tumor diameters ≤8 cm. These criteria, based on explant histology and subsequently validated by radiological imaging, obtained results comparable to patients within Milan criteria in terms of DFS (90% vs. 94%, respectively) and risk of pretreatment tumor understaging (29% vs. 20%, respectively) [15]. In a subsequent study by the group from Milan, it was demonstrated that the wider the expansion of morphology criteria for selecting LT candidates with HCC is, the lower is the expected posttransplant survival outcome. Patients fulfilling the "up-to-7" criteria (7 cm being the sum of the maximum tumor diameter and the number of nodules) with no microvascular invasion achieve 5-year survival comparable to patients within Milan criteria, suggesting that a more accurate patient selection based on biologic aggressiveness rather than pure morphologic criteria may enlarge the proportion of transplant candidates, without compromising survival outcomes [16]. With this respect AFP levels have been proposed as a surrogate of aggressive biology and microvascular invasion.

As 20–25% of surgical patients with HCC are both resectable and transplantable, another treatment approach is "salvage LT," in which LR is performed as first step and LT is proposed only in case of deterioration of liver function or intrahepatic HCC recurrence [17]. Although the applicability of such approach in daily practice may be as low as 10–20%, LR in the light of LT represents a useful selection tool. Based on the presence of vascular invasion or tumor satellites in the surgical specimens, resected patients can be stratified according to the risk of recurrence and therefore offered LT as a preemptive, de principe procedure.

To compensate for donor shortage, living donor liver transplantation (LDLT) can be proposed [18]. Indications for LDLT should not differ from those ones for cadaveric LT, but size and number limits considered suitable to LDLT are less restrictive as compared with cadaveric LT, since the reduction of expected survival in LDLT is felt acceptable if organ donation is considered a personal gift rather than a resource to be distributed in the community (Fig. 9.2).

Concerns also include ethical issues, higher complication rate especially at the biliary reconstruction (>30%), and the low but persistent risk of donor death (0.5%).

A new generation of direct antiviral agents (DAAs) reduce the risk of postoperative liver failure and late recurrence from "de novo" HCC in HBV- and HCV-related tumors undergoing LR

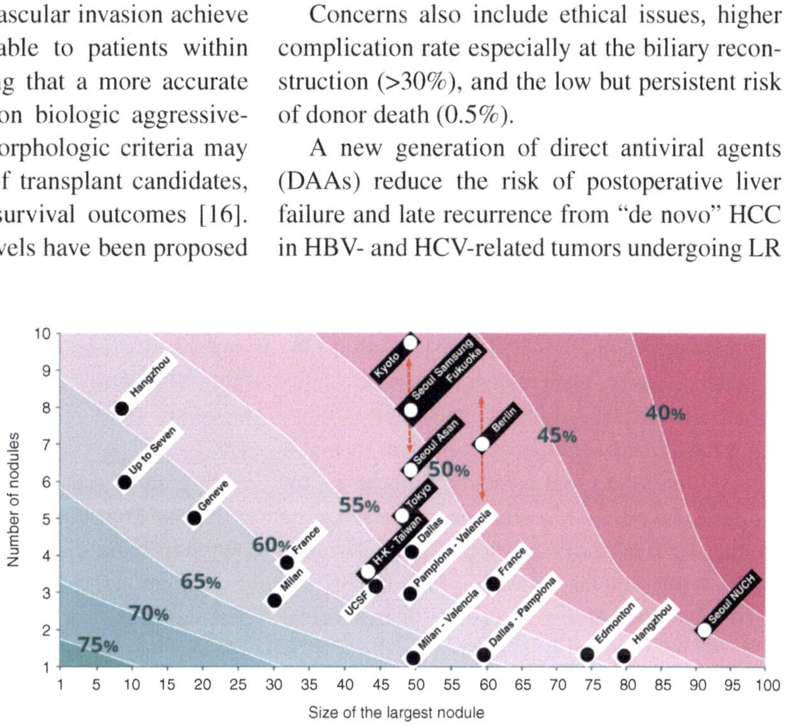

Fig. 9.2 Diagram rapresenting expected survival according to size and number of the principle selecting criteria for liver transplantation

or local ablation. In transplanted patients, DAAs are useful for prevention and treatment of HCV recurrence, which heavily affects graft failure rate and early mortality following LT [19, 20].

9.4.2 Intermediate HCC

Patients at intermediate stage (BCLC B) have multifocal HCC within the liver, but good performance status and no signs of impending liver failure. This population shows high variability and heterogeneity of tumor presentation, confirmed by the wide range of available treatments and consequent expected survival rates [21].

According to guidelines, BCLC B patients are not considered for LR, but there could be a subset of patients (i.e., multifocal disease within Milan criteria, limited to a single hepatic lobe) who may benefit from LR, with comparable survival benefit as locoregional treatments [22, 23].

TACE (transarterial chemoembolization) is the first-line option for intermediate-stage patients, but large variability exists in treatment protocols, schedule, devices, and indications among different centers. Generally, a good performance status with preserved liver function is required. Best candidates to TACE are patients with well-preserved liver function (Child-Pugh score ≤ 7) and no ascites. Main contraindications to TACE are liver failure, refractory ascites, encephalopathy, bilirubin level > 3 mg/dL, renal failure, platelet count <50,000/mL, prothrombin time < 50%, portal hypertension, main portal venous thrombosis, severely reduced or hepatofugal portal flow, hepatic artery thrombosis, and severe atheromatosis [24]. Several randomized trials and meta-analyses have confirmed the value of TACE in intermediate-stage HCC, with significant benefit in terms of survival, doubling that achieved with best supportive care (HR 0.53). However, the range of median survival may vary significantly, from 8 to 50 months. Local recurrence rate of TACE is as high as 60% at 1 year. The 2-year survival rate of patients with progressive disease is 5–8%, while in patients with complete or partial response it increases to 20–25% [25].

TACE may be performed with chemotherapeutic agents emulsified with Lipiodol as embolic agents (conventional TACE or c-TACE) or with embolic microspheres of different size preloaded with chemotherapeutic agents [drug-eluting beads-TACE (DEB-TACE)].

TACE can be scheduled at fixed intervals or "on demands." Prospective comparative studies between the two schedules are lacking, but this last option is likely more effective at reducing the exposure of patients to the toxic effects of the treatment, thus increasing compliance. When c-TACE is used, radiological assessment of tumor by means of MRI may provide better accuracy, as CT evaluation is frequently hindered by artifacts caused by Lipiodol retention.

It is not established how many times TACE can be repeated, but, according to the "treatment shift paradigm" within the BCLC scheme, the offered treatment at any stage of HCC can be shifted to those recommended for the following level of tumor advancement, therefore from TACE to sorafenib.

In current practice, the assessment of tumor response should be performed after at least two cycles of TACE. Conversely, TACE should be discontinued when a deterioration of the performance status or liver function occurs [23].

Noteworthy, TACE can be also used as a downstaging treatment aimed at reducing tumor burden within Milan criteria in patients eligible for LT.

In field practice, about 33% of transplant candidates with HCC show tumor progression during the waiting period, and if this occurs under TACE treatment the risk of posttransplant recurrence is significantly increased. HCCs presenting with high AFP serum level and poorly differentiated histology (G3) tend to have low responses to TACE.

In case of paucinodular intrahepatic tumors, TACE may be combined with percutaneous ablation to increase disease control. RFA, MWA, and laser ablation (LA) are the most widely employed percutaneous treatments combined with TACE. Combination therapies are not considered in Western guidelines, but several experiences in the East have shown that intermediate HCC can be approached with ablation alone in selected cases, with complete response achievable in more than 90% of nodules ≤3 cm. Other candidates to percutaneous local ablation are patients with centrally located HCC in borderline liver function, for whom very high response rates have been reported.

Transarterial radioembolization (TARE) is a relatively novel treatment for intermediate and advanced HCC, consisting of hepatic intra-arterial infusion of radioactive β-emitting yttrium-90 isotope integrated in glass or resin microspheres. Comparable median survival and toxic effects of TACE and TARE have been described, while cost-benefit considerations and quality of life results speak in favor of radioembolization in the large majority of studies. Randomized prospective trials are still missing.

The role of TARE in the management of intermediate stage is less defined than in advanced stage, especially in HCC with portal vein thrombosis (PVT). However, significant increase in TARE treatment and expertise is growing worldwide, with evidences showing consistent control of intrahepatic progression of HCC associated with survival benefit [25].

9.4.3 Advanced HCC

Advanced HCC is characterized by the presence of portal vein thrombosis, extrahepatic tumor spread, or symptoms related to cancer. The standard of care in the presence of preserved liver function (Child-Pugh A) is the systemic agent, multikinase inhibitor sorafenib, the only agent that has been proven to extend survival in advanced HCC [26]. The efficacy of sorafenib was demonstrated in two large phase 3 trials in both Western and Eastern population (SHARP and Asia-Pacific, respectively) [27]. Treatment with sorafenib offers survival outcomes around 11 months. Systemic toxicity is a relevant issue, and up to 30% of patients undergo treatment discontinuation because of adverse events. Side effects include hand-foot skin reaction, diarrhea, and fatigue. In case of progression or intolerance, best supportive care or enrolment in clinical trials is indicated.

In patients progressing under sorafenib while tolerating it, second-line treatment with regorafenib has proven significant survival advantage with respect to placebo.

A less evidence-based alternative for advanced intrahepatic HCC in patients maintaining good liver function is TARE. Phase 2 trials in patients with intermediate to advanced HCC proved radioembolization to be competitive with sorafenib, with median survival of 15 months and a median time to progression of 11 months [28].

Several phase 2 and 3 trials have been conducted in the last decade to evaluate the efficacy of new targeted agents inhibiting either the same pathway as sorafenib or others, both in the first- and second-line setting. However, due to the intrinsic heterogeneity of HCC and toxicity issues related to the association with chronic liver disease, most of these trials did not meet their primary end points [29].

Hopes are placed on immunotherapy, as significant tumor responses have been registered in phase 1–2 studies. Altered peritumoral liver microenvironment by means of locoregional or systemic therapies has fostered prospective trials on use of immunomodulating agents alone or in combination with other systemic or locoregional therapies. It is likely that a subgroup of immune-sensitive HCCs will be the specific target of new treatment associations and better patient and tumor selection tools.

9.4.4 End-Stage HCC

If cancer-related symptoms are present and liver function is severely impaired (Child-Pugh C stage), patients are defined in terminal stage. Survival in this context is extremely poor (around 3 months), and there is no specific treatment available except for best supportive care. However, it should be noted that selected patients with very advanced liver cirrhosis associated with small tumor within conventional criteria (see above) still can be considered for LT and therefore for a curative treatment alternative.

Key Points

- HCC is the fifth most frequent cancer in the world and the second leading cause of cancer-related death worldwide. Liver cirrhosis is the main associated condition; other relevant risk factors are HCV and HBV infections, chronic alcohol intake and metabolic syndrome.
- Diagnosis of HCC is mainly based on imaging. Depending on the nodule size, the diagnostic workup includes ultrasound, CEUS, CT scan and MRI. Atypical lesions <1 cm are best managed with close follow-up. Lesions >1cm with atypical findings require 2 imaging modalities. Needle biopsy is rarely indicated but increasingly practiced.
- Management of HCC depends on tumor stage, liver function and performance status. Patients with early-stage, single HCC and compensated cirrhosis are best treated with liver resection and local ablation especially when <3 cm in size. When portal hypertension and increased bilirubin is present liver transplantation should be considered according to Milan criteria. Expanded criteria are various, being the most promising based on alpha-fetoprotein level and grade of response to loco-regional therapies (tumor downstaging).
- Intra-arterial therapies offer a survival benefit in intermediate-stage HCC and are the recommended treatment. None of the intra-arterial embolo-therapies, including TAE, TACE, DEB-TACE or TARE offer clear advantages over the other ones, although DEB-TACE may have less systemic toxicity. TARE can be offered also to patients with portal vein thrombosis, where all the other approaches are contraindicated.
- The standard of care for patients with advanced HCC is systemic treatment with the multikinase inhibitor sorafenib. Selected patients can benefit from radioembolization. Regorafenib is now recognized as second-line treatment. Targeted therapies against several signalling pathways involved in HCC carcinogenesis are being tested in phase 2 and 3 trials. Immunotherapy is a promising treatment option.

References

1. International Agency for Research on Cancer, WHO. Globocan 2012: estimated cancer incidence, mortality and prevalence worldwide. 2012.
2. Choo SP, Tan WL, Goh BKP, Tai WM, Zhu AX. Comparison of hepatocellular carcinoma in eastern versus western populations. Cancer. 2016;122:3430–46.
3. Balogh J, Victor D III, Asham EH, Gordon Burroughs S, Boktour M, et al. Hepatocellular carcinoma: a review. J Hepatocell Carcinoma. 2016;3:41–53.
4. Italian Association for the Study of the Liver (AISF). Position paper of the Italian association for the study of the liver (AISF): the multidisciplinary clinical approach to hepatocellular carcinoma. Dig Liver Dis. 2013;45:712–23.
5. Llovet JM, Brú C, Bruix J. Prognosis of hepatocellular carcinoma: the BCLC staging classification. Semin Liver Dis. 1999;19(3):329–38.
6. Farinati F, Sergio A, Baldan A, Giacomin A, Di Nolfo MA, et al. Early and very early hepatocellular carcinoma: when and how much do staging and choice of treatment really matter? A multi-center study. BMC Cancer. 2009;9(1):33.
7. Hasegawa K, Kokudo N, Imamura H, Matsuyama Y, Aoki T, et al. Prognostic impact of anatomic resection for hepatocellular carcinoma. Ann Surg. 2005;242(2):252–9.
8. Citterio D, Facciorusso A, Sposito C, Rota R, Bhoori S, Mazzaferro V. Hierarchic interaction of factors associated with liver decompensation after resection for hepatocellular carcinoma. JAMA Surg. 2016;151(9):846–53.
9. Cucchetti A, Sposito C, Pinna AD, Citterio D, Cescon M, Bongini M, et al. Competing risk analysis on outcome after hepatic resection of hepatocellular carcinoma in cirrhotic patients. World J Gastroenterol. 2017;23(8):1469–76.
10. Sasaki A, Iwashita Y, Shibata K, Matsumoto T, Ohta M, Kitano S. Improved long-term survival after liver resection for hepatocellular carcinoma in the modern era: retrospective study from HCV-endemic areas. World J Surg. 2006;30(8):1567–78.
11. Imamura H, Matsuyama Y, Tanaka E, Ohkubo T, Hasegawa K, Miyagawa S, et al. Risk factors contributing to early and late phase intrahepatic recurrence of hepatocellular carcinoma after hepatectomy. J Hepatol. 2003;38(2):200–7.
12. Sala M, Llovet JM, Vilana R, Bianchi L, Solé M, Ayuso C, et al. Initial response to percutaneous ablation predicts survival in patients with hepatocellular carcinoma. Hepatology. 2004;40(6):1352–60.
13. Livraghi T, Meloni F, Di Stasi M, Rolle E, Solbiati L, Tinelli C, Rossi S. Sustained complete response and complications rates after radiofrequency ablation of very early hepatocellular carcinoma in cirrhosis: is resection still the treatment of choice? Hepatology. 2008;47(1):82–9.

14. Mazzaferro V, Regalia E, Doci R, Andreola S, Pulvirenti A, Bozzetti F, et al. Liver transplantation for the treatment of small hepatocellular carcinomas in patients with cirrhosis. N Engl J Med. 1996;334(11):693–9.
15. Yao FY, Xiao L, Bass NM, Kerlan R, Ascher NL, Roberts JP. Liver transplantation for hepatocellular carcinoma: validation of the UCSF-expanded criteria based on preoperative imaging. Am J Transplant. 2007;7(11):2587–96.
16. Llovet JM, Fuster J, Bruix J. Intention-to-treat analysis of surgical treatment for early hepatocellular carcinoma: resection versus transplantation. Hepatology. 1999;30(6):1434–40.
17. Cherqui D, Laurent A, Mocellin N, Tayar C, Luciani A, Van Nhieu JT, et al. Liver resection for transplantable hepatocellular carcinoma: long-term survival and role of secondary liver transplantation. Ann Surg. 2009;250(5):738–46.
18. Todo S, Furukawa H, Japanese Study Group on Organ Transplantation. Living donor liver transplantation for adult patients with hepatocellular carcinoma: experience in Japan. Ann Surg. 2004;240(3):451–61.
19. Mazzaferro V, Romito R, Schiavo M, Mariani L, Camerini T, Bhoori S, et al. Prevention of hepatocellular carcinoma recurrence with alpha-interferon after liver resection in HCV cirrhosis. Hepatology. 2006;44(6):1543–54.
20. Wu C-Y, Chen Y-J, Ho HJ, Hsu YC, Kuo KN, Wu MS, Lin JT. Association between nucleoside analogues and risk of hepatitis B virus–related hepatocellular carcinoma recurrence following liver resection. JAMA. 2012;308(18):1906–14.
21. Bolondi L, Burroughs A, Dufou JF, Galle PR, Mazzaferro V, Piscaglia F, et al. Heterogeneity of patients with intermediate (BCLC B) hepatocellular carcinoma: proposal for a subclassification to facilitate treatment decisions. Semin Liver Dis. 2012;32(04):348–35.
22. Giannini EG, Moscatelli A, Pellegatta G, Vitale A, Farinati F, Ciccarese F, et al. Application of the intermediate-stage subclassification to patients with untreated hepatocellular carcinoma. Am J Gastroenterol. 2016;111:70–7.
23. Lobo L, Yakoub D, Picado O, Ripat C, Pendola F, Sharma R, et al. Unresectable hepatocellular carcinoma: radioembolization versus chemoembolization: a systematic review and meta-analysis. Cardiovasc Intervent Radiol. 2016;39:1580–8.
24. Liang H, Cui P, Guo Q, Mao X, Wen F, Sun W, Shan M, Lu Z. Prognostic factors of hepatocellular carcinoma patients with portal vein tumor thrombosis treated with transcatheter arterial chemoembolization. Asia Pac J Clin Oncol. 2017. https://doi.org/10.1111/ajco.12606.
25. Pesapane F, Nezami N, Patella F, Geschwind JF. New concepts in embolotherapy of HCC. Med Oncol. 2017;34(4):58.
26. Llovet JM, Ricci S, Mazzaferro V, Hilgard P, Gane E, Blanc JF, et al. Sorafenib in advanced hepatocellular carcinoma. N Engl J Med. 2008;359(4):378–90.
27. Cheng AL, Kang YK, Chen Z, Tsao CJ, Qin S, Kim JS, et al. Efficacy and safety of sorafenib in patients in the Asia-Pacific region with advanced hepatocellular carcinoma: a phase III randomised, double-blind, placebo-controlled trial. Lancet Oncol. 2009;10(1):25–34.
28. Rognoni C, Ciani O, Sommariva S, Facciorusso A, Tarricone R, Bhoori S, Mazzaferro V. Trans-arterial radioembolization in intermediate-advanced hepatocellular carcinoma: systematic review and meta-analyses. Oncotarget. 2015;7(44):72343–55.
29. Ribeiro de Souza A, Reig M, Bruix J. Systemic treatment for advanced hepatocellular carcinoma: the search of new agents to join sorafenib in the effective therapeutic armamentarium. Expert Opin Pharmacother. 2016;17(14):1923–36.

10 Medical Devices for Radioembolization

Anna Bogni and Claudio Pascali

Abstract

Microspheres of the proper size injected into the hepatic artery lodge themselves preferentially in and around tumours as a result of both the increased vascularity of tumours and the fact that blood from the hepatic artery flows preferentially to malignancies. Thus, radioembolization with microspheres labelled with β^--emitter radionuclides has become a well-established and powerful tool for the treatment of liver malignancies, since it adds to the embolization effect the deposition of lethal doses of radiation to the tumour cells.

Two commercially available medical devices of this type labelled with yttrium-90 (^{90}Y) are presently authorized for human use. Although both are reportedly effective, they have key dissimilarities strictly related to their chemical form and manufacturing method. The aim of this chapter is to examine these factors in terms of pro and cons and how they can affect the use and biodistribution of radiolabelled microspheres.

Last, the need to have good *in vivo* imaging during pretreatment procedure, as well as during and/or after administration of the dose, has encouraged to explore alternative radionuclides to ^{90}Y able to fulfil this requirement, such as holmium-166 (^{166}Ho) and rhenium-186 and rhenium-188 ($^{186}Re/^{188}Re$). These, together with the development of different microsphere matrixes, will be also discussed.

10.1 Introduction

Yttrium-90 (^{90}Y) microspheres are increasingly applied to the therapy of primary and metastatic liver tumours. Their use is based on early studies reporting how liver tumours are well vascularized and, unlike healthy liver tissue, receive their blood supply mainly from the hepatic artery rather than the portal vein [1]. Thus, regional

A. Bogni (✉) • C. Pascali
Fondazione IRCCS "Istituto dei Tumori", Nuclear Medicine Unit, Milan, Italy
e-mail: Anna.Bogni@istitutotumori.mi.it; Claudio.Pascali@istitutotumori.mi.it

E. Bombardieri et al. (eds.), *Clinical Applications of Nuclear Medicine Targeted Therapy*,
https://doi.org/10.1007/978-3-319-63067-0_10

administration of agents (chemotherapy drugs, radioactive microsphere) via the hepatic artery is one strategy that has been developed to maximize the effect to the tumour while sparing toxicity to the surrounding healthy liver.

By this procedure microspheres of the appropriate size will lodge in and around the tumour microvasculature, blocking the vessels supplying oxygen and nutrients to the tumour, therefore causing a bland embolization. At the same time, if these microspheres are labelled with radionuclides emitting β^--particles of high energy, they will deposit over a very short range (mm) a high radiation dose to the tumour cells. From the two combined effects derives indeed the term radioembolization applied to this treatment.

These microspheres can be based on polymers, polymeric resins, albumin or an inorganic material such as glass.

Ideally, for reasons that will be briefly explained over the text, radiolabelled microspheres for hepatic radionuclide therapy should have the following characteristics:

- Density closer to the blood to prevent premature settling and suboptimal distribution.
- Uniform spherical size of 25–30 μm. Arterioles feeding liver tumours in humans average 15–35 μm in diameter. Larger microspheres would not reach the capillary bed, while smaller ones might pass through the tumour capillaries and reach the neighbouring organs, especially the lungs [2]. Spherical particles reduce or prevent the formation of particle clusters within peripheral vessels [3].
- Labelled with high-energy β^--emitters having a sufficiently long half-life ($T_{1/2}$). High energy, i.e. high tissue range, is required in order to reach the interior of large tumours.
- Easily prepared/good availability.
- High specific activity (GBq/sphere).
- Resistance to radiation damage, particularly during neutron irradiation. From this point of view, glass is the most resistant matrix, while polymeric and resin-based microsphere undergoes changes in molecular weight and morphology [4].
- Very low levels of radionuclidic impurities.
- No radionuclide release.
- Biocompatible and biodegradable, although with sufficiently long *in vivo* stability to fully deposit its radiation dose to the tumour. Since multicycle treatment might be more effective, [5] biodegradability, and thus clearance of the vascular occlusion within the tumour, is a prerequisite for homogeneous distribution within the tumour [6].
- Possibility to predict and follow their distribution by imaging techniques.

Among the radioisotopes used for labelling are yttrium-90, rhenium-186/rhenium-188 ($^{186}Re/^{188}Re$) and holmium-166 (^{166}Ho).

Yttrium-90, with its average β^- energy of 0.94 MeV, a mean tissue penetration of 2.5 mm and a decay to stable zirconium-90 with a half-life of 2.67 days, was among the first candidates for this task.

Hepatic radioembolization with ^{90}Y-microspheres was first described in the early 1960s, and the very first studies were troubled by a large leaching of yttrium and a somewhat not optimal microsphere size. These problems were overcome over the years, leading to a gradual investigation in humans [7, 8].

Currently, two different types of ^{90}Y-microspheres are commercially available and authorized by the US Food and Drug Administration (FDA): TheraSphere®, for radiation treatment of unresectable hepatocellular carcinoma (HCC) or as neoadjuvant to surgery or liver transplantation in patients, and SIR-Spheres® for the treatment of unresectable metastatic liver tumours from primary colorectal cancer. In Europe, both devices have a CE marking for the treatment of patients with either primary or metastatic liver cancer. These two devices differ in many respects, but no randomized trial has been conducted so far to determine which one is clinically superior, although there seems to be a general agreement on the effectiveness of both products when properly selected according to the patients' needs.

Properties and characteristic of TheraSphere® and SIR-Spheres® will be herein briefly summarized[1] and their differences highlighted and discussed.

[1] As it is often the case with products covered by patent, detailed and clear information is not always available. Where this was missing, second-hand data available from literature was used.

Table 10.1 Most common radionuclides used/proposed for radioembolization

Isotope	Half-life (h)	Emission	Average/max beta-energy (MeV)	Average/max range in tissue (mm)	Imaging
^{90}Y	64.2	99.9% β^-	0.94/2.28	2.5/12	Bremsstrahlung SPECT and PET
		0.003% β^+			
^{166}Ho	26.8	93.3% β^-	0.66/1.85	2.2/10.2	SPECT and MRI
		6.7% γ (81 keV)			
^{188}Re	17	84.9% β^-	0.76/2.12	3.8/11	SPECT
		15.1% γ (155 keV)			
^{186}Re	89.3	91% β^-	0.35/1.08	1/4.5	
		9% γ (137keV)			

Despite the unequivocal success of the therapy, many aspects of radioembolization remain challenging. These include determination of embolic distribution, microdosimetry and post-implantation dosimetry.

Thus, ^{166}Ho and ^{186}Re/^{188}Re were introduced to cope with these issues since, as opposed to the pure β^--emitter ^{90}Y (Table 10.1), they both have also a γ component that can be exploited for nuclear imaging.[2] In addition to the nuclear characteristic, holmium is highly paramagnetic and can consequently be visualized by magnetic resonance imaging (MRI) [9].

Concomitant to the introduction of these new radionuclides is also the development of different microsphere materials aimed to overcome some of the drawbacks associated to the existing glass and resin microspheres.

On the whole, these advances open the way for second-generation technologies, allowing for more unfailing administration as well as predictable and reliable response.

[2]Microsphere distribution after treatment commonly exploits the bremsstrahlung radiation produced by the decelerating β^-. Unfortunately, ^{90}Y-bremsstrahlung post-therapy imaging is not optimal for precise evaluation and dose calculation of radioactive sphere deposition within tumour lesion. However, since ^{90}Y decay is accompanied also by a 0.003% positron emission, the recent development of highly sensitive tomographs has made feasible the imaging also by positron emission tomography (PET).

10.2 ^{90}Y Glass Microspheres (TheraSphere®, Nordion, Ottawa, Canada; Distributed by BTG Int., London, UK)

This medical device consists of ^{90}Y embedded into glass microspheres.

Although the term "glass" is commonly associated to the well-known transparent material used in everyday life and of which exists several types according to the composition, scientifically speaking, "glass" denotes a solid, obtained by solidification of a liquid, having a non-crystalline structure. This irregular lattice allows the presence of interstices in which metal impurities, often desired, can be accommodated.

TheraSphere production can be split in two main stages:

- Incorporation of the stable isotope ^{89}Y into glass microspheres. This is achieved by melting at 1500–1600 °C a mixture of yttrium-89 oxide ($^{89}Y_2O_3$), aluminium oxide (Al_2O_3) and silicone dioxide (SiO_2). After cooling, the mixture (the "glass"; composition $17Y_2O_3$-$19Al_2O_3$-$64SiO_2$ mol% or $40Y_2O_3$-$20Al_2O_3$-$40SiO_2$ wt%) [10] is crushed and then passed through a flame sprayer with the purpose to give a more spherical size to the glass particles. A final passage of these particles through sieves consents to single out those having a mean diameter of 25 ± 10 μm diameter.

– Neutron bombardment in a nuclear reactor of the above glass microspheres to convert ^{89}Y to ^{90}Y through the $^{89}Y(n,\gamma)^{90}Y$ nuclear reaction.

The composition of TheraSphere® has been adjusted in order to maximize the content of yttrium, reduce the melting temperature and get rid of possible undesired radionuclides (see below).

The embedding technique explains the extremely low release (0.02–0.13%) of ^{90}Y observed in an early study *in vitro* after a 6-week incubation at 37 °C in water or saline [11].

Conversely, the neutron irradiation step can pose a problem in terms of radionuclidic impurities.

In fact, apart from the desired $^{89}Y(n,\gamma)^{90}Y$ reaction, also the (2n,γ) and (n,2n) reactions commonly occur leading to ^{91}Y (half-life 58.5 days) and ^{88}Y (half-life 106.6 days), respectively [12].

In addition, while the stables ^{27}Al, ^{26}Mg and ^{30}Si are activated to ^{28}Al, ^{27}Mg and ^{31}Si having relatively short half-lives (2.2 min, 9.5 min and 2.6 h, respectively), any extra element present in the starting oxides might undergo a nuclear transformation as well.

To reduce this possibility, particular attention is given in using only high-purity raw materials in the manufacture of the glass, so that ^{90}Y is yet by far the main radionuclide (>99.999%) in the glass microspheres at the date of calibration.

The product specification for gamma-emitting by-products is less than 1.11 MBq/50 mg at 60-day post calibration and since January 2010 has typically been <0.185 MBq/50 mg with the predominant radionuclides being ^{91}Y, ^{88}Y and ^{51}Cr (half-life 27.7 days). Other nuclides which may be present as by-products are (in order of decreasing probability of detection): ^{46}Sc, ^{124}Sb, ^{60}Co, ^{59}Fe, ^{152}Eu, ^{181}Hf, ^{233}Pa, ^{58}Co, ^{141}Ce, ^{192}Ir, ^{134}Cs, ^{54}Mn, ^{65}Zn, ^{86}Rb, ^{110m}Ag and ^{22}Na (BTG, personal communication). Dose calculations have indicated that the quantities of radiocontaminants are low enough to meet regulatory safety limits. Nevertheless, the presence of long half-life isotopes such as yttrium-88 and, even if in much smaller amount, cobalt-60 (5.3 years) and europium-152 (13.6 years) is enough to cause some concern on radioactive waste management.

To decrease the presence of longer-lived contaminants, short-intense thermal neutron flux is preferred to longer irradiation time with less neutron flux [13].

Radiation dose from ^{90}Y-labelled microsphere is limited in range, with roughly 50% of the adsorbed dose within 2.5 mm of the microsphere [14]. While this short-range minimizes the amount of radiation reaching healthy liver tissue, it dictates final positioning of the microspheres close to their intended target and stresses the need for predictable distribution for maximum effect. To this end, factors thought to be significant include number, size and density of the particles and the degree to which they mix with the blood during administration.

The relatively high content of ^{89}Y embedded into glass microsphere together with their robustness to neutron bombardment allows to achieve a high ratio of radioactivity per microsphere (often indicated as specific activity) in the amount of 2500 Bq/sphere at the time of calibration. High specific activities are deemed an advantage since they consent to administer a smaller number of microspheres, thus reducing the risks of both macroembolic effects and stasis/retrograde flow during administration. Besides, although not yet supported by literature, it seems reasonable to expect fewer microspheres of high specific activity to be preferable in case of small-volume tumours.

Generally speaking, particle density becomes particularly important for applications that require microspheres to be suspended in a fluid, as it is the case for radioembolization where the fluid is blood. It is critical that the density of microspheres is matched as close as possible to the density of the fluid at the correct temperature, particularly so when a long-term suspension of microspheres is required. Settling time is proportional to the density mismatch, which means that matching the density of the particle to the density of the liquid (blood) is very important for minimizing settling velocity and maximizing the time microspheres spend in suspension.

Density of TheraSphere® (3.3–3.6 g/mL) is reported to be much higher than blood (1.06 g/mL), something which authors [15, 16] highlight as a possible cause of premature intravascular settling and even suboptimal distribution, since the need to inject more forcefully may lead to microspheres achieving velocities' rate greater than the native artery velocity. However, considering the very short time required to reach the target, this difference in density does not appear to be so relevant, as reported in other works [17–19].

TheraSphere® is supplied in a 1.0-mL vial containing 0.6 mL of sterile water. According to the instructions for use reported in the leaflet, the sealed vial cannot be altered in any way, which means that the content cannot be fractionated. Consequently, a washing procedure of vial and delivery line is prescribed to ensure the complete transfer of the intended activity. However, customers can choose among six standard activity sizes for delivery: 3, 5, 7, 10, 15 and 20 GBq. Custom dose size are also available in 0.5 GBq increments. Besides, calibration time can vary according to weekday dispensing. Overall, the combination of these factors allows for some flexibility when it comes to select the dose to be administered. Nevertheless, the inability to make "last minute" changes to a treatment plan can be limiting.

Given the low number of microspheres infused, the entire vascular bed is never completely saturated, and continuous fluoroscopic guidance during infusion is not necessary.

10.3 ^{90}Y Resin Microspheres (SIR-Spheres®, SIRTeX Medical Ltd., Sydney, Australia)

As it often happens when patents are involved, not much is known on the exact composition and preparation of this medical device [20]. According to the patent:

> Yttrium (^{90}Y) labelled microspheres are made in the form of a sterile, pyrogen free suspension of resin beads labelled with yttrium (^{90}Y) phosphate. The resin beads consist of sulphuric acid groups attached to a styrene divinylbenzene copolymer lattice. Symmetrical microspheres of ion exchange resin (Aminex 50W-X4 cation exchange resin; supplied by 'Bio-Rad Cat # 1474313') with a diameter of approximately 30 to 35 microns are added to water (Water for Injections BP) to form a slurry that is then transferred into a reaction vessel. Yttrium (^{90}Y) sulphate solution is added to the reaction vessel and the mixture stirred at a speed sufficient to ensure homogeneity to absorb the yttrium-90 (^{90}Y) solution into the resin-based microspheres. Tri-sodium phosphate solution (1.25% w/v) is then added to the reaction vessel with further stirring to precipitate the radionuclide as yttrium (^{90}Y) phosphate. The microspheres are then washed with a phosphate buffer solution until the pH of the wash solution is less than 9 and preferable less than 8.5. Following washing of the microspheres with water (Water for Injection BP), the microspheres are resuspended and diluted (if necessary) with water (Water for Injections BP) to give a light brown suspension

It is also said that "...the yttrium-90 is precipitated as yttrium phosphate, for example, by addition of trisodium phosphate solution, to stably incorporate the yttrium-90 into the microspheres". This sentence has been often interpreted as a step to enhance the embedding of ^{90}Y into the resin (!) while it is probably just a mean to remove any lousy bound yttrium and, possibly, other unwanted cations.[3] No matter the reason, according to the manufacturer, the resin-based yttrium microspheres produced by the above method have shown a 0.01–0.4% unbound ^{90}Y when incubated at 37 °C for 20 min in water at pH 7.0. As mentioned, ion exchange is a reversible process, and so the use of an ionic solution like saline instead of water might have yielded to the release of yttrium.

However, it has been observed that only a 0.064% of the total activity was excreted in the urine during the first 12 h following treatment (0.003% in the case of TheraSphere®) [21, 22].

As for the source of ^{90}Y, the production method described allows for the use of alternate sources.

Similarly to what is seen for glass microspheres, ^{89}Y can first be bound to the resin and next transformed in ^{90}Y by neutron bombardment. The organic nature of the resin—and thus the lack of metal impurities—should help to prevent or reduce the side production of radiocontaminants.

[3] A support to this opinion is the fact that, as pointed out later in the text, the use of saline should be avoided since it could release ^{90}Y by a cation-exchange process, something that should be irrelevant in case of yttrium phosphate.

However, since a major disadvantage of polymer-based microspheres is their inability to withstand high thermal neutron fluxes, a more convenient approach to highly pure ^{90}Y is its extraction from the parent nuclide strontium-90 (^{90}Sr, half-life 28.8 years; it is a fission product of uranium in nuclear reactors) and using this extracted ^{90}Y to prepare the soluble yttrium-90 sulphate that is then incorporated into the polymeric matrix of the microspheres. In this case, as efficient as it might be the chemical separation of ^{90}Y from ^{90}Sr, the latter radionuclide would still likely be present as a radionuclidic impurity in the ^{90}Y-microspheres.

Nevertheless, regardless of the origin of ^{90}Y, the levels of detectable radiocontaminants, particularly those with long half-lives, were reported to be very low [12, 23], posing a problem, at worst, only in terms of waste disposal.

Even though not clearly stated by the manufacturer, ^{90}Y extraction from ^{90}Sr seems to be the route followed for the production of SIR-Spheres®.

According to SIRTeX, SIR-Spheres® have a density of 1.6 g/mL, while the specific activity, which initially varied from 37.5 up to 75 Bq/sphere according to the number of submitted orders, has been recently fixed to 75 Bq/sphere at the time of calibration, regardless of the batch size.

As mentioned earlier, a lower value of specific activity means a higher number of particles infused. This aspect, while it ensures an adequate coverage for very large tumours, definitely increases the risks of stasis or retrograde flow, thus limiting the complete administration of the desired activity, although a 2009 study on 680 patients infused with SIR-Spheres® in water reported that the median injected activity was ca. 92% of the drawn activity [24].

Anyhow, given the higher embolic load associated to SIR-Spheres® and the risk of unintended delivery into other organs, the infusion must be performed slowly (<5 mL/min) and alternating or mixing with a contrast medium to allow direct monitoring of the treatment, something which is not required with TheraSphere® [21].

The SIR-Spheres® delivery vial contains 3 GBq ± 10% of ^{90}Y resin microspheres at the time of calibration in 5 mL of water. In contrast to TheraSphere®, it is possible to fractionate the activity of SIR-Sphere microspheres, although this can result in an increased exposure of the operator because of the supplementary manual operations required.

The need to avoid any possible release of ^{90}Y ions from the resin by ion exchange with sodium ions is the reason behind the use of water rather than saline for the delivery vial as well as for the following infusion process. On the other hand, because of the physiologic effect of sterile water on the vasculature [25], it was thought that this might be the reason—or one of the reasons—for the changes in flow observed during administration of even a small aliquot of SIR-Spheres®. To overcome this problem, SIRTeX has suggested the use of 5% dextrose in water (D5W), a solution isotonic with plasma. Infusion utilizing D5W has a significantly lower rate of stasis than water and results in a more complete dose delivery [26]. The procedure was approved by the FDA in 2014.

Up to date there have been no clinical trials demonstrating superiority or inferiority of glass or resin microspheres in regard to changes in blood flow during radioembolization.

A recent study investigating the influence of material density, flow and viscosity on microsphere distribution within an *in vitro* vascular flow model designated to simulate flow condition within hepatic arteries reached the conclusion that glass and resin microspheres demonstrate a similar distribution in a range of clinical relevant flow conditions [17].

For a more direct comparison between TheraSphere® and SIR-Spheres®, a summary of their properties is reported in Table 10.2.

10.4 ^{166}Ho Poly-L-Lactic Acid (PLLA) Microsphere (QuiremSpheres®, Quirem Medical, Deventer, Netherlands)

^{90}Y has two major disadvantages as a radioisotope for therapy:

- The small thermal neutron section (1.28 barn) of ^{89}Y for the reaction $^{89}Y(n,\gamma)^{90}Y$ means that

Table 10.2 Summary of registered medical devices for radioembolization

	SIR-Spheres® (CE marking in 2002)	TheraSphere® (CE marking in 2014)	QuiremSpheres® (CE marking in 2015)
Composition	Cation-exchange sulphuric acid groups attached to a styrene divinylbenzene copolymer	Glass ($17Y_2O_3$-$19Al_2O_3$-$64SiO_2$ mol%)	Poly-L-Lactic-acid (PLLA)
	Not biodegradable	Not biodegradable	Biodegradable
Radiolabelling	^{90}Y is attached to the resin matrix through ion exchange of sodium for yttrium	The ^{89}Y glass microspheres are made radioactive by neutron activation in a nuclear reactor	The ^{165}Ho-PLLA microspheres are made radioactive by neutron activation in a nuclear reactor
Release of radionuclide	Trace amounts (25–50 kBq/L) of urinary excretion are a possibility in the first 24 h after implantation (SIRTeX operating manual)	*in vitro*, less than 0.13% after 6 weeks of incubation in water or saline	*in vitro*, 0.3% after 270 h in isotonic buffer Stability in human plasma: 93.5% after 72 h
Radionuclidic impurities	With reactor-produced ^{90}Y: ^{88}Y ($T_{1/2}$ = 106 days) and ^{91}Y ($T_{1/2}$ = 58.5 days) With generator-produced ^{90}Y: ^{90}Sr ($T_{1/2}$ = 28.78 year)	Besides ^{88}Y and ^{91}Y, derived from the neutron bombardment of ^{89}Y, there is presence of ^{154}Eu ($T_{1/2}$ = 8.8 year), ^{152}Eu ($T_{1/2}$ = 136 year), ^{57}Co ($T_{1/2}$ = 271 days) and ^{60}Co ($T_{1/2}$ = 5.3 year) originating from neutron bombardment of impurities in the glass	^{166m}Ho (1200 year)
Density (blood = 1.05 g/mL)	1.6 g/mL	3.6 g/mL	1.4 g/mL
Diameter	20–60 μm	20–30 μm	15–60 μm
Specific activity (at calibration time)	75 Bq/sphere	ca. 2500 Bq/sphere	Max 450 Bq/sphere
Vial size and number of microspheres	3 GBq/vial	Six activity sizes: 3, 5, 7, 10, 15 and 20 GBq in 0.6 mL of sterile water. Custom dose size are also available in 0.5 GBq increments	Customized dose, max 15 GBq/vial
	Each vial contains 40 million microspheres	A 3-GBq vial contains ca. 1.2 million microspheres	Each vial contains 33 million microspheres
Delivering	Mondays through Thursdays, calibration on the day following delivery and can be used up to 24 h after calibration	Mondays (calibrated the prior Sunday) or Wednesdays and Thursdays (calibrated the following Sunday). Can be used up to 12 days following calibration (extended shelf life)	Data not available
Administration	The dose can be fractionated	The dose cannot be fractionated	The dose cannot be fractionated
Medium	Sterile water or 5% dextrose in water	Saline	Saline

long neutron activation times (>2 weeks) are required to achieve therapeutic amount of ^{90}Y.

- The biodistribution of ^{90}Y-microsphere is difficult to monitor since ^{90}Y is an almost pure β^- emitter.

^{166}Ho is an attractive alternative to ^{90}Y for what concerns radioembolization with microspheres since, in addition to high-energy β^- particles, it has also a γ-ray emission which, while allowing nuclear imaging, contributes only to a 1.1% of the overall adsorbed dose [27]. Moreover, owing to its paramagnetic properties, ^{166}Ho can be visualized also by MRI.

On the other hand, the lower β^- energy and shorter half-life of ^{166}Ho compared to ^{90}Y result that, for an equivalent radiation dose on tissue, roughly three times the amount of radioactivity of ^{166}Ho has to be administered compared to ^{90}Y [28]. Even so, in ^{166}Ho radioembolization, considerably less microspheres are used compared to resin-based ^{90}Y-microspheres. That, combined with the near-plasma density of ^{166}Ho microspheres (1.4 g/mL), results in a lower risk of stasis or backflow during infusion [29]. Furthermore, the shorter half-life of ^{166}Ho leads to deposition of a radiation dose in a shorter time than with ^{90}Y, which is deemed to be advantageous for the radiobiological effect on tumour [30].

^{166}Ho-PLLA microspheres were originally developed at the University Medical Center Utrecht (Netherlands) (Nijsen et al. 1999) and then produced by a spin-off company (Quirem Medical) with the commercial name of QuiremSpheres®, which received in 2015 the European CE mark for quality and safety.

They are prepared from stable holmium-165 chloride ($^{165}HoCl_3$) which is treated with acetylacetone (AcAc) at pH 8 in water. The crystallized complex of holmium acetylacetonate ($Ho(AcAc)_3$) is dried and then mixed with PLLA in chloroform. This solution is combined with an aqueous solution of polyvinyl alcohol and stirred, causing the precipitation of the microspheres. Stirring rate and percentage of polyvinyl alcohol plays an important role in determining the average particle size. After separation from the solvent, the microspheres are washed first with diluted hydrochloric acid to remove any unincorporated holmium and then with deionized water to remove the hydrochloric acid itself. After drying, a final filtration ensures an average particle size of 30 ± 5 μm (15–60 μm). As the last step, microspheres are made radioactive by neutron activation in a nuclear reactor. Quite conveniently, ^{165}Ho has a natural abundance of 100%, a fact which contributes to reduce the risk of collateral production of undesired radionuclides.

Nevertheless, during the ^{165}Ho activation process, ^{166m}Ho (half-life = 1200 year, 3.1 barn) will always be produced, but to a considerably lesser extent than ^{166}Ho (64 barn), so that its presence will be a concern only in terms of waste management. As usual, target purity is important to avoid radionuclidic impurities after irradiation since any other element present on ^{165}Ho-PLLA will be activated, too. The possible contaminants of holmium targets are rare earths such as ytterbium, lutetium, lanthanum and cerium.

Because of the relatively short half-life of ^{166}Ho, separate neutron irradiation of each patient dose is needed. For the same reason, a good reactor-to-hospital logistic is of key importance. The vial used during the bombardment is used also for the administration. The content, due to the high radiation dose received during neutron bombardment, is considered sterile, and it has no residual organic solvent (namely, chloroform) [31].

While the activity, according to the parameters of bombardment, can reach up to 15 GBq, the amount of microspheres in the vials is kept fixed to 600 mg (33 million microspheres), which brings to a maximum specific activity value of 450 Bq/sphere [29].

Once injected, glass and resin microspheres remain in the liver as permanent implant. On the opposite, a major advantage of the polymer-based QuiremSpheres® is that these degrade to insoluble holmium lactate, which retains the holmium after degradation. In fact, hydrolysis of ester bonds in poly(lactic acid) results in the formation of soluble lactic acid oligomers which are ultimately converted into lactic acid. By this hydrolytic process,

PLLA microspheres disintegrate and finally dissolve in time. *In vitro* studies showed that neutron-irradiated Ho-PLLA microspheres disintegrated after 52 weeks of incubation in buffer at 37 °C, with the formation of insoluble holmium lactate microcrystals [32]. Hardly any holmium (0.3%) was released from the microspheres into isotonic phosphate buffer after 270 h. [31]. Also, ^{166}Ho-PLLA microspheres showed great stability (93.5%) up to 72 h in human plasma [33].

In spite of the particles' low density, the administration procedure, which consists in administering the radioactive macrospheres in a 50% mixture of saline and non-ionogenic contrast, is performed under fluoroscopic guidance to instantly visualize retrograde flow [34].

Recent trials have shown ^{166}Ho microsphere to be safe and effective for the treatment of advanced liver cancer [35, 36]. The first clinical case with commercial QuiremSpheres® has been reported on the company website while this chapter was being written.

As a result of ^{166}Ho-PLLA distinctive features, a new concept, that of "scout dose", has been introduced. It consists in using a small dose (250 MBq, 60 mg) of the same ^{166}Ho microspheres of a low specific activity to predict the distribution of the treatment dose [37]. Compared to technetium-99m macroaggregated albumin (^{99m}Tc-MAA), which is the gamma-emitter tracer usually employed for this task, ^{166}Ho-PLLA is expected to better simulate treatment because it shares the same density, size distribution and morphology with the treatment dose. It has been shown that a ^{166}Ho scout dose is a more reliable predictor of lung shunting than ^{99m}Tc-MAA [38].

However, it has been pointed out how this procedure should be thoroughly assessed in terms of safety, since even a low unwanted extrahepatic deposition of activity dose may induce ulceration and inflammation of abdominal organs [39]. In order to replace ^{99m}Tc-MAA in clinical practice, the risk of extrahepatic deposition of a ^{166}Ho scout dose should be known, although theoretic analysis of the potential risk of a 250-MBq ^{166}Ho scout dose resulted in a low incidence (1.3%) of potentially harmful extrahepatic deposition [37].

10.5 ^{186}Re/^{188}Re Microspheres

Rhenium-186 and rhenium-188 have been proposed as alternatives to ^{90}Y for the labelling of microspheres on account of their dual β^- and γ emission (see Table 10.1) [40–42].

Both glass and PLLA were suggested as matrix for the microspheres, with stable rhenium incorporated in non-radioactive form and subsequently activated by neutron bombardment, analogously to what is done with yttrium and holmium. Unfortunately, as an outcome of the isotopic composition of the naturally occurring rhenium (37.4% ^{185}Re and 62.6% ^{187}Re), an indivisible mixture of ^{186}Re and ^{188}Re is produced. Obviously, the presence of two radionuclides of different energies and half-lives poses serious problems on dosimetric calculation. Moreover, an unexpected setback came from Re-PLLA which was reported to undergo damage during neutron irradiation.

As a result, no human studies have been reported so far.

In addition to the nuclear reactor production, ^{188}Re alone can be conveniently obtained from an alumina-based ^{188}W/^{188}Re generator. Compared to ^{90}Y, this feature makes ^{188}Re cheaper and more readily available (no more nuclear reactor shutdowns or somewhat unreliable overseas transports) and overcomes the need of careful advance planning for the required dose, allowing a prompt response to clinical demands.

On the other hand, preparation of ^{188}Re-labelled microspheres of the glass, resin or PLLA type is quite complex to carry out, even more so because of the shorter half-life of ^{188}Re when compared to ^{90}Y. As a consequence, ^{188}Re-human serum albumin (^{188}Re-HSA) microspheres were proposed as a more feasible alternative.

^{188}Re-HSA microspheres were prepared by adding generator-produced, carrier-free ^{188}Re perrhenate ($^{188}ReO_4^-$) to human serum albumin microspheres, followed by a reduction step of perrhenate with tin (II) [43]. Quite conveniently—and similarly to what is done for ^{99m}Tc-HSA—the labelling was carried out adapting a commercial kit, with some changes introduced in order to increase both radiochemical yield and radiochemical purity. The original publication is somewhat unclear on these two parameters, reporting the percentage of rhenium reacted (97%) and the purity of the supernatant (97–98%) but without ever mentioning the need of applying a filtration or centrifugation to the product vial, as instead acknowledged by other authors [44].

^{188}Re-HSA microspheres were found to be stable *in vitro* in human plasma, blood and saline for 30 h as >88% of the ^{188}Re was still bound to the microspheres. Their diameter between 14 and 40 μm (mean value 22 μm) is smaller than those of ^{90}Y and ^{166}Ho microspheres. Major advantage is their biocompatibility and *in vivo* degradability, so that the occlusion of blood vessels following intraarterial application is only temporary.

Similar to ^{166}Ho, four- to fivefold higher ^{188}Re activity needs to be administered to obtain an equivalent absorbed dose as ^{90}Y.

Currently there are few publications on the use of ^{188}Re-HSA microspheres in patients with advanced primary and secondary liver cancer. Preliminary results showed that their infusion was well tolerated, with evidence of symptomatic response in many patients [44].

Key Points

- Microspheres of the proper size injected into the hepatic artery lodge themselves preferentially in and around tumours. Thus, radioembolization with microspheres labelled with β^--emitter radionuclides is a powerful tool for the treatment of liver malignancies, because it adds to the embolization effect the deposition of lethal doses of radiation to the tumour cells.
- Three commercial radiolabelled microspheres are currently available: ^{90}Y glass microspheres (TheraSphere®), ^{90}Y resin microspheres (SIR-Spheres®) and, more recently, ^{166}Ho poly-L-lactic acid microspheres (QuiremSpheres®).
- Crucial features in the choice of radiolabelled microspheres are density closer to the blood, homogeneous spherical size of 25–30 μm, energy and half-life of the β^- emitter, high specific activity, very low levels of radionuclidic impurities, negligible in vivo radionuclide release, good availability, resistance to radiation damage, biocompatibility/biodegradability and possibility to predict and follow their distribution by imaging techniques.
- High specific activities are deemed an advantage since they consent to administer a smaller number of microspheres, thus reducing the risks of both macroembolic effects and stasis/retrograde flow during administration. On the other hand, a very small number of microspheres might not ensure an adequate coverage for very large tumours.
- ^{166}Ho is an attractive alternative to ^{90}Y for what concern radioembolization with microspheres since it has a γ-ray emission which allows nuclear imaging. Owing to its paramagnetic properties, ^{166}Ho can be visualized also by MRI.
- In addition, while glass and resin microspheres once injected remain in the liver as permanent implant, a major advantage of the polymer-based ^{166}Ho QuiremSpheres® is that these degrade to insoluble holmium lactate, which retains the holmium after degradation.
- ^{188}Re-HSA microspheres can be conveniently prepared from an alumina-based ^{188}W/^{188}Re generator and human serum albumin microspheres by adapting a commercial kit, making them more readily available than the above-mentioned microspheres. Major advantage is their biocompatibility and in vivo degradability.
- Similar to ^{166}Ho, four- to fivefold higher ^{188}Re activity needs to be administered to obtain an equivalent absorbed dose as ^{90}Y.

References

1. Breedis C, Young G. The blood supply of neoplasms in the liver. Am J Pathol. 1954;30(5):969–85.
2. Van de Wiele C, Maes A, Brugman E, D'asseler Y, De Spiegeleer B, Mees G, Stellamans K. SIRT of liver metastases: physiological and pathophysiological considerations. Eur J Nucl Med Mol Imaging. 2012;39:1646–55.
3. Laurent A. Microspheres and nonspherical particles for embolization. Tech Vasc Interv Rad. 2007;10:248–56.
4. Nijsen JFW, Zonnenberg BA, Woittiez JRW, Rook DW, Swildens-van Woudenberg IA, van Rijk PP, van het Schip AD. Holmium-166 poly lactic microspheres applicable for intra-arterial radionuclide ther-

apy of hepatic malignancies: effects of preparation and neutron activation techniques. Eur J Nucl Med. 1999;26:699–704.
5. Cremonesi M, Ferrari M, Bartolomei M, Orsi F, Bonomo G, Aricò D, et al. Radioembolization with 90Y-microspheres: dosimetric and radiobiological investigation for multi-cycle treatment. Eur J Nucl Med Mol Imaging. 2008;35(11):2088–96.
6. Wunderlich G, Schiller E, Bergmann R, Pietzsch HJ. Comparison of the stability of Y-90-, Lu-177- and Ga-68- labeled human serum albumin microspheres (DOTA-HSAM). Nucl Med Biol. 2010;37:861–7.
7. Burton MA, Gray BN, Klemp PF, Kelleher DK, Hardy N. Selective internal radiation therapy: distribution of radiation in the liver. Eur J Cancer Clin Oncol. 1989;25(10):1487–91.
8. Lau WY, Ho S, Leung TWT, Chan M, Ho R, Johnson PJ, Li AKC. Selective internal radiation therapy for nonresectable hepatocellular carcinoma with intraarterial infusion of ^{90}Yttrium microspheres. Int Radiat Oncol Biol Phys. 1998;40(3):583–92.
9. Van de Maat GH, Seevinck PR, Elschot M, Smits MLJ, de Leeuw H, van het Schip AD, et al. MRI-based biodistribution assessment of holmium-166 poly (L-lactic acid) microspheres after radioembolization. Eur Radiol. 2013;23:827–35.
10. Aspasio RD, Borges R, Marchi J. Biocompatible glasses for cancer treatment. In: Marchi J, editor. Biocompatible glasses: from bone regeneration to cancer treatment. Cham: Springer; 2016. p. 267–84.
11. Erbe EM, Day DE. Chemical durability of Y2O3-Al2O3-SiO2 glasses for the *in vivo* delivery of beta radiation. J Biomed Mater Res. 1993;27(10):1301–8.
12. Metyko J, Williford JM, Erwin W, Poston J, Jimenez S. Long-lived impurities of ^{90}Y-labeled microspheres, Thera Sphere and SIR-Spheres, and the impact on patients dose and waste management. Radiat Saf J. 2012;103(2):S204–8.
13. Day DE, Ehrhardt GJ. Glass microspheres. United States Patent number 4789501. 1988.
14. Morgan B, Kennedy AS, Lewington V, Jones B, Sharma RA. Intra-arterial brachytherapy of hepatic malignancies: watch the flow. Nat Rev Clin Oncol. 2011;8:115–20.
15. Basciano CA, Kleinstreuer C, Kennedy AS. Computational fluid dynamics modeling of ^{90}Y microspheres in human hepatic tumors. J Nucl Med Radiat Ther. 2011. https://doi.org/10.4172/2155-9619.1000112.
16. Wagner HN, Rhodes BA, Sasaki Y, Ryan JP. Studies of the circulation with radioactive microspheres. Investig Radiol. 1969;4(6):374–86.
17. Caine M, McCafferty MS, McGhee S, Garcia P, Mullett WN, Zhang X, et al. Impact of Yttrium-90 microspheres density, flow dynamics, and administration technique on spatial distribution: analysis using an *in vitro* model. J Vasc Interv Radiol. 2017;28:260–8.
18. Ibrahim S, Lewandowski RJ, Ryu RK, Sato KT, Gates VL, Mulcahy MF, et al. Radiographic response to yttrium-90 radioembolization in anterior versus posterior liver segments. Cardiovasc Intervent Radiol. 2008;31:1124–32.
19. Salem R, Mazzaferro V, Sangro B. Yttrium-90 radioembolization for the treatment of hepatocellular carcinoma: biological lesson, current challenges, and clinical perspectives. Hepatology. 2013;58(6):2188–97.
20. Gray BN. Polymer based radionuclide containing particulate material. Patent application WO 02/34300 A1. 2002.
21. Giammarile F, Bodei L, Chiesa C, Flux G, Forrer F, Kraeber-Bodere F, et al. EANM procedure guidelines for the treatment of liver metastases with intra-arterial radioactive compounds. Eur J Nucl Med Mol Imaging. 2011;38(7):1393–406.
22. Lambert B, Mertens J, Ravier M, Blanken T, Defreyne L, Van Vlierberghr H, et al. Urinary excretion of Yttrium-90 following intra-arterial microspheres treatment for liver tumours. J Nucl Med. 2011;52(Supplement 1):1744.
23. Nelson K, Vause PE, Koropova P. Post-mortem considerations of yttrium-90 (^{90}Y) microspheres therapy procedures. Health Phys. 2008;95(5):S156–61.
24. Kennedy AS, McNeille P, Dezarn WA, Nutting C, Sangro B, Wertman WA, et al. Treatment parameters and outcome in 680 treatments of internal radiation with resin 90Y-microspheres for unresectable hepatic tumors. Int J Radiat Oncol Biol Phys. 2009;74(5):1494–500.
25. Rother RP, Bell L, Hillmen P, Gladwin MT. The clinical sequelae of intravascular hemolysis and extracellular plasma hemoglobin: a novel mechanism of human disease. JAMA. 2005;293(13):1653–62.
26. Koran ME, Stewart S, Baker JC, Lipnik AJ, Banovac F, Omary RA, Brown DB. Five percent dextrose maximizes dose delivery of yttrium-90 resin microspheres and reduces rates of premature stasis compared to sterile water. Biomed Rep. 2016;5:745–8.
27. Turner JH, Claringbold PG, Klemp PF, Cameron PJ, Martindale AA, Glancy RJ, et al. 166Ho-microsphere liver radiotherapy: a preclinical SPECT dosimetry study in the pig. Nucl Med Commun. 1994;15(7):545–53.
28. Vente MA, Hobbelink MG, van Het Schip AD, Zonnnenberg BA, Nijsen JF. Radionuclide liver cancer therapies: from concept to current clinical status. Anticancer Agent Med Chem. 2007;7(4):441–59.
29. Smits MLJ, Nijsen JFW, van der Bosch MAAJ, Lam MGEH, Vente MAD, Huijbregts JE, et al. Holmium-166 radioembolization for the treatment of patients with liver metastases: design of the phase I HEPAR trial. J Exp Clin Cancer Res. 2010;29:70. http://www.jeccr.com/content/29/1/70
30. Dale RG. Dose-rate effects in targeted radiotherapy. Phys Med Biol. 1996;41:1871–84.
31. Zielhuis SW, Nijsen JFW, de Roos R, Krijger GC, van Rijk PP, Hennink WE, van het Schip AD. Production of GMP-grade radioactive holmium loaded poly(L-lactic acid) microspheres for clinical application. Int J Pharm. 2006;311:69–74.
32. Zielhuis SW, Nijsen JFW, Krijger GC, van het Schip AD, Hennink WE. Holmium-loaded poly (L-lactic

acid) microspheres: *in vitro* degradation study. Biomacromolecules. 2006;7(7):2217–23.
33. Yavari K, Yeganeh E, Abolghasemi H. Production and characterization of 166Ho polylactic acid microspheres. J Label Compd Radiopharm. 2016;59:24–9.
34. Vente MAD, de Wit TC, van den Bosch MAAJ, Bult W, Seeninck PR, Zonnenberg BA, et al. Holmium-166 poly(l-lactic acid) microsphere radioembolization of the liver: technical aspects studied in a large animal model. Eur Radiol. 2010;20:862–9.
35. Prince JF. Holmium radioembolization: efficacy and safety. PhD thesis. 2016. ISBN 978–90–393-6489-5.
36. Smits MLJ, Nijsen JFW, van der Bosch MAAJ, Lam MGEH, Vente MAD, Mali WP, et al. Holmium-166 radioembolisation in patients with unresectable, chemorefractory liver metastases (HEPAR trial): a phase 1, dose escalation study. Lancet Oncol. 2012;13:1025–34.
37. Prince JF, van Rooij R, Bol GH, de Jong HWAM, van den Bosch MAAJ. Safety of a scout dose preceding hepatic radioembolization with ^{166}Ho microspheres. J Nucl Med. 2015;56:817–23.
38. Elschot M, Nijsen JFW, Lam MGEH, Smits MLJ, Prince JF, Viergever MA, et al. ^{99m}Tc-MAA overestimates the absorbed dose to the lungs in radioembolization: a quantitative evaluation in patients treated with ^{166}Ho-microspheres. Eur J Nucl Med Mol Imaging. 2014;41:1965–75.
39. Cosimelli M. The evolution of radioembolization. Lancet Oncol. 2012;13:965–6.
40. Hafeli UO, Casillas S, Dietz DW, Pauer GJ, Rybicki LA, Conzone SD, et al. Hepatic tumor radioembolization in a rat model using radioactive rhenium (^{186}Re/^{188}Re) glass microspheres. Int J Radiat Oncol Biol Phys. 1999;44(1):189–99.
41. Hafeli UO, Roberts WK, Pauer GJ, Kraeft SK, Macklis RM. Stability of biodegradable radioactive rhenium (Re-186 and Re-188) microspheres after neutron-activation. Appl Radiat Isot. 2001;54:869–79.
42. Wunderlich G, Pinkert J, Andreeff M, Stintz M, Knapp FF, Kropp J, Franke WG. Preparation and biodistribution of rhenium-188 labeled albumin microspheres B20: a promising new agent for radiotherapy. Appl Radiat Isot. 2000;52:63–8.
43. Wunderlich G, Drews A, Kotzerke J. A kit for labeling of [^{188}Re]human serum albumin microspheres for therapeutic use in nuclear medicine. Appl Radiat Isot. 2005;62:915–8.
44. Nowicki ML, Cwikla JB, Sankowski AJ, Shcherbinin AJ, Grimes J, Celler A, et al. Initial study of radiological and clinical efficacy radioembolization using ^{188}Re-human serum albumin (HSA) microspheres in patients with progressive, unresectable primary or secondary lung cancers. Med Sci Monit. 2014;20:1353–62.

11

HCC Radioembolization with Yttrium-90 Glass Microspheres (TheraSphere)

Marco Maccauro, Gianluca Aliberti, Carlo Chiesa, and Carlo Spreafico

Abstract

Intraarterial radioembolization (RE) using microspheres labelled with the high-energy beta-emitter yttrium-90 (90Y) is an innovative local therapy for hepatocellular carcinoma (HCC). This procedure allows the tumour to be irradiated with a dose higher than that allowed by whole-liver external beam radiation treatment. The TheraSphere (TheraSphere_BTG®) consist of glass microspheres labelled with 90Y as an integral component of glass. The mean diameter of glass sphere is 20–30 μm, and a high specific activity per sphere at calibration is 2500 Bq. The recommended TheraSphere® Dose to the hepatic lobe is 120 Gy (80–150 Gy). It is possible to choose 35 dose size options, between 3 GBq and 20 GBq in 0.5 GBq increments, a dosing flexibility and an individualized patient treatment. Yttrium-90 glass microspheres are indicated for the treatment in early-stage HCC to the downstaging or bridging to liver transplantation or in patients with intermediate to advanced HCC. BCLC B patients refractory to transarterial chemoembolization (TACE) or BCLC C patients with branch portal vein thrombosis (PVT). Considering the favourable tumour response and long-term outcomes, this treatment is an option for unresectable HCC.

M. Maccauro (✉) • G. Aliberti • C. Chiesa
Nuclear Medicine, Istituto Nazionale Tumori (National Cancer Institute) IRCCS Foundation, Milan, Italy
e-mail: marco.maccauro@istitutotumori.mi.it

C. Spreafico
Radiology 1, Istituto Nazionale Tumori (National Cancer Institute) IRCCS Foundation, Milan, Italy

11.1 Introduction

Primary liver cancer is the second most common cause of cancer-related death [1] and sixth most common cancer. The incidence is more in the Southern European countries that in the Northern European countries. In Europe, the incidence of HCC is growing, and its pattern of occurrence is heterogeneous [2]. About 83% of cases occurred in less-developed countries.

E. Bombardieri et al. (eds.), *Clinical Applications of Nuclear Medicine Targeted Therapy*,
https://doi.org/10.1007/978-3-319-63067-0_11

Fewer than 10% of patients with hepatocellular carcinoma (HCC) are candidates for radical treatment, the majority being unsuitable due to advanced stage at presentation, presence of hepatic dysfunction or presence of comorbidities. Local treatment, such as radiofrequency ablation or transarterial chemoembolization (TACE), and systemic therapy with cytotoxic drugs are alternative palliative treatments in patients with non-resectable disease. Because of their characteristic blood supply, primarily from the hepatic artery, and their hypervascularization—supplies 80–100% of blood flow to liver tumours and only 25% of blood flow to normal liver tissue—liver lesions are suitable for locoregional therapy by intraarterial administration of drugs.

Several techniques have been developed to selectively target liver tumours; these include administration of cytostatic drugs or intraarterial embolization techniques. Intraarterial radioembolization (RE) using microspheres labelled with the high-energy beta-emitter yttrium-90 (90Y) is an innovative local therapy for conditions in which, to date, systemic therapy was the only option [2]. This procedure allows the tumour to be irradiated with a dose higher than that allowed by whole-liver external beam radiation treatment, in which doses are limited to 30–40 Gray (Gy).

Three microsphere products are available: 90Y glass spheres, 90Y resin spheres and holmium-166 spheres.

The radioembolization is a two-step procedure:

- *Treatment planning phase* that is the heart of the procedure and consists of *CT/MRI* to evaluate the tumour, *angiography* to study the tumour perfusion and to embolize where needed and to identify the best point for the infusion of microspheres and *^{99m}Tc-MAA* scan with SPECT/TC to visualize extrahepatic shunts (lung and gastrointestinal) and to perform the dosimetric calculation.
- *Treatment phase* that consists an intraarterial microsphere angiography infusion, reproducing the exact catheter position of previous *angiography*.

The TheraSphere (TheraSphere_BTG®) consist of glass microspheres containing native, nonradioactive yttrium-89 which is then converted to 90Y by neutron irradiation and with 90Y as an integral component of glass. The mean diameter of glass sphere is 20–30 μm, and a high specific activity per sphere at calibration is 2500 Bq; 1 GBq in tissue delivers 50 Gy/kg. It is specifically engineered to be minimally embolic due to its high activity (2500 Bq/sphere) and small diameter (20–30 μm) of glass spheres [3]; minimized the risk of stasis, reflux and gastric ulceration; and preserve the tissue aeration useful to increase the efficacy of yttrium radiations and its killing potency. The use of Yttrium is favourable because it is 100% pure beta-emitter, the physical half-life is 64.1 h (2.67 days), and the tissue penetration range of 90Y beta radiation is 2.5 mm (max. 11 mm), 94% of radiation delivered within 11 days. TheraSphere® glass microspheres are infused via transfemoral or brachial catheterization of hepatic artery, penetrate and lodge within the tumour arteriolar capillaries, and emit beta radiation with an average tissue penetration range of 2.5 mm.

11.2 Clinical Indications

TheraSphere® is indicated for the treatment of hepatic neoplasia in the absence of any contraindication to transarterial radioembolization. Chronic liver disease and cirrhosis remain the most important risk factors for the development of HCC of which viral hepatitis and excessive alcohol intake are the leading risk factors worldwide. Many HCC treatments have adverse effects on liver function, which are compounded on a cirrhotic background: HCC is a complex and heterogeneous disease, with several factors affecting prognosis and treatment [2], like tumour stage, liver function and performance status.

90Y radioembolization is not yet included in BCLC algorithm as a potential treatment modality. Many studies may be competitive with sorafenib or TACE and may be used as part of a strategy for bridging patients to curative therapies such as transplantation or to downstage patients so that they may be considered candidates for transplantation [4–6].

90Y radioembolization approach changes according to the stage of HCC.

Some authors suggest the use of TheraSphere® in early-stage HCC can be curative, because it allows:

- Downstaging HCC and bridging to transplantation [3, 7]

In 2009 Lewandowski et al. [8] demonstrated *in 75 p*atients with stage T3 unresectable HCC, *43 patients* treated with TheraSphere® and 35 with TACE, that downstaging from T3 to T2 was achieved in more patients treated with TheraSphere® (58 vs 31%) and prolonged TTP for patients treated with TheraSphere® (33.3 vs 12.8 months). This long TTP suggests that TheraSphere® may be effective in bridging T2 patients to transplantation.

In 2011 Salem et al. [7] proved a prolonged TTP in BCLC A HCC patients who had received TheraSphere® (n = 123) than patients who had received TACE (n = 122). The median time to progression in BCLC A patients was 8.8 months for TACE patient group vs 25.1 months for TheraSphere® patient group; this result suggests that TheraSphere® may be effective in bridging to transplantation.

- Reach tumour ablation with segmentectomy

In a study of 84 patients with unresectable HCC with angiographically isolatable tumours, Riaz et al. [9] demonstrated feasibility of radiation segmentectomy with TheraSphere®. It was delivered as localized, high-dose radiation to target tumour tissue while minimizing exposure of normal tissue with a mean tumour dose of 1214 Gy and a mean normal parenchymal dose of 210 Gy. A median overall survival of 26.9 months was found. The overall response rate assessed using WHO was 59%, using EASL was 81% and was associated with low toxicity and absence of radiation-induced liver disease.

Vouche et al. [10] demonstrated in a multicenter study good results in selective delivery of high-dose radiation to tumour tissue while minimizing exposure to normal hepatic parenchyma.

In 102 patients with solitary HCC lesions of ≤5 cm, not amenable to resection or RFA, mRECIST showed a complete response in 47%, partial response in 39% and stable disease in 12% and a median time-to-disease progression of 33.1 months.

Other authors suggest the use of TheraSphere® in patients with advanced HCC and who have higher risk of normal tissue complications, such as patients with Child-Pugh B disease status and Branch PVT within treated segment. In this condition, the treatment can be considered palliative.

Extensive data demonstrate the safety and efficacy of TheraSphere® in treating HCC in the palliative setting, for patients with intermediate to advanced HCC (BCLC B and C).

In a prospective study with 291 patients with primarily intermediate to advanced HCC treated with TheraSphere®, Salem et al. highlight a favourable survival outcomes particularly in BCLC A and B patients and was most beneficial to Child-Pugh A patients.

In an observational study with 108 patients with advanced HCC (BCLC C), or early-intermediate HCC (BCLC A and B) and ineligible for cTACE, Hilgard et al. [11] showed an overall median survival of 16.4 months, PVT absent for 16.4 months, 1 PVT present for 10.0 months, BCLC B of 16.4 months, BCLC C NA, CR 6%, RP 35%, SD 48n% and PD 10%.

Salem et al. [12] in a retrospective, comparative, effectiveness analysis trial studied 245 patients with HCC, 123 received TheraSphere® and 122 TACE. Median overall survival was 20.5 months for a patient who received TheraSphere® and 17.4 months for patients who received TACE. With BCLC C stratification, the median overall survival was 21.1 months for TheraSphere® group and 9.3 months for TACE group. A statistically significant difference in median overall survival was seen in BCLC C patients.

In a prospective, phase II trial, Mazzaferro et al. [13] studied 52 patients with intermediate HCC (without PVT) or advanced HCC (with PVT) and well-compensated cirrhosis who

Table 11.1 Patient selection in the palliative setting

BCLC B patients	Refractory or intolerant to TACE
BCLC B or C patients	Large tumours, multifocal disease
BCLC C patients	With PVT

were ineligible to receive conventional curative therapy. The median overall survival was 15 months, 18 months for patients without PVT and 13 months for patients with PVT.

The patient characteristics, if it is a palliative aim, are summarized in Table 11.1.

11.3 Calculating the Required TheraSphere® Activity

The parameters to consider when calculating required TheraSphere® activity are the optimal therapeutic radiation dose, the target liver volume—not tumour volume—and the lung shunt fraction.

Amount of radioactivity required to deliver the dose to the target liver volume is:

Activity required (GBq) = (Desired Dose)(Liver Mass)/50 (1-LSF)(1-R)

Liver Mass is the lobe target measured by CT slices.

LSF is the lung shunt; R is the estimated percent residual dose in the administration system.

The lung shunt fraction has to be individually measured on ^{99m}TcMAA scan as lung counts/(lungs + liver counts). Count in each organ should be preferably obtained using geometrical mean of anterior and posterior counts, correct at least for the attenuation.

The limit dose for the lung is 30 Gy for a single administration and 50 Gy for cumulative administrations.

Recommended TheraSphere® Dose to the liver is 80–150 Gy (nominal 120 Gy) (*TheraSphere® Yttrium-90 Glass Microspheres—Biocompatibles UK Ltd—a BTG International group company*)

Dose adjustments may be necessary based on patient characteristics:

- Perfused liver volume/liver mass by CT or ultrasound scan
- Lesion size and location
- Tumour hypervascularity determined by angioscintigraphy
- Tumour radiopharmaceutical uptake determined by ^{99m}TcMAA scan
- Healthy liver radiopharmaceutical uptake determined by ^{99m}TcMAA scan
- Lung shunt fraction (LSF) determined by ^{99m}TcMAA scan
- Treatment window—considering the required yttrium-90 activity at administration time, the different dose size options based on a preferred treatment time and the microsphere quantity

The TheraSphere supply 35 dose size options to meet individual patient needs, for example, size of tumour, and allow to choose between 3 GBq and 20 GBq in 0.5 GBq increments (Table 11.2).

The TheraSphere® 90Y glass microspheres shelf life allows patient treatment to be planned for the first or second week after the calibration date. This provides more treatment options based on the number of spheres desired.

In particular conditions as low tumour vascularity, underlying liver performance, poor ECOG PS, high pulmonary dose, prior systemic therapy having vascular impact and uptake in healthy liver, it is possible to reduce the dose. Instead in conditions of high tumour vascularity, good underlying liver performance, superselective injection and no uptake in healthy liver, in accordance with internal protocol, there is a possibility to plan an increase dose. This dosing flexibility allows to perform individualized patient treatment.

Table 11.2 Different activity and number of spheres for a vial

Dose vial	Number of microspheres
3 GBq	1.2 million
5 GBq	2 million
7 GBq	2.8 million
10 GBq	4 million
15 GBq	6 million
20 GBq	8 million

11.4 Dosimetric Aspects

The other focal point of 90Y radioembolization is the dosimetric aspect. This aspect is particularly crucial with TheraSphere®, thanks to the possibility to administer different activities and different number of spheres (Table 11.1). Dosimetry can be easily calculated before the treatment, using the ^{99m}Tc-MAA SPECT/CT images of the simulation session, and after the therapeutic administration as confirmation, using either 90Y bremsstrahlung SPECT or more quantitatively accurate 90Y positron emission tomography (PET) images. The relationship between the ^{99m}Tc-MAA SPECT-based tumour absorbed dose and tumour response is reported in several studies investigating the possibilities of treatment optimization by individualized ^{99m}Tc-MAA SPECT-based dose planning. All published studies found a dose-efficacy correlation with glass spheres. Garin et al. [14] found that the minimum dose for an EASL response was 205 Gy, while in Milan cohort [15] it was 217 Gy with excellent agreement (Fig. 11.1).

Concerning toxicity limits, from the dosimetric point of view, Garin et al. [16] determined that more than 120 Gy to a portion larger than 70% is a risk factor for liver toxicity, defined with a more restrictive end point than ours. Their limits correspond to a mean parenchyma dose of 120 Gy × 70%/100% = 84 Gy, which is not so far from Milan group [15], and 75 Gy for 15% toxicity risk, obtained using a wider acceptance toxicity definition.

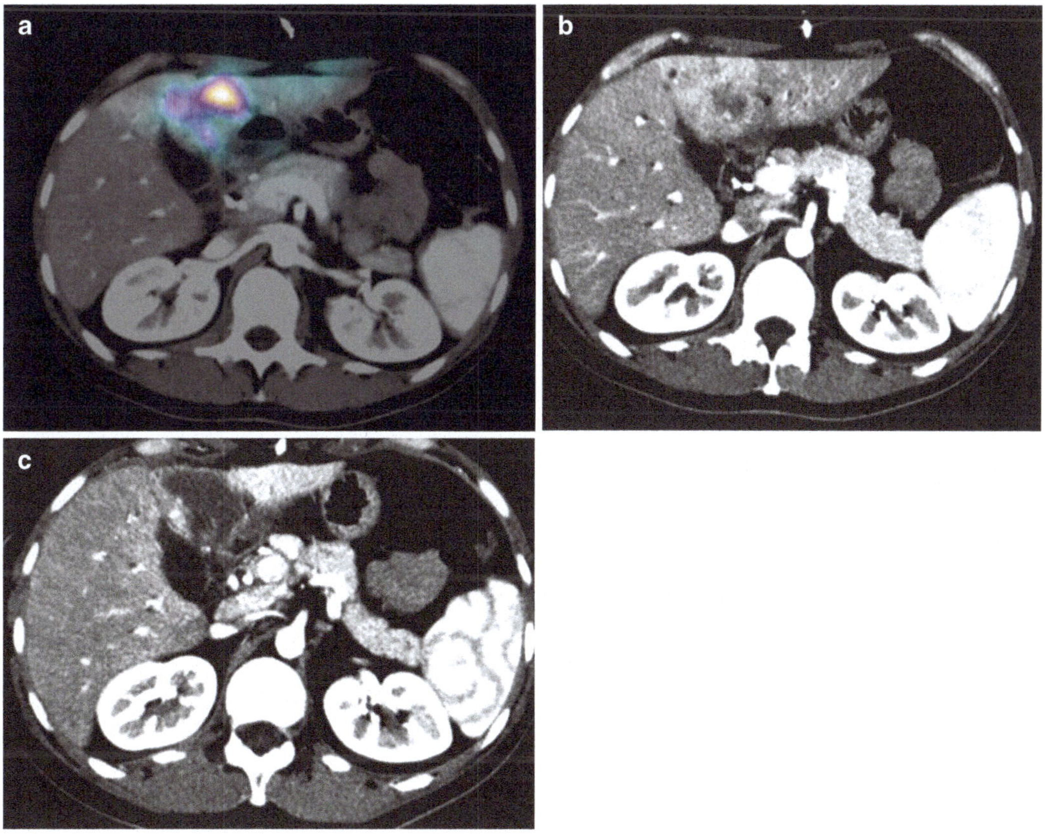

Fig. 11.1 (**a**) ^{99m}Tc MAA SPECT/TC of liver lesion. (**b**) Pretherapeutic contrast-enhanced CT of liver lesion. (**c**) Contrast-enhanced CT of liver lesion 3 months post radioembolization showing excellent response

Table 11.3 Treatment considerations

Whole HCC liver treatment	Is contraindicated
Bilobar or unilobar treatment	Based on tumour characteristics
Sequential treatments in different segments but in the same lobe	Wait 1 or 2 weeks to treat the other segment or treat in the same therapeutic section
Sequential treatments in bilobar disease	Treating one lobe and then the other in separate sessions, a 30–45-day interval is generally accepted
Catheter placement and haemodynamics	Proximal infusion allows wide distribution
Catheter placement and haemodynamics	Distal infusion allows targeted distribution
Dosing flexibility	Dose reduction for child B
Dosing flexibility	Dose reduction in hepatectomy patients
Dosing flexibility	Dose reduction if the healthy liver dose is high

11.5 Treatment Considerations

In conclusion to perform a correct planning treatment, it is mandatory to do some treatment considerations that are summarized in Table 11.3.

Conclusion

Y90 radioembolization with glass spheres is not an embolic therapy but is a radiotherapy. This therapy minimizes stasis and reflux and allows to deliver a high radioactive dose to the tumour while limiting normal tissue toxicity. Considering the favourable tumour response and long-term outcomes, this treatment is an option for unresectable HCC.

Key Points

- The mean diameter of glass sphere (20–30 μm) and a high specific activity per sphere at calibration (2500 Bq) minimize the risk of stasis, reflux and gastric ulceration and preserve the tissue aeration useful to increase the efficacy of yttrium radiations and its killing potency.
- Recommended TheraSphere® Dose to the liver is 80–150 Gy (nominal 120 Gy); dose adjustments may be necessary based on patient characteristics: perfused liver volume, lesion size and location, tumour radiopharmaceutical uptake, healthy liver radiopharmaceutical uptake, LSF and treatment window.
- The TheraSphere supply 35 dose size options to choose between 3 GBq and 20 GBq in 0.5 GBq increments.
- The glass spheres can be used to downstage HCC and bridge to transplantation and in the palliative setting for BCLC B patients (refractory or intolerant to TACE), BCLC B or C patients (large tumours, multifocal disease) and BCLC C patients (with PVT).
- The relationship between the ^{99m}Tc-MAA SPECT-based tumour absorbed dose and tumour response is reported, allowing the possibilities of treatment optimization by individualized ^{99m}Tc-MAA SPECT-based dose planning.

References

1. GLOBOCAN. Liver Cancer. Estimated incidence, mortality and prevalence worldwide in 2012. 2012. http://globocan.iarc.fr/old/FactSheets/cancers/liver-new.asp. Accessed 10 Sept 2015.
2. European Association for the Study of the Liver, European Organisation for Research and Treatment of Cancer. EASL-EORTC clinical practice guidelines: management of hepatocellular carcinoma. J Hepatol. 2012;56(4):908–43.
3. Atassi B, Bangash AK, Bahrani A, et al. Multimodality imaging following 90Y radioembolization: a comprehensive review and pictorial essay. Radiographics. 2008;28(1):81–99.
4. Llovet JM, Di Bisceglie AM, Bruix J, et al. Design and endpoints of clinical trials in hepatocellular carcinoma. J Natl Cancer Inst. 2008;100(10):698–711.
5. Yang T, Lau WY, Zhang H, et al. Grey zone in the Barcelona Clinic Liver Cancer Classification for hepatocellular carcinoma: surgeons' perspective. World J Gastroenterol. 2015;21(27):8256–61.
6. National Comprehensive Cancer Network. NCCN practice guidelines in oncology. Hepatobiliary cancers, V2.2015.
7. Salem R, Lewandowski RJ, Kulik L, et al. Radioembolization results in longer time-to-progression and reduced toxicity compared with chemoembolization in patients with hepatocellular carcinoma. Gastroenterology. 2011;140(2):497–507.
8. Lewandowski RJ, Kulik LM, Riaz A, et al. A comparative analysis of transarterial downstag-

ing for hepatocellular carcinoma: chemoembolization versus radioembolization. Am J Transplant. 2009;9(8):1920–8.
9. Riaz A, Gates VL, Atassi B, et al. Radiation segmentectomy: a novel approach to increase safety and efficacy of radioembolization. Int J Radiat Oncol Biol Phys. 2011;79(1):163–71.
10. Vouche M, Habib A, Ward TJ, et al. Unresectable solitary hepatocellular carcinoma not amenable to radiofrequency ablation: multicenter radiology-pathology correlation and survival of radiation segmentectomy. Hepatology. 2014;60(1):192–201.
11. Hilgard P, Hamami M, Fouly AE, et al. Radioembolization with yttrium-90 glass microspheres in hepatocellular carcinoma: European experience on safety and long-term survival. Hepatology. 2010;52(5):1741.
12. Salem R, Lewandowski RJ, Mulcahy MF, et al. Radioembolization for hepatocellular carcinoma using Yttrium-90 microspheres: a comprehensive report of long-term outcomes. Gastroenterology. 2010;138(1):52–64.
13. Mazzaferro V, Sposito C, Bhoori S, Romito R, Chiesa C, Morosi C, Maccauro M, Marchiano A, Bongini M, Lanocita R, Civelli E, Bombardieri E, Camerini T, Spreafico C. Yttrium90 radioembolization for intermediate-advanced hepatocarcinoma: a phase II study. Hepatology. 2013;57:1826–37.
14. Garin E, Lenoir L, Rolland Y, Edeline J, Mesbah H, Laffont S, et al. Dosimetry based on 99mTc-macroaggregated albumin SPECT/CT accurately predicts tumor response and survival in hepatocellular carcinoma patients treated with 90Y-loaded glass microspheres: preliminary results. J Nucl Med. 2012;53:255–63.
15. Chiesa C, Mira M, Maccauro M, Spreafico C, Romito R, et al. Radioembolization of hepatocarcinoma with (90)Y glass microspheres: development of an individualized treatment planning strategy based on dosimetry and radiobiology. Eur J Nucl Med Mol Imaging. 2015;42(11):1718–38. https://doi.org/10.1007/s00259-015-3068-8. (Epub 2015 Jun 27)
16. Garin E, Lenoir L, Edeline J, Laffont S, Mesbah H, Porée P, et al. Boosted selective internal radiation therapy with 90Y-loaded glass microspheres (B-SIRT) for hepatocellular carcinoma patients: a new personalized promising concept. Eur J Nucl Med Mol Imaging. 2013;40:1057–68. https://doi.org/10.1007/s00259-013-2395-x.

HCC Radioembolization with Yttrium-90 Polymer Beads (SIR-Spheres)

12

Marcello Rodari and Riccardo Muglia

Abstract

Introduction: Transarterial radioembolization (TARE) is a form of brachytherapy in which microspheres loaded with the radioactive isotope yttrium-90 (^{90}Y) are injected selectively to the tumor-feeding arteries through a catheter using fluoroscopic guidance. The use of ^{90}Y microspheres leads to tumor necrosis by delivering a high radiation dose (>70 Gy, tumoricidal threshold) directly to HCC nodules, sparing the non-tumoral liver, and with little or no embolic effect on the vessels. Resin ^{90}Y microspheres are 20–60 μm in size, carry approximately 50 Bq/sphere, and contain 40–80 million microspheres per 3 GBq (1 vial).

Indications: TARE is a suitable first-line therapy for intermediate-stage patients with locally advanced disease and those who are poor candidates for transarterial chemoembolization (TACE). Surgery and thermal ablation are precluded due to lesion size or amount. TARE is a valid treatment option also for patients with HCC and portal vein tumor thrombosis (PVTT), which is commonly recognized as a relative contraindication to other transarterial therapies.

Selection Criteria: To be considered for TARE, patients with HCC should have liver-only or liver-dominant disease, a life expectancy >12 weeks, and ECOG performance status <2 or Karnofsky performance index ≥60%. Preserved liver function is essential. Kidney function and blood coagulation are other important parameters to assess.

Administration: The majority of TAREs are performed by calculating the injected activity based on empiric formulas suggested by the manufac

M. Rodari (✉)
Department of Nuclear Medicine, Humanitas Research Hospital, Rozzano, Italy
e-mail: marcello.rodari@cancercenter.humanitas.it

R. Muglia
Resident in Radiology,
Humanitas University, Pieve Emanuele, Italy
e-mail: riccardo.muglia@humanitas.it

E. Bombardieri et al. (eds.), *Clinical Applications of Nuclear Medicine Targeted Therapy*,
https://doi.org/10.1007/978-3-319-63067-0_12

turers instead of following a scrupulous dosimetric algorithm. Three methods of activity estimation are suggested in the manufacturer's user manual for resin microspheres: body surface area (BSA), empiric, and partition.

Pre-TARE Imaging: HCC can be evaluated through different techniques: US, contrast-enhanced CT, and contrast-enhanced MRI (gold standard for HCC nodules).

Treatment Procedure: All patients scheduled for TARE have to undergo initial hepatic and gastrointestinal angiography to evaluate the amount of resin microspheres that could inadvertently pass from the artery site of injection to the systemic blood circulation. During angiography, contrast media is administered intra-arterially followed by administration of 150 MBq of ^{99m}technetium-labeled macroaggregated albumin (^{99}Tc; eluted in 5 mL of saline; ^{99}Tc-MAA) at the same site. The ^{99}Tc-MAA microparticles act as good surrogate for ^{90}Y resin microspheres due to the similarities in average diameter and density. One hour after administration of ^{99}Tc, a SPECT is performed in order to assess the percentage of radioactive spheres shunted to the systemic circulation, particularly to the lungs and extrahepatic abdominal organs. Patients may undergo TARE only if <20% of ^{99}TC albumin macroaggregates are shunted to the lungs and if the ^{90}Y dose does not exceed 30 Gy in single administration or 50 Gy in cumulative doses for all planned infusions. TARE is then performed retracing the tumor-feeding arteries and administering the ^{90}Y resin microspheres.

Follow-up: Follow-up comprises a complete liver function test, a complete blood count, tumor marker analysis, and contrast-enhanced CT 40 or 60 days after TARE.

Post-procedural Assessments: Radionecrosis is demonstrated by a hypointense area with absence of contrast enhancement on CT. Response is classified according to modified Response Evaluation Criteria in Solid Tumors (mRECIST).

Adverse Events: The most common adverse event experienced by patients following TARE is postembolization syndrome (PES), which encompasses symptoms of nausea, vomiting, fatigue, fever, and mild abdominal pain, especially in the right hypochondrium. Rare but serious complications of TARE have been reported and include gastrointestinal ulceration/bleeding, cholecystitis, pancreatitis, and radiation pneumonitis.

Conclusions: To summarize, TARE is a well-tolerated procedure that shows comparable or better outcomes and toxicities to those reported for other intra-arterial therapies.

12.1 Introduction

Hepatocellular carcinoma (HCC) is the most common primary tumor of the liver and by its nature is sensitive to radiotherapy. To obtain a tumoricidal effect with conventional external beam radiotherapy, the radiation dose administered should exceed 70 Gy [1]. However, at an administered radiation dose over 35 Gy [2], liver parenchyma starts showing severe harmful effects such as anicteric hepatomegaly, elevated liver enzymes, and ascites occurring between 2 weeks and 3 months after irradiation [3]. Hence, external beam radiotherapy has historically played a very limited role in the treatment of patients with HCC and is rarely considered a treatment option for this patient population.

Transarterial radioembolization (TARE; also known as selective internal radiation therapy) is a form of brachytherapy in which microspheres loaded with the radioactive isotope yttrium-90 (^{90}Y) are injected selectively to the tumor-feeding arteries through a catheter using fluoroscopic guidance. ^{90}Y is a beta radiation emitter with a short half-life (2.67 days) and short-range penetration in human tissue (mean 2.5 mm, maximum 11 mm) [4].

The use of ^{90}Y microspheres leads to tumor necrosis by delivering a high radiation dose (>70 Gy, tumoricidal threshold) directly to HCC nodules, sparing the non-tumoral liver, and with little or no embolic effect on the vessels [5].

Two types of microspheres loaded with ^{90}Y are available and are either made from resin (SIR-Spheres®; Sirtex Medical Limited, North Sydney, NSW, Australia) or glass (TheraSpheres®, MDS Nordion, Toronto, Ontario, Canada) [6]. This section reviews the use of resin microspheres for the administration of ^{90}Y TARE in patients with HCC. Resin ^{90}Y microspheres are 20–60 μm in size, carry approximately 50 Bq/sphere, and contain 40–80 million microspheres per 3 GBq (1 vial) [4].

Once the ^{90}Y microspheres are injected, they lodge within the tumor-feeding arteries (whose diameter is approximately 50 μm), where they become entrapped and deliver their therapeutic effect via radiation necrosis.

12.2 Indications

According to the Barcelona Clinic Liver Cancer (BCLC) staging classification, TARE is a suitable first-line therapy for intermediate-stage patients with locally advanced disease and those who are poor candidates for transarterial chemoembolization (TACE). In these patients, surgery is typically precluded due to lesion size or amount, and thermal ablation is usually unsuitable for the same reasons.

Clinical evidence supports TARE as a valid treatment option, particularly for patients with HCC and portal vein tumor thrombosis (PVTT), which is commonly recognized as a relative contraindication to other transarterial therapies [7]. Moreover, results from several new studies have suggested that TARE could be useful for downstaging patients classified slightly outside the criteria for liver transplantation [8] and can also be applied as a second-line treatment in patients with progressive disease following TACE or sorafenib [4].

However, there are four main contraindications for the use of TARE in patients with HCC: (1) excessive amounts of arteriovenous shunts in the liver; (2) pre-assessment angiogram demonstrating abnormal vascular anatomy that would result in significant reflux of hepatic arterial blood to the stomach, pancreas, or bowel; (3) pregnancy or breastfeeding; and (4) use of capecitabine within 8 weeks before TARE [9].

12.3 Selection Criteria

Employing an interdisciplinary team to evaluate candidates is crucial during the selection of eligible patients for TARE [4]. Clinical members of the interdisciplinary team are usually interventional radiologists; nuclear medicine physicians; hepatologists; medical, surgical, and radiation oncologists; and transplant surgeons [4].

To be considered for TARE, patients with HCC should have liver-only or liver-dominant disease, a life expectancy >12 weeks, and ECOG performance status <2 or Karnofsky performance index ≥60% [10, 11]. Moreover, preserved liver function is essential; in particular, it is important to maintain bilirubin below 2 mg/dL, aspartate aminotransferase (AST) and alanine aminotransferase (ALT) less than five times normal values, and albumin above 3 g/dL [11]. Kidney function (creatinine) and blood coagulation (platelets, international normalized ratio) are other important parameters to assess in a patient under consideration for TARE [11].

On the other hand, the presence of ascites (or other signs of clear liver failure) is a categorical exclusion criterion, whereas additional exclusion criteria can be debated on a case-by-case basis: (1) previous radiation therapy to the liver, (2) excessive tumor burden with limited hepatic reserve, (3) abnormal bone marrow function (leukocytes <2500/dL; absolute neutrophil count <1500/dL; platelet count <60,000/dL), (4) abnormal liver function (according to AST and ALT >5× normal, bilirubin >2 mg/dL with absence of evident cause, and albumin <3 g/dL), and (5) creatinine >2.5 mg/dL. A combination of any of the aforementioned relative exclusion criteria can dramatically increase the risk of severe complications [10, 11].

12.4 Administration

The administered radiation dose corresponds to the activity of the injected microspheres and to the distribution of these microspheres in different tissues [4]. Calculation of required activity, tailored for every treatment, is therefore a crucial aspect of dosimetric planning and delivery of TARE. However, dose optimization is frequently unattainable [4]. For this reason, the majority of TAREs are performed by calculating the injected activity based on empiric formulas suggested by the manufacturers instead of following a scrupulous dosimetric algorithm.

Three methods of activity estimation are suggested in the manufacturer's user manual for resin microspheres: body surface area (BSA), empiric, and partition (Table 12.1) [12].

In some cases, the BSA method and empiric method may overestimate the radiation dose that can be delivered to the patient [13], while the partition method can determine absorbed dose with a satisfying accuracy [14], although the latter method has been misapplied on occasion. Therefore, none of these methods is the "best" option for calculating the optimal administered radiation dose, rather clinical skills and personal experience of the clinician serve as important guides in reaching the best decision for the patient.

12.5 Pre-TARE Imaging

Preoperative imaging assessment is central to the success of the TARE procedure. Ultrasound (US) is the first-line strategy for evaluation of an HCC nodule. This technique is widespread, and rapidity of access renders US suitable for first detection or follow-up after diagnosis.

HCC is typically visualized as an iso-hypoechoic round nodule under US, usually in a pattern of cirrhotic liver [15]. Major limitations of US, however, are low sensitivity in operators with limited experience and bowel gas superimposition. In B-mode US, detection sensitivity is around 60–70% [16]. Techniques such as color Doppler, power Doppler, or contrast-enhanced ultrasound (CEUS) have been invaluable in enhancing US detection rates [17].

Nevertheless, US is not an ideal sole technique for diagnosing HCC and should be accompanied in a stepwise process by computed tomography (CT) and/or magnetic resonance imaging (MRI). Biphasic imaging of the liver in both arterial and portal venous phases can be considered as the standard CT protocol in current diagnostic strategies [12], although literature suggests that CT may be somewhat inferior for detecting and characterizing malignant nodules (especially

Table 12.1 Methods of microsphere activity estimation

Method	Formula
BSA	BSA calculation: BSA [m^2] = 0.20247 × (height [m])$^{0.725}$ × (weight [kg])$^{0.425}$ GBq to administer: A [GBq]$_{resin}$ = (BSA − 0.2) + (% of tumor involvement/100)
Empiric	Relates tumor burden to LTM, estimated by CT triphasic scan: Tumor <25% of LTM = 2 GBq whole liver delivery Tumor 25%< x <50% of LTM = 2.5 GBq whole liver delivery Tumor >50% of LTM = 3 GBq whole liver delivery
Partition	Tissue radiation dose [Gy] = (49670 × total ^{90}Y activity in liver [GBq])/mass of liver [g]

CT computed tomography, *LTM* total mass of the liver

for nodules <1 cm in size) when compared with gadolinium-enhanced MRI [18]. The characteristic appearance of HCC under contrast-enhanced CT is a solid nodule, sometimes accompanied by little satellites, which is iso- or hypodense to surrounding parenchyma [19]. As contrast media enters the liver, HCC lesions demonstrate a quick wash-in in the arterial phase, followed by a quick washout in later phases as a result of prevalent arterial hypervascularization.

Currently, MRI is the gold standard imaging for detecting and characterizing HCC nodules. MRI provides good image quality together with the advantages of the availability of multiple sequences and contrast agents. However, notable limitations of MRI are motion or respiratory artifacts (frequent in uncooperative patients [20]) and longer time to image acquisition compared with CT. HCC behavior on T1-weighted (T1W) MRI sequences is dependent on its fibrous content, whereas mild hyperintensity is observed for HCC malignancies on T2-weighted (T2W) sequences [21].

Two types of liver-specific contrast agents are available for use with MRI: (1) iron-oxide particles target Kupffer cells and lead to a decreased intensity in the appearance of normal liver on T2W sequences; and (2) hepatobiliary contrast agents target hepatocytes, thereby enhancing the signal of liver and benign lesions on T1W images [22]. Following contrast media application, HCC nodules appear hyperintense with iron-oxide contrast agents and hypointense with hepatobiliary contrast media [22, 23].

12.6 Treatment Procedure

The aim of treatment with TARE is to inject radioactive microspheres into selected hepatic arteries in order to enable accumulation near to or within HCC lesions and to facilitate consequent radionecrosis. It is imperative that resin microspheres are concentrated in the nodule, thereby avoiding systemic migration.

Liver vascular anatomy is extremely variable and therefore the possibility of arteriovenous shunts is high. Hence, all patients scheduled for TARE have to undergo initial hepatic and gastrointestinal angiography to evaluate the amount of resin microspheres that could inadvertently pass from the artery site of injection to the systemic blood circulation. Lung shunting of (2–7 GBq of Y^{90} microspheres could result in radiation pneumonitis and other side effects [24].

During angiography, contrast media is administered intra-arterially followed by administration of 150 MBq of ^{99m}technetium-labeled macroaggregated albumin (^{99}Tc; eluted in 5 mL of saline; ^{99}Tc-MAA) at the same site (Figs. 12.1 and 12.2).

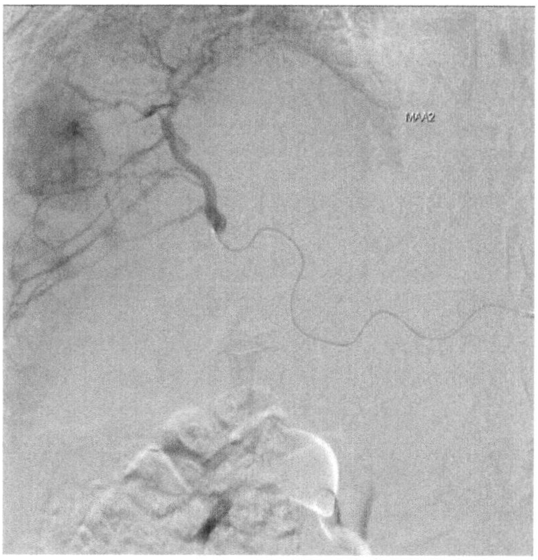

Fig. 12.1 ^{99}Tc-MAA injection site in right hepatic artery. Angiography did not show any aberrant vascularization

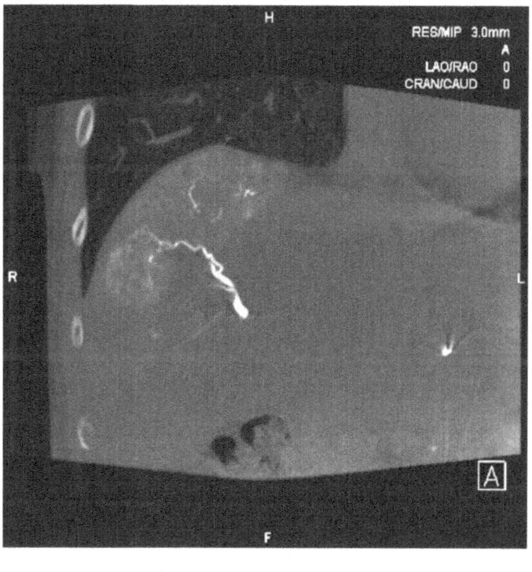

Fig. 12.2 ^{99}Tc-MAA injection site in right hepatic artery. An intraprocedural Cone Beam CT did not show any aberrant vascularization

As the only preoperative procedure, a vial of potassium perchlorate is given 1 hour before angiography to saturate iodine receptors and therefore avoid false-positive accumulations of the radiopharmaceuticalf.

The ^{99}Tc-MAA microparticles act as good surrogate for ^{90}Y resin microspheres due to the similarities in average diameter 20–40 μm and 30–35 μm, respectively, and density 1.3 g/cm^3 and 1.6 g/cm^3, respectively. Although the number of ^{99}Tc-MAA microparticles and ^{90}Y resin microspheres injected is markedly different, it is reasonable to assume the distribution of the two microparticle types will be similar within the liver and tumor compartments [25]. Several studies have shown that the intrahepatic distribution of ^{99}Tc-MAA is correlated with intrahepatic distribution of ^{90}Y resin microspheres [24–28]. There is a good correlation between intended tumor mean doses determined from ^{99}Tc-MAA angiography and actual delivered doses of ^{90}Y resin microspheres, and the dose-response relationship for ^{90}Y resin microspheres has been demonstrated [29, 30] (Fig. 12.5).

Therefore, 1 hour after administration of ^{99}Tc, a SPECT is performed in order to assess the percentage of radioactive spheres shunted to the systemic circulation, particularly to the lungs and extrahepatic abdominal organs (Figs. 12.3, 12.4 and 12.5). It is important to occlude eventual aberrant arteries with embolizing agents to prevent radionecrosis of nontarget tissues [31]. The use of ^{99}Tc also enables calculation of the total pulmonary dose. Consequently, patients may undergo TARE only if <20% of ^{99}TC albumin macroaggregates

Fig. 12.3 Total body planar scintigraphy shows ^{99}Tc-MAA uptake in the right lobe of liver

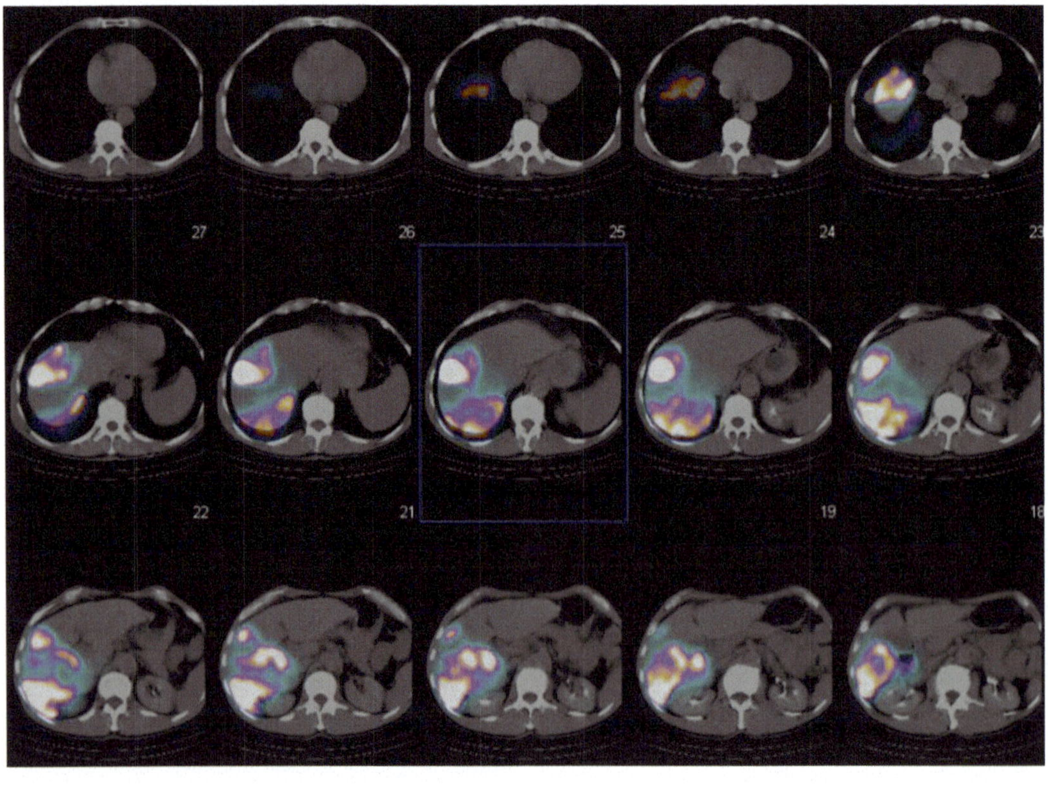

Fig. 12.4 A SPECT-CT confirming the uptake in the right lobe of liver, without extrahepatic deposition of particles

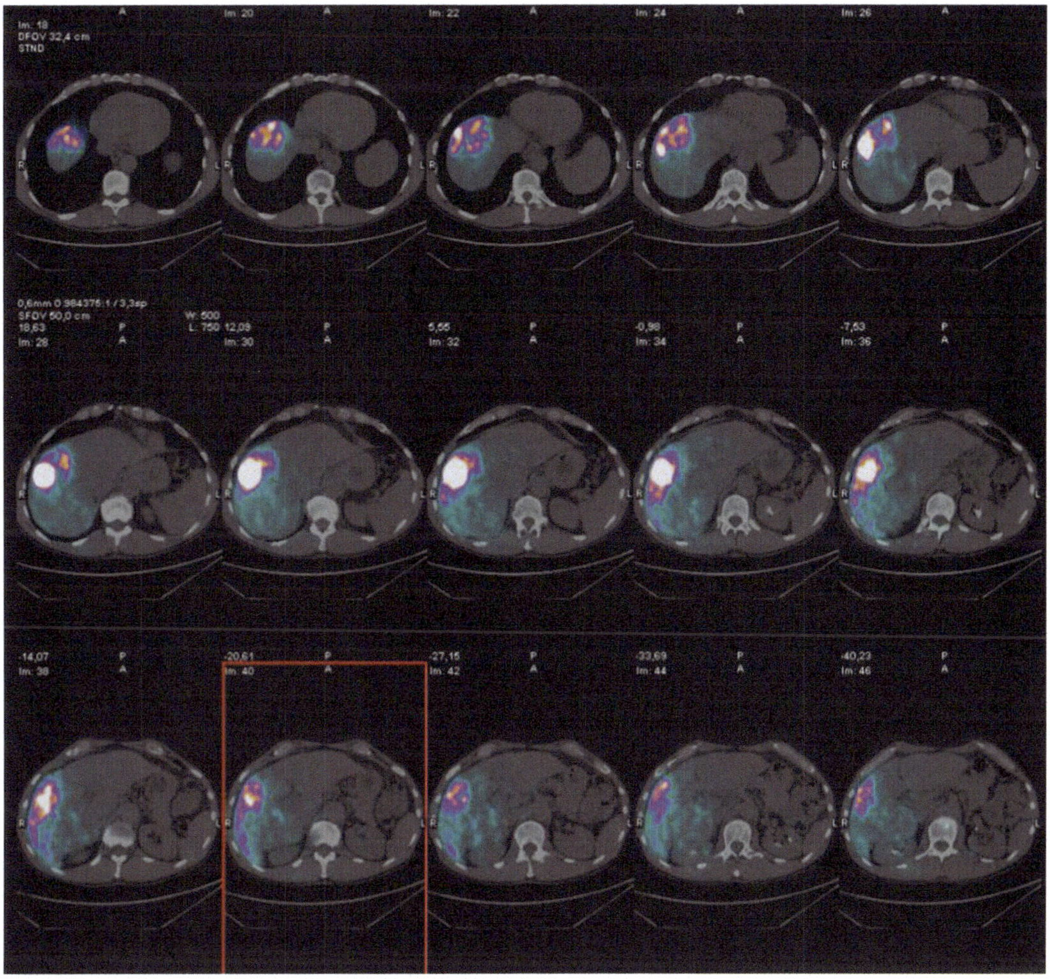

Fig. 12.5 90Y-SIR-Spheres biodistribution PET/TC image confirms high uptake in VIII hepatic segment lesion

are shunted to the lungs and if the ^{90}Y dose does not exceed 30 Gy in single administration or 50 Gy in cumulative doses for all planned infusions [14, 32]. As soon as technically feasible after angiography, TARE is performed by the same operator, who retraces the tumor-feeding arteries previously visualized during angiography and administers the ^{90}Y resin microspheres.

12.7 Follow-Up

Follow-up comprises a complete liver function test, a complete blood count, tumor marker analysis, and contrast-enhanced CT [4] 40 or 60 days after TARE. If treatment is successful, a contrast-enhanced CT is performed every 3 months. On the other hand, a new TARE can be rescheduled at least 6 months later if follow-up analyses show incomplete radioembolization of HCC lesions.

In recent years, more attention has been directed toward new techniques for pre- or post-treatment assessment. For example, the functional and metabolic, rather than anatomic, information provided by diffusion-weighted MRI and choline positron emission tomography has resulted in increasing use of these methods in patients. More studies need to be performed, but preliminary data are encouraging for the inclusion of these newer techniques for follow-up assessment of TARE-treated patients [33, 34].

12.8 Post-procedural Assessments

Response to TARE is assessed with contrast-enhanced CT in patients with HCC and is generally performed 40–60 days after the procedure. Radionecrosis is demonstrated by a hypointense area with absence of contrast enhancement. Response is classified according to modified Response Evaluation Criteria in Solid Tumors (mRECIST): (a) complete response, the disappearance of any intratumoral arterial enhancement in all target lesions; (b) partial response, at least a 30% decrease in the sum of diameters of viable (contrast enhancement in the arterial phase) target lesions, taking as reference the baseline sum of the diameters of target lesions; (c) progressive disease, an increase of at least 20% in the sum of the diameters of viable (enhancing) target lesions, taking as reference the smallest sum of the diameters of viable (enhancing) target lesions recorded since the treatment started; and (d) stable disease, any cases that do not qualify for either partial response or progressive disease [35, 36] (Figs. 12.6 and 12.7).

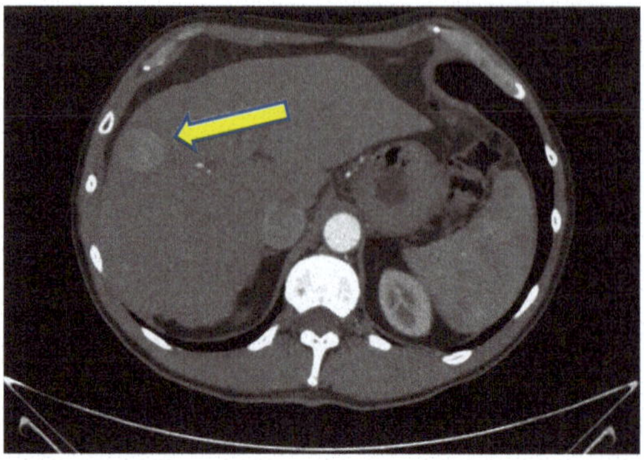

Fig. 12.6 CT performed before a SIR therapy demonstrates a large hypervascular nodule and adjacent satellites

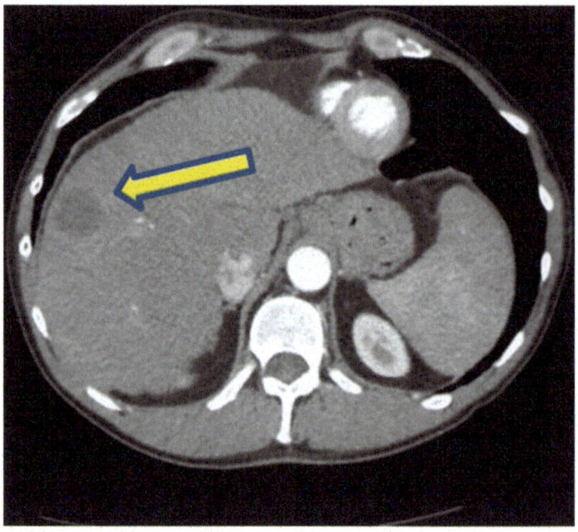

Fig. 12.7 CT performed 45 days after SIR therapy demonstrates full radiological response of the large nodule and adjacent satellites

12.9 Adverse Events

The most common adverse event experienced by patients following TARE is postembolization syndrome (PES), which encompasses symptoms of nausea, vomiting, fatigue, fever, and mild abdominal pain, especially in the right hypochondrium [37]. Depending on the administering center, a combination of paracetamol, ketorolac, and metoclopramide may be given minutes before the embolization, in order to relieve symptoms of PES. Laboratory toxicities associated with TARE include derangements of alkaline phosphatase, albumin, and transaminases [37]. Rare but serious complications of TARE have been reported and include gastrointestinal ulceration/bleeding, cholecystitis, pancreatitis, and radiation pneumonitis [38]. Most of these serious events occur when microspheres are inadvertently deposited in excessive amounts in organs other than the liver, but the risk of such complications can be minimized or avoided with accurate patient selection and meticulous pretreatment dose assessments [39].

Conclusions

To gain maximum clinical benefit from TARE, four fundamental management aspects should be borne in mind: (1) selection of the right patient, (2) pretreatment angiography or embolization and SPECT evaluation, (3) dose assessment, and (4) appropriate follow-up.

To summarize, TARE is a well-tolerated procedure that shows comparable or better outcomes and toxicities [40, 41] to those reported for other intra-arterial therapies.

References

1. Dawson LA, et al. Escalated focal liver radiation and concurrent hepatic artery fluorodeoxyuridine for unresectable intrahepatic malignancies. J Clin Oncol. 2000;18:2210–8.
2. Lawrence TS, et al. Hepatic toxicity resulting from cancer treatment. Int J Radiat Oncol Biol Phys. 1995;31:1237–48.
3. Klein J, Dawson LA. Hepatocellular carcinoma radiation therapy: review of evidence and future opportunities. Int J Radiat Oncol Biol Phys. 2013;87: 22–32.
4. Cappelli A, Pettinato C, Golfieri R. Transarterial radioembolization using yttrium-90 microspheres in the treatment of hepatocellular carcinoma: a review on clinical utility and developments. J Hepatocell Carcinoma. 2014;1:163–82.
5. Bilbao JI, et al. Biocompatibility, inflammatory response, and recannalization characteristics of non-radioactive resin microspheres: histological findings. Cardiovasc Intervent Radiol. 2009;32:727–36.
6. Sato K, et al. Treatment of unresectable primary and metastatic liver cancer with yttrium-90 microspheres (TheraSphere): assessment of hepatic arterial embolization. Cardiovasc Intervent Radiol. 2006;29:522–9.
7. Lau W-Y, et al. Treatment for hepatocellular carcinoma with portal vein tumor thrombosis: the emerging role for radioembolization using yttrium-90. Oncology. 2013;84:311–8.
8. Parikh ND, Waljee AK, Singal AG. Downstaging hepatocellular carcinoma: a systematic review and pooled analysis. Liver Transpl. 2015;21:1142–52.
9. Murthy R, Kamat P, Nuñez R, Salem R. Radioembolization of yttrium-90 microspheres for hepatic malignancy. Semin Interv Radiol. 2008;25:48–57.
10. Kennedy A, et al. Recommendations for radioembolization of hepatic malignancies using yttrium-90 microsphere brachytherapy: a consensus panel report from the radioembolization brachytherapy oncology consortium. Int J Radiat Oncol Biol Phys. 2007;68:13–23.
11. Hoffmann R-T, Jakobs TF, Reiser MF. In: Bilbao JI, Reiser MF, editors. Liver radioembolization with 90Y microspheres. Heidelberg: Springer; 2008. p. 11–4. https://doi.org/10.1007/978-3-540-35423-9_2.
12. Bilbao JI, Reiser MF, editors. Medical radiology. Heidelberg: Springer; 2014. https://doi.org/10.1007/978-3-642-36473-0.
13. Kennedy AS, et al. Dose selection of resin 90Y-microspheres for liver brachytherapy: a single center review. Brachytherapy. 2006;5:103–4.
14. Ho S, et al. Clinical evaluation of the partition model for estimating radiation doses from yttrium-90 microspheres in the treatment of hepatic cancer. Eur J Nucl Med. 1997;24:293–8.
15. Badea R, Ioanitescu S. In: Julianov A, editor. Liver tumors. Rijeka: InTech; 2012. https://doi.org/10.5772/31137.
16. Choi BI, et al. Small hepatocellular carcinoma: detection with sonography, computed tomography (CT), angiography and Lipiodol-CT. Br J Radiol. 1989;62:897–903.
17. Hosoki T, et al. Visualization of tumor vessels in hepatocellular carcinoma. Power Doppler compared with color Doppler and angiography. Acta Radiol. 1997;38:422–7.
18. Semelka RC, Martin DR, Balci C, Lance T. Focal liver lesions: comparison of dual-phase CT and multisequence multiplanar MR imaging including dynamic gadolinium enhancement. J Magn Reson Imaging. 2001;13:397–401.
19. Cartier V, Aubé C. Diagnosis of hepatocellular carcinoma. Diagn Interv Imaging. 2014;95:709–19.
20. Kim BS, Lee KR, Goh MJ. New imaging strategies using a motion-resistant liver sequence in uncooperative patients. Biomed Res Int. 2014;2014:142658.
21. Hennedige T, Venkatesh SK. Imaging of hepatocellular carcinoma: diagnosis, staging and treatment monitoring. Cancer Imaging. 2013;12:530–47.
22. Kim SH, Lee WJ, Lim HK, Park CK. SPIO-enhanced MRI findings of well-differentiated hepatocellular carcinomas: correlation with MDCT findings. Korean J Radiol. 2009;10:112–20.
23. Albiin N. MRI of focal liver lesions. Curr Med Imaging Rev. 2012;8:107–16.
24. Ho S, et al. Partition model for estimating radiation doses from yttrium-90 microspheres in treating hepatic tumours. Eur J Nucl Med. 1996;23:947–52.
25. Gulec SA, Mesoloras G, Dezarn WA, McNeillie P, Kennedy AS. Safety and efficacy of Y-90 microsphere treatment in patients with primary and metastatic liver cancer: the tumor selectivity of the treatment as a function of tumor to liver flow ratio. J Transl Med. 2007;5:15.
26. Lau WY, et al. Diagnostic pharmaco-scintigraphy with hepatic intra-arterial technetium-99m macroaggregated albumin in the determination of tumour to non-tumour uptake ratio in hepatocellular carcinoma. Br J Radiol. 1994;67:136–9.
27. Cremonesi M, et al. Radioembolisation with 90Y-microspheres: dosimetric and radiobiological investigation for multi-cycle treatment. Eur J Nucl Med Mol Imaging. 2008;35:2088–96.
28. Campbell JM, et al. Early dose response to yttrium-90 microsphere treatment of metastatic liver cancer by a patient-specific method using single photon emission computed tomography and positron emission tomography. Int J Radiat Oncol Biol Phys. 2009;74:313–20.
29. Kao YH, et al. Image-guided personalized predictive dosimetry by artery-specific SPECT/CT partition modeling for safe and effective 90Y radioembolization. J Nucl Med. 2012;53:559–66.
30. Kao Y-H, et al. Post-radioembolization yttrium-90 PET/CT – part 2: dose-response and tumor predictive dosimetry for resin microspheres. EJNMMI Res. 2013;3:57.
31. Covey AM, Brody LA, Maluccio MA, Getrajdman GI, Brown KT. Variant hepatic arterial anatomy revisited: digital subtraction angiography performed in 600 patients. Radiology. 2002;224:542–7.
32. Mosconi C, Cappelli A, Pettinato C, Golfieri R. Radioembolization with Yttrium-90 microspheres

in hepatocellular carcinoma: role and perspectives. World J Hepatol. 2015;7:738–52.
33. Schelhorn J, et al. Does diffusion-weighted imaging improve therapy response evaluation in patients with hepatocellular carcinoma after radioembolization? Comparison of MRI using Gd-EOB-DTPA with and without DWI. J Magn Reson Imaging. 2015;42:818–27.
34. Hartenbach M, et al. Evaluating treatment response of radioembolization in intermediate-stage hepatocellular carcinoma patients using 18F-fluoroethylcholine PET/CT. J Nucl Med. 2015;56:1661–6.
35. Lencioni R, Llovet JM. Modified RECIST (mRECIST) assessment for hepatocellular carcinoma. Semin Liver Dis. 2010;30:52–60.
36. Seyal AR, et al. Reproducibility of mRECIST in assessing response to transarterial radioembolization therapy in hepatocellular carcinoma. Hepatology. 2015;62:1111–21.
37. Bhangoo MS, et al. Radioembolization with Yttrium-90 microspheres for patients with unresectable hepatocellular carcinoma. J Gastrointest Oncol. 2015;6:469–78.
38. Vente MAD, et al. Yttrium-90 microsphere radioembolization for the treatment of liver malignancies: a structured meta-analysis. Eur Radiol. 2009;19:951–9.
39. Salem R, et al. Technical aspects of radioembolization with 90Y microspheres. Tech Vasc Interv Radiol. 2007;10:12–29.
40. Kooby DA, et al. Comparison of yttrium-90 radioembolization and transcatheter arterial chemoembolization for the treatment of unresectable hepatocellular carcinoma. J Vasc Interv Radiol. 2010;21:224–30.
41. Carr BI, Kondragunta V, Buch SC, Branch RA. Therapeutic equivalence in survival for hepatic arterial chemoembolization and yttrium 90 microsphere treatments in unresectable hepatocellular carcinoma: a two-cohort study. Cancer. 2010;116:1305–14.

13 Dosimetry in the Treatment of Liver Malignancies with Microspheres

Carlo Chiesa

Abstract

The goal and the importance of dosimetry in the treatment of liver malignancies with radioactive microspheres are presented. A single acquisition is enough to provide the necessary information for the dosimetric calculations. This unique feature among all the other radiopharmaceuticals, together with the initial indications about the clinical impact of absorbed dose calculation, manifests in two interesting new phenomena in nuclear medicine therapy. From one side, dosimetry in radioembolization is adopted to plan the treatment in many more centers with respect to all the other radiopharmaceuticals. Second, this is the first and unique kind of therapy where all the microsphere producers are undertaking substantial efforts in order to implement dosimetry. This kind of dosimetry is extremely simple from the side of the technical methodology and on that of the calculation. The only problem is the potential discrepancy between the simulator particles (^{99m}Tc-MAA or trace administration of ^{166}Ho microspheres) and the actual distribution of therapeutic particles.

13.1 Goal and Importance of Dosimetry in Radioembolization

The first remarkable issue of dosimetry in radioembolization is that it can be performed before the treatment, differently from many other important agents (radiopeptides, mIBG), where this is either impossible or impractical. This possibility, given by the simulator (^{99m}Tc-macro aggregates of albumine, ^{99m}Tc-MAA), enlightens the main goal of dosimetry in general: optimize the treatment. The application of the optimization principle to nuclear medicine therapy as a kind of radiation therapy was already required by the directive EURATOM 97/43 and inserted in the national laws of the member countries. The new directive 2013/59, to be translated in the national legislation within 6th February 2018, renews the requirement of optimization. Moreover, it explicitly adds the need of post-therapy verification of absorbed dose to target and nontarget

C. Chiesa
Nuclear Medicine, Foundation IRCCS Istituto Nazionale Tumori, Milan, Italy
e-mail: Carlo.Chiesa@istitutotumori.mi.it

E. Bombardieri et al. (eds.), *Clinical Applications of Nuclear Medicine Targeted Therapy*,
https://doi.org/10.1007/978-3-319-63067-0_13

volumes. Both these evaluations are possible with microspheres.

The possibility of predicting the absorbed dose to lesions and to non-tumoral tissue is extremely important in this kind of treatments since, in most of patients, therapy is intended to be delivered in a single administration, except in case of bilobar disease or recurrence. By sure microsphere therapy is not conceived as a sequence of repeated administrations like radioiodine for metastatic differentiated thyroid cancer or radiopeptides for neuroendocrine tumors. As mentioned previously [1], the importance of treatment planning goes in parallel with the aggressiveness of the disease, measured in overall survival (OS) or progression-free survival (PFS). This factor usually leads also to the aggressiveness of the therapy. In thyroid carcinoma, the median OS is of the order of decades, even without radioiodine administration, with a reduction to about 5 years for cases with distant metastases [2]. Patients with somatostatin-receptor-positive advanced midgut neuroendocrine tumors show PFS of about 8 months if treated with non-radiolabeled octreotide, while median PSF after ^{177}Lu-DOTATATE-repeated administrations was not reached yet at 28 months (more than 2 years) [3]. In both these classes of tumors, there is plenty time to repeat several therapeutic administrations. In my center experience, cases with more than ten repetitions are known, both with thyroid cancer and neuroendocrine tumor. There is also a broad safety margin for repetition, since, with the fixed activity schedule presently adopted, hematological toxicity is uncommon and reversible [3], and the only other potential toxicity is the irreversible renal impairment, only after ^{90}Y-DOTATOC administration [4] and not after ^{177}Lu-DOTATATE [5].

For liver neoplasm the overall survival is different. In patients affected by unresectable colorectal cancer liver metastases, the median OS is 6–12 months if the patients are not treated and improves to 18–24 months after chemotherapy. In the SHARP trial for advanced primary hepatocarcinoma (HCC) patients, the median overall survival was 7.9 months (placebo group) and 10.7 months after biological therapy with sorafenib, which became the standard of care thanks to that trial [6]. Radioembolization is delivered only once to the largest majority of patients. In the prospective phase II study accomplished in the National Tumor Institute of Milan, only 6 HCC patients over 52 (11%) received a second administration [7]. A third administration is reported in the literature but is extremely rare. The possibility of repeating several microsphere administration is prevented both by the lack of time and by safety reasons. With the presently adopted activity, radioembolization is effective but, for the same reason, potentially aggressive. The maximum energy of the beta rays emitted by ^{90}Y is 2280 keV, the highest among the nuclide used for present nuclear medicine applications. The experimental ^{166}Ho-labeled microspheres have also highly energetic beta rays (1855 keV). For a comparison, consider that the most intense beta emission from ^{131}I has a maximum beta energy of 606 keV, while ^{177}Lu has 498 keV (https://www-nds.iaea.org/relnsd/vcharthtml/VChartHTML.html#dcy1). Differently from all other radiopharmaceuticals, radioactivity is concentrated in one organ, thanks to the locoregional administration and to the fact that microspheres are designed to be permanently trapped in microcapillaries, with absolute absence of clearance. The mean absorbed dose reached with ^{90}Y microspheres in a single administration to normal parenchyma is about ten times higher than those delivered to the kidney with ^{90}Y-DOTATOC.

In addition to that, and again differently to almost all other radiopharmaceuticals, the target organ is also the critical one, i.e., the tissue that first shows radiation damage increasing the administered activity. For other radiopharmaceuticals, the red marrow is the most common critical organ, and it is the target organ only in case of bone marrow involvement. The kidney is the critical organ in ^{90}Y-DOTATOC administration, but it is never the target organ.

The aggressiveness of microsphere therapy raises the important concern about its life-threatening feature. Kennedy et al. first report 28 cases of death over 515 patients after ^{90}Y resin microsphere administration (21 in a single center based on the empirical tumor involvement planning method) [8]. Strigari et al. report 8/73 (11%) HCC patients with G4 toxicity (death related to treatment) after resin administration of resin microsphere planned with body surface area method [9]. Mazzaferro et al. report 19/52 cases of liver decompensation after radioembolization with glass microspheres, leading to death in 12 of them [7]. A more detailed review of papers reporting treatment-related deaths is given by the review paper by Cremonesi et al. [10]. It is nontrivial to attribute the imputability of this symptom to the treatment, since HCC patients are usually affected by liver infections (HBV, HCV), cirrhosis, and cancer. Liver decompensation may also be observed as natural history of these diseases. However, the treatment should not anticipate its manifestation. Dosimetry should be therefore first focused to prevent liver toxicity. On the efficacy side, according to the multivariate analysis of Garin et al. [11], lesion absorbed dose is the only factor associated with prolonged overall survival in HCC. Dosimetry has then been used to predict also lesion absorbed dose to provide a prognostic evaluation of survival.

13.1.1 Producer Indications for the Choice of Therapeutic Activity

^{90}Y resin spheres were approved with three possible methods for the choice of the activity to be administered [12]:

(a) Tumor involvement (activity depends on the percentage tumoral volume in the liver)
(b) Body surface area method, corrected for the tumor volume
(c) Compartmental model, which considers the tumor-to-non-tumor (TNT) concentration ratio

Only the last method is truly dosimetric, i.e., provides a differentiated evaluation between tumoral and non-tumoral tissue. It however has to be improved in cases where several lesions show different TNT.

^{90}Y glass microsphere should be administered in order to deliver between 80 Gy and 150 Gy to the "liver" (https://www.btg-im.com/getattachment/Therasphere/Products/Indications/10093509-Rev8_English-searchable.pdf.aspx), where "liver" is generally interpreted as "the injected lobe." The prescription is not truly dosimetric, though expressed in terms of gray, since it does not differentiate between tumoral and non-tumoral tissue.

For ^{166}Ho-labeled microspheres, a single phase I study is available, where absorbed dose escalation reached 80 Gy to the liver, without tumor-vs-non-tumor differentiation [13].

While speaking of "dosimetry," we mean here the separate dosimetric evaluation of tumor and non-tumor, with multiple evaluations in case of multiple lesions, up to a reasonable number. This dual evaluation is ordinarily performed in external beam treatment planning, and it is explicitly required by the present EURATOM directive 2013/59, in article 56 (optimization).

13.2 The Practical Implementation of Dosimetry in Liver Radioembolization

Dosimetry in radioembolization is based on three hypotheses:

1. Permanent trapping of microspheres in arterial microcapillaries
2. Identity of biodistribution between the simulator and the therapeutic particles
3. Patient relative calibration

The first two were adopted by all authors in the field. The third is very convenient though somebody adopts an absolute system calibration.

13.2.1 Permanent Trapping of Microspheres

There is only another radiopharmaceutical where biological clearance was assumed to be absent in uptake regions: the bone-seeking agent ^{153}Sm-EDTMP [14]. This assumption is much more reliable for microsphere, though it was never explicitly investigated. The simplification enters in the determination of the cumulative activity $\tilde{A}$

in a volume of interest (VOI), for instance, in a liver tumor. Mathematically, $\tilde{A}$ is the integral over time of the activity $A(t)$ in the VOI:

$$\tilde{A} = \int A(t)\,\mathrm{d}t \qquad (13.1)$$

The behavior of the activity in a tumor along the time may be complex for other radiopharmaceuticals. This requires a sampling at several time points through several scintigrams or PET scans. Permanent trapping, i.e., the absence of biological uptake and clearance phase, makes this curve the simplest possible, i.e., a pure monoexponential, where the half-life is the physical half-life of the radionuclide (64.2 h for ^{90}Y and 26.8 h for ^{166}Ho). In this situation the solution of Eq. (13.1) is well known:

$$\tilde{A} = \int A(t)\,\mathrm{d}t = A/\lambda = A T_{1/2}^{\mathrm{phys}} / \ln 2 \qquad (13.2)$$

A is the initial activity in the VOI.

For ^{90}Y microspheres, remember the basic MIRD equation for self-irradiation with non-penetrating radiations (beta rays) in a mass M, with Snider factor S:

$$D = \tilde{A} S \qquad (13.3)$$

From Eqs. (13.2) and (13.3), we can group all the constant values and obtain an approximated equation very useful in practice for the mean absorbed dose D_{VOI} [Gy] calculation in a volume of interest (VOI) of mass M which contains an initial activity A_{VOI} [GBq]:

$$D_{\mathrm{VOI}}[\mathrm{Gy}] = 50\, A_{\mathrm{VOI}}[\mathrm{GBq}] / M[\mathrm{kg}] \qquad (13.4)$$

This holds as long as the VOI dimension is large with respect to ^{90}Y beta range (90% if energy is deposited within 4.9 mm).

Apart from mathematics, permanent trapping has the utmost practical consequence that microsphere dosimetry can be calculated starting from a single tomographic scan: ^{99m}Tc-MAA or ^{166}Ho scout dose SPECT for planning and ^{90}Y PET or ^{166}Ho SPECT for peri-therapeutic verification. Since holmium is paramagnetic, the therapeutic amount injected for therapy is enough to obtain also magnetic resonance imaging, offering this modality for post-therapy dosimetry.

13.2.2 Identity of Biodistribution Between the Simulator and the Therapeutic Particles

While permanent trapping is an undeniable advantage, the correspondence of the particle biodistribution between the simulation and the therapy session is the weak point of microspheres dosimetry with respect to dosimetry of other radiopharmaceuticals. Radiolabeled agents are taken up thanks to metabolic or receptor mechanism, which in principle are the same after the tracer or the therapeutic administration (biochemistry is unfortunately not so simple. Deviations may occur also with radiopharmaceuticals). With microspheres, the link between simulation and therapy is much less direct. More variables are involved. Therapeutic particles are positioned by an interventional radiologist, through a blood stream. Identical catheter tip position both longitudinally and laterally in the two sessions is the first critical factor, above all in proximity of an arterial bifurcation [15, 16]. The kind of microspheres plays also a role. Size, number, and specific weight are three important physical parameters in reproducibility of biodistribution.

Initial evidence is available about the importance of particle size. Elschot et al. demonstrated that MAA escape to the lung in larger amount than ^{166}Ho particles injected both in tracer amount for simulation and in therapeutic amount [17]. The reason is that a fraction of MAA has a size of 10 μm, smaller than ^{166}Ho microspheres (about 28 ± 5 μm) [18]. ^{90}Y microspheres have diameters similar to ^{166}Ho particles: 32 ± 2.5 μm of resin and 25 ± 5 μm of glass microspheres. We could then extrapolate the same problem of lung shunt MAA overestimation for ^{166}Ho to ^{90}Y microspheres. Actually this marked overestimation was observed for most of patients showing lung shunt at ^{99m}Tc-MAA SPECT and then verified after glass microsphere administration with ^{90}Y PET (PHILIPS GEMINI 64 TF and GE Discovery 710) in the National Tumor Institute, Milan (Fig. 13.1).

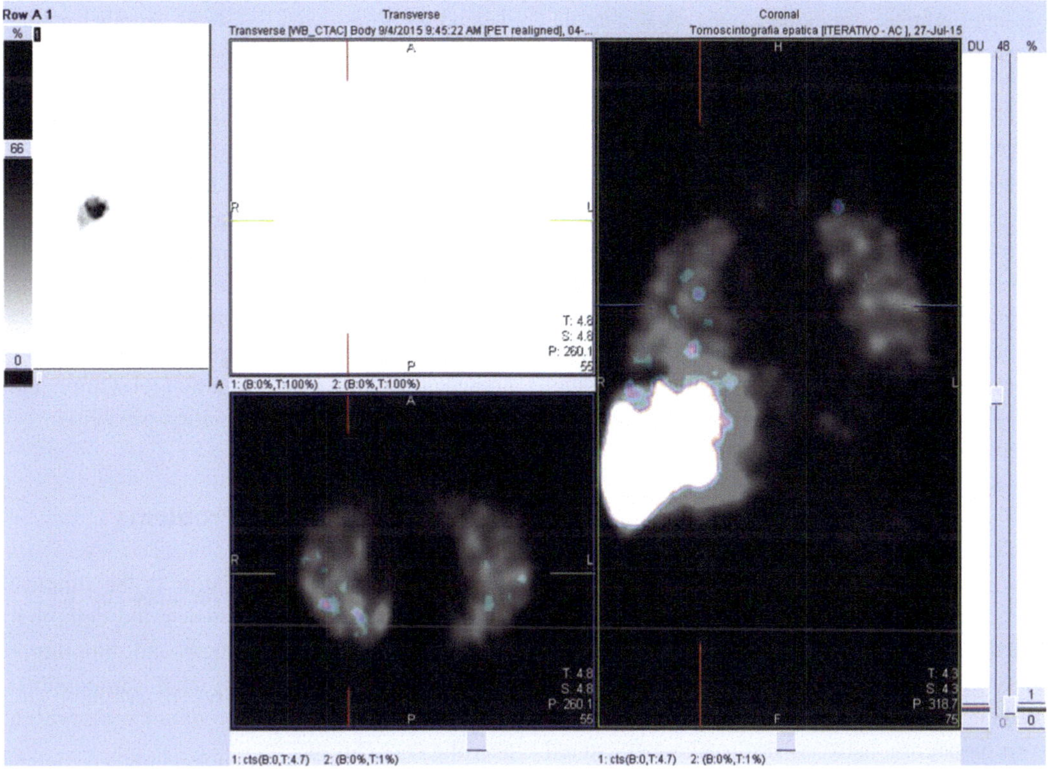

Fig. 13.1 Example of overestimation of lung shunt in ^{99m}Tc-MAA SPECT (in gray level) compared to ^{90}Y PET (color)

The number of microspheres seems to be responsible of the stasis or backflow phenomenon reported with ^{90}Y resin microspheres, and not with ^{90}Y glass microspheres. A typical injection involves tenths of millions of the former versus some millions of the latter. Seeing the limited intracapillary available volume, we may have therefore an embolic effect with a high number of resin microspheres, while glass microspheres injected in the first week after the treatment are non-embolic. Stasis may then stop the injection of resin spheres, with a consequent discrepancy of therapeutic biodistribution from the simulated one. However, the use of 5% glucose solution instead of sterile water markedly reduces the rate of stasis and backflow with resin microspheres, showing that the kind of washing solution is important [19].

Note however that if the kind of particles impact on their biodistribution, we should not focus on the differences among resin, glass, and ^{166}Ho microspheres, but rather to the fact that MAA are markedly different in size and in the administered number with respect to all the therapeutic particles. The typical MAA injection involves less than one million of particles, which moreover have a fraction with small size (10 μm). This is probably at the origin of the observed discrepancy between simulation and therapy reported with resin, glass, and ^{166}Ho microspheres, not only in the lung [20].

The last item to be considered is the possibility of temporary ischemia of vessels induced by long angiographic procedure, above all during the search for the optimal position during the simulation session [Garin and Rolland, private communication]. This phenomenon is the most difficult to be investigated, and there is no study available yet.

As a conclusion about predictive power of pretreatment dosimetry, the ideal treatment planning method obviously needs a perfect prevision of the therapeutic biodistribution of microspheres. This would require a perfect reproducibility of angiographic procedure, an ideal simulator, and no vessel spasm. The correspondence of the catheter tip position can be checked longitudinally, not laterally. The present simulator, MAA, showed some limitation. Even the use of a tracer dose with ^{166}Ho is not free of limitations, as seen in the large difference in the number of particles between simulation and therapy. Spasm should be avoided. Despite these points that can be improved (use of new kind of catheter, development of a new simulator, short angiographic procedure), the last paragraph will show the success of dosimetry in this field and the possible improvement of patient outcome.

13.2.3 Patient Relative Calibration and Imaging

The quantification step in radioembolization can be very simple if the patient relative calibration method is adopted. This consists in setting a correspondence between the total administered or intended ^{90}Y activity $A_{TOT}(^{90}Y)$ and the total counts C_{TOT} in the tomographic image (SPECT or ^{90}Y PET). Joined with the identity of biodistributions, this can be expressed mathematically by a simple proportion:

$$A_{VOI}\left(^{90}Y\right) : A_{TOT}\left(^{90}Y\right) = C_{VOI} : C_{TOT} \quad (13.5)$$

We can easily solve for A_{VOI}:

$$A_{VOI}\left(^{90}Y\right) = \left[A_{TOT}\left(^{90}Y\right) / C_{TOT}\right] \times C_{VOI} \quad (13.6)$$

The term in brackets gives the conversion between counts and activity, i.e., it is the patient and ^{90}Y activity-dependent calibration factor CF:

$$CF\left(^{90}Y\right) = \left[A_{TOT}\left(^{90}Y\right) / C_{TOT}\right] \quad (13.7)$$

In this calibration method, each patient is the calibration phantom for himself. The advantage is that the total activity is fully recovered by definition. This is not the case adopting an absolute calibration based on ^{90}Y phantom scan [21]. The accuracy limit of this method is given by the fact that in a SPECT or PET scan, the total counts depend on the adopted threshold. Another potential limit is the accuracy on $A_{TOT}(^{90}Y)$, which in cases of stasis with uncomplete administration should be accurately determined.

Apart from second-order problems, all the ingredients for dosimetry are in the previous equations. Once VOI is drawn on tumoral and non-tumoral liver, C_{VOI} and mass M are obtained; Eq. (13.6) gives activity in each region, and Eq. (13.4) gives the mean absorbed dose. Dosimetry can be calculated in a simple spreadsheet. The nontrivial point is the definition of tumor and normal liver border (segmentation problem).

13.2.4 Segmentation Problems

While the dosimetric calculation is the simplest among all radionuclide therapies, the definition of the border between tumor and non-tumor region may be difficult, and often it is impossible. Often HCC shows as a large tumor mass with a necrotic core (Fig. 13.2).

Two segmentation methods are possible: SPECT-based method, using a threshold on counts, which includes only the perfused tumor region, or CT-based method, which includes in the VOI the whole CT lesion volume. According to the analysis of our group [22], the SPECT-based segmentation gives better correlation between the absorbed dose and response. This can be understood since the response was evaluated with Hounsfield density variation (Choi method), which is maximal over the active tumor region. No density variation takes place within the necrotic core. On the other side, it goes without saying that necrosis is not a part of a functional liver and should be excluded from the functional volume. Therefore, both segmentation methods are required to properly define the active lesion portion (^{99m}Tc-MAA SPECT) and the functional liver volume (CT). At a more refined investigation, this approach might appear oversimplified. An elegant method is proposed by Lam et al. [23]. It is based on the fact that sulfur colloid (SC) labeled with ^{99m}Tc (TcSC) is taken up by hepatocytes, and not by liver lesions. The drawback of this method is the need of two sequential SPECT scans: the first after ^{99m}TcSC administra-

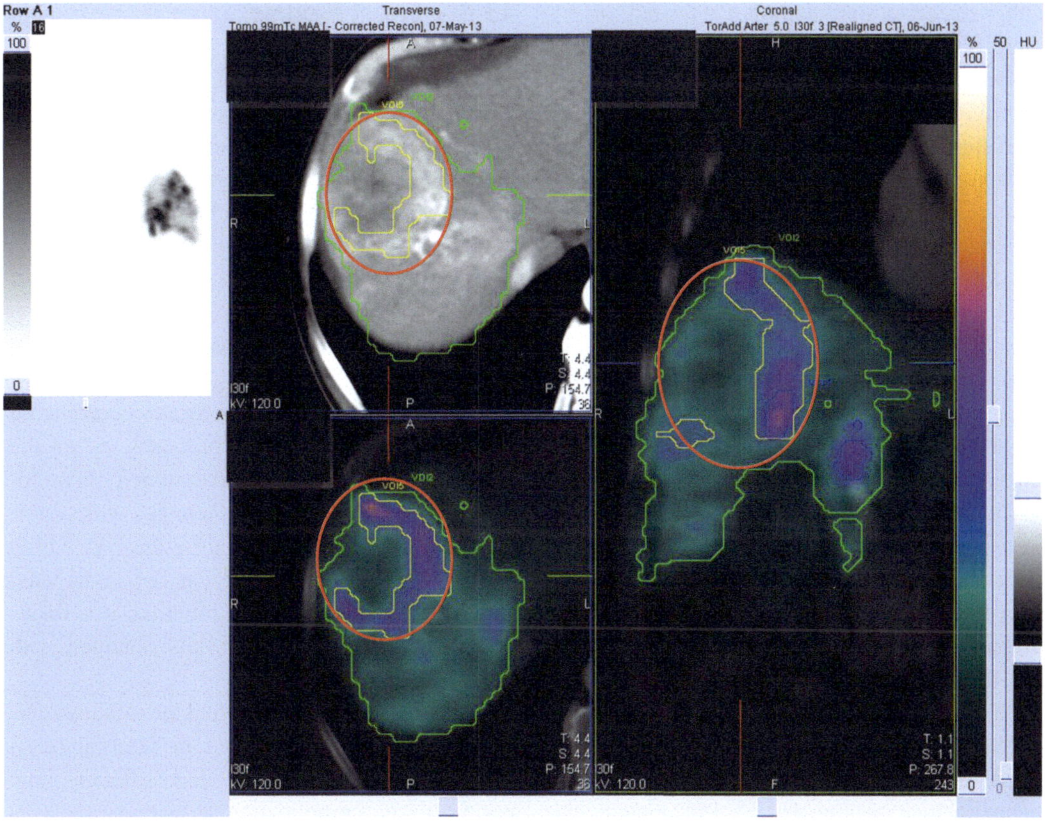

Fig. 13.2 Two possible segmentation methods for an HCC lesion with a necrotic core. The yellow line shows the perfused region (SPECT with threshold). The red line shows the CT-based morphological volume

tion and the second after ^{99m}Tc-MAA administration, with the patient in the same position on the couch. SPECT images have then to be coregistered and subtracted.

Infiltrative lesions cannot be segmented, since often not even CT is able to distinguish between tumoral and non-tumoral tissue. In these cases, an MRI-based segmentation is proposed [24]. FDG PET is not indicated in HCC, but it can be conveniently used to define metastases border, followed by a coregistration of FDG-PET images with ^{99m}Tc-MAA SPECT or ^{90}Y PET images [25].

13.3 Feasibility in the Routine

As suggested before, dosimetry in microsphere treatment is easily doable, both to plan and to verify the treatment.

The pretreatment SPECT is normally acquired for clinical reasons. The additional workload is only for medical physicists. Planning of ^{90}Y microspheres requires at least a SPECT taken short time after the angiographic injection of 160 MBq of ^{99m}Tc-MAA, to avoid the well-known radionuclide detachment from MAA [26]. Low-energy high-resolution collimators are suggested, with 3° angular step and 20 s per projection. Iterative reconstruction for dosimetry may be different that for diagnostic. It has suggested a higher number of iterations and no additional filter to reach higher spatial resolution to preserve recovery of small objects. SPECT-CT is advised. If not, reconstruction of attenuation-corrected SPECT with CT from diagnostic department is feasible on workstations of some vendor. Non-attenuation-corrected SPECT gives approximated quantification but allows better planning with respect to the methods indicated in ^{90}Y microspheres. Coregistration with CT is strongly advised not only for quantification but also for careful check of extrahepatic depositions. ^{166}Ho microspheres injected in tracer dose allow to plan the treatment thanks to the emission of 81 keV photons (6.7% photon abundance). Despite the low energy of emitted photons, Smits et al. [13] adopted medium-energy collimators to reduce the background generated by bremsstrahlung photons, with a sacrifice of spatial resolution.

Posttreatment imaging is strongly advised, since inadvertent gastroduodenal depositions might take place. A prompt realization of this misplacement allows pharmaceutical administration in order to reduce the future radiation damage symptoms. Moreover it gives time to plan a surgery intervention, which is challenging for the surgeon radiation dose to hands, up to 2 weeks after treatment. As for the pretreatment case, once post-therapy images are available, dosimetry is just a matter of region copying and of repeating the same calculation.

An important difference between ^{90}Y SPECT bremsstrahlung imaging and ^{90}Y PET imaging has to be remarked. It is extremely difficult to obtain quantitative bremsstrahlung SPECT. Special algorithm, noncommercially available, is needed, inclusive of Monte Carlo modeling of the SPECT system. For this reason, posttreatment ^{90}Y microsphere dosimetry requires ^{90}Y PET, possibly with time of flight. The infinitesimal positron emission from ^{90}Y (32 positrons per million of decay) requires 15 min per bed position. From the logistic organization, such verification scans can be performed at the beginning of the FDG routine, during the uptake time. ^{166}Ho post-therapy dosimetry can be done by waiting 3 days after administration, when the therapeutic activity gives no saturation in gamma camera, unless the newest SPECT dead-time correction software is available. Unique feature of holmium is the possibility of using MRI for dosimetry, but, until today, only post therapy, since the NMR signal from a tracer administration seems too low.

Softwares required for dosimetry are a SPECT-CT or PET-CT coregistration and display tool and a segmentation tool to draw contour slice by slices. Calculations can be done on a spreadsheet. Commercial softwares speeds up the process.

13.4 Short Review

Dosimetry in ^{90}Y microsphere treatment is so easy that in one decade more dosimetric results were published than for all other kinds of nuclear medicine therapy in the previous 60 years. For an extensive review, see the work by Cremonesi et al. [10]. Here we give only some hints.

13.4.1 Dosimetry to Prevent Toxicity

A foreword to the dose-toxicity correlation studies is that there is no consensus yet on the definition of radio-induced liver toxicity in radioembolization. In particular, there is a wide variation among authors of the time interval within which the decompensation can be considered treatment related (1, 2, 3, 6 months). It is therefore difficult to compare results obtained with different endpoint definitions.

Strigari et al. [9] first applied the radiobiological models currently applied in external beam radiotherapy to nuclear medicine therapy. The normal tissue complication probability (NTCP) curve and the tumor control probability (TCP) curve were determined on 73 HCC patients treated with resin spheres using post-therapy bremsstrahlung SPECT. Obtaining such curves is just a matter of interpolating an experimental histogram with the proper available radiobiological curve. Figure 13.3 shows an example of such histogram for HCC patients treated with glass microspheres. Each bar represents the ratio of the number of patients who showed liver decompensation and of the number of patients that received a parenchyma absorbed dose within predefined intervals (0–35 Gy, 35–70 Gy, etc.).

Figure 13.4 shows the interpolation of a re-elaboration of such histogram [22] with the radiobiological model by Lyman [28]. The re-elaboration consisted in the fact that we applied the concept of imputability of liver decompensation, reporting as treatment-related toxicity only in cases without evident concomitant tumor progression [29]. The problem of imputability of liver toxicity complicates the dose-toxicity analysis, since organ impairment in HCC may derive from tumor progression, cirrhosis progression,

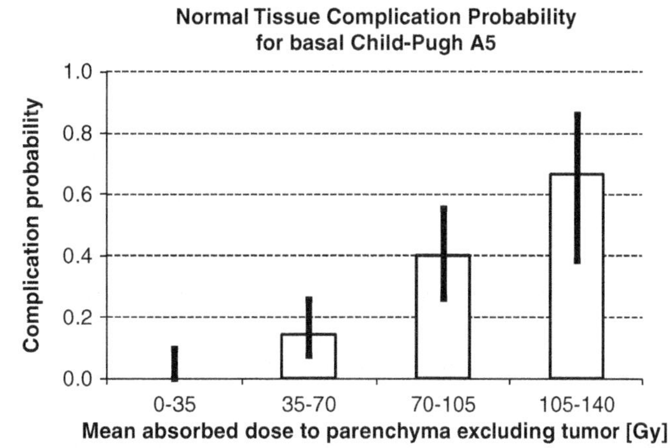

Fig. 13.3 Normal tissue complication probability histogram for HCC Child-Pugh A5 patient treated with glass microspheres shows the increase of the observed risk of liver decompensation versus whole parenchyma absorbed dose. Reprinted from Chiesa et al. [27] with permission of Minerva Medica

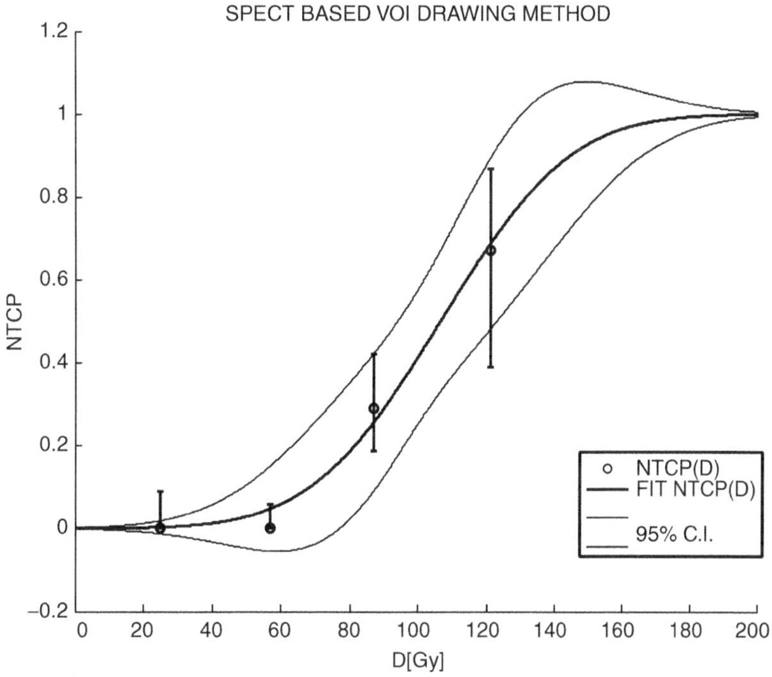

Fig. 13.4 Normal tissue complication probability as a function of the mean absorbed dose D averaged over parenchyma, including nonirradiated regions, excluding tumor (SPECT-based VOI drawing method)

or irradiation. This happens because the target region and the organ at risk are the same, differently from most of other nuclear medicine therapies.

The Lyman model with $n = 1$ (pure parallel organ) indicates that the tolerated absorbed dose depends on the dose averaged over the organ, and it is inversely proportional to the irradiated fraction:

$$\mathrm{TD}_{50}\left(V_f\right) = \mathrm{TD}_{50}\left(\text{whole liver}\right) / V_f \quad (13.8)$$

TD_{50} is the absorbed dose that gives the 50% risk in NTCP curve (Fig. 13.4). In this way the volume effect, well studied in external beam radiotherapy on liver, is taken into account. The smaller is the irradiated volume fraction, the higher is the absorbed dose tolerance. The indication of glass microsphere producer disregards this important effect. 120 Gy delivered to a single segment, to a left lobe, to a right lobe, or to the whole liver are four completely different levels of risk. In the Lyman framework, delivering 120 Gy to half of the parenchyma corresponds to a 60 Gy whole liver injection. 120 Gy to a segment occupying ¼ of the organ corresponds to 30 Gy whole liver injection. The risk is reduced according to the NTCP curve shown in Fig. 13.4.

Note that the NTCP analysis is a pure univariate approach. It probably can be applied as long as the clinical liver condition is not too compromised. The NTCP needs stratification when additional risk factors are present: high basal bilirubin value (Child-Pugh B) and complete obstruction of the main trunk of the portal vein [30].

Lung toxicity was observed with ^{90}Y resin microspheres [31], and the absorbed dose limit to the lung was set at 30 Gy for single administration and 50 Gy for cumulative administrations. The same limit was transposed to ^{90}Y glass microspheres. However, Salem et al. treated 58 patients and followed up 53 of them, with MAA-predicted lung absorbed dose larger than those limits. Only ten developed mild lung toxicity [32]. The key is probably in the large MAA overestimation of the actual lung shunt fraction.

13.4.2 The Importance of the Number of Microspheres

The Lyman model is the simplest one, and probably it underestimates the tolerance for small volume fractions. According to the external beam experience and to a more refined model by Walrand et al. [33], an irradiated volume fraction lower than 40% would allow the tolerance of an arbitrarily high absorbed dose. No confirmation of this 40% threshold is however available in radioembolization of cirrhotic patients. It is very important to note that TD_{50} (whole liver) obtained by Strigari et al. with resin spheres on HCC was 53 Gy [9], while for Chiesa et al. with glass spheres on the same kind of patients, it was about 100 Gy [22]. This marked difference of dose-toxicity relationship, found also in the dose-response correlation, enlightens the fact that a lower number of particles per GBq gives a less uniform irradiation at microscopic scale and a lower biological effect (toxicity and efficacy) for a fixed absorbed dose value [34]. For this reason the tolerance to resin spheres (20 million of particles per GBq) is of 40 Gy according to Sangro et al. [35] and of 70 Gy to glass spheres injected 4 days after reference time (1 million per GBq) according to Chiesa et al. [22].

Garin et al. proposed for glass spheres a limit of 120 Gy to the lobe if the injected lobe volume fraction is larger than 0.7. Averaging 120 Gy to 0.7 over the whole volume gives 120 Gy * 0.7 = 84 Gy, which is not so different from the 70 Gy, if we remember that Garin et al. considered toxicity events as only irreversible liver decompensations, differently from Chiesa et al. [22].

13.4.3 Dose-Response Correlation

The dose-response correlation analysis is much simpler than the dose-toxicity study, since response may derive from treatment only. However, the manifold of response evaluation criteria available may raise some confusion in the comparison of published results. In HCC the same factors that make the segmentation difficult make also the response evaluation difficult. HCC is not suitable for FDG PET imaging. HCC is often infiltrative. HCC treated with microspheres does not shrink, at least in the first months following the treatment. For this reason, pure dimensional criteria (RECIST, WHO) are definitely not suitable to monitor the response of HCC to radioembolization. mRECIST or EASL is proposed, which considers the largest dimensions in the arterial phase. According to the experience of the Milan group, densitometric criteria (Choi) seem more suitable. The debate is ongoing [36]. In metastases the situation seems simpler, since secondary lesions are avid of FDG, and metabolic imaging may be used to early monitor the response. mRECIST is also generally accepted. The best timing to ascertain the response is linked to the choice of the response criteria. Metabolic response happens usually earlier than the radiological response. Dimensional reduction, if it takes place, is the last step of the response process.

The number of studies reporting dose-response correlations is much higher than the dose-toxicity studies [10]. We may say that, apart from one study with insufficient number of patients, all authors found dose-response correlation, with both resin and glass microspheres and both for HCC and colorectal metastases [10]. Strigari et al. [9] obtained the tumor control probability for HCC treated with resin spheres, evaluated with EASL criteria, with a 50% probability of response (TCP_{50}) at about 150 Gy. Chiesa et al. [22] studied the dose-response correlation (Fig. 13.5) and obtained the TCP curves, which however were markedly different after stratification on lesion size (Fig. 13.6). Tumors lighter than 10 g have TCP_{50} at about 250 Gy, while lesions

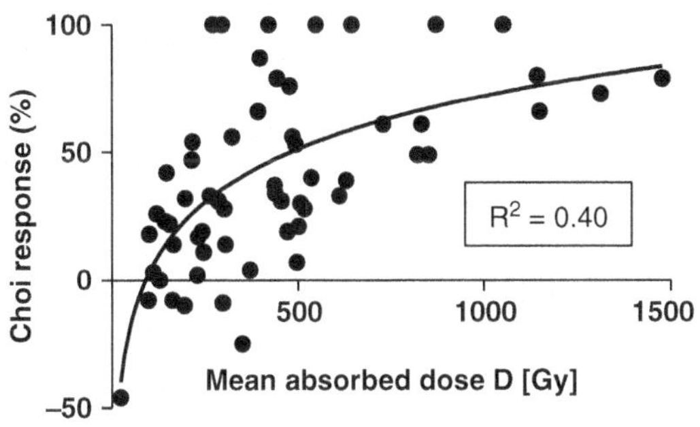

Fig. 13.5 Dose-response correlation of HCC lesions with diameter larger than 1.8 cm treated with ^{90}Y glass spheres. Dose was evaluated on ^{99m}Tc-MAA SPECT. Response was defined as Hounsfield unit variation larger than 50% (Choi criteria)

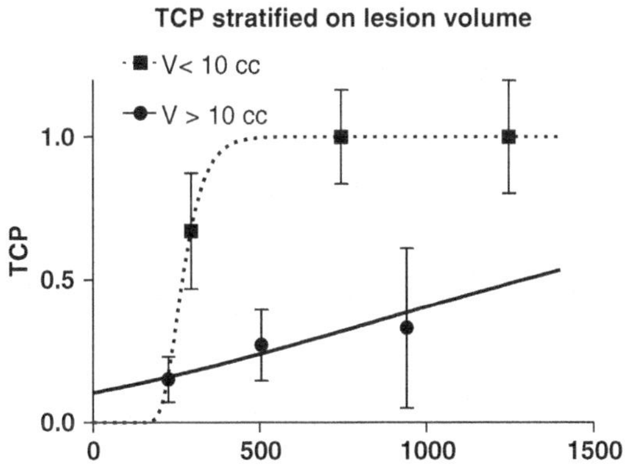

Fig. 13.6 Tumor control probability of HCC lesions with diameter larger than 1.8 cm treated with ^{90}Y glass spheres. Dose was evaluated on ^{99m}Tc-MAA SPECT. Response was defined as Hounsfield unit variation larger than 50% (Choi criteria)

larger than 10 g have TCP_{50} at about 1300 Gy. This is the limit of the radioembolization. The larger is the lesion, the larger is the probability of having non-perfused and therefore nonirradiated island. The marked difference between TCP_{50} of resin and glass microspheres confirms the importance of the number of particles per GBq also for lesions [37].

For colorectal metastases, the efficacy threshold seems lower than HCC, around 50 Gy, as found by two studies conducted with resin spheres. Flamen et al. [38] monitored the response of 39 lesions of 8 patients with FDG PET, adopting as endpoint a TLG reduction >50% at 1.5 and 3 months. Lesion absorbed dose was evaluated on ^{99m}Tc-MAA SPECT. van den Hoven et al. [39] studied 133 lesions of 30 patients with TLG at 1 month after treatment. Dosimetry was performed on post-therapy ^{90}Y PET images, to avoid the problem of possible MAA-^{90}Y microsphere biodistribution mismatch. Their result is in agreement with the previous study. The interesting fact is that the lesions with higher basal TLG need a higher absorbed dose to respond. This finding could be in agreement with the lesion size behavior of Fig. 13.6 for HCC, if the SUV_{mean} of the studied colorectal metastases was approximately the same for all lesions. Under this hypothesis, higher TLG means higher volume.

13.4.4 Dose-Survival Correlation

The most exciting result about dosimetry in radioembolization is about the prognostic value of lesion absorbed dose on overall survival.

Garin et al. [30] modified the therapeutic activity according to predictive ^{99m}Tc-MAA SPECT dosimetry on some of 71 intermediate and 33 advanced (i.e., patients with portal vein thrombosis, PVT) HCC patients. Similarly the improvement in the time to progression (TTP) for intermediate and advanced patients was associated to lesion absorbed dose >205 Gy (Fig. 13.7). For PVT patients, a statistically significant longer overall survival was obtained if dose to tumor was >205 Gy

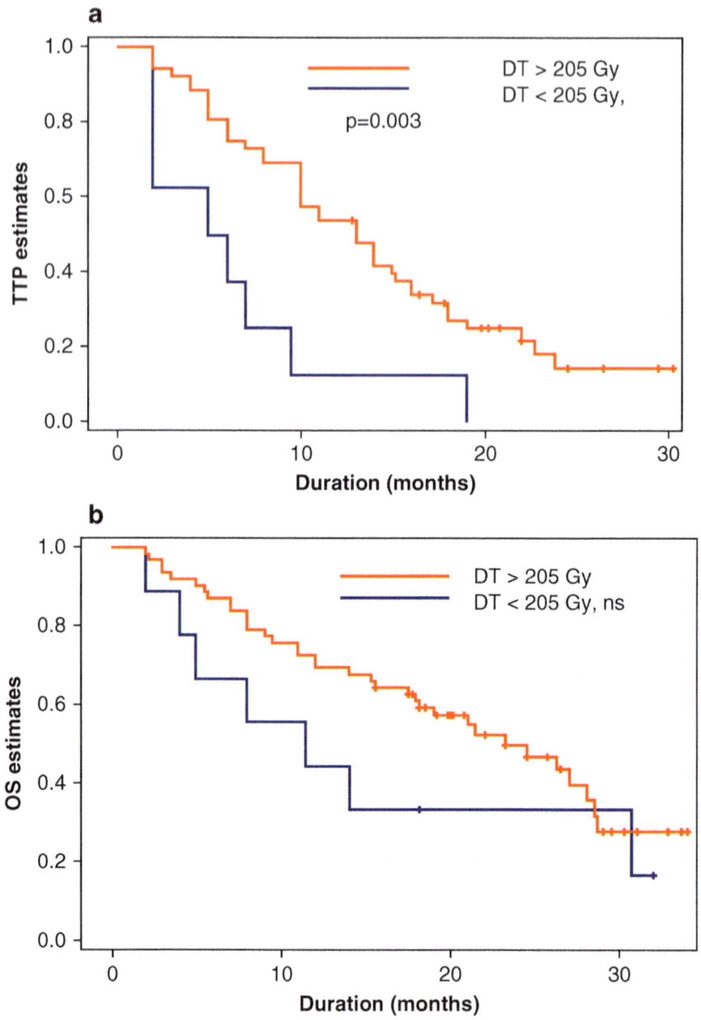

Fig. 13.7 The prognostic value of lesion dosimetry on time to progression TTP, upper panel (**a**) and overall survival (OS, lower panel (**b**) in intermediate and advanced HCC patients. Difference in lower panel **b** is not statistically significant, but the trend is clear [30]

In the paper collecting their whole experience with HCC treated with glass spheres, the same group [11] performed the unique available multivariate analysis of overall survival. For the whole population, the lesion absorbed dose larger than 205 Gy is the only significant factor associated with prolonged survival. For the restricted PVT population, the good or poor PVT perfusion at ^{99m}Tc-MAA SPECT is the only factor affecting survival.

Garin's group usually select nodular lesion patients for radioembolization. Kokabi et al. [24] studied the overall survival of advanced infiltrative HCC depending on the lesion absorbed dose (dose cutoff of 100 Gy). They segmented lesions on MRI and used glass spheres and post-therapy bremsstrahlung dosimetry. Median OS was 4.6 versus 13.2 months ($p < 0.001$) for doses lower and higher than the cutoff.

13.5 Author's Results [40]

The individualized dosimetry in the radioembolization of HCC with ^{90}Y glass microspheres was introduced in the National Tumor Institute of Milan since 2009 to plan treatment with glass microspheres as in external beam radiotherapy, after a first series treated with the standard "120 Gy to lobe" prescription.

The planning paradigm for Child-Pugh A patients [22] aimed to deliver 70 Gy averaged over the non-tumoral tissue, if the predicted lesion absorbed dose was high (curative intent). The 70 Gy limit should have kept the liver decompensation incidence below 15% obtained on Child A patients with the "120 Gy to lobe" prescription and considered acceptable. A lower parenchyma absorbed dose was prescribed if the predicted tumor dose was low (palliative intent). Planning was applied to 116 patients. With respect to the standard 120 Gy to lobe indication, administered activity was, on the average, doubled in half of patients and reduced of 50% in a quarter of patients. The decompensation incidence was maintained below 15%, as planned. After stratification of patients with/without portal vein thrombosis, comparing the PVT subgroups, where lesions had the same size distribution, treatment planning improved median survival from 8 to 12 months, close to significance with Mantel-Cox test ($p = 0.067$). In the NO PVT subgroups, the median survival was 17 vs 15 months (n.s.), i.e., maintained, despite twice tumor sizes.

13.6 Conclusion and Future Perspectives

In the history of nuclear medicine therapy there were well-known examples of studies denying the usefulness of dosimetry (for instance with ^{90}Y-ibritumomab tiuxetan) remarking the absence of correlation between absorbed dose and effects. Producers of radiopharmaceuticals also were not interested to dosimetry, seen as an additional cost limiting the diffusion on the market. Producers of software were also not interested in nuclear medicine therapy.

The fact that only one scan is enough to perform dosimetry brought a revolution in the field. All producers of microspheres made substantial investments in dosimetry [13, 21] (https://www.btg-im.com/en-GB/Simplicit90Y/Home). Plenty of commercial software were developed both by one producer of microspheres and by other companies. From a recent EANM survey about nuclear medicine therapy planning criteria, about 80% of responding centers perform dosimetry on a regular basis to plan radioembolization treatments versus an average of 25% for the other kinds of therapy [41]. All scientists reported dose-response correlation, despite the possible MAA-microsphere biodistribution mismatch. Dose-toxicity and dose-survival associations are less studied but reported.

Dosimetry in microsphere treatment gives therefore an outstanding clinical impact on therapy outcome. For these reasons it should be used to plan the first and maybe the unique possible treatment on each patient. It should be used also to verify each treatment, seen the possible mismatch between MAA and microspheres.

Key Points

- Pretreatment and peri-treatment dosimetry in liver radioembolization with microsphere are greatly simplified with respect to other nuclear medicine agents thanks to the permanent trapping of injected particles. This allows to calculate the absorbed dose using only one tomographic scan.
- A second advantage of this kind of dosimetry is that pretreament SPECT imaging is required for clinical reasons (check of absence of gastroduodenal deposition). These images can be used as simulation to perform a real treatment planning.
- A weak point in planning is the possible mismatch between biodistribution obtained in the simulation and in the therapeutic session. This may derive first on the catheter tip mispositioning but also on the different sizes of macro aggregates of albumin, which have a fraction remarkably smaller that therapeutic microspheres, leading to a higher MAA penetrability through arterial capillaries. Temporary vessel spasm may also cause differences between prediction and therapy.
- Despite such weak point, dose-response correlation was reported by all authors who accomplished such investigation. Much more evidence of this correlation for ^{90}Y microspheres was collected in 10 years than in 60 years for all radiopharmaceutical. Few papers report also dose-toxicity correlation. The most exciting point is that some group reported and confirmed dose-survival correlation. On the other side, several authors reported deaths from treatment-related liver decompensation.

- Such kind of therapy, aggressive against one of the most aggressive cancers, should be therefore properly planned. The balance between dosimetry cost and benefits is the most favorable among all nuclear medicine treatments. Moreover, the short life expectancy of liver cancer patients (roughly one year) requires an optimized therapeutic approach, having only one or two administration chances.

References

1. Chiesa C, Lassmann M. Dosimetry in nuclear medicine therapy. Q J Nucl Med Mol Imaging. 2011;55:2–4.
2. Wada N, Nakayama H, Suganuma N, Masudo Y, Rino Y, Masuda M, Imada T. Prognostic value of the sixth edition AJCC/UICC TNM classification for differentiated thyroid carcinoma with extrathyroid extension. J Clin Endocrinol Metab. 2007;92(1):215–8.
3. Strosberg J, El-Haddad G, Wolin E, et al. Phase 3 trial of ^{177}Lu-dotatate for midgut neuroendocrine tumors. N Engl J Med. 2017;376:125–35.
4. Barone R, Borson-Chazot F, Valkema R, Walrand S, Chauvin F, Gogou L, Kvols LK, Krenning LP, Jamar F, Pauwels S. Patient-specific dosimetry in predicting renal toxicity with ^{90}Y-DOTATOC: relevance of kidney volume and dose rate in finding a dose–effect relationship. J Nucl Med. 2005;46:99S–106S.
5. Bergsma H, Konijnenberg M, van der Zwan WA, Kam BLR, Teunissen JJM, Kooij PP, Mauff KAL, Krenning EP, Kwekkeboom DJ. Nephrotoxicity after PRRT with 177Lu-DOTA-octreotate. Eur J Nucl Med Mol Imaging. 2016;43(10):1802–11.
6. Llovet JM, Ricci S, Mazzaferro V, Hilgard P, Gane E, Blanc JF, de Oliveira AC, Santoro A, et al. Sorafenib in advanced hepatocellular carcinoma. N Engl J Med. 2008;359(4):420–2.
7. Mazzaferro V, Sposito C, Bhoori S, Romito R, Chiesa C, Morosi C, et al. Yttrium90 radioembolization for intermediate-advanced hepatocarcinoma: a phase II study. Hepatology. 2013;57:1826–37.
8. Kennedy AS, McNeillie P, Dezarn WA, Nutting C, Sangro B, Wertman D, Garafalo M, Liu D, Coldwell D, Savin M, Jakobs T, Rose S, Warner R, Carter D, Sapareto S, Nag S, Gulec S, Calkins A, Gates VL, Salem R. Treatment parameters and outcome in 680 treatments of internal radiation with resin 90Y-microspheres for unresectable hepatic tumors. Int J Radiat Oncol Biol Phys. 2009;74:1494–500.
9. Strigari L, Sciuto R, Rea S, Carpanese L, Pizzi G, Soriani A, Iaccarino G, Benassi M, Ettorre GM, Maini CL. Efficacy and toxicity related to treatment of hepatocellular carcinoma with 90Y SIR spheres: radiobiological considerations. J Nucl Med. 2010;51:1377–85.
10. Cremonesi M, Chiesa C, Strigari L, Ferrari M, Botta F, Guerriero F, De Cicco C, Bonomo G, Orsi F, Bodei L, Di Dia A, Grana CM, Orecchia R. Radioembolization of hepatic lesions from a radiobiology and dosimetric perspective. Front Oncol. 2014;4:210.
11. Garin E, Rolland Y, Pracht M, Le Sourd S, Laffont S, Mesbah H, Haumont LA, Lenoir L, Rohou T, Brun V, Edeline J. High impact of macroaggregated albumin-based tumour dose on response and overall survival in hepatocellular carcinoma patients treated with ^{90}Y-loaded glass microsphere radioembolization. Liver Int. 2017;37:101–10.
12. SIR-Spheres. Yttrium-90 microspheres [package insert]. Sirtex Medical, Lane Cove. 2004. http://www.sirtex.com/files/US20Package20Insert1.pdf.
13. Smits ML, Nijsen JF, van den Bosch MA, Lam MG, Vente MA, Mali WP, van Het Schip AD, Zonnenberg BA. Holmium-166 radioembolisation in patients with unresectable, chemorefractory liver metastases (HEPAR trial): a phase 1, dose-escalation study. Lancet Oncol. 2012;13:1025–34.
14. Bianchi L, Baroli A, Marzoli L, Verusio C, Chiesa C, Pozzi L. Prospective dosimetry with ^{99m}Tc-MDP in metabolic radiotherapy of bone metastases with ^{153}Sm-EDTMP. Eur J Nucl Med Mol Imaging. 2009;36:122–9.
15. Jiang M, Fishman A, Nowakowski FS, Heiba S, Zhang Z, Knesaurek K, Weintraub J, Machac J. Segmental perfusion differences on paired Tc-99m macroaggregated albumin (MAA) hepatic perfusion imaging and yttrium-90 (Y-90) bremsstrahlung imaging studies in SIR-sphere radioembolization: associations with angiography. J Nucl Med Radiat Ther. 2012;3:1.
16. Wondergem M, Smits ML, Elschot M, de Jong HW, Verkooijen HM, van den Bosch MA, Nijsen JF, Lam MG. 99mTc-macroaggregated albumin poorly predicts the intrahepatic distribution of 90Y resin microspheres in hepatic radioembolization. J Nucl Med. 2013;54:1294–301.
17. Elschot M, Nijsen JFW, Lam MGEH, et al. 99mTc-MAA overestimates the absorbed dose to the lungs in radioembolization: a quantitative evaluation in patients treated with 166Ho-microspheres. Eur J Nucl Med Mol Imaging. 2014;41:1965–75.
18. Zielhuis SW, Nijsen JFW, de Roosa R, Krijger GC, van Rijk PP, Hennink WE, van het Schip AD. Production of GMP-grade radioactive holmium loaded poly(l-lactic acid) microspheres for clinical application. Int J Pharm. 2006;311:69–74.
19. Ahmadzadehfar H, Meyer PCC, Bundschuh R, Muckle M, Gärtner F, Essler SHH. Evaluation of the delivered activity of yttrium-90 resin microspheres using sterile water and 5% glucose during administration. EJNMMI Res. 2015;5:54.
20. Gnesin S, Canetti L, Adib S, Cherbuin N, Silva Monteiro M, Bize P, Denys A, Prior JO, Baechler

S, Boubaker A. Partition model-based ^{99m}Tc-MAA SPECT/CT predictive dosimetry compared with 90Y TOF PET/CT posttreatment dosimetry in radioembolization of hepatocellular carcinoma: a quantitative agreement comparison. J Nucl Med. 2016;57(11):1672–8.
21. Willowson KP, Tapner M, QUEST Investigator Team, Bailey DL. A multi-centre comparison of quantitative 90Y PET/CT for dosimetric purposes after radioembolization. Eur J Nucl Med Mol Imaging. 2015;42(8):1202–22.
22. Chiesa C, Mira M, Maccauro M, Romito R, Spreafico C, Morosi C, Camerini T, Carrara M, Pellizzari S, Negri A, Aliberti G, Sposito C, Bhoori S, Facciorusso A, Civelli E, Lanocita R, Padovano B, Migliorisi M, Seregni E, Marchianò A, Crippa F, Mazzaferro V. Radioembolization of hepatocarcinoma with 90-Y glass microspheres: development of an individualized treatment planning strategy based on dosimetry and radiobiology. Eur J Nucl Med Mol Imaging. 2015;42:1718–38.
23. Lam MG, Goris ML, Iagaru AH, Mittra ES, Louie JD, Sze DY. Prognostic utility of 90Y radioembolization dosimetry based on fusion 99mTc-macroaggregated albumin-99mTc-sulfur colloid SPECT. J Nucl Med. 2013;54(12):2055–61.
24. Kokabi N, Galt JR, Xing M, Camacho JC, Barron BJ, Schuster DM, Kim HS. A simple method for estimating dose delivered to hepatocellular carcinoma after yttrium-90 glass-based radioembolization therapy: preliminary results of a proof of concept study. J Vasc Interv Radiol. 2014;25:277–87.
25. D'Arienzo M, Chiaramida P, Chiacchiararelli L, Coniglio A, Cianni R, Salvatori R, Ruzza A, Scopinaro F, Bagni O. 90Y PET-based dosimetry after selective internal radiotherapy treatments. Nucl Med Commun. 2012;33:633–40.
26. Giammarile F, Bodei L, Chiesa C, Flux G, Forrer F, Kraeber-Bodere F, Brans B, Lambert B, Konijnenberg M, Borson-Chazot F, Tennvall J, Luster M. EANM procedure guidelines for the treatment of liver cancer and liver metastases with intra-arterial radioactive compounds. Eur J Nucl Med Mol Imaging. 2011;38(7):1393–406.
27. Chiesa C, Mira M, Maccauro M, Romito R, Spreafico C, Sposito C, Bhoori S, Morosi C, Pellizzari S, Negri A, Civelli E, Lanocita R, Camerini T, Bampo C, Carrara M, Seregni E, Marchianò A, Mazzaferro V, Bombardieri E. A dosimetric treatment planning strategy in radioembolization of hepatocarcinoma with ^{90}Y glass microspheres. Q J Nucl Med Mol Imaging. 2012;56:503–8.
28. Lyman JT. Complication probability as assessed from dose-volume histograms. Radiat Res. 1995;104:13–9.
29. Garin E, Rolland Y, Laffont S, Edeline J. Clinical impact of 99mTc-MAA SPECT/CT-based dosimetry in the radioembolization of liver malignancies with 90Y-loaded microspheres. Eur J Nucl Med Mol Imaging. 2016;43:559–75.
30. Garin E, Lenoir L, Edeline J, Laffont S, Mesbah H, Porée P, Sulpice L, Boudjema K, Mesbah M, Guillygomarc'h A, Quehen E, Pracht M, Raoul JL, Clement B, Rolland Y, Boucher E. Boosted selective internal radiation therapy with 90Y-loaded glass microspheres (B-SIRT) for hepatocellular carcinoma patients: a new personalized promising concept. Eur J Nucl Med Mol Imaging. 2013;40:1057–68.
31. Leung TW, Lau WY, Ho SK, Ward SC, Chow JH, Chan MS, Metreweli C, Johnson PJ, Li AK. Radiation pneumonitis after selective internal radiation treatment with intraarterial 90yttrium-microspheres for inoperable hepatic tumors. Int J Radiat Oncol Biol Phys. 1995;33:919–24.
32. Salem R, Parikh P, Atassi B, Lewandowski RJ, Ryu RK, Sato KT, Gates VL, Ibrahim S, Mulcahy MF, Kulik L, Liu DM, Riaz A, Omary RA, Kennedy AS. Incidence of radiation pneumonitis after hepatic intra-arterial radiotherapy with yttrium-90 microspheres assuming uniform lung distribution. Am J Clin Oncol. 2008;31:431–8.
33. Walrand S, Hesse M, Jamar F, Lhommel R. A hepatic dose-toxicity model opening the way toward individualized radioembolization planning. J Nucl Med. 2014;55(8):1317–22.
34. Walrand S, Hesse M, Chiesa C, Lhommel R, Jamar F. The low hepatic toxicity per gray of 90Y glass microspheres is linked to their transport in the arterial tree favoring a nonuniform trapping as observed in posttherapy PET imaging. J Nucl Med. 2014;55:135–40.
35. Sangro B, Gil-Alzugaray B, Rodriguez J, Sola I, Martinez-Cuesta A, Viudez A, Chopitea A, Iñarrairaegui M, Arbizu J, Bilbao JI. Liver disease induced by radioembolization of liver tumors: description and possible risk factors. Cancer. 2008;112:1538–46.
36. Gavanier M, Ayav A, Sellal C, Orry X, Claudon M, Bronowicki JP, Laurent V. CT imaging findings in patients with advanced hepatocellular carcinoma treated with sorafenib: alternative response criteria (Choi, European association for the study of the liver, and modified Response Evaluation Criteria in Solid Tumor (mRECIST)) versus RECIST 1.1. Eur J Radiol. 2016;85(1):103–12.
37. Pasciak AS, Bourgeois AC, Bradley YC. A microdosimetric analysis of tumor absorbed-dose as a function of the number of microspheres per unit volume in yttrium-90 radioembolization. J Nucl Med. 2016;57(7):1020–6.
38. Flamen P, Vanderlinden B, Delatte P, et al. Corrigendum: multimodality imaging can predict the metabolic response of unresectable colorectal liver metastases to radioembolization therapy with yttrium-90 labeled resin microspheres. Phys Med Biol. 2014;59:2549.
39. van den Hoven AF, Rosenbaum CE, Elias SG, de Jong HW, Koopman M, Verkooijen HM, Alavi A, van den Bosch MA, Lam MG. Insights into the dose-response relationship of radioembolization with resin 90Y-microspheres: a prospective cohort study

in patients with colorectal cancer liver metastases. J Nucl Med. 2016;57(7):1014–9.
40. Chiesa C. The individualized dosimetry in the radioembolization of hepatocarcinoma with 90Y microspheres. Phys Med. 2016;32:169–70. http://www.physicamedica.com/pb/assets/raw/Health%20Advance/journals/ejmp/1stECMP_abstracts_EJMP32S3.pdf
41. Sjögreen Gleisner K, Spezi E, Solny P, Gabina PM, Cicone F, Stokke C, Chiesa C, Paphiti M, Brans B, Sandström M, Tipping J, Konijnenberg M, Flux G. Variations in the practice of molecular radiotherapy and implementation of dosimetry: results from a European survey. EJNMMI Phys. 2017;4:28. doi 10.1186/s40658-017-0193-4.

14 The Clinical Challenge of Liver Metastasis

Stefano Cappato, Federica Brena, Michela Squadroni, Rosalba Barile, Davide Piccinali, Annalisa Mancin, Giorgio Quartierini, Orlando Goletti, and Giordano Beretta

Abstract

The treatment of liver metastases is generally considered as a palliative approach. A large body of literature refers to the experience gained in colorectal metastases, and surgery remains the cornerstone of treatments with a 40% survival at 5 years. Comparable results are attainable in the treatment of patients with neuroendocrine liver metastases. However, only a small proportion of these patients are suitable candidates for hepatic resection. Furthermore, there is limited data referring to the management of non-colorectal, non-neuroendocrine liver metastases, and most of the reports refer to smaller, retrospective case series with scarce information on treatment carried out during the patient's journey. In this chapter, we present current perspectives on the management of liver metastases, with a focus on state-of-the-art resection, by drawing on clinical data provided in the medical literature.

14.1 Molecular Mechanisms of Cancer Metastasis

Tumor cells have genetic alterations which allow them to colonize distant organ [1, 2]. Liver is one of the most common sites of hematogenous metastases. If we considered patients affected by colorectal cancer, 20% present liver metastases at diagnosis [3], 13% of patients with NETs have liver synchronous disease, and 50% of metastatic patients with breast cancer develop liver metastases during their disease history [4]. Cancer cells invade surrounding tissues, intravasate into blood vessels, survive in circulation, extravasate into distant organs, and expand to macrometastasis. Recent studies demonstrated that chemokine receptor system is a potential mechanism of tumor metastasis by promoting cancer cell migration, invasion, survival, and angiogenesis and by recruiting distal stromal cells to facilitate tumor invasion and metastasis [3]. The tropism of metastatic tumor cells for specific organ can be aided by interactions between chemokine receptors on cancer cells and their ligands in target organs [3–6]. The formation of metastasis is an

S. Cappato • D. Piccinali • A. Mancin • G. Quartierini
O. Goletti (✉)
Department of General, Microinvasive and Oncological Surgery, Humanitas Gavazzeni, Bergamo, Italy
e-mail: orlando.goletti@gavazzeni.it

F. Brena • M. Squadroni • R. Barile • G. Beretta
Department of Oncology, Humanitas Gavazzeni, Bergamo, Italy

E. Bombardieri et al. (eds.), *Clinical Applications of Nuclear Medicine Targeted Therapy*,
https://doi.org/10.1007/978-3-319-63067-0_14

extremely complex, multistep, and multifunctional biological event [7]. It is the result of a cascade of events: (1) local invasion of cancer cells through surrounding extracellular matrix (ECM) and stromal cells, (2) intravasation into the lumina of blood vessels, (3) survival in the circulation, (4) arrest at a distant organ site, (5) extravasation into the parenchyma of distant tissues, (6) formation of micrometastasis through survival in foreign microenvironment, and (7) metastatic colonization by carcinoma cells to form macroscopic metastasis [8] (Fig. 14.1).

14.1.1 Local Invasion

In order to invade the stroma, carcinoma cells must first breach the basement membrane (BM), a specialized ECM (extracellular matrix) that plays vital roles in organizing epithelial tissues. The ECM contains growth factor molecules that can be liberated by carcinoma-secreted proteases. BM also plays crucial roles in signal transduction events. In cancers, various types of cell migration can be found to different degrees and in different mixes. For example, at the invasive front, colorectal cancer cells disseminate as solitary, actively migrating cells, and once they have reached their target organ, they redifferentiate to form secondary tumors with a phenotype that is comparable to that of the primary tumor [7, 9]. In contrast squamous cell carcinoma invades predominantly by collective cell migration, with cone-shaped or sheetlike invasion fronts [10]. Cancer cells use morphogenetic developmental programs to control their migratory and invasive abilities [7]. The entry of neoplastic cells into the stroma provides abundant opportunities for tumor cells to directly access the systemic circulation and then disseminate to distant sites.

14.1.2 Intravasation

Carcinoma cells enter into the lumina of lymphatic or blood vessels. Intravasation can be facilitated by molecular changes that promote the ability of

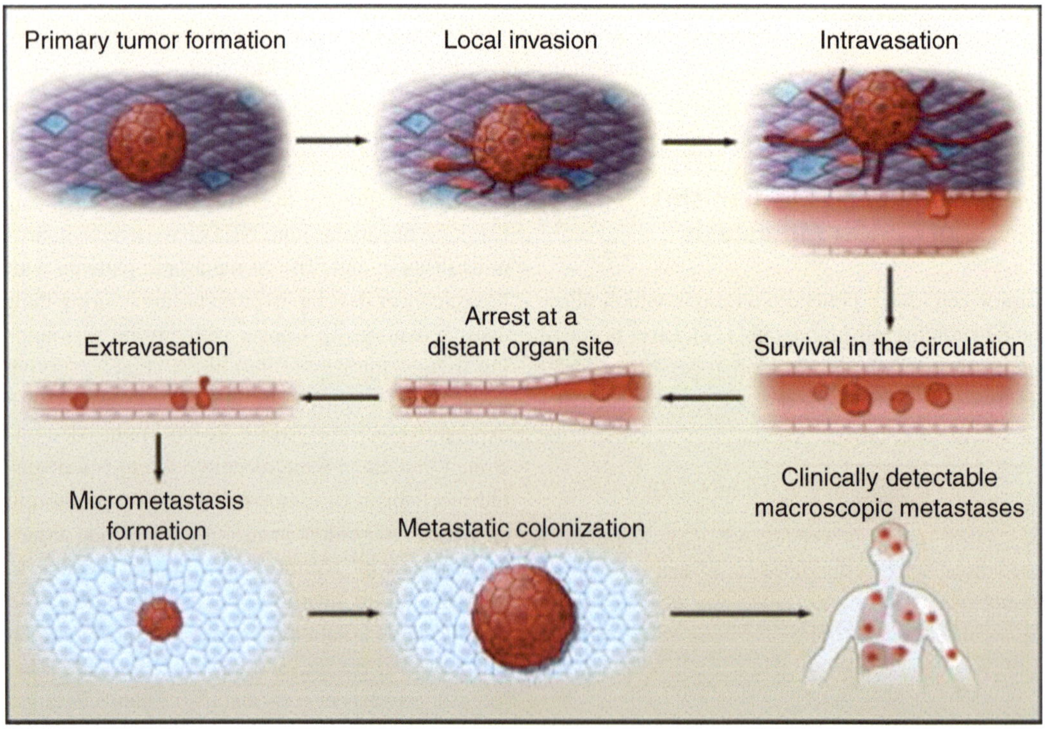

Fig. 14.1 The invasion-metastases cascade from Valastyan et al.: tumor metastasis—molecular insight and evolving paradigms [8]

carcinoma cells to cross the pericyte and endothelial cell barriers that form the walls of microvessels. The mechanics of intravasation are likely to be strongly influenced by the structural features of tumor-associated blood vessels. Through a variety of mechanisms, tumor cells stimulate the formation of new blood vessels present in normal tissues. These vessels are tortuous and leak.

14.1.3 Survival in Circulation

Carcinoma cells can disseminate widely through the venous and arterial circulation. Circulating tumor cells (CTCs) represent the intermediates between primary tumor and sites of dissemination. It is not known how long cancer cells linger in circulation. Circulating tumor cells have to survive to immune system, specifically natural killer cells. Tumor cells can evade immune detection [11].

14.1.4 Arrest at Distant Organ Sites

Individual carcinoma types form metastasis only in a limited subset of target organs [2]. It is unresolved if tissue tropism simply reflects a passive process in which CTCs arrest in capillary beds or indicates a capacity of CTCs to actively home to specific organs through ligand-receptor interactions. The anatomical layout of the vasculature precludes the arrest of carcinoma cells within the capillary beds. The trapping of colorectal carcinoma cells in the liver is dictated by the portal vein that drains the mesenteric circulation directly into the liver [12]. CTCs may elude this trapping because of their unusual plasticity or passing through arteriovenous shunts. The other hypothesis is that CTCs have predetermined predilections to lodge in certain tissues. For example, colorectal cells into hepatic microvasculature can initiate a pro-inflammatory cascade that results in Kupffer cells being triggered to chemokines that upregulate vascular adhesion receptors, enabling adhesion of CTCs in the microvasculature of the liver [13].

14.1.5 Extravasation

The term extravasation describes the passage of tumorigenic cells together with immune cells and serum from vessels to tissues, in order to initiate secondary metastatic outgrowth. The site of a tumor metastasis is influenced by both the primary tumor cell and the distant microenvironment into which it spreads. Extravasation of cancer cells is a highly dynamic process that involves the modulation of tumor cell adhesion to the endothelium and intravascular cell migration along the luminal surface of the vascular wall [14]. Circulating tumor cells, as with leukocytes, can use endothelial cell-specific adhesion molecules to interact with these cells before they touch the underlying BM in the further course of their extravasation. Neutrophils and platelets regulate metastasis development through physical interactions and anchoring of the circulation tumor cells to the endothelium [15].

14.1.6 Micrometastasis Formation

In order to form micrometastases, extravasated cells must survive in the foreign microenvironment that they encounter in the parenchyma of distant tissues. The microenvironment at the metastatic locus usually differs from that present in the site of primary tumor formation. There are predisposing changes that convert distant microenvironments into more hospitable sites for future settling by disseminated tumor. Tumor cells have complex mechanisms to modify foreign microenvironments in order to initially survive at these ectopic locations and form small micrometastases.

14.1.7 Metastatic Colonization

In the event that disseminated carcinoma cells survive their initial encounter with the microenvironment of a foreign tissue and succeed in persisting, they still are not guaranteed to proliferate and form large macroscopic metastases – the process of metastatic colonization. Instead, it seems that the vast majority of disseminated tumor cells suffer either slow attrition over periods of weeks and months or persist as microcolonies in a state of apparent long-term dormancy, retaining viability in the absence of any net gain or loss in overall cell number. In fact, these occult micrometastases may persist in one of two ways. The disseminated tumor cells may be largely quiescent, with their proliferation at metastatic sites greatly impaired due to incompatibilities with the foreign microenvironments that surround them. Alternatively, the cancer cells in occult micrometastases may proliferate continuously; however, a net increase in their overall number may not occur due to the counterbalancing effects of a high apoptotic rate [16]. The appreciation that disseminated tumor cells often encounter significant obstacles as they attempt to reactivate their growth machinery at metastatic sites is hardly a new concept. More than 120 years ago, Stephen Paget articulated his "seed-and-soil" hypothesis of metastatic outgrowth. From autopsy records, Paget observed preferential metastasis of a given type of cancer to one or more particular distant organ sites, which led him to posit that while tumor cells are broadly disseminated during the course of malignant progression, detectable metastases only develop at those sites ("soils") where the tumor cells ("seeds") are suitably adapted for survival and proliferation [2]. Consistent with the seed-and-soil hypothesis, evidence from a number of laboratories has documented that specific organ microenvironments are indeed intrinsically more or less hospitable for the

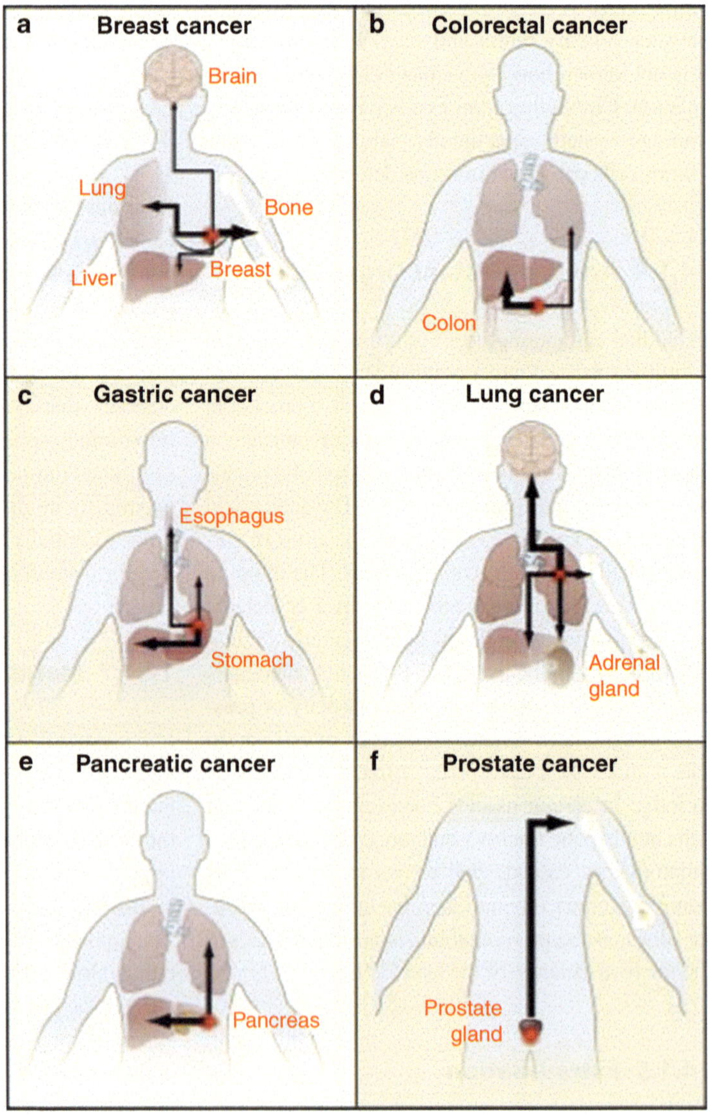

Fig. 14.2 Metastatic tropism. From Valastyan et al.: tumor metastasis – molecular insight and evolving paradigms [8]

proliferation and survival of certain types of disseminated tumor cells (Fig. 14.2).

14.2 The Diagnosis of Liver Metastases

14.2.1 Clinical Presentation

Most liver metastases are clinically silent and detected with cross-sectional imaging. When they are symptomatic, the disease is most often at an advanced stage and the prognosis is poor. Metastasis from hormonally active tumors may present with symptoms related to the hormonally active metabolites secreted by the metastatic cells [17].

14.2.2 Biochemistry

In order to diagnose liver disease, biochemistry can be useful.

- Enzymes that are found in the liver, including alanine transaminase (ALT) and aspartate transaminase (AST)
- Total protein and albumin
- Bilirubin, alkaline phosphatase, and gamma-glutamyl transpeptidase
- Prothrombin time and platelet count
- Serum cholinesterase

14.2.3 Imaging

Liver magnetic resonance imaging (MRI) is becoming the gold standard in liver metastasis detection and treatment response assessment. The most sensitive magnetic resonance sequences are diffusion-weighted images and hepatobiliary phase images. Peripheral ring enhancement, diffusion restriction, and hypointensity on hepatobiliary phase images are all marks of liver metastases. In patients with normal ultrasonography, computed tomography (CT), and positron emission tomography (PET)-CT findings and high clinical suspicion of metastasis, MRI should be performed for diagnosis of unseen metastases. In melanoma, colon cancer, and neuroendocrine tumor metastases, MRI allows confident diagnosis of treatment-related changes in the liver and enables differential diagnosis from primary liver tumors. Focal nodular hyperplasia-like nodules in patients who received platinum-based chemotherapy, hypersteatosis, and focal fat can mimic metastasis. In cancer patients with fatty liver, MRI should be preferred to CT. Although the first-line imaging for metastases is CT, MRI can be used as a problem-solving method. MRI may be used as the first-line method in patients who would undergo curative surgery or metastasectomy. Current limitation of MRI is low sensitivity for metastases smaller than 3 mm [17].

14.3 The Treatment of Liver Metastasis

14.3.1 Colorectal Cancer

Colorectal cancer (CRC) is the third leading cause of cancer death in the world [18]. The liver is the most frequent site of metastases from CRC cancer, and overall close to 50% of patients will develop liver metastases during the course of the disease. Indeed, for nearly one third of the patients with CRC, the liver is the only site of metastatic disease [19].

14.3.1.1 Operable Disease

Hepatic resection is the gold standard in the treatment of colorectal liver metastases and currently is the only curative treatment with a 40% survival at 5 years and almost 25% to 10 years in specialized centers [20, 21]. Results from a survey involving 13,334 patients from 330 centers who underwent surgery for liver metastases show a better survival outcome in patients who undergo first resection [22]. Furthermore a systematic review of 142 studies published in 1999–2010 confirmed these results [23]. Unfortunately, the majority of patients with CRC liver metastases are not amenable to surgery initially [24], and in those who undergo resection, almost 60% will develop recurrent disease, either in the liver or elsewhere [25]. The optimal treatment strategies for patients with colorectal liver metastases are evolving with improved clinical outcomes being achieved, especially when the multidisciplinary approach is used [26]. The multidisciplinary model is a patient-centered approach, requiring a team of specialists (surgeons, oncologists, radiologists, and pathologists at least), which is mandatory to finding the best strategy, the main objective of which is to achieve surgical resection. The strategy should be directed toward achieving complete resection, with both oncological and technical criteria being considered. The technical definition of resectability has evolved over time, with the current consensus proposing that liver metastases can be resectable as long as complete macroscopic resection is feasible while maintaining at least 30% of liver parenchyma (in patients with normal functioning liver). The oncological criteria provide prognostic information. Attention should be paid to the preoperative evaluation of extrahepatic disease, as these patients have a significantly worst prognosis [27]. However the presence of a limited number of lung metastases, without mediastinal node involvement, is no more considered a contraindication for resection of liver metastases, as resection of lung metastases can prolong survival [28]. Although patients with metachronous liver metastases have a better survival compared with patients with synchronous metastases, a 5-year survival of up to 31% can be obtained by resection of synchronous metastases [29]. One of the controversial issues is the optimal timing of liver resection; traditionally colorectal cancer and liver metastases have been approached with staged resection. Recently this paradigm has begun to change, and no increase of morbidity or mortality for simultaneous surgical removal, in selected cases, has been showed [30]. Finally, repeat hepatectomy is advised for patients with recurrent liver disease, if technically feasible. In these patients, surgery is safe and prolongs survival [31]. For patients with initially resectable disease, with good prognostic factors, one approach is an immediate surgical resection and another is perioperative chemotherapy. For patients who are resectable, the advantages of neoadjuvant chemotherapy may be to decrease the tumor size, control the micrometastatic disease, and assess the activity of chemotherapy in order to identify a group of patients who may benefit most from liver resection [32, 33]. The multi-institutional, intergroup, randomized prospective trial of the European Organization for Research and Treatment of Cancer (EORTC protocol 40983) studied the impact of pre- and postoperative 5-fluorouracil (5-FU)/leucovorin and oxaliplatin treatment on disease-free and overall survival in patients with resectable metastases. The major finding of this study was that overall survival was not significantly greater in patients who received perioperative FOLFOX4 than in those who received surgery only [34]. The role of adjuvant systemic chemotherapy after curative hepatic resection is unclear [35, 36]. The use of biological agent cetuximab in addition to chemotherapy is detrimental [37].

14.3.1.2 Initially Unresectable Liver Metastases

Only a minority of patients with liver metastases are susceptible to surgery. Some studies have showed how neoadjuvant chemotherapy (*conversion* chemotherapy) can make some metastases resectable [38]. Neoadjuvant therapy with irinotecan combined with 5-FU/FA enabled a significant proportion of patients with initially unresectable liver metastases to undergo surgical resection [39, 40]. Patients whose disease converted to operable disease have significant survival benefit compared with those who did not undergo surgery [41]. The addition of cetuximab to chemotherapy improved the objective response and resection rates, conferring a potential survival benefit, compared to chemotherapy alone or in combination with bevacizumab [42].

14.3.1.3 Unresectable Disease

For unresectable disease, the only possible approach is systemic treatment. 5-Fluorouracil plus leucovorin (FU/Lv) is the hinge of colorectal cancer (CRC) therapy [41]. FU/Lv in combination with either oxaliplatin [43] or irinotecan can increase progression-free survival and overall survival. Monoclonal antibodies targeting cancer cells (bevacizumab, cetuximab) are used in recent years and have effects on overall survival and progression-free survival only in combination with chemotherapy when used in advanced CRC [44–47]. The choice of treatment should always be based on patient safety, with regard to drug toxicity and other side effects, and patient agreement. The biological agents that target the epidermal growth factor receptor (EGFR) or vascular endothelial growth factor (VEGF) have proven clinical benefits in the treatment of patients with metastatic CRC. Anti-EGFR agents, including cetuximab [48] and panitumumab [49], as well as anti-VEGF agents, including bevacizumab, aflibercept, and ramucirumab, have been shown to extend survival in combination with cytotoxic chemotherapy. In particular, the addition of anti-EGFR agents has demonstrated significant efficacy in patients with the RAS wild-type metastatic CRC. In the future, building a personalized treatment strategy, according to the clinical characteristics and biologic features of patients with unresectable or metastatic CRC, will be necessary [42].

14.3.2 Neuroendocrine Liver Metastasis

Neuroendocrine tumors (NETs) are a heterogeneous group of neoplasms composed of carcinoid tumors and pancreatic NETs. The majority are characterized by a relatively indolent rate of growth and a propensity to produce and secrete a variety of hormones and other vasoactive substances that are linked with a clinical syndrome (diarrhea and flushing). Carcinoid tumors arise from enterochromaffin endocrine cells of gastrointestinal tract and airways [50]. Tumor growth rates also correlate with the site of origin. Treatment options for metastatic NETs have evolved in recent years. Somatostatin analogs octreotide and lanreotide, with their antiproliferative role, can stabilize tumor growth in metastatic neuroendocrine tumors [51]. Recent data have demonstrated the antiproliferative effect of many agents, including interferon alfa, mTOR inhibitors, and angiogenesis inhibitors [50]. For patients who have predominantly metastatic to the liver disease, locoregional approach can be considered. Forty-six percent of patients with neuroendocrine tumors (NETs) suffer from liver metastases [52, 53]. Their clinical course is variable, some NETS having an aggressive behavior with rapid progression to liver metastases. The prognosis and the approach to NETs are guided according to the histological classification: tumors with grade 3, mitotic count exceeding 20/10 high-powered fields, and/or Ki-67 proliferative index exceeding 20% represent malignant disease [54]. Hepatic involvement is an important prognostic factor, regardless of the site of primary tumor. Moreover the presence of liver metastases is closely related to the appearance or aggravation of symptoms because the metastases lead to reduced metabolization of NET peptides [55]. Surgery remains the only potential for cure in patients with liver metastases. In patients who underwent resection, a 5-year survival has been shown to be greater than 60% [56]. But although an aggressive surgical approach is considered to prolong survival and contribute to better symptom control, the criteria for patient selection are still ill-defined. In 2007, the European Neuroendocrine Tumor Society (ENETS) proposed guidelines for surgical resection based on three distinct patterns of involvement: (1) simple pattern when metastases are located in one or two contiguous lobes, (2) complex pattern where there is one major focus and other lesions are in the contralateral lobe, and (3) diffuse disease in both lobes [57]. In simple and complex patterns, surgery can be proposed; on the contrary, patients with diffuse liver metastases are not candidates for resection, and cytoreductive surgery can be helpful only for selected patients (Fig. 14.3). However, due to the rarity of the disease, the number of prospective studies is limited, and most recommendations represent expert opinions. The analyses from retrospective studies showed that high-grade tumors (G3) had a worse postsurgical

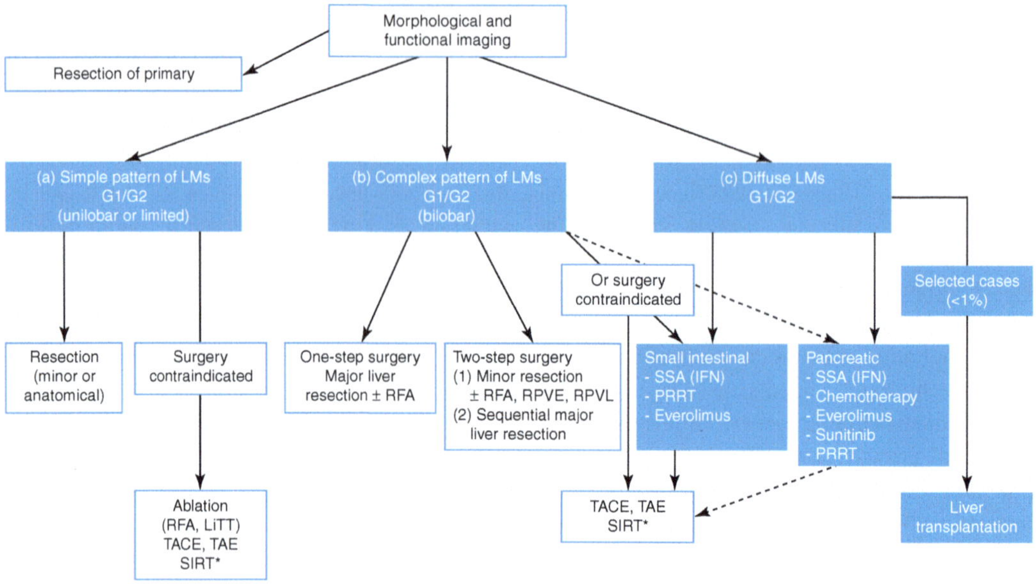

Fig. 14.3 ENETS Consensus Guidelines 2016 on treatment of liver metastases

outcome when compared to low-grade tumors [58]; therefore, G3 patients are candidates for chemotherapy that includes streptozocin- and temozolomide-based regimes.

14.3.3 Non-colorectal Non-neuroendocrine Liver Metastasis

If liver resection for metastatic colorectal and neuroendocrine tumors is a recognized approach which has consolidated in the last 20 years, the clinical utility of resection for non-colorectal non-neuroendocrine liver metastases has still many controversies. Defining the benefits of resection of isolated non-colorectal non-neuroendocrine liver metastases has been difficult because outcome data published using multi-institutional registries include a myriad of primary sites with little data on specific tumor types. Data on individual histologic subtypes come from small case series. So, defining benefits of liver resection for individual patients is difficult. Selection for resection should be a multidisciplinary decision, considering the histology of the primary tumor, the biologic history of the tumor in the individual patient, and the response to chemotherapy. There is no real evidence that surgery brings a survival benefit, and for these patients, systemic chemotherapy is generally recommended [59]. Recently liver resection has become a realistic treatment option for metastatic sarcomatous lesions, particularly gastrointestinal stromal tumors (GIST). Selected studies [60, 61] report a 5-year survival rate of 49% after hepatic metastasectomy. The introduction of tyrosine kinase inhibitors (TKI) has revolutionized the treatment of metastatic GIST, since it targets the specific molecular abnormalities [62]. Patients with primary unresectable liver metastases are clearly candidates for TKI neoadjuvant therapy. However, for resectable patients, the role and the setting of TKI are unclear. Vassos in 2015 published a retrospective analysis [63] on 87 patients treated within a period of 10 years, showing that TKI in the neoadjuvant setting may improve the survival. In light of the current evidence, it is recommended that all patients with hepatic metastases be treated aggressively with both surgery and TKI in neoadjuvant and adjuvant setting [64]. In all patients, a multidisciplinary approach is the mainstay of the management [65]. The likelihood of finding favorable isolated liver metastases, fit for surgery and for non-colorectal, non-neuroendocrine, non-sarcoma tumors, is low, and current literature is plagued with problems including the heterogeneity of primary tumor types, small sample size, as well as a lack of prospective studies. In this setting of patients, oncologic selection criteria must predominate, as the ability to control systemic disease is generally more limited. Determination of prognostic factors has therefore been attempted in some studies [66]. Favorable indicators include genitourinary, breast and soft tissue primaries, metachronous metastases, and curative resection. In 2006, Earle [67] showed that a longer interval between the diagnosis of the primary tumor and the diagnosis of liver metastases was predictive of survival. A prolonged disease-free interval is thought to be a surrogate marker for favorable tumor biology. Moreover there is a growing evidence that hepatectomy offered to patients who have shown response to chemotherapy yields better results [68]. A multidisciplinary approach is however necessary for the treatment of these patients.

References

1. Weinberg RA. The biology of cancer. New York: Garland Science; 2007.
2. Fidler IJ. The pathogenesis of cancer metastasis: the 'seed and soil' hypothesis revisited. Nat Rev Cancer. 2003;3:453–8.
3. Kawada K, Hasegawa S, Murakami T, et al. Molecular mechanisms of liver metastasis. Int J Clin Oncol. 2011;16:464–72.
4. Page AJ, Weiss MJ, Pawlik TM, et al. Surgical management of noncolorectal cancer liver metastases. Cancer. 2014;15:3111–21.
5. Mueller A, Homey B, Soto H, et al. Involvement of chemokine receptors in breast cancer metastasis. Nature. 2001;410:50–6.
6. Wang JM, Deng X, Gong W, et al. Chemokines and their role in tumor growth and metastasis. J Immunol Methods. 1998;220:1–17.
7. Spano D, Heck C, De Antonellis P, et al. Molecular networks that regulate cancer metastasis. Semin Cancer Biol. 2012;22:234–49.
8. Valastyan S, Weinberg RA. Tumor metastasis: molecular insight and evolving paradigms. Cell. 2011;147:275–92.
9. Brabletz T, Jung A, Spaderna S, Hlubek F, Kirchner T. Opinion: migrating cancer stem cells-an integrated concept of malignant tumor progression. Nat Rev Cancer. 2005;5:744–9.
10. Wicki A, Christofori G. The potential role of podoplanin in tumor invasion. Br J Cancer. 2007;96:1–5.
11. Joyce JA, Pollard JW. Microenvironmental regulation of metastasis. Nat Rev Cancer. 2009;9:239–52.
12. Gupta GP, Massaguè J. Cancer metastasis: building a framework. Cell. 2009;127:679–95.
13. Auguste P, Fallavollita L, Wang N, et al. The host inflammatory response promotes liver metastasis by increasing tumor cell arrest and extravasation. Am J Pathol. 2007;170:1781–92.
14. Stoletov K, Kato H, Zardouzian E, et al. Visualizing extravasation dynamics of metastatic tumor cells. J Cell Sci. 2010;123:2332–41.
15. Erpenbeck L, Schön MP. Deadly allies: the fatal interplay between platelets and metastasizing cancer cells. Blood. 2010;115:3427–2436.
16. Chambers AF, Groom AC, MacDonald IC. Dissemination and growth of cancer cells in metastatic sites. Nat Rev Cancer. 2002;2(8):563–72.
17. Karaosmanoglu AD, Onur MR, Ozmen NM, et al. Magnetic resonance imaging of liver metastasis. Semin Ultrasound CT MRI. 2016;37:533–48.
18. Ferlay J, Shin HR, Bray F, et al. GLOBOCAN 2008, VERSION 1.2, cancer incidence and mortality worldwide. IARC CancerBase No. 10. http://globocan.iarc.fr.
19. Weiss L, Grundmann E, Torhost J, et al. Haematogenous metastatic patterns of colonic carcinoma : an analysis of 1541 necropsies. J Pathol. 1986;150:195–203.
20. Adam R, De Gramont A, Figueras J, et al. The oncosurgery approach to managing liver metastases from colorectal cancer: a multidisciplinary international consensus. Oncologist. 2012;17:1225–39.
21. Rees M, Tekkis PP, Welsh FK, et al. Evaluation of long term survival after hepatic resection for metastatic colorectal cancer. A multifactorial model of 929 patients. Ann Surg. 2008;247:125–35.
22. LiverMetSurvey. International registry of patients operated for colorectal liver metastases. Available at http:// livermetsurvey.org.
23. Taylor A, Kanas G, Langerberg W, et al. Survival after surgical resection of hepatic metastases from colorectal cancer: a systematic review and meta-analysis. Ann Oncol. 2010;21(Suppl 8):632.
24. Scheele J, Stange R, Altendof-Hoffman A, et al. Resection of colorectal liver metastases. World J Surg. 1995;19:59–71.
25. De Jong MC, Pulitano C, Ribero D, et al. Rates and pattern of recurrence following curative intent surgery for colorectal liver metastases: an international multi-institutional analysis of 1669 patients. Ann Surg. 2009;250:440–8.
26. Fennell ML, Das IP, Clauser S, et al. The organization of multidisciplinary care teams: modeling internal and external influences on cancer care quality. J Natl Cancer Inst Monogr. 2010;2010:72–80.

27. Fong Y, Fortner J, Sun RL, et al. Clinical score for predicting recurrence after hepatic resection for metastatic colorectal cancer: analysis of 1001 consecutive cases. Ann Surg. 1999;230:309–18.
28. Mineo TC, Ambrogi V, Tonini G, et al. Long term results after resection of simultaneous and sequential lung and liver metastases from colorectal carcinoma. J Am Coll Surg. 2003;197:386–91.
29. Fujita S, Akasu T, Moriya Y. Resection of synchronous liver metastases from colorectal cancer. Jpn J Clin Oncol. 2000;30:7–11.
30. Capussotti L, Ferrero A, Viganò L, et al. Timing of resection of liver metastases synchronous to colorectal tumor: proposal for prognosis–based decisional model. Ann Surg Oncol. 2007;14:1143–50.
31. Adam R, Bismuth H, Castaing D, et al. Repeat hepatectomy for colorectal liver metastases. Ann Surg. 1997;225:51–60.
32. Juez I, Rubio C, Figueras J. Multidisciplinary approach of colorectal liver metastases. Clin Transl Oncol. 2011;13:721–7.
33. Gruenberger B, Scheithauer W, Punzengruber B, et al. Importance of response to neoadjuvant chemotherapy in potentially curable colorectal cancer liver metastases. BMC Cancer. 2008;8:120.
34. Nordliger B, Sorbye H, Glimelius B, et al. Perioperative FOLFOX4 chemotherapy and surgery versus surgery alone for resectable liver metastases from colorectal cancer (EORTC 40983): long-term results of a randomised, controlled, phase 3 trial. Lancet Oncol. 2013;14(12):1208–15.
35. Langer B, et al. Fluorouracil plus leucovorin versus observation after potentially curative resection of liver or lung metastases from colorectal cancer (CRC): results of the ENG (EORTC/NCIC CTG/GIVo) randomized trial. Proc Am Soc Clin Oncol. 2002;21:149a.
36. Portier G, Elias D, Bouche O, et al. Multicenter randomized trial of adjuvant fluorouracil and folinic acid compared with surgery alone after resection of colorectal liver metastases: FFCD ACHBTH AURC 9002 trial. J Clin Oncol. 2006;24:4976–82.
37. Primrose J, Falk S, Finch-Jones M, et al. Systemic chemotherapy with or without cetuximab in patients with resectable colorectal liver metastasis: the new EPOC randomised controlled trial. Lancet Oncol. 2014;15:601–11.
38. Adam R, Delvart V, Pascal G, et al. Rescue surgery for unresectable colorectal liver metastases downstaged by chemotherapy: a model to predict long-term survival. Ann Surg. 2004;240:644–57.
39. Pozzo C, Basso M, Cassano A, et al. Neoadjuvant treatment of unresectable liver disease with irinotecan and 5-fluorouracil plus folinic acid in colorectal cancer patients. Ann Oncol. 2004;15:933–9.
40. Barone C, Nuzzo G, Cassano A, et al. Final analysis of colorectal cancer patients treated with irinotecan and 5-fluorouracil plus folinic acid neoadjuvant chemotherapy for unresectable liver metastases. Br J Cancer. 2007;97:1035–9.
41. Venook A, Niedzwiecki D, Blanke C, et al. CALGB/SWOG 80405: analysis of patients undergoing surgery as part of treatment strategy. *ESMO* 2014. Proffered paper session (ref LBA10).
42. Barone C, Basso M, Dadduzio V, et al. Conversion chemotherapy for technically unresectable colorectal liver metastases. Medicine. 2016;95(20):e3722.
43. De Gramont A, Figer A, Seymour M, et al. Leucovorin and fluorouracil with or without oxaliplatin as first-line treatment in advanced colorectal cancer. J Clin Oncol. 2000;18:2938–47.
44. Hurwitz H, Fehrenbacher L, Novotny W, et al. Bevacizumab plus irinotecan, fluorouracil, and leucovorin for metastatic colorectal cancer. NEJM. 2004;350:2335–42.
45. Saltz LB, Clark S, Dìaz-Rubio E, et al. Bevacizumab in combination with oxaliplatin-based chemotherapy as first-line therapy in metastatic colorectal cancer: a randomized phase III study. J Clin Oncol. 2008;26:2013–9.
46. Huwitz H, Fehrenbacher L, Novotny W, et al. Bevacizumab in combination with fluorouracil and leucovorin: an active regimen for first-line metastatic colorectal cancer. J Clin Oncol. 2005;23:3502–8.
47. Cunningham D, Lang I, Marcuello E, et al. Bevacizumab plus capecitabine versus capecitabine alone in elderly patients with previously untreated metastatic colorectal cancer (AVEX): an open-label, randomized phase 3 trial. Lancet Oncol. 2013;14:1077–85.
48. Van Cutsem E, Köhne CH, Hitre E, et al. Cetuximab and chemotherapy as initial treatment for metastatic colorectal cancer. NEJM. 2009;360:1408–17.
49. Douillard JY, Siena S, Cassidy J, et al. Randomized, phase III trial of panitumumab with infusional fluorouracil, leucovorin, and oxaliplatin (FOLFOX4) versus FOLFOX4 alone as first-line treatment in patients with previously untreated metastatic colorectal cancer: the PRIME study. J Clin Oncol. 2010;28(31):4697–705.
50. Strosberg JR, Cheema A, Kvols LK, et al. A review of systemic and liver-directed therapies for metastatic neuroendocrine tumors of the gastroenteropancreatic tract. Cancer Control. 2011;18(2):127–37.
51. Strosberg JR, Kvols L. Antiproliferative effect of somatostatin analogs in gastroenteropancreatic neuroendocrine tumors. World J Gastroenterol. 2010;16:2963–70.
52. Frilling A, Sotiropoulos GC, Li J, et al. Multimodal management of neuroendocrine liver metastases. HPB. 2010;12:361–79.
53. Ramage J, Davies A, Ardill J, et al. Guidelines for the management of gastroenteropancreatic neuroendocrine tumors (NETs). Gut. 2012;61:6–32.
54. Gu P, Wu J, Newman E, et al. Treatment of liver metastases in patients with neuroendocrine tumors of gastroesophageal and pancreatic origin. Int J Hepatol. 2012;2012:1.

55. Lee E, Pachter HL, Sarpel U. Hepatic arterial embolization for the treatment of metastatic neuroendocrine neoplasms. Int J Hepatol. 2012;2012:471203.
56. Schurr PG, Strate T, Rese K, et al. Aggressive surgery improves long term survival in neuroendocrine pancreatic tumors. Ann Surg. 2007;245:273–81.
57. Steinmuller T, Kianmanesh R, Falconi M, et al. Consensus guidelines for the management of patients with liver metastases from digestive neuroendocrine tumors: foregut, midgut, hindgut and unknown primary. Neuroendocrinology. 2007;87:47–62.
58. Harring T, Nguyen N, Gross JA, et al. Treatment of liver metastases in patients with neuroendocrine tumors: a comprehensive review. Int J Hepatol. 2011;2011:154541. 11 pages
59. Neri F, Ercolani G, Di Gioia P, et al. Updat Surg. 2015;67:223–33.
60. Rehders A, Peiper M, Stoeklein NH, et al. Hepatic metastasectomy for soft tissue sarcomas: is it justified? World J Surg. 2009;33:111–7.
61. Turley RS, Peng PD, Reddy SK, et al. Hepatic resection for metastatic gastrointestinal stromal tumors in the tyrosine kinase inhibitor era. Cancer. 2012;118:3571–8.
62. Zhu J, Yang Y, Zhou L, et al. A long term follow up of the imatinib mesylate treatment for the patients with recurrent gastrointestinal stromal tumors (GIST): the liver metastasis and the outcome. BMC Cancer. 2010;10:199.
63. Vassos N, Agaimy A, Hohenberger W, et al. Management of liver metastases of gastrointestinal stromal tumors (GIST). Ann Hepatol. 2015;14:531–9.
64. Seesing MFJ, Tielen R, van Hillegersberg R, van Coevorden F, de Jong KP, Nagtegaale ID, Verhoeff C, de Wilt JHW, Dutch Liver Surgery Working Group. Eur J Surg Oncol. 2016;42:1407.
65. Radkani P, Ghersi MN, Paramo JC, et al. A multidisciplinary approach for the treatment of GIST liver metastasis. World J Surg Oncol. 2008;6:46.
66. Adam R, Chiche L, Aloia T, et al. Hepatic resection for noncolorectal non neuroendocrine liver metastases: analysis of 1452 patients and development of a prognostic model. Ann Surg. 2006;244:524–35.
67. Earle SA, Perez EA, Gutierrez JC, et al. Hepatectomy enables prolonged survival in selected patients with isolated noncolorectal liver metastases. J Am Coll Surg. 2006;203:436–46.
68. Schmelzie M, Eisenberg CF, Matthaei M, et al. Non-colorectal, non-neuroendocrine, and non-sarcoma metastases of the liver: resection as a promising tool in the palliative management. Langenbeck's Arch Surg. 2010;395:227–34.

15 Radioembolization of Hepatic Metastases with ^{90}Y-Microspheres: Indications and Procedure

Rosa Sciuto, Sandra Rea, Giuseppe Pizzi, Giulio E. Vallati, and Lidia Strigari

Abstract

Radioembolization using ^{90}Y-microspheres (^{90}Y-RE) represents a safe and efficacy technique for treating metastatic liver malignancies with a growing number of ongoing trials and clinical experience in different types of tumors. ^{90}Y-RE is treatment modality that needs to be adapted to the individual patient, every step of the way. The appropriate patient selection for selection of patients to the treatment requires a multidisciplinary discussion to provide a benefit with acceptable risk. Pre-therapy workup, therapy planning and intra-arterial infusion of ^{90}Y-microspheres procedure require an experienced and synergic team formed by nuclear medicine physician, interventional radiologist and medical physicist. A personalized therapeutic plan with a tailored target volume and prescribed dose should be developed for each patient after analysis of all clinical, laboratory and multimodality imaging data. Both efficacy and safety will result improved as the patient's selection will be more appropriate and delivery technique accurate.

R. Sciuto (✉) • S. Rea
Nuclear Medicine Unit, Department of Research, Advanced Diagnostic and Innovation Technology, Regina Elena National Cancer Institute, Rome, Italy
e-mail: rosa.sciuto@ifo.gov.it; sandra.rea@ifo.gov.it

G. Pizzi • G.E. Vallati
Interventional Radiology Unit, Department of Research, Advanced Diagnostic and Innovation Technology, Regina Elena National Cancer Institute, Rome, Italy
e-mail: giuseppe.pizzi@ifo.gov.it; giulio.vallati@ifo.gov.it

L. Strigari
Laboratory of Medical Physics and Expert Systems, Department of Research, Advanced Diagnostic and Innovation Technology, Regina Elena National Cancer Institute, Rome, Italy
e-mail: lidia.strigari@ifo.gov.it

15.1 Introduction

The management of hepatic metastases is a significant clinical problem due to their high morbidity and mortality. Surgical resection of metastatic liver cancer, with or without adjuvant chemotherapy, is the most effective method for enhancing survival; however, only a small percentage of patients (less than 30%) are suitable candidates for surgery. In recent years, the clinical management of metastatic liver cancer has become more aggressive, including an increasing rate of major hepatectomy procedures and more multidisciplinary, including various nonsurgical interventions.

E. Bombardieri et al. (eds.), *Clinical Applications of Nuclear Medicine Targeted Therapy*, https://doi.org/10.1007/978-3-319-63067-0_15

New treatment options such as interventional liver-directed therapies have been proposed in addition to the standard approach of resection and chemotherapy. Liver-directed therapies include transarterial approaches, such as chemoembolization and radioembolization (RE) as well as a multitude of different ablative techniques, such as radiofrequency and microwave ablation as well as irreversible electroporation. Radioembolization (RE) using yttrium-90 (^{90}Y)-microspheres (^{90}Y-RE) is one effective and safe transarterial treatment option for patients with liver-only or liver-dominant disease [1, 2].

^{90}Y-RE is currently known by a variety of titles including mostly selective internal radiation therapy (SIRT), transarterial radioembolization (TARE) or, sometimes, intra-arterial radionuclide therapy and involves the catheter-based infusion of ^{90}Y-microspheres into the hepatic arterial circulation, from which approximately 80–100% of liver tumor blood flow derives. This minimal invasive treatment modality combines the advantages of internal radiation therapy, owing to intratumoral ^{90}Y radiation dose delivered, and embolic effect of β-emitting particles by way of deposit of millions of no biodegradable microspheres in the neoplastic microvasculature. The assumption of the intra-arterial placement of microspheres arises from anatomic and physiological aspects of the liver tissue. The technology takes advantage of the fact that healthy liver tissue derives over 70% of its blood supply from the portal vein, while metastatic liver tumors >3 mm derive 90% of their blood supply from the hepatic artery [3]. Placing the ^{90}Y-labelled microspheres into branches of the hepatic artery, a high-dose radiotherapy can be delivered to the tumor with minor radiation-induced hepatic damage [2, 4, 5].

Two distinctively different types of ^{90}Y-microspheres for RE are commercially available: resin microspheres or SIR-Spheres® (Sirtex Medical Sydney, Australia) and glass microspheres or TheraSphere® (MDS Nordion, Ottawa, Canada). SIR-Spheres® were approved in 2002 in the United States for treating colorectal cancer metastatic (mCRC) of the liver in combination with floxuridine hepatic arterial chemotherapy. TheraSphere® were approved in 1999 in the United States for the treatment of unresectable hepatocellular carcinoma (HCC). Both microspheres are currently approved in the Europe and other countries for the treatment of unresectable liver tumors. Resin microspheres are mostly used in the setting of liver metastasis both in current practice and in clinical trial. Different properties of resin and glass microspheres are illustrated in Table 15.1. Both resin and glass microspheres are loaded with the same β-emitter ^{90}Y having optimal characteristics for therapy (half-life, 64.2 h; average energy, 0.94 MeV; maximum and mean penetration ranges in soft tissue, 11 and 4 mm, respectively) [6].

Efficacy and safety of ^{90}Y-RE depend on numerous patients' factors, including the hepatic arterial flow distribution, vascularity of the target tumor, functional integrity of uninvolved liver parenchyma and relative radio sensitivities of both tissues. However, two other impor-

Table 15.1 Main characteristics of resin and glass ^{90}Y-microspheres

Characteristics	Resin microspheres	Glass microspheres
Trade name	SIR-Spheres®	TheraSphere®
Diameter of microsphere (μm)	20–60	20–30
Specific gravity (g/mL)	1.6	3.6
Specific activity (Bq/sphere)	40–70	2500
Number of microspheres per vial	60 million/3 GBq	1.2 million/3 GBq
Material	Resin with bound yttrium	Glass with yttrium in matrix
Embolic effect	Moderate	Mild
Splitting one vial for two or more patients	Possible	Not possible
Activity available (GBq)	3	3, 5, 7, 10, 15, 20

TheraSphere® obtained from BTG, London, UK and SIR-Spheres® from Sirtex Medical Limited, NSW, Australia

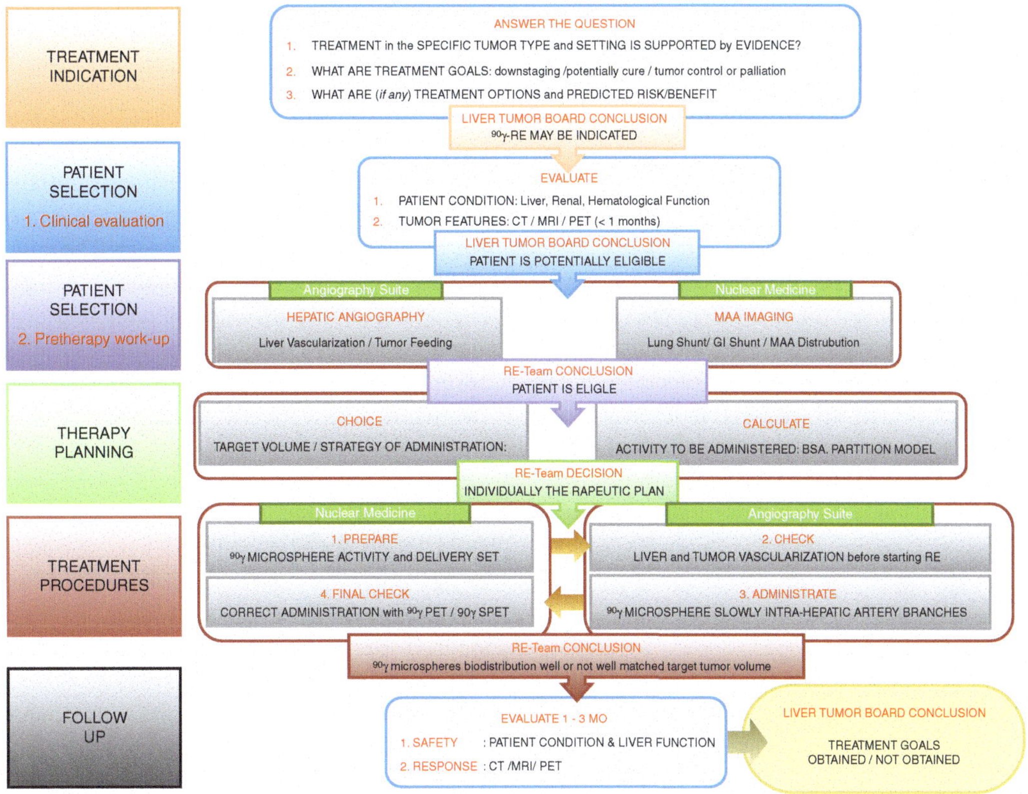

Fig. 15.1 Diagnostic-therapeutic path of ^{90}Y-radioembolization is illustrated outlining sequential decisional and operative steps. *MAA* technetium-99m-labelled macroaggregated albumin scintigraphy, *CT* computed tomography, *MRI* magnetic resonance imaging, *PET* positron emission tomography, *^{90}Y-RE* radioembolization with yttrium-90 resin microspheres

tant factors, not to underestimate for treatment to be successful, are represented by a multidisciplinary approach across all patients' clinical path and a well-trained and synergistic treatment team, including nuclear medicine physician, interventional radiologist and medical physicist. Therefore, treatment should be reserved to tertiary referral centres with documented experience and facilities.

^{90}Y-RE diagnostic-therapeutic path includes several phases: (1) treatment indications; (2) patients' selection, including clinical evaluation and pretreatment workup; (3) therapy planning; (4) treatment procedures; and (5) follow-up, including response monitoring and safety evaluation (Fig. 15.1).

This chapter describes all the phases of ^{90}Y-RE clinical framework from patient selection to follow-up collating the published evidence and personal clinical experience with the aim to propose a practical guide when planning and performing ^{90}Y-RE treatment with resin microspheres of liver metastases.

15.2 Treatment Indications

Clinical management of unresectable hepatic metastases in the last 10 years is gradually evolving from an empiric chemotherapy approach to an individually tailored approach. Currently, the best treatment possible is periodically selected in the perspective of a care continuum. Accordingly, ^{90}Y-RE appropriate indications in hepatic metastases have to be evaluated in the clinical context and confirmed in a multidisciplinary liver tumor board setting. Although the indications for treatment vary widely depending on the type of tumor and patient clinical status, currently ^{90}Y-RE may be considered as a treatment option for unresectable liver metastases or in patients unfit for surgery with most common accepted use of a salvage therapy in almost any kind of primary tumors [1, 2].

The most ^{90}Y-RE experience is currently based on treatment of mCRC to the liver in which it can be combined with modern chemotherapy or administered as a monotherapy, either during a chemotherapy holiday, in a salvage setting or as an alternative to local chemotherapy. Considering available clinical trial results [7–16] and current guidelines for the management of patients with mCRC from the European Society of Medical Oncology (*ESMO*) [17], ^{90}Y-RE with resin microspheres may be indicated in the following setting:

- *Salvage setting* for patients with liver-limited or liver-dominant metastases failing the available chemotherapeutic options. In this setting radioembolization with ^{90}Y-resin microspheres has been shown to prolong the time to tumor progression in the liver, based on a small randomized phase III study [14], and may be considered indicated (ESMO 2016, *recommendation II,B*).
- *Adjuvant or consolidation setting* as a first- or second-line treatment of mCRC in combination with or as an alternative to available biological agents. A number of studies are ongoing to further explore this indication that is currently accepted only in a clinical trial setting.
- *Neoadjuvant setting*: ^{90}Y-RE may also currently be a good alternative in patients who are potential candidates for resection but display a small functional liver residual volume with the aim to induce contralateral liver hypertrophy. The combination of antitumoral effect and simultaneous hypertrophy induction of the non-embolized segments has clear advantages over standard portal vein embolization (PVE) in terms of tumor control and morbidity [18].
- *Conversion to resectable disease*: this is a promising emerging ^{90}Y-RE indication that could shift treatment goal from palliation towards curative setting. Patient initially unfit for surgery due to tumor extension may be downstaged to curative surgery. The combination of selective tumor treatment and the induction of hypertrophy of untreated segments make ^{90}Y-RE an appealing strategy even only limited published studies are available [19].

However, in mCRC there is an increasing amount of data and several ongoing clinical phase III trials are likely to broaden the currently accepted indications. In particular, results of FOXFIRE [20] trial are soon awaited, as is the combined overall survival data from SIRFLOX, FOXFIRE and FOXFIRE Global [21].

The use of radioembolization for treatment of liver metastases from different primary cancers is also expanding [22, 23]. More clinical experience is reported for liver metastases of neuroendocrine tumors (mNETs) and breast cancer (mBC). In liver metastases of mNETs, overall studies have demonstrated that in patients with treatment-refractory disease as either first-line treatment or salvage therapy for liver metastases, ^{90}Y-resin microspheres are efficacious and associated with good tolerability and improvements in health-related quality of life (QoL) [24–36]. mNETs are particularly well-matched to this treatment approach as these tumors are well arterialized and thus an ideal target for transarterial therapies similarly to HCC. Treatment goal in these patients is control of symptoms as well as survival. However, there are no RCTs on any of these entities, and further data is needed to confirm these encouraging results.

In mBC resin microspheres have shown efficacy in the treatment of chemotherapy-refractory metastatic disease and in the treatment of liver progression during a treatment hiatus. Overall,

86% of patients with chemotherapy-refractory liver metastases from breast cancer or with liver progression during a treatment hiatus after first- or second-line chemotherapy were alive 14 months after receiving ^{90}Y-resin microspheres [37]. The use of ^{90}Y-resin microspheres in chemorefractory mBC is further supported by a high proportion of patients with partial response (25–56%) or stable disease (39–63%) [37–41]. Less experience has been reported in other tumor types including metastases from uveal melanoma, sarcoma, oesophageal, endometrial, lung, ovarian and squamous cell carcinoma of the anus [42–45]. Most relevant studies in mCRC and other tumors are summarized, respectively, in Tables 15.2 and 15.3.

In our own practice, we have noted a wide variety of treatment responses to ^{90}Y-RE, ranging from progressive disease to a significant partial response (unpublished data). This wide range of response may reflect both genetic heterogeneity in clinical setting and tumor target than technical factors influencing ^{90}Y-microspheres biodistribution [46, 47]. It is probable that in the future, molecular profiling of the tumor will allow greater patient selection and more targeted use of ^{90}Y-RE.

Key Points

^{90}Y-RE represents a safe and efficacy technique for treating metastatic liver malignancies. The current data justifies its clinical use in mCRC and mNET, while its role outside a salvage setting needs to be identified for liver metastases from other tumor entities. However, considering ongoing trials and the increasing clinical experience, a growing role of ^{90}Y-RE in metastatic liver disease has to be expected in the next years.

A multidisciplinary approach in a setting of liver tumor board is mandatory to identify appropriate indications to ^{90}Y-RE for patients with liver metastases and to integrate this treatment with all the available therapy options in the perspective of a strategy based on a care continuum.

Strategic treatment goals and therapy setting (potentially improve overall survival, increase the time to progression, downstage tumors for liver resection or provide palliation of symptoms) for each patient should be always clearly stated when treatment is indicated.

Table 15.2 Summary of most relevant studies in liver metastases from colorectal cancer

Reference	Pts N	Micro-spheres	Study design	Setting	Regimen	ORR (%)	SD (%)	Median OS months
Gray et al. [10]	74	Resin	RCT	First-line	FUDR-HA ± SIR-Spheres	44.4	8.3	17 months
Van Hazel et al. [9]	21	Resin	RCT	First-line	5FU/LV ± SIR-Spheres	90.1	9.9	29.4
Sharma et al. [15]	20	Resin	Prospective single arm	First-line	FOLFOX + SIR-Spheres	90	10	nr
Lim et al. [11]	30	Resin	Prospective single arm	Second-line	5FU/LV + SIR-Spheres	33	27	nr
Van Hazel et al. [12]	25	Resin	Prospective single arm	Second-line	Irinotecan + SIR-Spheres	48	39	12.2
Cosimelli et al. [8]	50	Resin	Prospective single arm	Salvage therapy	SIR-Spheres	24	24	12.6
Hendlisz et al. [14]	44	Resin	RCT	Salvage therapy	5FU ± SIR-Spheres	10	76	10
Seidensticker et al. [13]	58	Resin	Matched-pair, retrospective control	Salvage therapy	SIR-Spheres vs. BSC	41.4	17.2	8.3
Sofocleous et al. [16]	19	Resin	Prospective single arm	Salvage therapy	SIR-Spheres	5	53	12.7

FUDR-HA floxuridine given by hepatic artery infusion, *5FU* 5 fluorouracil, *LV* leucovorin

Table 15.3 Summary of most relevant studies in liver metastases form various tumor types

Reference	Pts N^	Micro-spheres	Tumor type	Study design	Setting	ORR	SD	Median OS months
Saxena et al. [25]	48	Resin	NET	Retrospective	Salvage	55%	23%	35
Cao et al. [26]	58	Resin	NET	Retrospective	Mixed	39.2%	27.5%	36
Paprottka et al. [27]	42	Resin	NET	Retrospective	Mixed	22.5%	75%	NA
Memon et al. [28]	40	Glass	NET	Retrospective	Mixed	63.9%	32.5%	34.4
Peker et al. [34]	30	Resin	NET	Retrospective	Mixed	40%	43%	39
Kennedy et al. [35]	148	Resin	NET	Retrospective	Mixed	63.2%	22.7%	70
King et al. [24]	34	Resin	NET	Retrospective	Mixed	50%	14.7%	59.0% alive at 35.2 months
Ceelen et al. [30]	45	Resin	NET	Retrospective	Mixed	13%	82%	NR
Ezziddin et al. [31]	23	Resin	NET	Retrospective	Salvage	30.4%	60.9%	29
Barbier et al. [32]	40	Resin	NET	Retrospective	Salvage	54%	41%	24.7
Filippi et al. [33]	15	Resin	NET	Retrospective	Salvage	47%	53%	31
Haug et al. [39]	58	Resin	Breast	Retrospective	Salvage	25%	63%	10.8
Cianni et al. [37]	52	Resin	Breast	Retrospective	Salvage	56%	35%	11.5
Saxena et al. [40]	40	Resin	Breast	Retrospective	≥1 Line	31%	39%	13.6
Coldwell et al. [38]	44	Resin	Breast	Retrospective	Treatment hiatus or salvage	47%	47%	NR
Michl et al. [42]	19	Resin	Pancreas	Retrospective	Mixed	64.3%	0	9
Gonsalves et al. [43]	32	Resin	Uveal melanoma	Retrospective	Salvage	6%	56%	10
Eldredge-Hindy et al. [44]	71	Resin	Uveal melanoma	Retrospective	Mixed	8%	52%	23.9
Klingenstein et al. [45]	13	Resin	Uveal melanoma	Retrospective	Mixed	62%	15%	19

15.3 Patients Selection

Patient selection is a critical phase to provide a benefit with acceptable risk. Each patient referred for ^{90}Y-RE should be discussed individually in a multidisciplinary setting to assess the appropriateness for the treatment considering both efficacy and safety and defining the treatment intention. Multidisciplinary setting (if possible a dedicated Liver Tumor Board) should include both a "technique ^{90}Y-RE treatment team", formed by nuclear medicine physician, interventional radiologist and medical physicist who are experienced in the procedure (*RE-Team*), and a panel of clinical liver specialist mainly comprising liver surgeon, medical oncologist, gastroenterologist/hepatologist, pathologist and diagnostic radiology.

Patient selection includes two different steps: the first step or *clinical evaluation* consists of physical examination together with imaging and laboratory analysis evaluation, whereas the second step, commonly named *pre-therapy workup*, includes hepatic angiography and scintigraphy with technetium-99m-labelled macroaggregated albumin (^{99m}Tc-MAA imaging). Therefore, the final confirmation of patient eligibility for treatment will be only at the end of pre-therapy workup and will require a careful evaluation of all the acquired elements in both the steps.

15.3.1 Clinical Evaluation

Clinical evaluation involves all the specialists of Liver Tumor Board in a joint analysis of many factors aimed to establish tumor characteristics and disease extension, patient clinical conditions and liver function, alternative therapy options and, finally, the goals of the proposed treatment, i.e. treatment intention (Fig. 15.1).

Independent from the underlying disease, candidates for ^{90}Y-RE should have:

- A life expectancy greater than 3 months
- Good performance status (i.e. Eastern Cooperative Oncology Group – ECOG ≤2)
- Unresectable liver metastases or no fit for surgery (the exact confirmation of unresectability preferably should be documented by expert liver surgeon)
- Liver-limited or liver-predominant disease (oligometastatic-extrahepatic disease may be accepted after multidisciplinary discussion)
- No contraindication for selective angiography, including adequate renal function (low impairment may be corrected by medical therapy) and no significant allergy to iodinated contrast medium (mild allergy may be compensated by adequate steroid therapy)
- Adequate liver function (bilirubin level <2.0 mg/dL, albumin >2.5 g/dL, alanine aminotransferase and aspartate aminotransferase levels lower than five times the upper limit)

Safety is of utmost priority and hence it is important to note the limitations and conditions from which patients must be excluded. In particular, liver, renal and haematological functions have to be accurately assessed to identify absolute or relative contraindications. Liver reserve might be (often is) affected owing to neoplastic replacement and prior hepatotoxic treatments. Alanine transaminase-aspartate transaminase and alkaline phosphatase-gamma glutamyl transferase are the markers for acute and subacute hepatocellular and biliocanalicular injury, respectively. More difficult to evaluate is the real "functional liver volume" (FLV) in the anatomically intact appearing liver region(s). Bilirubin is a composite marker of liver reserve and has been widely used in many classification systems as a predictive measure. A bilirubin level more than 2 mg/dL with the absence of correctable obstructive aetiology precludes ^{90}Y-RE [48].

Taking into account these issues, absolute contraindications to ^{90}Y-RE are:

- Significant intractable or refractory ascites
- Hepatic encephalopathy
- Presence of clinical liver for best clarity abnormal synthetic and excretory liver function tests
- bleeding diathesis not correctable by therapy signs; INR > 2
- Severe peripheral vascular disease that would preclude arterial catheterization
- Disseminated extrahepatic malignant disease
- Extensive bilateral liver involvement (more than 70%)

Along with these strict inclusion and exclusion criteria, many other clinical conditions should be checked as relative contraindications and be carefully evaluated for each patient in the specific clinical context (age, performance status, life expectancy, alternative options, aim of the therapy and possible corrective interventions) before confirming ^{90}Y-RE eligibility:

- Extensive bilateral liver involvement or infiltrative pattern (50–70%).
- Severe portal hypertension.
- Previous external beam radiotherapy to major volume of the liver.

- Platelet values <50,000; haemoglobin values <9.5; leucocytes <2500. It is needed to monitor the trend and eventually provide appropriate blood replacement or stimulating factors.
- Creatinine >1.8 mg/dL. It is usually enough an appropriate hydration and medical therapy support to have value normalization.
- Previous treatment with angiogenesis inhibitors could affect the quality of the blood vessels and induce complication during angiography. A washout period of at least 4 weeks should be planned before ^{90}Y-RE.

Another important aspect of the clinical evaluation is multimodality imaging to assess the baseline disease characteristics and specifically:

- Multiphase CT or MRI or both need to assess extent of disease and the tumor burden within the liver (size, multifocality, infiltrative pattern) whether there is major vascular and biliary tract invasion by the tumor as well as to assess the anatomical localization of the tumor with regard to availability of access via hepatic arteries. Also, radiological imaging is essential to estimate the tumor volume and liver volume needed to calculate the required activity for the desired effect.
- ^{18}F-FDG PET/CT imaging also is necessary to assess whether there is extrahepatic disease and, if there is, whether they appear as oligometastatic or polymetastatic disease. Another benefit of performing a pre-therapy ^{18}F-FDG PET/CT scan is that it serves as a baseline imaging modality to assess therapy response as early as 4–6 weeks post-therapy, which is almost impossible to achieve with other imaging modalities. Recent studies have indicated that consecutive 18F-FDG PET imaging in patients with liver metastases before and after ^{90}Y-RE was more predictive of survival than assessment with CT imaging [49].

Ideally, all imaging studies should be performed within 1 month from treatment planning in the same centre where ^{90}Y-RE will be planned and carefully evaluated by experienced radiologist and nuclear medicine of the *RE-Team*.

15.3.2 Pre-therapy Workup

The patients meeting the criteria of the first-step evaluation, after receiving both written and verbal information about the procedure, undergo second-step evaluation that consists of hepatic angiography and ^{99m}Tc-MAA imaging.

These two procedures represent a true "treatment simulation" and are done at the same day, usually performing an overnight patient admission, to definitively confirm or reject patient eligibility to the treatment. While in the clinical evaluation step all liver experts are involved to point out the intention to treat, in this very technical phase, the main actor is the *RE-Team* consisting of nuclear medicine physician, interventional radiologist and medical physicist.

Treatment simulation is essential for:

- Confirming the appropriateness of the patient for treatment
- Preparing the liver for ^{90}Y-RE
- Planning the treatment procedure itself (either a whole-liver or more selective approach)
- Ensuring the optimum and safe delivery of ^{90}Y-resin microspheres to liver tumor(s), while limiting the impact of RE on healthy tissue
- Calculating the appropriate activity of ^{90}Y-resin microspheres to be administered

15.3.2.1 Hepatic Angiography

Pre-therapy hepatic angiography is essential for two main issues:

- To delineate an accurate road map of vascular anatomy, evidencing all possible abdominal arteries to feed the liver and the tumor that allows the interventional radiologist to identify technique criticisms and solve them avoiding complications
- To predict, together with ^{99m}Tc-MAA imaging, the ultimate ^{90}Y deposition and to decide strategy of administration and the position of the catheter that will be used for the treatment phase (selective to tumor, segmental, lobar or hepatic)

A meticulous map of vascular anatomy is crucial for a safe delivery of ^{90}Y-microspheres and good treatment outcome. Three main issues, which might require specific intervention to avoid inadequate delivery of microspheres, need to be identified by hepatic angiography: the arterial anatomy of the liver and potential arterial variants, tumor feeders and extrahepatic branches coming off the hepatic arteries.

Arterial Anatomy and Potential Arterial Variants

Anatomic variants of the hepatic arterial vasculature are common, and correct identification of these variants during hepatic angiography is essential as it is related to two main concerns:

- Vascular anomalies may prevent appropriate placement of the catheter into the hepatic artery for the delivery of microspheres.
- These anomalies, if not identified properly, may lead to microspheres lodging in excess amounts in the hepatic parenchyma or other nontarget organs in the gastrointestinal tract [50, 51].

In the standard vascularization condition, the celiac trunk gives three branches as common hepatic, splenic and left gastric artery. The common hepatic artery becomes, after the gastroduodenal artery has branched off, the proper hepatic artery that continues towards the hilar plate, where it splits into the right and left hepatic arteries (Fig. 15.2). Conventional anatomy, represented by a single proper hepatic artery, vascularizing the whole liver originating from the celiac trunk, is only encountered in 60% of patients [52]. This means that in 40% at least two different arteries vascularize the liver.

The most common variants are the so-called replaced right hepatic artery coming off the superior mesenteric artery and the replaced left hepatic artery coming from the left gastric artery. Furthermore, in some patients, any liver segment may have another arterial source along with the proper hepatic artery and this aberrant artery is called *accessory hepatic artery*. If such accessory arteries are overlooked during angiography, then it would be more probable for ^{90}Y-microspheres to shunt into gastrointestinal region when they are selectively injected through the segmentary artery without the knowledge of accessory arteries.

In these cases, if a patient has bilobar tumors and multiple hepatic arteries, an option is to redistribute the blood flow in order to have the

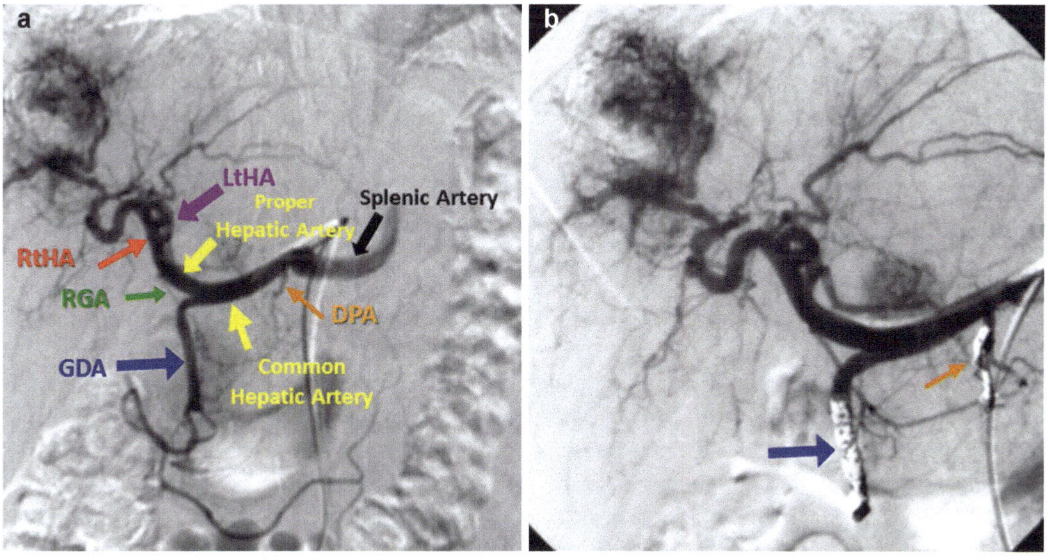

Fig. 15.2 Angiogram digital subtraction showing normal liver vascularization (**a**) and prophylactic embolization of gastroduodenal and dorsal pancreatic arteries (**b**). *RtHA* right hepatic artery, *LtHA* left hepatic artery, *GDA* gastroduodenal artery, *RGA* right gastric artery, *DPA* dorsal pancreatic artery

whole liver vascularized by only one artery like for intra-arterial chemotherapy [53]. The concept of vascular redistribution (i.e. occluding intrahepatic vessels before radioembolization to induce redistribution of flow) has been developed to simplify treatment and potentially avoid gastric vessels. For example, in the case of a replaced left hepatic artery originating from a left gastric artery, the gastrohepatic trunk is embolized to redistribute flow to the left from the right hepatic artery. Obviously, it must be aware that this technique of redistribution must be carefully done. Another option is to separately catheterize each artery to implant the microsphere.

Tumor Feeding from Parasitizing Arteries

In up to 37% of cases, tumor vascular supply comes from an extrahepatic artery usually feeding adjacent structures. The most frequent ones, commonly defined parasitized extrahepatic arteries, are the inferior phrenic artery, taking part of the vascularization of right-sided liver tumors, and intercostal, omental and internal mammary arteries [54]. These branches must be recognized before treatment using catheter-directed CT with direct injection of contrast medium into the hepatic artery at the beginning of hepatic angiography procedure. This is particularly important in tumors located close to the hepatic dome or to the falciform ligament.

Two different solutions have been proposed by some authors to overcome this criticism: the first is to embolize those parasitizing arteries before ^{90}Y-RE using particles and coils [55], while the second solution is to perform ^{90}Y-RE from these arteries when possible [54].

Extrahepatic Branches Coming Off the Hepatic Arteries

Angiography also can show whether there is extrahepatic arterial shunting due to extrahepatic branches coming off the hepatic arteries and going to gastrointestinal region mostly via gastroduodenal, right gastric or other accessory arteries. Significant extrahepatic depositions are found mostly within the distribution of three distinct side branches: the gastroduodenal artery, cystic artery and right gastric artery [52]. Obviously, any possible arterial shunt to gastrointestinal region must be avoided to protect especially the stomach and the small intestines from undesired effects of radiation due to unintended access of ^{90}Y-microspheres to those organs. The general assumption is that if there is a branch feeding an extrahepatic territory downstream of the final catheter position for beads injection, this branch must be embolized (prophylactic embolization) to minimize the risk of delivering radioactive beads in digestive or pancreatic branches. This is particularly true for the right gastric artery which origin is usually located distally to the gastroduodenal artery (Fig. 15.2).

In recent years, however, the prophylactic embolization of extrahepatic branches has been debated, and standard rigorous occlusion of all side branches of the hepatic arteries has been progressively abandoned [50]. Many cases of collateral vessel formation have been observed following gastroduodenal and right gastric artery embolization, and these collateral vessels are exceedingly difficult to embolize [56, 57]. Moreover, numerous disadvantages are related to the angiography procedure itself: increased procedure complexity, additional radiation dose, potential vessel damage and complications of coil deployment. Another problem may be unnecessary prophylactic coiling in patients who may be later disqualified on the basis of unfavourable dosimetry.

Thus, the choice to perform prophylactic embolization of extrahepatic vessels (e.g. gastroduodenal artery, right gastric artery) is largely operator-dependent and varies considerably across institutions. At present, most experienced centres, exploiting new-generation antireflux microcatheters and multimodality imaging as intra-arterial catheter-directed CT, try to avoid prophylactic coil embolization and assess potential culprit vessels individually. Catheter-directed CT (e.g. C-arm cone-beam CT or hybrid angiography/CT), in addition to digital subtraction angiography (CdHA), is now routinely used intra-procedurally to better determine vascular supply to the tumor and detect potential extrahepatic vessels. It allows for visualization of tumor as well as intra-procedural guidance to position microcatheters in the appropriate vessels for targeting [58, 59].

It has been recently recommended by the Society of Interventional Radiology Standard of Practice Committee [60] that new users have a low threshold to perform prophylactic embolization of extrahepatic vessels before radioembolization while, many experienced, high-volume centres equipped with CdHA have to move away from routine prophylactic embolization of the gastroduodenal artery and right gastric artery. Obviously, angiogram must be assessed by a physician skilled in scan interpretation with a view to identifying any anomalous vessels leading to other organs. New users need of a period of clinical proctoring to address all the issues concerning the identification of such vessels.

Finally, once the interventional radiologist is satisfied with the hepatic angiography and the catheter in good position, a standard dose (111–185 MBq) of ^{99m}Tc-MAA is slowly injected in close collaboration with nuclear medicine physician. After the ^{99m}Tc-MAA injection, all catheters, wires and the sheath are removed and appropriately disposed of in nuclear waste bags, and haemostasis of the common femoral artery is secured. The patient will then be sent in the Nuclear Medicine Unit to perform ^{99m}Tc-MAA imaging.

15.3.2.2 ^{99m}Tc-MAA Imaging

After injection of ^{99m}Tc-MAA at the end of angiography, the patient should undergo scintigraphy preferably within 1 h from the injection. Imaging time is of great importance, because some amount of in vivo degradation of ^{99m}Tc-MAA may occur by time and produce free ^{99m}Tc uptake in thyroid and more importantly the stomach, so mimicking an arterial shunt from the liver to the stomach. Macroaggregated albumin (MAA) is a particulate form of albumin with an average size of 20–40 μm with a density close to that of resin microspheres. For this reason, labelled with Tc-99m, MAA constitutes a "reasonable" surrogate diagnostic radiopharmaceutical to simulate ^{90}Y-microsphere distribution when injected in the hepatic artery. ^{99m}Tc-MAA imaging must include both standard anterior-posterior planar images of the chest and the abdomen than SPET or SPET /CT images of the upper abdomen.

After image acquisitions, the study must be accurately evaluated in order to obtain the following data:

- Quantification of lung shunt
- Visualization of any shunt to gastrointestinal (GI) region even when shunting occurs via very small accessory arteries which may not appear on angiography clearly
- Simulation of the biodistribution of ^{90}Y-microspheres within the liver and determination of the blood flow ratio of the tumor to normal hepatic parenchyma (T/N) which is the major determinant of degree of "selectivity" of RE

Lung Shunt

A common feature of the neoplastic vasculature within hepatic tumors is the formation of abnormal hepatic arterial to hepatic venous (arteriovenous) anastomoses, otherwise known as shunts.

The ratio of lung shunting in percentages is calculated by drawing regions of interests on the chest and liver planar ^{99m}Tc-MAA images (Fig. 15.3).

Geometrical mean of lung and liver counts from anterior and posterior chest planar images is used to calculate the lung shunt ratio according to the following formula:

$$\text{Lung shunt ratio} = \frac{(\text{Geometrical mean of lung counts})}{(\text{Geometrical mean of lung counts}) + (\text{Geometrical mean of the liver counts})} \times 100$$

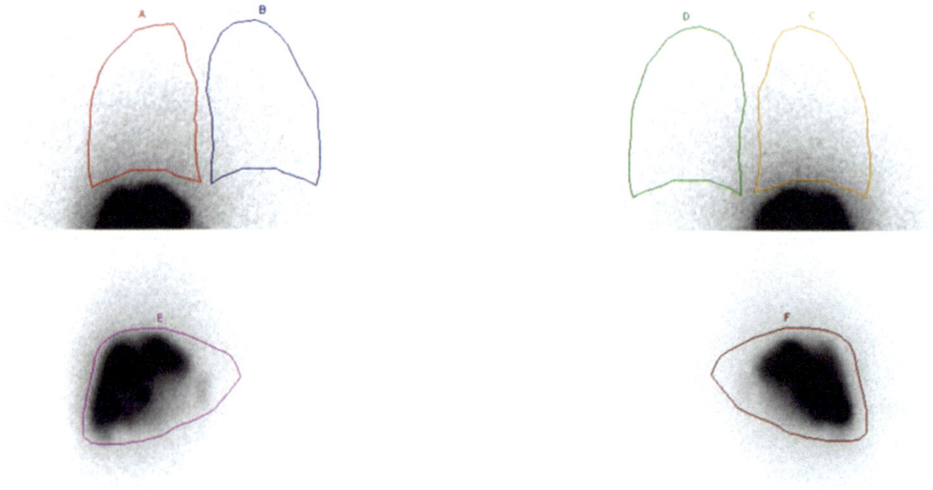

Fig. 15.3 Anterior and posterior planar images of the thorax (top) and upper abdomen (bottom) obtained after intrahepatic artery injection of technetium-99m-labelled macroaggregated albumin (^{99m}Tc-MAA). Regions of interest are drawn on the lung and liver to calculate lung shunt

Lung shunting could potentially result in radiation pneumonitis after radioembolization [61]. At low shunt fractions, the amount of radiation reaching the lung has minimal clinical sequelae and is acceptable in relation to the potential benefit from RE. At higher shunt fractions, it may be necessary to reduce the prescribed activity of microspheres so that the known upper radiation dose limit from ^{90}Y-microspheres of 25 Gy to the lungs is not exceeded. Even such shunts are more common in hepatocellular carcinoma, there will always be some degree of shunting from the arteriolar to the venous circulation also in metastatic tumors to liver (Fig. 15.4).

Therefore, the degree of liver-lung shunting must be quantified prior to treatment with microspheres and the ^{90}Y prescribed activity modified according to the resin microspheres manufacturer instructions [62].

If the lung shunt ratio is:

- Below 10% there is no need to reduce the therapy dose.
- Between 10% and 20%, dose reduction is recommended (20–40% reduction).
- Over 20% there is a relative contraindication to therapy.

However, this method is based on planar imaging and is operator and institution-dependent. Overall, an absolute threshold (in Gy) is preferred over a relative one. SPET/CT leads to more accurate calculation of lung shunt absorbed dose than does planar imaging.

The highest tolerable lung shunt absorbed dose was defined as 30 Gy after a single treatment and up to 50 Gy after repeated treatments; in analogy with external beam radiation therapy

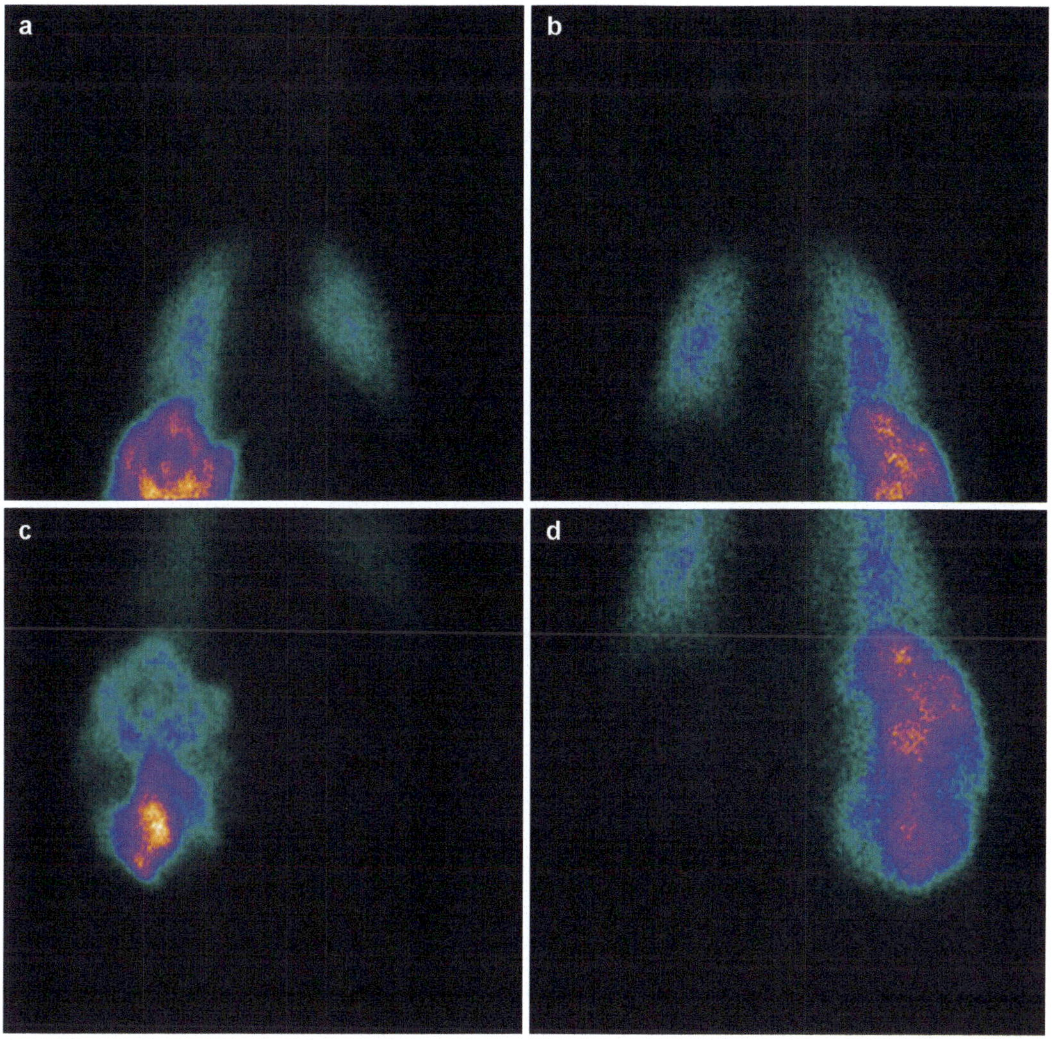

Fig. 15.4 ^{99m}Tc-MAA lung shunt evaluation in a patient with pancreatic NET and voluminous liver metastases. Anterior (**a**, **c**) and posterior (**b**, **d**) planar images of the thorax (top) and upper abdomen (bottom) showing a high lung shunt fraction (33%). *^{99m}Tc-MAA* technetium-99m-labelled macroaggregated albumin, *NET* neuroendocrine tumors

of the liver [63, 64], even resin microsphere manufacturers recommend lower limits (<25 Gy for both first than repeated treatment).

Gastrointestinal Shunt

Any extrahepatic activity in GI region is highly suspicious for unrecognized hepatofugal vascular runoff and is named gastrointestinal shunting. In about 15% of patients, there can be small vessels that are very small and hard to see on an angiogram and which pass from the liver to the gut. These are the cause of most of the problems with gastro-duodenitis. GI uptake should be further evaluated in detail with the help of SPET or better with SPET/CT to assess the exact localization. As SPET/CT imaging provides both functional and anatomical information at the same time, any gastrointestinal arterial shunting activity can easily be seen and more precisely localized than SPET alone imaging.

Once any shunt is detected in the stomach or intestines on scintigraphy imaging, more options can be evaluated depending on case complexity:

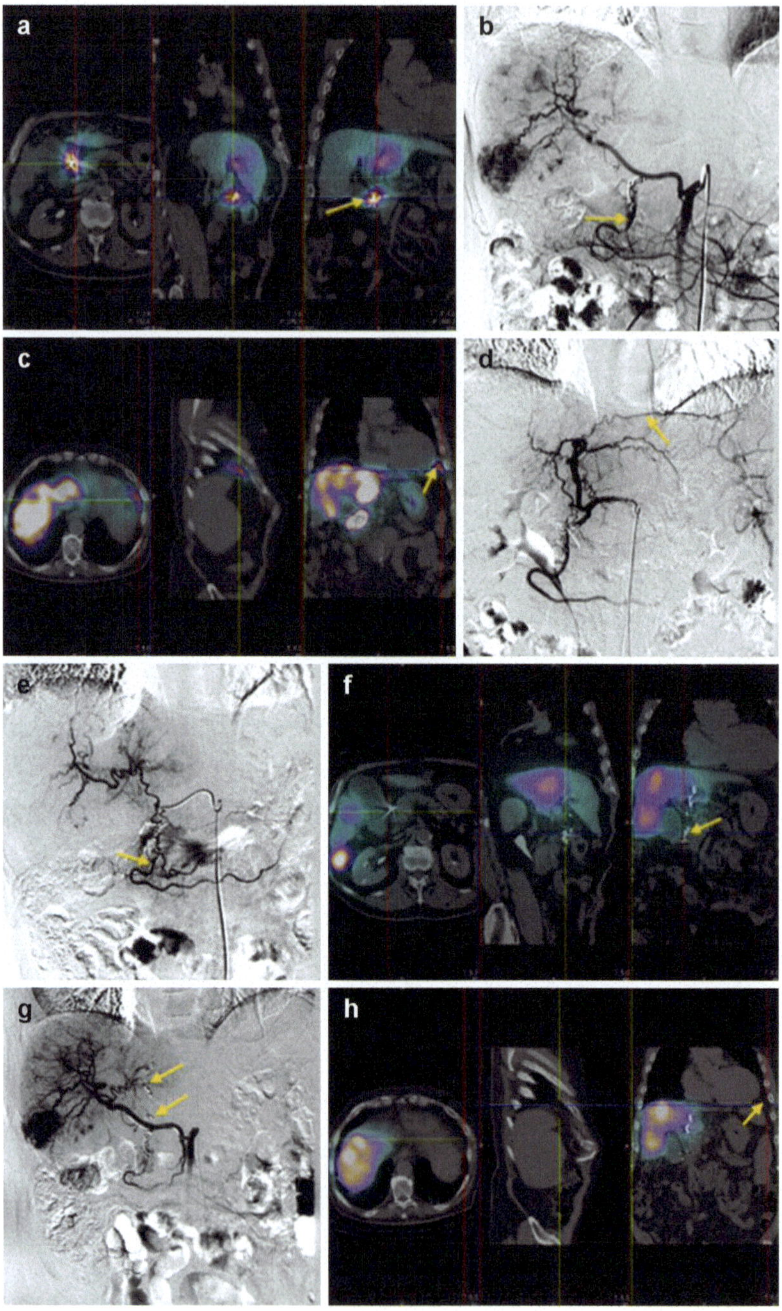

Fig. 15.5 Pre-therapy (top) and post-therapy (bottom) workup in a patient with multiple hepatic metastases. Pre-therapy ^{99m}Tc-MAA SPET/CT showing a focal extrahepatic uptake in the right hypochondrium at coil deployment site (**a**) and in the left hypochondrium in correspondence of the diaphragm (**c**). Angiography survey, re-evaluated on the basis of ^{99m}Tc-MAA SPET findings, that showed a replaced GDA in right hypochondrium (**b**) and a falciform artery with phrenic artery in left hypochondrium (**d**). Therapy angiography showing the further embolization of anatomic variants identified with microcoils: GDA embolization (**e**) and phrenic embolization (**g**). Post-therapy ^{90}Y SPET/CT showing a correct biodistribution without any extrahepatic shunt both in in the right hypochondrium (**f**) and in the left hypochondrium (**h**). *GDA* gastroduodenal artery, *^{99m}Tc-MAA* technetium-99m-labelled macroaggregated albumin

- Patient could be considered no fit for ^{90}Y-RE, when a significant and not correctable reflux of hepatic arterial blood to the stomach, pancreas or bowel is visualized and a potential significant damage could be predicted.
- Patient could still be eligible for ^{90}Y-RE planning a corrective intervention directly during treatment procedures if it is possible. In these cases coil-embolizing the culprit vessel, a more distal position of the catheter or super-selective catheterization will be performed during ^{90}Y-RE, rendering 91–96% of the prior selected patients eligible for radioembolization [65] (Fig. 15.5).

- Patient could undergo a second exploratory hepatic angiography with reinjection of ^{99m}Tc-MAA to find and coil-embolize the shunting artery before planning RE to make the patient eligible [66].

The choice of the best option is based on a series of factors and varies among centres according to experience. In any case it is most important to interpret ^{99m}Tc-MAA and angiography imaging very precisely. A careful review of both imaging by nuclear medicine physician and interventional radiologist with a discussion of relevant findings is very important, particularly if there is extrahepatic deposition of ^{99m}Tc-MAA.

Simulation of the Predicted Biodistribution of Microspheres Within the Liver

Because MAA particles are intended to replicate the distribution of the ^{90}Y-microspheres, the ^{99m}Tc-MAA biodistribution on SPET imaging of the upper abdomen should match that planned for subsequent ^{90}Y-microsphere administration.

^{99m}Tc-MAA planar and SPET images also allow the estimation of total ^{90}Y activity likely to accumulate in both the neoplastic and the parenchymal microvasculature. This tumor/normal tissue (T/N) ratio aids in the assessment of the safety margin for resin microsphere infusion [67]. The T/N ratio will not correlate with the baseline volume of the liver or tumor nor with the proportion of neoplastic involvement. However, a ratio of 2.0 has generally been taken as the lower threshold for safe ^{90}Y-microsphere administration [67, 68]. Other authors using a cut-off value of 1 for the MAA-tumor-to-normal uptake ratio demonstrated that a significant metabolic response could be predicted after Y-90 treatment [69].

^{99m}Tc-MAA SPET/CT gives a more detailed biodistribution of radioactivity within the liver with anatomical references allowing to evidence adequacy of target embolization and can be analysed to verify the correspondence between lesion documented by CT, MRI or PET/CT (Fig. 15.6). ^{99m}Tc-MAA SPET/CT volume measurements are accurate and reproducible [70]. Therefore, it can be used to adjust therapy dose more precisely compared to SPET alone, allowing a better therapy plan definition.

In conclusion, ^{99m}Tc-MAA imaging should play an important role in safety assessment and therapy plan definition and should, therefore, be undertaken for every patient, regardless of the activity planning method used [71].

15.3.2.3 Eligibility Confirmation

At the end of the second step, the following further contraindications to therapy may be evidenced:

- Pathological lung shunting (>20%) assessed by 99mTc-MAA scan or fraction potentially causing a lung dose of ≥30 Gy in a single application

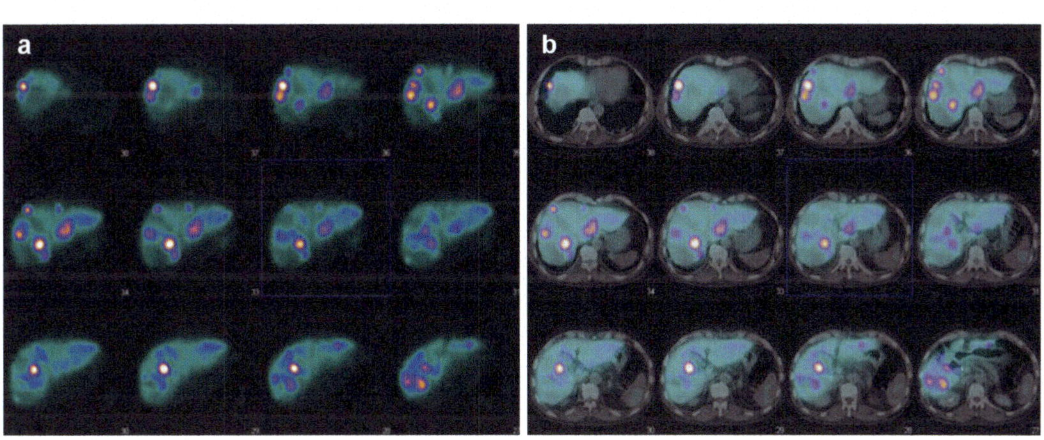

Fig. 15.6 Comparison of ^{99m}Tc-MAA SPET imaging (**a**) versus ^{99m}Tc-MAA SPET/CT imaging (**b**) in multifocal liver metastases from colorectal cancer. SPET/CT localize with a better definition ^{99m}Tc-MAA focal uptake giving anatomical references. *^{99m}Tc-MAA* technetium-99m-labelled macroaggregated albumin

- No correctable abnormal vascular anatomy that would result in significant reflux of hepatic arterial blood to the stomach, pancreas or bowel
- Nontarget embolization that cannot be avoided by adequate transarterial embolization

However, pre-therapy workup, in addition to confirm or exclude the treatment, provides a number of important elements that are necessary to set up a proper treatment plan and represents the basis for the treatment outcome.

Key Points
Selection of patients requires a multidisciplinary discussion of a number of factors both clinical and technique imaging based. Eligibility needs a carefully evaluation, in addition to standard indications and inclusion criteria, of clinical context and treatment intention.

Pre-therapy workup, including hepatic angiography and ^{99m}Tc imaging, is a crucial step and requires an experienced and synergic *RE-Team* to definitively confirm or reject therapy.

Modern multimodality imaging as CdHA and ^{99m}Tc-MAA SPET/CT allows an accurate assessment of target liver volumes and radiation planning. A well-made preliminary workup is a solid foundation for the future treatment outcome: it's like walking on a well-lit road and with a route already highlighted.

15.4 Therapy Planning

Once the pre-therapy workup/simulation phase is completed and eligibility to ^{90}Y-RE is confirmed, it is possible to plan therapy and specifically:

- The patient will be rescheduled for the treatment phase (on average 1–2 weeks later) that is usually performed in 2 or 3 days admission to nuclear medicine ward depending on the local expertise and regulatory issues.
- ^{90}Y-microspheres order will be submitted to manufacturers.

In addition, this is a crucial step in decisional path leading to the strategy definition that includes:

- The choice of hepatic target volume: whole-liver, lobar, segmental or selective
- The calculation of ^{90}Y activity to be administered

A personalized therapeutic plan is so developed for each patient by the *RE-Team* based on the analysis of all clinical, imaging and laboratory collected data and the treatment goals (extend overall survival, increase the time to progression, potentially downsize or downstage, provide palliation of symptoms).

In the next future, it is likely ^{90}Y-RE will be as a suit is to a tailor: uniquely adapted to the patient, every step of the way.

15.4.1 Hepatic Target Volume Choice

The decision to use whole-liver, lobar, segmental (i.e. two or fewer hepatic segments perfused) or selective (target tumor vascularization) approaches is dependent on the patient's baseline laboratory values, clinical characteristics, ^{99m}Tc-MAA SPET/CT biodistribution and vascular anatomy.

In general, patients with better performance status, adequate liver function and lack of previous treatment tend to tolerate treatment of larger hepatic target volumes. In select situations, especially in the setting of metastatic liver tumors in which no underlying liver disease is present, whole-liver infusion can be performed (via separate lobar injections in a single session). However, it is always best to avoid it as much as possible a whole-liver treatment and sparing as much liver as possible by sequential treatment with super-selective catheterization [72, 73].

Lobar infusion is currently the most common approach for multifocal disease. For whole-liver therapy, sequential lobar injections (typically separated by 6–8 weeks) are the most common method [74]. Segmental radioembolization, whereby one or two hepatic segments are treated, can be considered in patients with isolated tumor burden and may allow higher administered dose because most segments of the liver would remain unaffected by treatment. In the case of a tumor that dominates a single hepatic segment (e.g. single nodule), the treatment approach may be modified to "radiation segmentectomy". In this case, super-selective SIRT may be performed, thus sparing numerous non-tumorous liver segments in both the ipsilateral and contralateral lobes [75].

15.4.2 Calculation of ^{90}Y Activity to be Administered

Optimal prescribed ^{90}Y activity should deliver an adequate radiation dose to tumor cells (tumor dose) while sparing the total absorbed radiation dose in healthy liver parenchyma, also called the non-tumor dose.

In the absence of significant extrahepatic activity, the only true dosimetric limitation left is the non-tumor dose. Little is known about the maximum tolerable non-tumor dose in radioembolization. It varies between patients depending on multiple variables (e.g. previous treatment and patient comorbidities), including distribution of radiation within the healthy liver parenchyma. A non-tumor dose limit of less than 70 Gy has been proposed for hepatic metastases (with a limit of less than 50 Gy depending on liver reserve) [69, 76] although these limits seem quite arbitrarily defined and need to be confirmed in prospective studies. A dose response model of normal tissue complication probability has been proposed in literature suggesting an increase of toxicity rate with the dose delivered to liver [77].

A tumoricidal dose for resin microspheres is considered to be 120 Gy, and when lesions are of small dimensions, little benefit is gained from exceeding this threshold, especially because it increases unnecessary parenchymal exposure [68, 69, 78]. With an average dose of 120 Gy to the tumor, the observed and estimated rates of complete or partial response were 80% and 60% of patients according to the EASL guideline and RECIST, respectively [77].

When calculating dose is also necessary to consider the target volume and modality of administration, i.e. lobar or selective [62]:

- If "radiation lobectomy" is planned, thus sparing the non-tumorous liver segments in the contralateral lobe, a maximum of 70 Gy for uninvolved parenchyma in the affected lobe is suggested, and an activity reduction is not *usually* required.
- If both lobes are involved (whole-liver approach) and it is not possible to spare any liver segments from exposure to radiation, the ^{90}Y-microsphere radiation doses should not be >50 Gy either bilobar or sequential unilobar approach. Where possible, this limit should be calculated for each lobe individually and not averaged across the liver.
- In the case of a tumor that dominates a single hepatic segment and a "radiation segmentectomy" is feasible, thus sparing numerous non-tumorous liver segments in both the ipsilateral and contralateral lobes, dose limits are unnecessary. If sub-segmental treatment is indicated, none of the currently available activity calculation methods could provide a reliable estimation because the mathematical modelling breaks down for extremely small and extremely large tumor volumes.

Another consideration to be kept in mind is that many patients with liver metastases from colorectal or breast cancer receive biologic or chemotherapy agents before—or concurrent with—^{90}Y-RE. Exposure to systemic therapy could compromise hepatic vessel morphology, patency and neogenesis in both neoplastic and uninvolved tissue. For instance, both irinotecan and oxaliplatin can produce sinusoidal obstruction syndrome, even without radioembolization

[79]. Whatever activity planning method is used, previous systemic therapy should be considered equivalent to functional liver impairment when setting the parenchymal safety limits.

There are two methods for calculating the prescribed activity of resin microspheres: the body surface area (BSA) and the partition model method. A third method, which is the earliest and empirical method, is no longer recommended.

15.4.2.1 BSA Method

The BSA method is the most commonly used worldwide because it is simple to apply and has been historically successful. This method has a conservative tendency to underdose sacrificing efficacy for safety. BSA method is described in the manufacture documentation [62] and is also formalized and simplified in the SIR-Spheres Microspheres Activity Calculator (SMAC), available at http://apps01.sirtex.com/smac.

The BSA method requires for activity calculation:

- The patient's body surface area to be calculated from the patient's weight and height
- The percentage of the liver that is replaced with tumor as calculated from the baseline CT scan
- The percentage of liver-lung shunting, determined during the nuclear medicine study with Tc-99m-labelled macroaggregated albumin (99mTc-MAA)

The following formula is used for whole-liver treatment:

$$\text{Activity}(\text{GBq}) = \text{BSA} - 0.2 + \left\{\frac{\text{Tumor volume}}{\text{Total liver volume}}\right\}$$

where:

- Tumor volume is the volume of tumor present in the liver.
- Total liver volume is the total volume of the liver including the tumor.
- BSA is the body surface area (m^2).

In patients who receive lobar or segmental treatment with resin microspheres, the prescribed activity must be reduced in accordance with the size of the portion of the liver being treated and the following formula:

$$\text{Activity}_L(\text{GBq}) = \left[\text{BSA} - 0.2 + \left\{\frac{\text{Tumor volume}_L}{\text{Total volume}_L}\right\}\right] \times \left[\frac{\text{Tumor volume}_L}{\text{Total liver volume}_L}\right]$$

where:

- Activity L is the prescribed activity for the lobe.
- Tumor volume L is the volume of tumor present in the lobe.
- Total volume L is the total volume of the lobe including the tumor in the lobe.
- Total liver volume is the total volume of the liver including the tumor.
- BSA is the body surface area (m^2).

The BSA method has been used safely in many clinical trials and is generally strongly recommended during the early experience phase of a new user's of resin microspheres. It was developed to calculate safe treatment activities, but it does not incorporate a target tumor-absorbed dose, nor does it account for interindividual differences in microsphere distribution. Achievable tumor-absorbed doses may consequently be suboptimal and impair treatment efficacy. Its main limitation is the absence of target volume in the calculation method, which can result in undertreatment (small patient with large liver) or overtreatment (large patient with small liver) [80, 81]. Furthermore, it does not correct for the individual intrahepatic distribution differences, calculated by the so-called T/N ratio, which is to the disadvantage of patients with hyper- or hypo-vascular tumors. The T/N ratio is a critical parameter that numerically describes the extent of preferential microsphere implantation within the target arterial territory that can vary significantly between patients. Therefore, using this simple method, the effective tumor-absorbed dose remains uncertain (reported range 66–495 Gy) [82].

Nowadays, in the face of widespread availability of hybrid tomographic scintigraphy, the ethics of subjecting patients to a decade-old semi-empiric treatment paradigm is questionable. The modern era of personalized medicine demands the measurement of patient-specific biophysical parameters to individualize treatment and to maximize the desired effect while minimizing toxicity. Single-photon emission tomography with integrated CT (SPET/CT) and positron emission tomography with integrated CT (PET/CT) overcome many of the technological limitations which have traditionally plagued planar and single-photon emission tomography (SPET), only scintigraphy to allow more accurate measurements of activity distribution, mandatory to assess the dose distribution. ^{90}Y-microsphere radioembolization is well placed to lead the science in personalized radionuclide therapy because the permanently implanted microspheres negate tedious time-activity measurements. Provided the angiographic conditions, especially catheter position, between exploratory angiography and radioembolization are identical, the ^{99m}Tc-MAA SPET/CT may be regarded as a "radiation simulation" study—a concept demonstrated for both resin and glass microspheres and may be used for a personalized predictive dosimetry by MIRD macrodosimetry models [82, 83].

15.4.2.2 Partition Model

The second method is the "partition model", which enables personalized radiation planning based on absorbed doses (Gy). This method, which applies MIRD macrodosimetry to resin microspheres [83], mathematically describes the biodistribution of microspheres in a typical patient considering three dosimetric compartments—tumor, non-tumorous liver and the lungs aiming to selecting safe radiation doses to the normal liver and lungs.

The method requires two measurements: (1) the volume of tumor and normal liver determined from a CT scan and (2) the proportions of ^{99m}Tc-MAA activity that lodges in the tumor, normal liver and lung as determined from scintigraphy. The ^{99m}Tc-MAA imaging analysis and derivative parameters such as the lung shunt fraction and the T/N ratio allow the estimation of the desired absorbed doses and activities in each of the three compartments. This enables predictive dosimetry to be performed for the tumor, normal liver and lungs prior to radioembolization. The radiation dose to the normal liver parenchyma should not exceed 70 Gy in patients with normal liver and 50 Gy in patients with impaired liver function. The dose to the lung should not exceed 25 Gy and preferably be less than 20 Gy. The dose received by the tumor has no upper limit, and the maximal dose to be delivered is determined fulfilling all the above normal tissue constraints.

With improvements in angiographic methods over the years, the original partition model has now evolved to take into account selective or super-selective radioembolization depending on the case-specific clinical, angiographic and dosimetric circumstances. This has developed into a "multi-partition" model where vascular territories are mapped by catheter-directed CT and the ^{99m}Tc-MAA biodistribution is tomographically mapped by SPET/CT. In addition, the multi-partition model improves radiation planning for large tumors that are supplied by multiple arteries by measuring the different T/N ratios for each arterial territory, allowing treatment personalization and absorbed dose optimization [83].

The partition model based on pretreatment ^{99m}Tc-MAA SPET/CT should be preferred by nuclear physicians and interventional radiologists, because lesion-based dosimetry on pretreatment ^{99m}Tc-MAA SPET/CT has been shown to correlate with response and survival [69, 77]. However, radiobiological guidance on this issue is scarce in the literature for both resin and glass microspheres, and further researches are ongoing. The partition model can only be used where the tumor mass is a discrete area within the liver. This is more likely patients with primary HCC where there is often a large single tumor mass. Patients with metastatic disease usually have multiple areas of metastatic spread that make difficult defining the tumor and normal parenchymal compartments.

Key Points
A personalized individually therapeutic plan should be developed for each patient by the *RE-Team* to optimize ^{90}Y-RE efficacy and toxicity in accordance to patient characteristics and the strategic treatment goals in the specific therapeutic window.

Treatment target volume and radiation prescribed dose have to be tailored as much as possible in order to calculate the appropriate ^{90}Y activity to be administered.

15.5 Therapy Procedures

Once therapeutic plan is well designed and confirmed, on the day of treatment, the following activities are performed: patient preparation, ^{90}Y-microsphere preparation, treatment administration and confirmation of correct administration (post-therapy workup).

15.5.1 Patients Preparation

After an overnight fast, on the day of the procedure, patient has to sign informed consent to treatment. Liver, renal and haematological function must be checked again the same day of treatment or the day before.

A peri-procedural supportive medical therapy is recommended:

- A proton-pump inhibitor (e.g. omeprazole or pantoprazole) or H2-blocker (e.g. ranitidine) should be started the day before treatment and continued for 4 weeks post-treatment to reduce gastric complications.
- Antiemetics (e.g. ondansetron or granisetron) for post-treatment nausea should be started in the morning of the day of treatment
- The use of empirical antibiotic prophylaxis is not routinely recommended and should be based upon assessment of each patient's individual infection risk.

15.5.2 ^{90}Y-Resin Microsphere Preparation

The ^{90}Y-resin microspheres are provided the scheduled day of the procedure in the Nuclear Medicine Unit. A specific administration set (delivery set) is supplied by manufactures including:

- A *shipping vial* containing ^{90}Y-resin microspheres suspended in pyrogen-free water for injection to a total of ~5 mL per 3 GBq with an activity of 3 GBq ± 10% at the calibration time and date. The microspheres may be used for up to 24 h post-calibration.
- A *v-vial*, in which the prescribed ^{90}Y-resin microsphere activity has to be placed.
- An acrylic *v-vial holder* for housing v-vial.
- A *syringe shield* for preparing the dose.
- Inlet and outlet connecting tubings and needles.

In addition, an acrylic Delivery Box needed to complete the set is provided from the manufactures at request. The components of the delivery set are illustrated in Fig. 15.7.

Dedicated accessories are designed to meet the general principles of radiation safety and to assist in the handling of ^{90}Y-resin microspheres. The vial containing the dose for each patient is packaged in an acrylic v-vial holder, which is designed to be seated in the acrylic box provided. A syringe shield is also provided for preparing the dose.

Yttrium-90 has two inherent safety features for staff and patients. These are:

- The minimal penetration depth of beta radiation emissions through tissue and air
- The relatively short half-life of 64.1 h

As the emission from yttrium-90 is high-energy beta, shielding is best provided with a low atomic number material such as acrylic. Acrylic shielding also reduces the amount of bremsstrahlung radiation produced. In addition, acrylic is optically clear and permits the physician to continually observe the product and procedure.

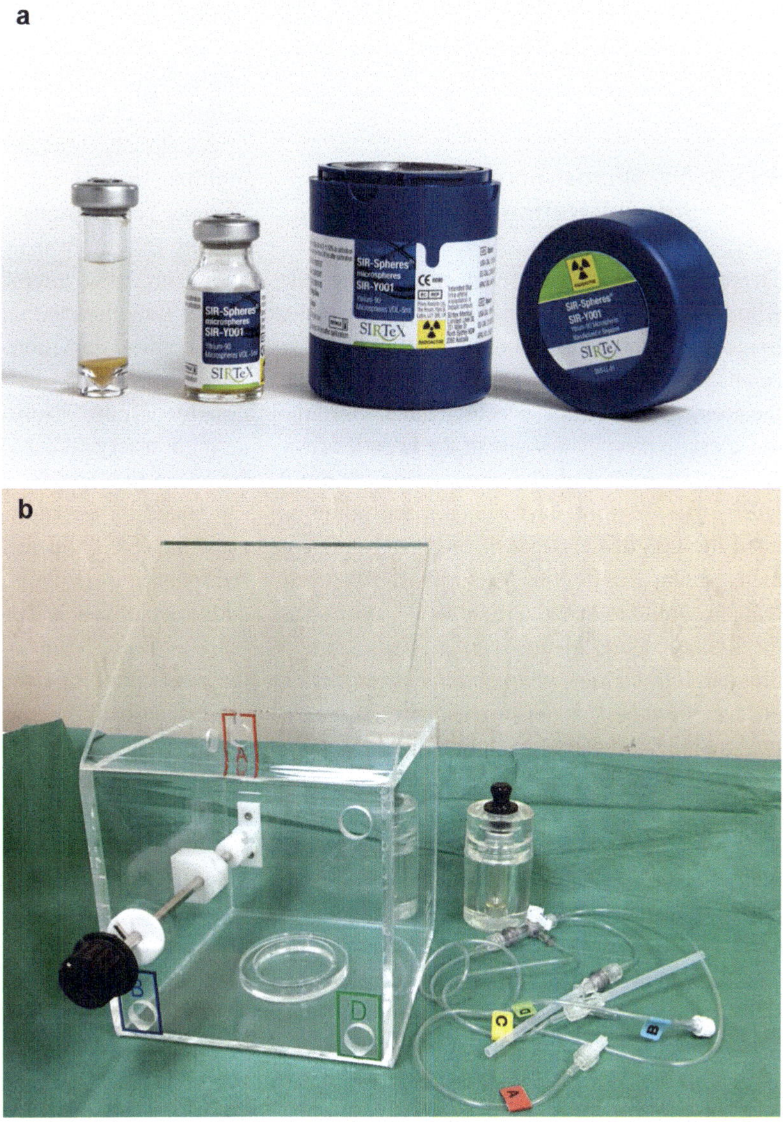

Fig. 15.7 ^{90}Y-microsphere radioembolization administration set. (**a**) ^{90}Y-microspheres vials and packages. From the right to the left: *V-vial* containing ^{90}Y-resin microsphere activity to be administered; the shipping vial containing the supplied ^{90}Y-resin microspheres suspended in pyrogen-free water and external shipping packages. (**b**) All the delivery set is shown including Delivery Box, an acrylic *v-vial holder* for housing v-vial, inlet and outlet connecting tubings and needles

The prescribed treatment dose is prepared in nuclear medicine radiopharmaceutical laboratory immediately before the treatment according to manufactures instruction and radio-pharmacy regulatory issues and afterward placed in the specific administration set. The patient-specific activity (as previously determined) is drawn from the shipping vial and placed into the v-vial. The v-vial is then placed into the acrylic v-vial holder and the v-vial holder is in turn placed into the acrylic Delivery Box.

Following the treatment vial placement into the Delivery Box, the radiation exposure from four sides of the administration set from equal distances is measured by a handheld radiation counter preferably by a physicist and recorded accordingly. This record is compared to post-infusion radiation exposure records that are done in the same way and serves as an indirect but a very practical method to understand whether the treatment dose has been administered completely following the infusion. At the end, all these data are collected in a specific record together with the prescribed activity.

The Delivery Box must be then transported to angiography suite where the patient will be treated and connecting tube is positioned according to manufacturer instructions and using aseptic technique.

15.5.3 ^{90}Y-Microspheres Administration

The procedure takes place in an angiography suite with patient under local anaesthetic. A specially trained interventional radiologist (IR) makes a small incision, usually into the femoral artery near the groin. A microcatheter is then guided through the artery to prespecified site in the hepatic artery (as identified during the pre-therapy workup) where the ^{90}Y-resin microspheres are administered through this catheter. It is strongly recommended that the IR who performs the baseline mapping angiogram is the same IR who performs the RE procedure, as the mapping angiogram is the most important pretreatment investigation prior to administering ^{90}Y-microspheres.

After the catheter is positioned in the exact position established during the simulation phase and according to therapy planning, the liver vasculature is again verified, and in case of any doubt, IR takes whatever steps are necessary to ensure that microspheres are never implanted if there is any possibility that they might enter these small aberrant vessels. Once the catheter position has been considered adequate, the proximal end of the catheter is connected to the delivery set that has been primed as outlined, and microspheres are then delivered into the trans-femoral catheter. The interventional radiologist should periodically check the position of the catheter to ensure it remains correctly sited during the delivery procedure. Microspheres must be delivered slowly at a rate of no more than 5 mL/min, as rapid delivery may cause flow stasis and reflux back down the hepatic artery into other nontarget organs. Flow stasis may sometimes result in incomplete delivery of the prescribed activity. Slow pulsatile administration of ^{90}Y-resin microspheres with water for injection (WFI) is associated with a low rate of stasis. It has been recently demonstrated that replacement of WFI with glucose 5% significantly reduces the need for peri-procedural analgesia. These data favour the use of glucose 5% for ^{90}Y-resin microsphere implantation in daily practice, especially in liver metastasis [84].

As already described, in case of tumors with multiple arterial supply, the ^{90}Y-RE strategies include two options: splitting the prescribed activity into more than one administrative setup and using new microcatheters for each injection or flow-directed microcatheter repositioning with contrast injection and coil embolization of other hepatic arteries allowing flow redistribution to permit ^{90}Y-microspheres injection from a single artery [85, 86]. The first option allows for more predictable absorbed dose delivery as calculated by the multi-partition model, as well as reduces the chance of contamination. Flow redistribution is unpredictable and introduces additional dosimetric uncertainty and is therefore the least preferred interventional technique from the perspective of radiation planning. When the prescribed activity is splitted according to target volumes, a simple one-third (left lobe) and two-thirds (right lobe) split is used by some centres, but most centres use the pretreatment CT scan for splitting the prescribed activity according to their manual liver segmentation. The most accurate method was proposed by Kao et al., who split the dose according to artery-specific SPET/CT-based liver segmentation, delineating an artery-specific target volume based on 99mTc-MAA distribution [83]. C-arm cone-beam CT may also be used for that particular goal.

At the conclusion of the procedure, which takes approximately an hour from starting to place the catheter, all wires, catheters and sheath are carefully removed and disposed of in nuclear waste bags. The medical physicist should measure the exposure rate due to the residual activity in the v-vial, the radiation exposure from the hands of administration team by a handheld radiation counter and also the environmental radiation monitoring should be done to confirm that no contamination exists. Patients are then moved to a recovery room for approximately 1 h before being transferred to the nuclear medicine ward, and a secure haemostasis of the groin by closure device is assured.

15.5.4 Post-therapy Workup

After the end of RE procedure, patient returns in nuclear medicine ward to undergo:

- Imaging procedures to confirm of correct ^{90}Y-microspheres administration
- Clinical post-therapy monitoring

15.5.4.1 Post-therapy Imaging

Usually, upper abdomen ^{90}Y bremsstrahlung SPET/CT or ^{90}Y PET is performed the same day or anyway within 30 h following infusion of spheres, to see the hepatic and extrahepatic distribution of microspheres and to confirm correct ^{90}Y-microsphere administration.

These assessments are relevant for two reasons.

First, ^{90}Y may unexpectedly be present outside the liver, despite a favourable distribution on the ^{99m}Tc-MAA scan. ^{90}Y-microspheres extrahepatic uptake will likely cause serious complications, like ulceration and bleedings in the GI tract. Therefore, severe pain after treatment should be early and aggressively managed to prevent development of more serious complications [87]. Second, the intrahepatic microsphere distribution and T/N rate are expected to be an important predictor of treatment efficacy (Fig. 15.8).

The SPET scan will detect the bremsstrahlung radiation from the yttrium-90 to confirm the placement of the microspheres in the liver. Bremsstrahlung images are broad-spectrum secondary gamma-ray emissions produced as a result of the interaction of the high-energy beta emissions with tissue. Per megabecquerel, approximately 23,000 bremsstrahlung photons with energy higher than 50 keV are produced by interaction of the beta particle with tissue requiring acquisition in a wide energy window to maximize sensitivity and image formation [88]. Also, ^{90}Y emits 32 positrons per second per megabecquerel, with a maximum energy of 758 keV allowing adequate PET imaging [89]. Although bremsstrahlung SPET/CT is a significant technological improvement from planar scintigraphy, the inherent problem of poor spatial resolution still remains. ^{90}Y PET, mostly with new time-of-light scanners, obtains high-resolution images for improved assessment of target and nontarget activity, superior to ^{90}Y bremsstrahlung SPET/CT. Diagnostic reporting guidelines for ^{90}Y PET/CT have recently been proposed [90].

15.5.4.2 Clinical Post-therapy Monitoring and Patient Management

Optimizing peri-procedural care and discharge planning of all patients is very important as most of these patients are treated in the palliative setting where quality of life is an important consideration.

After the ^{90}Y-RE procedure, patients should be kept under observation and vital signs monitored for few hours or longer according to clinical conditions. Most patients are discharged within 24–48 h post-^{90}Y-RE. The trans-femoral groin incision should be monitored for 24 h for haematoma formation. The patient should remain supine for approximately 6 h to reduce complications with the trans-femoral artery puncture wound, with full mobilization after 24 h. A liver, renal and haematological function assessment should be checked at 24 h and eventually repeated in the following days.

Most patients develop mild post-operative systemic symptoms as abdominal pain, nausea, vomiting, fatigue, anorexia and fever. This constellation of symptoms, named post-*radioembolization syndrome*, is a result of the radiation injury and embolic effect of the ^{90}Y-resin microspheres on the tumor neo-vasculature and may occur in up to 55% of patients, being more common with increasing number of administered microspheres. This short-term syndrome is self-limiting, lasting no longer than 2 weeks [91]. A passing elevation of liver enzymes, namely, in alkaline phosphatase, alanine transferase and bilirubin, is also normal early and transient post-treatment side effects. A supportive care is useful to reduce discomfort and improve the quality of life:

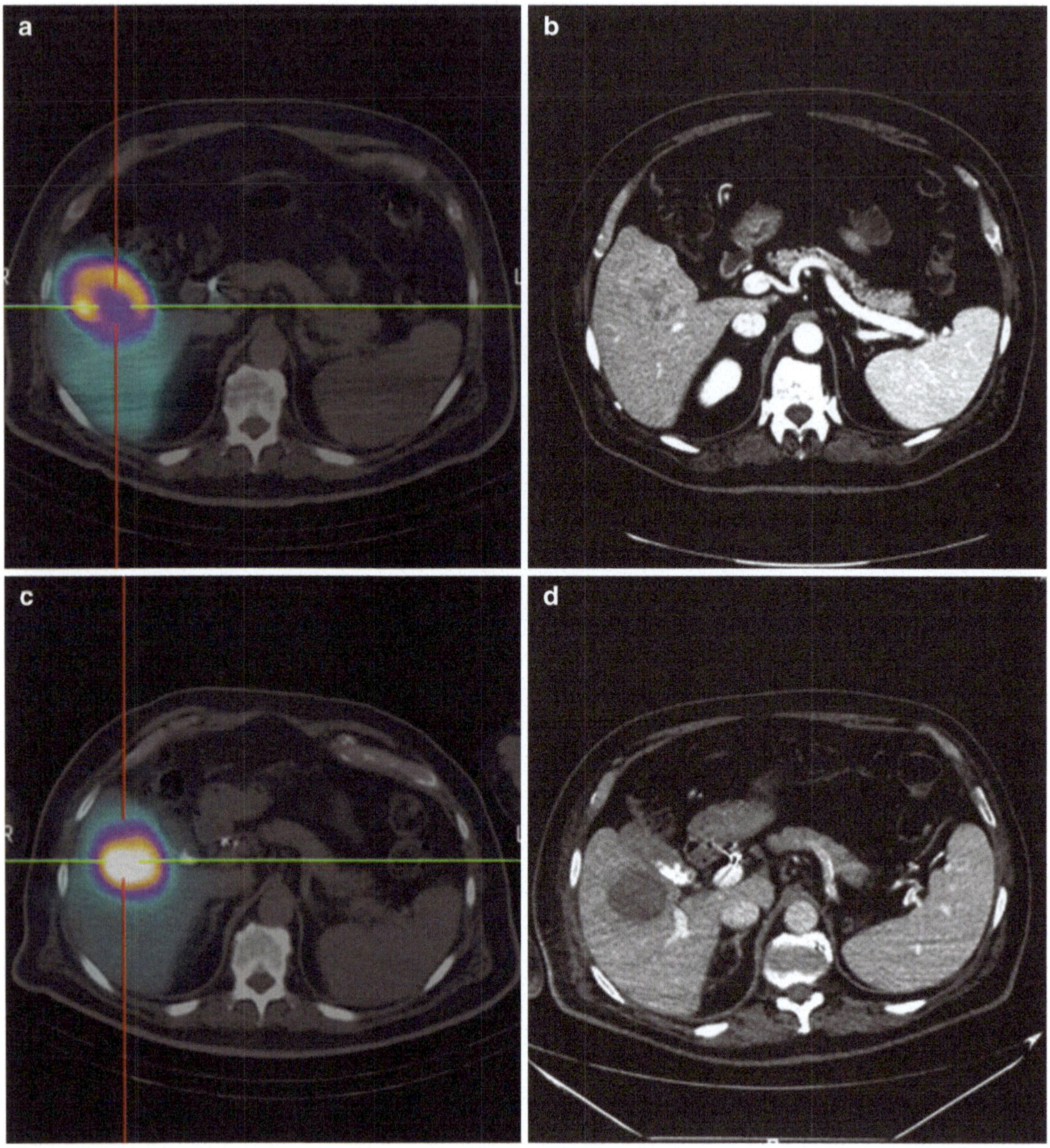

Fig. 15.8 Multimodality imaging in a patient with liver metastases from colorectal cancer treated with ^{90}Y-RE. Pre-therapy ^{99m}Tc-MAA SPET/CT showing a focal uptake with a high T/N ratio in right liver lobe (**a**) that well matched with pre-therapy CT (**b**) evidencing a 7 cm liver lesion in the V segment of the liver. Post-therapy ^{90}Y SPET (**c**) confirming a correct selective segmental procedure and a high focal ^{90}Y microspheres uptake on the target tumor volume. Post-therapy CT (**d**) performed at 3 months after ^{90}Y-RE evidenced a good objective response with all tumor volume replaced by necrosis. *^{99m}Tc-MAA* technetium-99m-labelled macroaggregated albumin, *T/N* tumor/not tumoral normal liver ratio, *^{90}Y-RE* radioembolization with yttrium-90 resin microspheres

- Oral or intravenous narcotic analgesia with or without oral steroids may be necessary for pain relief. Pain usually shrinks within an hour or so, but some patients may require oral analgesia for up to several days.
- Antiemetic agents such as ondansetron are usually required on the day of, and eventually also few days after, the treatment.
- Gastrointestinal prophylaxis with a proton-pump inhibitor (e.g. omeprazole or pantoprazole) or

H2-blocker (e.g. ranitidine) should be started before treatment and continued for 4 weeks post-treatment.

- The fever does not necessarily indicate sepsis but may be related to the embolic effect of the microspheres and the acute toxic effects on the tumor. So, antibiotic prophylaxis is not routinely required, but if there is any suspicion of bacterial infection, it is necessary to investigate and treat appropriately.
- Provided the patient is not diabetic—and oral steroids are not otherwise contraindicated—a tapering dose of oral corticosteroids (e.g. methylprednisolone or dexamethasone) may be useful. Also adequate hydration could be assured.

Anyway post-radioembolization syndrome is less severe than that observed after other embolic therapies (such as chemoembolization) in which fatigue and constitutional symptoms predominate [92].

Immediate, excessive and increasing over time abdominal pain after ^{90}Y-RE may indicate that microspheres have been inadvertently delivered to other organs such as the pancreas, stomach or duodenum. This will result in acute pancreatitis or peptic or duodenal ulceration. Post-treatment SPET/CT can determine if the microspheres have lodged in the pancreas or other organs, but additional tests such as serum amylase are also indicated if pancreatitis is diagnosed. If this were to occur, the patient should be treated using best standard practice, including pain relief and intravenous fluids. After the patients are discharged, total blood count and blood biochemistry tests should be monitored weekly, and any possible side effects are questioned on a weekly basis for the first months and monthly afterwards.

Key Points

Intra-arterial ^{90}Y-microspheres infusion must be performed by experienced *RE-Team.*

Post-therapy ^{90}Y bremsstrahlung SPET/CT or ^{90}Y PET imaging is of great importance for controlling the correct microspheres administration.

Post-procedural medical support is useful to reduce patient discomfort.

15.6 Follow-Up

The response to radioembolization in hepatic metastases may be evaluated by using imaging findings, changes in tumor markers and, sometimes, pathologic findings. The clinical impact and safety should be assessed as well, such as change in energy levels and pain palliation. Accordingly, a clinic visit is recommended with laboratory workup (including liver function tests) within 1 month of treatment. Multidisciplinary imaging and clinical re-evaluation is recommended at 1–3 months following treatment and at 3–6-month intervals thereafter to assess treatment response. Although early follow-up imaging at 1 month is often performed, mostly to assess absence of progression or treatment complication, one should interpret tumor response with caution at such an early time, as the effects of radioembolization occur over several months.

15.6.1 Response Evaluation

The imaging modality (i.e. CT, MRI, PET) should be consistent throughout the patient's care to best assess response to therapy [93]. It may be difficult in some situations to have patients receive the same imaging modality and temporal follow-up; if possible, standardization is recommended.

Tumor response can be measured on CT or MRI strictly based on size on radiological imaging by using the Response Evaluation Criteria In Solid Tumors (RECIST). RECIST criteria however can be misleading and may lead to an underestimation of the pathological tumor response, especially if determined early (<3 months). Imaging evaluation that incorporated necrosis indicators reported that response to treatment can become apparent earlier (1 month) [94]. According to the necrosis criteria, tumor response is assessed based on the amount of necrosis in the tumor following therapy. Non-enhancement is considered as a non-viable tumor according to the necrosis criteria. Various studies have stated that the necrosis criteria will identify responders earlier and with better accuracy than the RECIST criteria [95].

Positron emission tomography with ^{18}F-FDG (FDG PET) has an important clinical value as an adjunct to CT in patients with ^{18}F-FDG-avid tumors such as colorectal cancer as it detects response more rapidly and accurately. PET/CT is superior in response assessment to RECIST or tumor density measurements [96] and may also assist in differentiating viable neoplastic tissue from oedema, haemorrhage or fibrosis [97]. Prognostic value of change in metabolic volume or total lesion glycolysis evaluated on pre- and post-therapy PET has been also demonstrated [98, 99]. Predictive models using multimodality imaging approaches (PET/CT—SPET/CT image fusion algorithms) have been also proposed to better select patients for ^{90}Y-RE [100]. FDG PET/CT imaging can be performed at 4–6 weeks following the therapy to assess early therapy response, for the patients who had undergone baseline FDG PET/CT imaging before the therapy (Fig. 15.9).

15.6.1.1 Retreatment

For repeated radioembolization to the same arterial territory, the cumulative absorbed dose to healthy tissue and time interval between radioembolizations are important safety considerations.

Whether a repeat procedure is planned or opportunistic, the ^{90}Y-resin microsphere activity must be calculated a new for each ^{90}Y-RE. Not only will the patient's clinical status and treatment aims differ, but all three partitions—tumor, uninvolved liver and lung shunt fraction—continue to change qualitatively and quantitatively for 6–9 months after each radioembolization. However, the safety of repeated whole-liver radioembolization has not been firmly established yet [101, 102].

15.6.2 Safety Evaluation and Adverse Effects

The incidence of severe complications following ^{90}Y-RE is low if patient selection is appropriate

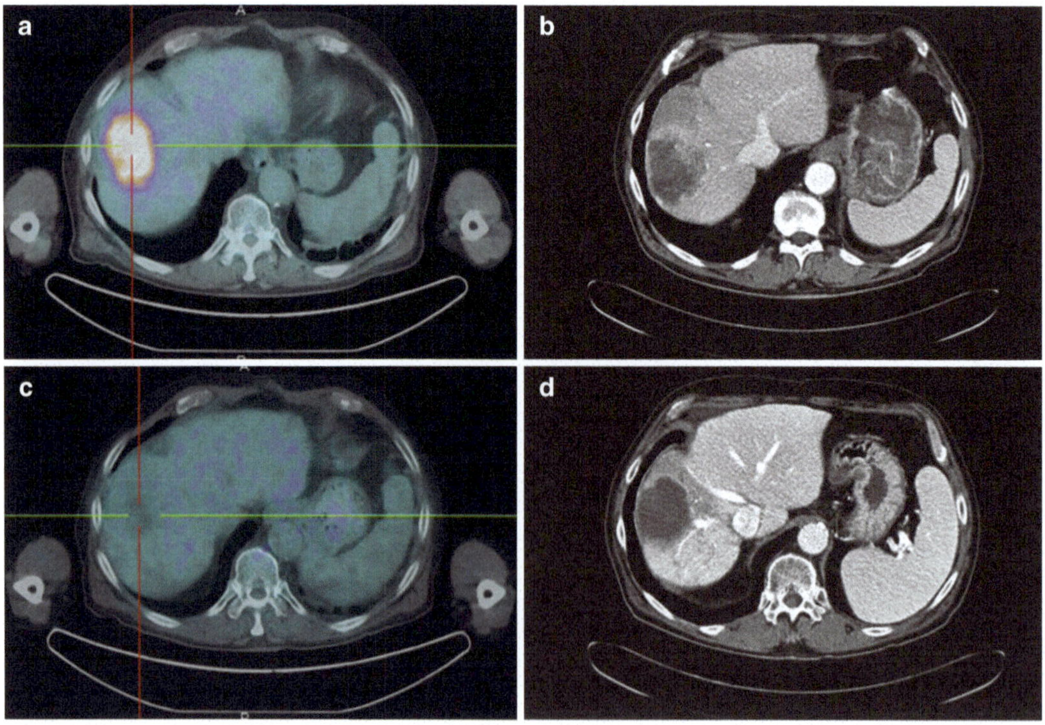

Fig. 15.9 Pre-therapy ^{18}F-FDG PET/CT (**a**) in a metastatic colorectal cancer showing an intense FDG uptake in correspondence of a 7 cm lesion of the VII segment evidenced at pre-therapy CT (**b**). Two month post-therapy PET (**c**) showing a complete response confirmed at a CT imaging (**d**) 1 month later

and delivery technique is accurate. The safety of resin microspheres in patients with inoperable liver-dominant metastatic colorectal cancer has been well established both as a monotherapy and in combination with systemic chemotherapy [7–10, 14].

Early side effects include rare complications of angiography (i.e. puncture site adverse events, vessel dissection) or systemic side effects (post-radioembolization syndrome) that have been previously described.

Delayed serious adverse events following radioembolization may occur as a result of a toxic dose to normal hepatic parenchyma or a toxic dose to extrahepatic tissue. Adverse events secondary to treatment delivery should be defined by using the National Cancer Institute Common Terminology Criteria for Adverse Events, version 4.03 [103]. Complications may occur despite careful pretreatment planning and require an expert multidisciplinary team approach in order to provide comprehensive care for patients.

15.6.2.1 Extrahepatic Adverse Effects

The most common relevant extrahepatic complications of RE include: radiation pneumonitis, radiation gastritis and gastrointestinal (GI) ulcers and cholecystitis.

Radiation Pneumonitis

Radiation pneumonitis is a very rare but worrisome complication that likely occurs from hepatic arterial-hepatic venous shunting, resulting in particle deposition to the lungs. It may occur 1–6 months after RE and is characterized by the appearance of restrictive ventilatory dysfunction and bilateral lung infiltrates. This may be suspected if patients develop a non-productive cough several days or weeks after the implantation of microspheres and is diagnosed by chest X-ray. Patients should be treated with systemic corticosteroids and supportive care until the disease has subsided. Strict adherence to the manufactures indicated lung dose limits largely prevents this complication with no reported cases in recent multicentre retrospective analyses of 606 patients with metastatic colorectal cancer (mCRC) [92].

Radiation Gastritis and Gastrointestinal Ulceration

Radiation-induced GI ulcerations are an uncommon complication of RE that presents usually 2–6 weeks after treatment with symptoms of acute epigastric pain, nausea, vomiting, dyspepsia and sometimes anorexia. Because patients may have difficulty eating, weight loss and poor nutritional status become a major concern, which may lead to fatigue and decrease in performance status. If this were to occur, the patient should be treated using best standard practice, including pain relief, gastric acid-blocking drugs and intravenous fluids. Treatment is the same as for any cause of acute peptic ulceration even radiation-induced GI ulceration is often poorly responsive to therapy. In case of treatment failure, surgery may be required. The incidence of GI ulcers ranges from 1.9 to 3.2% among patients with mCRC. Symptoms are usually mild to moderate and last for 4–10 months despite treatment, but full symptomatic and endoscopic recovery normally occurs. In the setting of metastatic disease, the use of biological agents is not recommended if gastrointestinal ulceration occurs. In addition, it may be necessary to withhold systemic chemotherapy agents to allow for healing.

Radiation-Induced Cholecystitis

Radiation-induced cholecystitis is a well-known adverse event when infusion is performed proximal to the cystic artery and occurs in as many as 2% of cases. Most instances of radiation-induced cholecystitis can be managed conservatively with hydration, pain control and antibiotic therapy. In rare cases, cholecystectomy or percutaneous cholecystostomy may be required; however, these measures should be reserved as a last option [104]. Prevention by administration of microspheres distal to the cystic artery should be attempted whenever feasible.

Other Rare Adverse Effects

Radiation-induced skin injury has been reported from microsphere deposition in the falciform artery [105]. Severe cases can manifest in dermatitis or even skin ulceration. Because of the exceedingly low incidence of severe adverse events from falciform artery uptake of ^{90}Y, it may not routinely require prophylactic embolization.

15.6.2.2 Hepatic Adverse Effects

Hepatic adverse events include liver failure, liver abscess, intrahepatic bilomas and liver infarction. The incidence of hepatic adverse events in the literature is highly variable as a result of diverse patient selection, duration of patient follow-up and definitions for grading toxicities.

Excessive irradiation of healthy liver parenchyma leads to the most serious and life-threatening complication after radioembolization that is called "radioembolization-induced liver disease" or REILD. In patients with metastatic liver tumors who received numerous lines of systemic chemotherapy, some of which may be hepatotoxic, liver function should be tested over time to assess their candidacy for ^{90}Y-RE and reduce REILD risk [72, 106–108].

Radioembolization-Induced Liver Disease (REILD)

REILD is characterized by a well-defined constellation of temporal, clinical, biochemical and histopathologic findings. It typically manifests approximately 4–8 weeks post-RE and is characterized clinically by jaundice and ascites in the absence of tumor progression or bile duct obstruction. The typical biochemical picture of REILD is an elevated bilirubin (>3 mg/dL) in almost all cases, elevated alkaline phosphatase (ALP) and gamma-glutamyl transpeptidase (GGT) in most cases, accompanied by virtually no change in the transaminases (AST and ALT). Although the incidence of REILD is relatively low (typically less than 4%), it can progress to liver failure and death [106]. Previous radioembolization, multiple lines of chemotherapy, abnormal baseline liver function, single-session whole-liver therapy and empiric model dosimetry with resin microspheres have been identified as risk factors for the development of REILD [72].

REILD resembles other forms of sinusoidal obstruction syndrome (SOS) that is caused by a vascular injury in the central vein with an eccentric wall thickening. Indeed in the most severe cases, liver biopsy shows veno-occlusive disease, the histological hallmark of SOS. Clinical "veno-occlusive disease" is characterized by development of portal hypertension, ascites and deterioration in liver function [107].

However, the radiomicrosphere-induced liver disease usually has a different pattern. Radiation from microspheres is deposited primarily in the region of the portal triad and away from the central vein, thus minimizing the damage pattern seen in radiation hepatitis from external beam sources. Microscopically, RE-induced liver disease is characterized by micro-infarcts and a chronic inflammatory infiltrate dominating at the portal areas [108]. Microspheres lodge preferentially in the growing rim of the tumor, as the centre may become necrotic and avascular as the tumor size increases. The highest dose exposure is at the zone immediately surrounding the tumor. The damage to this area of parenchyma is unavoidable. The remainder of the liver receives less radiation than would be predicted from assuming a homogeneous distribution of radiation dose throughout the parenchyma. Clinical veno-occlusive disease is then much less common with ^{90}Y-RE than after external beam radiotherapy.

Importantly, SOS may also occur in CRC patients that receive oxaliplatin- or irinotecan-based regimes, which is the clinical setting for many ^{90}Y-RE-treated patients. Prophylactic treatment with methylprednisolone and ursodeoxycholic acid starting on the day of ^{90}Y-RE and continued for 2 months may reduce the incidence of REILD [72]. In the treatment of REILD, low-molecular-weight heparin may also be considered, but both corticosteroids and heparin may only be useful if commenced very early in the course of the disease.

Thus preventing REILD is most important. Consequently selection of patients by liver function is crucial as deranged baseline hepatic function, presence of liver cirrhosis and administered radiation dose are the most important risk factors for developing REILD.

To avoid REILD, it may be useful to keep in mind some simple rules:

1. To limit the prescription of ^{90}Y-RE to multidisciplinary teams in tertiary centres working with experienced interventional radiologists and nuclear medicine specialists

2. To strictly respect the contraindications of RE especially, an elevated total bilirubin value at baseline (higher than 2 mg/dL)
3. To avoid whole-liver treatment and sparing as much liver as possible by sequential treatment with super-selective catheterization and an interval of 6–8 weeks between two procedures, especially for non-cirrhotic patients.

Other Hepatic Adverse Effects

Eventually radiation leads to fibrosis presenting with imaging signs of portal hypertension. Fortunately, these findings hardly ever have clinical consequences [109]. However, in neoadjuvant setting, the development of fibrosis in a treated lobe may be beneficial, as contralateral lobar hypertrophy may occur, facilitating an eventual surgical resection.

Biliary toxicity with biloma, abscess and radiation-induced cholecystitis occurs in ≤2% of patients [110]. Fortunately, many imaging findings indicative of biliary complications do not manifest clinically.

Systemic chemotherapeutic agents may render blood vessels fragile. Hence, vascular adverse events may occur more often following systemic chemotherapy for secondary liver tumors. Biological agents have been widely known to cause vascular adverse events during arteriography. Arterial dissection, vasoconstriction and poor vascular flow have been reported [111, 112]. The most common agent associated with vascular adverse events is bevacizumab, a monoclonal antibody to vascular endothelial growth factor commonly used in metastatic colon and breast cancer. Therefore, it is recommended that radioembolization proceed at least 4–6 weeks after the last dose of bevacizumab. Careful selection and manipulation of microcatheters and wires are mandatory in these situations.

Key Points

Hepatic and extrahepatic toxicity of ^{90}Y-RE is low if the patient selection and procedure are accurate.

REILD is the most serious effect and can be prevented checking liver function and performing an adequate therapeutic strategy.

References

1. Cosimelli M, Mancini R, Carpanese L, Sciuto R, Pizzi G, Pattaro G, et al. Integration of radioembolisation into multimodal treatment of liver-dominant metastatic colorectal cancer. Expert Opin Ther Targets. 2012;16(Suppl 2):S11–6. https://doi.org/10.1517/14728222.2011.647811.
2. Mahnken AH. Current status of transarterial radioembolization. World J Radiol. 2016;8(5):449–59. https://doi.org/10.4329/wjr.v8.i5.449.
3. Lien WM, Ackerman NB. The blood supply of experimental liver metastases. II. A microcirculatory study of the normal and tumor vessels of the liver with the use of perfused silicone rubber. Surgery. 1970;68(2):334–40.
4. Lewandowski RJ, Salem R. Yttrium-90 Radioembolization of hepatocellular carcinoma and metastatic disease to the liver. Semin Interv Radiol. 2006;23(1):64–72. https://doi.org/10.1055/s-2006-939842.
5. Geschwind JFH, Salem R, Carr BI, Soulen MC, Thurston KG, Goin KA, et al. Yttrium-90 microspheres for the treatment of hepatocellular carcinoma. J Gastroenterol. 2004;127:194–205. https://doi.org/10.1053/j.gastro.2004.09.034.
6. Giammarile F, Bodei L, Chiesa C, Flux G, Forrer F, Kraeber-Bodere F, et al. EANM procedure guideline for the treatment of liver cancer and liver metastases with intra-arterial radioactive compounds. Eur J Nucl Med Mol Imaging. 2011;38(7):1393–406. https://doi.org/10.1007/s00259-011-1812-2.
7. van Hazel GA, Heinemann V, Sharma NK, et al. SIRFLOX: randomized phase III trial comparing first-line mFOLFOX6 (plus or minus bevacizumab) versus mFOLFOX6 (plus or minus bevacizumab) plus selective internal radiation therapy in patients with metastatic colorectal cancer. J Clin Oncol. 2016;34:1723–31. https://doi.org/10.1200/JCO.2015.66.1181.
8. Cosimelli M, Golfieri R, Cagol PP, Carpanese L, Sciuto R, Maini CL, Italian Society of Locoregional Therapies in Oncology (SITILO), et al. Multicentre phase II clinical trial of yttrium-90 resin microspheres alone in unresectable, chemotherapy refractory colorectal liver metastases. Br J Cancer. 2010;103(3):324–31. https://doi.org/10.1038/sj.bjc.6605770.
9. Van Hazel G, Blackwell A, Anderson J, Price D, Moroz P, Bower G, et al. Randomised phase 2 trial of SIR-spheres plus fluorouracil/leucovorin chemotherapy versus fluorouracil/leucovorin chemotherapy alone in advanced colorectal cancer. J Surg Oncol. 2004;88(2):78–85. https://doi.org/10.1002/jso.20141.
10. Gray B, Van Hazel G, Hope M, Burton M, Moroz P, Anderson J, et al. Randomised trial of SIR-spheres plus chemotherapy vs. chemotherapy alone for treating patients with liver metastases from primary large bowel cancer. Ann Oncol. 2001;12(12):1711–20.

11. Lim L, Gibbs P, Yip D, Shapiro JD, Dowling R, Smith D, et al. A prospective evaluation of treatment with selective internal radiation therapy (SIR-spheres) in patients with unresectable liver metastases from colorectal cancer previously treated with 5-FU based chemotherapy. BMC Cancer. 2005;5:132. https://doi.org/10.1186/1471-2407-5-132.
12. Van Hazel GA, Pavlakis N, Goldstein D, Olver Ian N, Tapner MJ, Price D, et al. Treatment of fluorouracil-refractory patients with liver metastases from colorectal cancer by using yttrium-90 resin microspheres plus concomitant systemic irinotecan chemotherapy. J Clin Oncol. 2009;27:4089–95.
13. Seidensticker R, Denecke T, Kraus P, Seidensticker M, Mohnike K, Fahlke J, et al. Matched-pair comparison of radioembolization plus best supportive care vs. best supportive care alone for chemotherapy refractory liver-dominant colorectal metastases. Cardiovasc Intervent Radiol. 2012;35:1066–73.https://doi.org/10.1007/s00270-011-0234-7.
14. Hendlisz A, Van den Eynde M, Peeters M, Maleux G, Lambert B, Vannoote J, et al. Phase III trial comparing protracted intravenous fluorouracil infusion alone or with yttrium-90 resin microspheres radioembolization for liver-limited metastatic colorectal cancer refractory to standard chemotherapy. J Clin Oncol. 2010;28:3687–94. https://doi.org/10.1200/JCO.2010.28.5643.
15. Sharma RA, Van Hazel GA, Morgan B, Berry DP, Blanshard K, Price D, et al. Radioembolization of liver metastases from colorectal cancer using yttrium-90 microspheres with concomitant systemic oxaliplatin, fluorouracil, and leucovorin chemotherapy. J Clin Oncol. 2007;25(9):1099–106.
16. Sofocleous CT, Garcia AR, Pandit-Taskar N, Do KG, Brody LA, Petre EN, et al. Phase I trial of selective internal radiation therapy for chemorefractory colorectal cancer liver metastases progressing after hepatic arterial pump and systemic chemotherapy. Clin Colorectal Cancer. 2014;13(1):27–36. https://doi.org/10.1016/j.clcc.2013.11.010.
17. Van Cutsem E, Cervantes A, Adam R, Sobrero A, Van Krieken JH, Aderka D, et al. ESMO consensus guidelines for the management of patients with metastatic colorectal cancer. Ann Oncol. 2016;27:1386–422. https://doi.org/10.1093/annonc/mdw235.
18. Garlipp B, de Baere T, Damm R, Irmscher R, van Buskirk M, Stübs P, et al. Left-liver hypertrophy after therapeutic right-liver radioembolization is substantial but less than after portal vein embolization. Hepatology. 2014;59:1864–73. https://doi.org/10.1002/hep.26947.
19. Braat MN, Samin M, van den Bosch MA, Lam MG. The role of 90-Y radioembolization in downstaging primary and secondary hepatic malignancies: a systematic review. Clin Transl Imaging. 2016;4:283–95. https://doi.org/10.1007/s40336-016-0172-0.
20. Dutton SJ, Kenealy N, Love SB, Wasan HS, Sharma RA. FOXFIRE protocol: an open-label, randomised, phase III trial of 5-fluorouracil, oxaliplatin and folinic acid (OxMdG) with or without interventional selective internal radiation therapy (SIRT) as first-line treatment for patients with unresectable liver-only or liver-dominant metastatic colorectal cancer. BMC Cancer. 2014;14:497. https://doi.org/10.1186/1471-2407-14-497.
21. Virdee PS, Moschandreas J, Gebski V, Love SB, Francis EA, Phil D, et al. Protocol for combined analysis of FOXFIRE, SIRFLOX, and FOXFIRE-global randomized phase III trials of chemotherapy +/− selective internal radiation therapy as first-line treatment for patients with metastatic colorectal cancer. JMIR Res Protoc. 2017;6(3):e43. https://doi.org/10.2196/resprot.7201.
22. Zurkiya O, Ganguli S. Beyond hepatocellular carcinoma and colorectal metastasis: the expanding applications of radioembolization. Front Oncol. 2014;4:150. https://doi.org/10.3389/fonc.2014.00150.
23. Sato KT, Lewandowski RJ, Mulcahy MF, Atassi B, Ryu RK, Gates VL, et al. Unresectable chemorefractory liver metastases: radioembolization with 90Y microspheres-safety, efficacy, and survival. Radiology. 2008;247:507–15. https://doi.org/10.1148/radiol.2472062029.
24. King JMPH, Quinn RMB, Glenn DM, Janssen J, Tong D, Liaw W, et al. Radioembolization with selective internal radiation microspheres for neuroendocrine liver metastases. Cancer. 2008;113:921–9. https://doi.org/10.1002/cncr.23685.
25. Saxena A, Chua TC, Bester L, Kokandi A, Morris DL. Factors predicting response and survival after yttrium-90 radioembolization of unresectable neuroendocrine tumor liver metastases: a critical appraisal of 48 cases. Ann Surg. 2010;251:910–6. https://doi.org/10.1097/SLA.0b013e3181d3d24a.
26. Cao CQ, Yan TD, Bester L, Liauw W, Morris L. Radioembolization with yttrium microspheres for neuroendocrine tumor liver metastases. Br J Surg. 2010;97:537–43. https://doi.org/10.1002/bjs.6931.
27. Paprottka PM, Hoffmann RT, Haug A, Sommer WH, Raessler F, Trumm CG, et al. Radioembolization of symptomatic, unresectable neuroendocrine hepatic metastases using yttrium-90 microspheres. Cardiovasc Intervent Radiol. 2012;35(2):334–42. https://doi.org/10.1007/s00270-011-0248-1.
28. Memon K, Lewandowski RJ, Mulcahy MF, Riaz A, Ryu RK, Sato KT, et al. Radioembolization for neuroendocrine liver metastases: safety, imaging, and long-term outcomes. Int J Radiat Oncol Biol Phys. 2012;83(3):887–94. https://doi.org/10.1016/j.ijrobp.2011.07.041.
29. Kennedy AS, Dezarn WA, McNeillie P, Coldwell D, Nutting C, Carter D, et al. Radioembolization for unresectable neuroendocrine hepatic metastases using resin 90Y-microspheres: early results in

148 patients. Am J Clin Oncol. 2008;31(3):271–9. https://doi.org/10.1097/COC.0b013e31815e4557.
30. Ceelen F, Theisen D, de Albéniz XG, Auernhammer CJ, Haug AR, D'Anastasi M, et al. Towards new response criteria in neuroendocrine tumors: which changes in MRI parameters are associated with longer progression-free survival after radioembolization of liver metastases? J Magn Reson Imaging. 2015;41(2):361–8. https://doi.org/10.1002/jmri.24569.
31. Ezziddin S, Meyer C, Kahancova S, Haslerud T, Willinek W, Wilhelm K, et al. Biersack HJ90Y radioembolization after radiation exposure from peptide receptor radionuclide therapy. J Nucl Med. 2012;53(11):1663–9. https://doi.org/10.2967/jnumed.112.107482.
32. Barbier CE, Garske-Román U, Sandström M, Nyman R, Granberg D. Selective internal radiation therapy in patients with progressive neuroendocrine liver metastases. Eur J Nucl Med Mol Imaging. 2016;43(8):1425–31. https://doi.org/10.1007/s00259-015-3264-6.
33. Filippi L, Scopinaro F, Pelle G, Cianni R, Salvatori R, Schillaci O, et al. Molecular response assessed by (68)Ga-DOTANOC and survival after (90)Y microsphere therapy in patients with liver metastases from neuroendocrine tumors. Eur J Nucl Med Mol Imaging. 2016;43(3):432–40. https://doi.org/10.1007/s00259-015-3178-3.
34. Peker A, Çiçek O, Soydal Ç, Küçük NÖ, Bilgiç S. Radioembolization with yttrium-90 resin microspheres for neuroendocrine tumor liver metastases. Diagn Interv Radiol. 2015;21(1):54–9. https://doi.org/10.5152/dir.2014.14036.
35. Kennedy A, Bester L, Salem R, Sharma RA, Parks RW, Ruszniewski P, NET-Liver-Metastases Consensus Conference. Role of hepatic intra-arterial therapies in metastatic neuroendocrine tumors (NET): guidelines from the NET-liver-metastases consensus conference. HPB (Oxford). 2015;17(1):29–37. https://doi.org/10.1111/hpb.12326.
36. Fan KY, Wild AT, Halappa VG, Kumar R, Ellsworth S, Ziegler M, et al. Neuroendocrine tumor liver metastases treated with yttrium-90 radioembolization. Contemp Clin Trials. 2016;50:143–9. https://doi.org/10.1016/j.cct.2016.08.001.
37. Cianni R, Pelle G, Notarianni E, Saltarelli A, Rabuffi P, Bagni O, et al. Radioembolisation with (90)Y-labelled resin microspheres in the treatment of liver metastasis from breast cancer. Eur Radiol. 2013;23(1):182–9. https://doi.org/10.1007/s00330-012-2556-5.
38. Coldwell DM, Kennedy AS, Nutting CW. Use of yttrium-90 microspheres in the treatment of unresectable hepatic metastases from breast cancer. Int J Radiat Oncol Biol Phys. 2007;69(3):800–4. https://doi.org/10.1016/j.ijrobp.2007.03.056.
39. Haug AR, Tiega Donfack BP, Trumm C, Zech CJ, Michl M, Laubender RP, et al. 18F-FDG PET/CT predicts survival after radioembolization of hepatic metastases from breast cancer. J Nucl Med. 2012;53(3):371–7. https://doi.org/10.2967/jnumed.111.096230.
40. Saxena A, Kapoor J, Meteling B, Morris DL, Bester L. Yttrium-90 radioembolization for unresectable, chemoresistant breast cancer liver metastases: a large single-center experience of 40 patients. Ann Surg Oncol. 2014;21(4):1296–303. https://doi.org/10.1245/s10434-013-3436-1.
41. Fendler WP, Lechner H, Todica A, Paprottka KJ, Paprottka PM, Jakobs TF, et al. Safety, efficacy, and prognostic factors after Radioembolization of hepatic metastases from breast cancer: a large single-center experience in 81 patients. J Nucl Med. 2016;57(4):517–23. https://doi.org/10.2967/jnumed.115.165050.
42. Michl M, Haug AR, Jakobs TF, Paprottka P, Hoffmann RT, Bartenstein P, et al. Radioembolization with Yttrium-90 microspheres (SIRT) in pancreatic cancer patients with liver metastases: efficacy, safety and prognostic factors. Oncology. 2014;86(1):24–32. https://doi.org/10.1159/000355821.
43. Gonsalves CF, Eschelman DJ, Sullivan KL, Anne PR, Doyle L, Sato T. Radioembolization as salvage therapy for hepatic metastasis of uveal melanoma: a single-institution experience. AJR Am J Roentgenol. 2011;196(2):468–73. https://doi.org/10.2214/AJR.10.4881.
44. Eldredge-Hindy H, Ohri N, Anne PR, Eschelman D, Gonsalves C, Intenzo C, et al. Yttrium-90 microsphere brachytherapy for liver metastases from uveal melanoma: clinical outcomes and the predictive value of Fluorodeoxyglucose positron emission tomography. Am J Clin Oncol. 2016;39(2):189–95. https://doi.org/10.1097/COC.0000000000000033.
45. Klingenstein A, Haug AR, Zech CJ, Schaller UC. Radioembolization as locoregional therapy of hepatic metastases in uveal melanoma patients. Cardiovasc Intervent Radiol. 2013;36(1):158–65. https://doi.org/10.1007/s00270-012-0373-5.
46. Melucci E, Cosimelli M, Carpanese L, Pizzi G, Izzo F, Fiore F, Italian Society of Locoregional Therapies in Oncology (S.I.T.I.L.O.), et al. Decrease of survivin, p53 and Bcl-2 expression in chemorefractory colorectal liver metastases may be predictive of radiosensivity radiosensivity after radioembolization with yttrium-90 resin microspheres. J Exp Clin Cancer Res. 2013;32:13. https://doi.org/10.1186/1756-9966-32-13.
47. Dendy MS, Ludwig JM, Kim HS. Predictors and prognosticators for survival with Yttrium-90 radioembolization therapy for unresectable colorectal cancer liver metastasis. Oncotarget. 2017;8:37912. 10.18632/oncotarget.16007.
48. Gulec SA, Selwyn R, Weiner R, et al. Nuclear medicine guidelines for radiomicrosphere therapy using Y-90 microspheres in patients with primary and metastatic liver cancer. J Interv Oncol. 2009;2:26–39.

49. Fendler WP, Philippe Tiega DB, Ilhan H, Paprottka PM, Heinemann V, Jakobs TF, et al. Validation of several SUV-based parameters derived from 18F-FDG PET for prediction of survival after SIRT of hepatic metastases from colorectal cancer. J Nucl Med. 2013;54(8):1202–8. https://doi.org/10.2967/jnumed.112.116426.
50. Powerski MJ, Erxleben C, Scheurig-Münkler C, et al. Anatomic variants of arteries often coil-occluded prior to hepatic radioembolization. Acta Radiol. 2015;56:159–65. https://doi.org/10.1177/0284185114522148.
51. van den Hoven AF, Smits MLJ, de Keizer B, et al. Identifying aberrant hepatic arteries prior to intra-arterial radioembolization. Cardiovasc Intervent Radiol. 2014;37:1482–93. https://doi.org/10.1007/s00270-014-0845-x.
52. Favelier S, Germain T, Genson PY, et al. Anatomy of liver arteries for interventional radiology. Diagn Interv Imaging. 2014;96:537–46. https://doi.org/10.1016/j.diii.2013.12.001.
53. Bilbao JI, Garrastachu P, Herraiz MJ, et al. Safety and efficacy assessment of flow redistribution by occlusion of intrahepatic vessels prior to radioembolization in the treatment of liver tumors. Cardiovasc Intervent Radiol. 2010;33(3):523–53. https://doi.org/10.1007/s00270-009-9717-1.
54. Burgmans MC, Kao YH, Irani FG, et al. Radioembolization with infusion of yttrium-90 microspheres into a right inferior phrenic artery with hepatic tumor supply is feasible and safe. J Vasc Interv Radiol. 2012;23(10):1294–301. https://doi.org/10.1016/j.jvir.2012.07.009.
55. Abdelmaksoud MH, Louie JD, Kothary N, et al. Embolization of parasitized extrahepatic arteries to reestablish intrahepatic arterial supply to tumors before yttrium-90 radioembolization. J Vasc Interv Radiol. 2011;22(10):1355–62. https://doi.org/10.1016/j.jvir.2011.06.007.
56. Hamoui N, Minocha J, Memon K, et al. Prophylactic embolization of the gastroduodenal and right gastric arteries is not routinely necessary before radioembolization with glass microspheres. J Vasc Interv Radiol. 2013;24(11):1743–5. https://doi.org/10.1016/j.jvir.2013.07.011.
57. Abdelmaksoud MH, Hwang GL, Louie JD, et al. Development of new hepaticoenteric collateral pathways after hepatic arterial skeletonization in preparation for yttrium-90 radioembolization. J Vasc Interv Radiol. 2010;21:1385–95. https://doi.org/10.1016/j.jvir.2010.04.030.
58. Tacher V, Radaelli A, Lin M, Geschwind JF. How I do it: cone-beam CT during transarterial chemoembolization for liver cancer. Radiology. 2015;274:320–34. https://doi.org/10.1148/radiol.14131925.
59. Louie JD, Kothary N, Kuo WT, et al. Incorporating cone-beam CT into the treatment planning for yttrium-90 radioembolization. J Vasc Interv Radiol. 2009;20:606–13. https://doi.org/10.1016/j.jvir.2009.01.021.
60. Padia SA, Lewandowski RJ, Johnson GE, Sze DY, Ward TJ, Gaba RC, et al. Radioembolization of hepatic malignancies: background, quality improvement guidelines, and future directions. J Vasc Interv Radiol. 2016. https://doi.org/10.1016/j.ivir.2016.09.024.
61. Wright CL, Werner JD, Tran JM, et al. Radiation pneumonitis following yttrium- 90 radioembolization: case report and literature review. J Vasc Interv Radiol. 2012;23:669–74. https://doi.org/10.1016/j.jvir.2012.01.059.
62. Sirtex Medical Limited. North Sidney, Australia. SIR-spheres training program: physicians and institutions. version TRN-RW-05 (undated).
63. Salem R, Thurston KG. Radioembolization with 90yttrium microspheres: a state-of-the-art brachytherapy treatment for primary and secondary liver malignancies. Part 1: technical and methodologic considerations. J Vasc Interv Radiol. 2006;17:1251–78. https://doi.org/10.1097/01.RVI.0000233785.75257.9A.
64. Salem R, Parikh P, Atassi B, Lewandowski RJ, Ryu RK, Sato KT, et al. Incidence of radiation pneumonitis after hepatic intra-arterial radiotherapy with yttrium-90 microspheres assuming uniform lung distribution. Am J Clin Oncol. 2008;31:431–8. https://doi.org/10.1097/COC.0b013e318168ef65.
65. Barentsz MW, Vente MA, Lam MG, et al. Technical solutions to ensure safe yttrium-90 radioembolization in patients with initial extrahepatic deposition of 99mtechnetium-albumin macroaggregates. Cardiovasc Intervent Radiol. 2011;34:1074–9. https://doi.org/10.1007/s00270-010-0088-4.
66. Dudeck O, Wilhelmsen S, Ulrich G, et al. Effectiveness of repeat angiographic assessment in patients designated for radioembolization using yttrium-90 microspheres with initial extrahepatic accumulation of technitium-99m macroaggregated albumin: a single center's experience. Cardiovasc Intervent Radiol. 2012;35:1083–93. https://doi.org/10.1007/s00270-011-0252-5.
67. Ho S, Lau WY, Leung TW, Chan M, Ngar YK, Johnson PJ, et al. Partition model for estimating radiation doses from yttrium-90 microspheres in treating hepatic tumors. Eur J Nucl Med. 1996;23:947–52.
68. Ho S, Lau WY, Leung TW, Chan M, Chan KW, Lee WY, Johnson PJ, Li AK, et al. Tumor-to-normal uptake ratio of 90Y microspheres in hepatic cancer assessed with 99mTc macroaggregated albumin. Br J Radiol. 1997;70:823–8. https://doi.org/10.1259/bjr.70.836.9486047.
69. Flamen P, Vanderlinden B, Delatte P. Multimodality imaging can predict the metabolic response of unresectable colorectal liver metastases to radioembolization therapy with yttrium-90 labeled resin microspheres. Phys Med Biol. 2008;53:6591–603. https://doi.org/10.1088/0031-9155/53/22/019.
70. Garin E, Rolland Y, Lenoir L, Pracht M, Mesbah H, Porée P, Laffont S, Clement B, Raoul JL, Boucher E. Utility of quantitative Tc-MAA SPET/CT for

yttrium-labelled microsphere treatment planning: calculating vascularized hepatic volume and dosimetric approach. Int J Mol Imaging. 2011;2011:398051. https://doi.org/10.1155/2011/398051.
71. Dezarn WA. Quality assurance issues for therapeutic application of radioactive microspheres. Int J Radiat Oncol Biol Phys. 2008;71(Suppl. 1):S147–51. https://doi.org/10.1016/j.ijrobp.2007.05.094.
72. Gil-Alzugaray B, Chopitea A, Inarrairaegui M, et al. Prognostic factors and prevention of radioembolization-induced liver disease. Hepatology. 2013;57(3):1078–87. https://doi.org/10.1002/hep.26191.
73. Piana PM, Gonsalves CF, Sato T, et al. Toxicities after radioembolization with yttrium-90 SIR-spheres: incidence and contributing risk factors at a single center. J Vasc Interv Radiol. 2011;22(10):1373–9. https://doi.org/10.1016/j.jvir.2011.06.006.
74. Vouche M, Lewandowski RJ, Atassi R, et al. Radiation lobectomy: time-dependent analysis of future liver remnant volume in unresectable liver cancer as a bridge to resection. J Hepatol. 2013;59:1029–36. https://doi.org/10.1016/j.jhep.2013.06.015.
75. Riaz A, Gates VL, Atassi B, et al. Radiation segmentectomy: a novel approach to increase safety and efficacy of radioembolization. Int J Radiat Oncol Biol Phys. 2011;79:163–71. https://doi.org/10.1016/j.ijrobp.2009.10.062.
76. Lam MG, Goris ML, Iagaru AH, Mittra ES, Louie JD, Sze DY. Prognostic utility of 90Y radioembolization dosimetry based on fusion 99mTc-macroaggregated albumin-99mTc-sulfur colloid SPECT. J Nucl Med. 2013;54(12):2055–61. https://doi.org/10.2967/jnumed. 113.123257.
77. Strigari L, Sciuto R, Rea S, et al. Efficacy and toxicity related to treatment of hepatocellular carcinoma with 90Y-SIR spheres: radiobiologic considerations. J Nucl Med. 2010;51:1377–85. https://doi.org/10.2967/jnumed.110.075861.
78. Campbell AM, Bailey IH, Burton MA. Tumor dosimetry in human liver following hepatic yttrium-90 microsphere therapy. Phys Med Biol. 2001;46:487–98.
79. Morris-Stiff G, Tan YM, Vauthey JN. Hepatic complications following preoperative chemotherapy with oxaliplatin or irinotecan for hepatic colorectal metastases. Eur J Surg Oncol. 2008;34:609–14. https://doi.org/10.1016/j.ejso.2007.07.007.
80. Lam MG, Louie JD, Abdelmaksoud MH, Fisher GA, Cho-Phan CD, Sze DY. Limitations of body surface area-based activity calculation for radioembolization of hepatic metastases in colorectal cancer. J Vasc Interv Radiol. 2014;25:1085–93. https://doi.org/10.1016/j.jvir.2013.11.018.
81. Kao YH, Tan EH, Ng CE, Goh SW. Clinical implications of the body surface area method versus partition model dosimetry for yttrium-90 radioembolization using resin microspheres: a technical review. Ann Nucl Med. 2011;25:455–61. https://doi.org/10.1007/s12149-011-0499-6.
82. Cremonesi M, Chiesa C, Strigari L, et al. Radioembolization of hepatic lesions from a radiobiology and dosimetric perspective. Front Oncol. 2014;4:210. https://doi.org/10.3389/fonc.2014.00210.
83. Kao YH, Hock Tan AE, Burgmans MC, Irani FG, Khoo LS, Gong Lo RH, et al. Image-guided personalized predictive dosimetry by artery-specific SPET/CT partition modeling for safe and effective 90Y radioembolization. J Nucl Med. 2012;53:559–66. https://doi.org/10.2967/jnumed.111.097469.
84. Paprottka KJ, Lehner S, Fendler WP, Ilhan H, Rominger A, Sommer W, et al. Reduced periprocedural analgesia after replacement of water for injection with glucose 5% solution as the infusion medium for 90Y-resin microspheres. J Nucl Med. 2016;57:1679–84. https://doi.org/10.2967/jnumed.115.170779.
85. Karunanithy N, Gordon F, Hodolic M, Al-Nahhas A, Wasan HS, Habib N, et al. Embolization of hepatic arterial branches to simplify hepatic blood flow before yttrium90 radioembolization: a useful technique in the presence of challenging anatomy. Cardiovasc Intervent Radiol. 2011;34:287–94. https://doi.org/10.1007/s00270-010- 9951-6.
86. Ray CE Jr, Gaba RC, Knuttinen MG, Minocha J, Bui JT. Multiple arteries supplying a single tumor vascular distribution: microsphere administration options for the interventional radiologist performing radioembolization. Semin Intervent Radiol. 2014;31:203–6. https://doi.org/10.1055/s-0034-1373794.
87. Murthy R, Brown DB, Salem R, et al. Gastrointestinal complications associated with hepatic arterial yttrium-90 microsphere therapy. J Vasc Interv Radiol. 2007;18:553–62. https://doi.org/10.1016/j.jvir.2007.02.002.
88. Minarik D, Sjogreen GK, Ljungberg M. Evaluation of quantitative 90Y SPECT based on experimental phantom studies. Phys Med Biol. 2008;53:5689–703.
89. Nickles RJ, Roberts AD, Nye JA, et al. Assaying and PET imaging of yttrium-90: 1.34 ppm.0. In: Conference record of IEEE nuclear science symposium and medical imaging conference; 2004. p. 3412–4.
90. Kao YH, Steinberg JD, Tay YS, Lim GK, Yan J, Townsend DW, et al. Post-radioembolization yttrium-90 PET/CT – part 1: diagnostic reporting. EJNMMI Res. 2013;3:56. https://doi.org/10.1186/2191-219X-3-56.
91. Riaz A, Lewandowski RJ, Kulik LM, Mulcahy MF, Sato KT, Ryu RK, et al. Complications following radioembolization with yttrium-90 microspheres: a comprehensive literature review. J Vasc Interv Radiol. 2009;20:1121–30. https://doi.org/10.1016/j.jvir.2009.05.030.
92. Kennedy AS, Coldwell D, Nutting C, et al. Resin 90Y-microsphere brachytherapy for unresectable

colorectal liver metastases: modern USA experience. Int J Radiat Oncol Biol Phys. 2006;65:412–25. https://doi.org/10.1016/j.ijrobp.2005.12.051.
93. Memon K, Kulik L, Lewandowski RJ, et al. Radiographic response to locoregional therapy in hepatocellular carcinoma predicts patient survival times. Gastroenterology. 2011;141:526–35. https://doi.org/10.1053/j.gastro.2011.04.054.
94. Keppke AL, Salem R, Reddy D, Huang J, Jin J, Larson AC, et al. Imaging of hepatocellular carcinoma after treatment with yttrium-90 microspheres. AJR Am J Roentgenol. 2007;188(3):768–75. https://doi.org/10.2214/AJR.06.0706.
95. Bester L, Hobbins PG, Wang SC, Salem R. Imaging characteristics following 90yttrium microsphere treatment for unresectable liver cancer. J Med Imaging Radiat Oncol. 2011;55(2):111–8. https://doi.org/10.1111/j.1754-9485.2011.02241.x.
96. Zerizer I, Al-Nahhas A, Towey D, Tait P, Ariff B, Wasan H, Hatice G, Habib N, Barwick T. The role of early (18)F-FDG PET/CT in prediction of progression-free survival after (90)Y radioembolization: comparison with RECIST and tumor density criteria. Eur J Nucl Med Mol Imaging. 2012;39:1391–9. https://doi.org/10.1007/s00259-012-2149-1.
97. Miller FH, Keppke AL, Reddy D, et al. Response of liver metastases after treatment with yttrium-90 microspheres: role of size, necrosis and PET. AJR Am J Roentgenol. 2007;188:776–83. https://doi.org/10.2214/AJR.06.0707.
98. Obrzut S, McCammack K, Badran KW, Balistreri A, Ou E, Nguyen BJ, Hoh CK, Rose SC. Prognostic value of post-yttrium 90 radioembolization therapy 18F-fluorodeoxyglucose positron emission tomography in patients with liver tumors. Clin Imaging. 2017;42:43–9. https://doi.org/10.1016/j.clinimag.2016.11.009.
99. Sabet A, Meyer C, Aouf A, Sabet A, Ghamari S, Pieper CC, Mayer K, Biersack HJ, Ezziddin S. Early post-treatment FDG PET predicts survival after 90Y microsphere radioembolization in liver-dominant metastatic colorectal cancer. Eur J Nucl Med Mol Imaging. 2015;42:370–6. https://doi.org/10.1007/s00259-014-2935-z.
100. Tochetto SM, Rezai P, Rezvani M, Nikolaidis P, Berggruen S, Atassi B, Salem R, Yaghmai V. Does multidetector CT attenuation change in colon cancer liver metastases treated with 90Y help predict metabolic activity at FDG PET? Radiology. 2010;255:164–72. https://doi.org/10.1148/radiol.09091028.
101. Zarva A, Mohnike K, Damm R, et al. Safety of repeated radioembolizations in patients with advanced primary and secondary liver tumors and progressive disease after first selective internal radiotherapy. J Nucl Med. 2014;55:360–6. https://doi.org/10.2967/jnumed.113.127662.
102. Lam MG, Louie JD, Iagaru AH, Goris ML, Sze DY. Safety of repeated yttrium-90 radioembolization. Cardiovasc Intervent Radiol. 2013;36:1320–8. https://doi.org/10.1007/s00270-013-0547-9.
103. National Cancer Institute. Common terminology criteria for adverse events (CTCAE) v4.03. NIH Publication No. 09-5410. 2010. Available at: https://evs.nci.nih.gov/ftp1/CTCAE/CTCAE_4.03_2010-06-14_QuickRe ference_5x7.pdf. Accessed 27 October 2016.
104. Hickey R, Lewandowski RJ. Hepatic radioembolization complicated by radiation cholecystitis. Semin Intervent Radiol. 2011;28:230–3. https://doi.org/10.1055/s-0031-1280671.
105. Leong QM, Lai HK, Lo RG, Teo TK, Goh A, Chow PK. Radiation dermatitis following radioembolization for hepatocellular carcinoma: a case for prophylactic embolization of a patent falciform artery. J Vasc Interv Radiol. 2009;20:833–6. https://doi.org/10.1016/j.jvir.2009.03.011.
106. Sangro B, Gil-Alzugaray B, Rodriguez J, et al. Liver disease induced by radioembolization of liver tumors: description and possible risk factors. Cancer. 2008;112:1538–46.
107. Ingold JA, Reed GB, Kaplan HS, et al. Radiation hepatitis. Am J Roentgenol Radium Ther Nucl Med. 1965;93:200–8.
108. Gray BN, Burton MA, Kelleher D, et al. Tolerance of the liver to the effects of yttrium-90 radiation. Int J Radiat Oncol Biol Phys. 1990;18:619–23.
109. Nosher JL, Ohman-Strickland PA, Jabbour S, Narra V, Nosher B. Changes in liver and spleen volumes and liver function after radio- embolization with yttrium-90 resin microspheres. J Vasc Interv Radiol. 2011;22:1706–13. https://doi.org/10.1016/j.jvir.2011.08.017.
110. Atassi B, Bangash AK, Lewandowski RJ, et al. Biliary sequelae following radioembolization with yttrium-90 microspheres. J Vasc Interv Radiol. 2008;19:691–7. https://doi.org/10.1016/j.jvir.2008.01.003.
111. Wiggins E, Ibrahim SM, Lewandowski RJ, Sato KT, Omary RA, Salem R. Effect of chemotherapy on hepatic vasculature in patients undergoing Y-90radioembolization for metastatic disease. J Vasc Interv Radiol. 2008;19:S48–9. https://doi.org/10.1016/j.jvir.2007.12.138.
112. Murthy R, Eng C, Krishnan S, et al. Hepatic yttrium-90 radioembolotherapy in metastatic colorectal cancer treated with cetuximab or bevacizumab. J Vasc Interv Radiol. 2007;18:1588–91. https://doi.org/10.1016/j.jvir.2007.08.015.

16 Guidelines on Radioisotope Treatment of Liver Cancer and Liver Metastases with Intra-arterial Radioactive Compounds

Murat Fani Bozkurt and Laura Evangelista

16.1 Introduction

The present chapter has the aim to provide the current position of radioembolization (RE) for the treatment of primary and secondary liver lesions, in the main national and international clinical guidelines. In Table 16.1, a summary of clinical indications is reported.

16.2 Comments and Suggestions

The first three collected documents provided some procedural information on how to perform a 90Y-RE therapy in the liver (both in primary and metastatic lesions) [1–3]. Moreover, the Consensus Panel [2] dated back to 2007 explains why external radiotherapy (RT) is not sufficiently given to patients with hepatic tumors, due to certain limitations of severe toxicity. The principle of intra-arterial Y90 microsphere therapy is pointed out in order to emphasize its advantage over the other therapeutic approaches. Since at the time this guideline was written, there were only about 3000 patients who were treated with Y90 microspheres, and there were no extensive guidelines to follow; this report was aimed to set a standard approach to Y90 microsphere treatment in order to increase its usage worldwide. Radioembolization Brachytherapy Oncology Consortium (REBOC) which stated this report consisted of an independent group of experts from the fields of interventional radiology, radiation oncology, nuclear oncology, medical oncology, and surgical oncology who were dealing with RE using Y90 microspheres. It was clearly stated that all recommendations in this report are in Category 2A, which implies there is a panel report consensus based on lower-level evidence including clinical experience that therefore the recommendation is appropriate. The report stated that there has been no direct comparison of Y90 resin microspheres with Y90 glass microspheres with regard to efficacy and also stated differences in the approval of these two microspheres. The report explains in detail the procedures before the administration, how Y90 microspheres should be administered as well as after the administration. It gives a sample of "radiation safety discharge instructions" sheet, in order to inform the patient and the families about radiation protection mostly due to bremsstrahlung radiation. A satisfactory dosimetry and how the therapy dose should be calculated were also mentioned. The EANM procedural guidelines [3] cover not only the Y90

M.F. Bozkurt (✉)
Department of Nuclear Medicine, Hacettepe University Faculty of Medicine, Ankara, Turkey
e-mail: fanibozkurt@yahoo.com

L. Evangelista
Veneto Institute of Oncology IOV – IRCCS, Padua, Italy

E. Bombardieri et al. (eds.), *Clinical Applications of Nuclear Medicine Targeted Therapy*,
https://doi.org/10.1007/978-3-319-63067-0_16

Table 16.1 A schematic information about the available guidelines for the treatment of liver cancer and liver metastases with intra-arterial radioactive compounds

	Name of guidelines, Ref.	Year of Pub.	Useful link	Clinical indications	Level/grade of evidence
1.	Technical Methodologic Considerations-Salem, [1]	2006	https://www.ncbi.nlm.nih.gov/pubmed/16923973	TheraSphere: Hepatocellular carcinoma SIR-Spheres: Colorectal metastases	NA
2.	Consensus Panel Report-Kennedy, [2]	2007	https://www.ncbi.nlm.nih.gov/pubmed/17448867	Candidates for RE are patients with unresectable primary or metastatic hepatic disease with liver-dominant tumor burden and a life expectancy >3 months	Category 2A
3.	EANM procedure guidelines for the treatment of liver cancer and liver metastases, [3]	2011	http://eanm.org/publications/guidelines/EANM_liver_treatment_guidelines_2012.pdf	90Y-Microsphere: Unresectable liver cancers, both primary and metastatic 131I-Lipiodol: Palliative treatment of histologically confirmed, inoperable primary HCC	NA
4.	Research Reporting Standards-Radioembolization Salem, [4]	2011	https://www.ncbi.nlm.nih.gov/pubmed/21353979	Patients with unresectable/inoperable liver tumors and liver-dominant disease are candidates for RE. The indications and the absolute/relative contraindications may also be reported	NA
5.	AASLD practice guidelines: management of HCC, [5]	2011	https://www.aasld.org/sites/default/files/guideline_documents/HCCUpdate2010.pdf	Its value in the clinical setting has not been established and cannot be recommended as standard therapy for advanced HCC outside clinical trials	II
6.	EASL-EORTC clinical practice guidelines, management of HCC, [6]	2012	https://www.ncbi.nlm.nih.gov/pubmed/22424438	It cannot be recommended since there is no randomized clinical study testing the efficacy of Y90 microsphere therapy in comparison with TACE or sorafenib in patients with intermediate or advance stages	NA
7.	ESMO-ESDO clinical practice guidelines, [7]	2012	http://www.esmo.org/Guidelines/Gastrointestinal-Cancers/Hepatocellular-Carcinoma	RE may be competitive with sorafenib or TACE in subsets of patients, such as those with prior TACE failure, excellent liver function, macrovascular invasion, and the absence of extrahepatic disease	III/C
8.	BC Cancer Agency		http://www.bccancer.bc.ca/health-professionals/professional-resources/cancer-management-guidelines/gastrointestinal/liver#Liver-Primary-HepatOcellular-carcinoma-HCC	For inoperable HCC An alternative treatment for patients with contraindications to TACE, particularly portal venous thrombosis	NA

9.	CEPO HCC Review and clinical recommendation, [8]	2014	https://www.ncbi.nlm.nih.gov/pmc/articles/PMC4266441/	TARE is still in the investigation phase, and RCTs will be necessary to determine its place in the treatment of HCC. Because of its microembolic effect, TARE could, in theory, be the only local option to treat patients with portal vein thrombosis, especially in the absence of collateral irrigation. TARE could not be considered outside of a clinical trial setting	Grade B
10.	NET Liver Metastases Consensus Kennedy, [9]	2014	https://www.ncbi.nlm.nih.gov/pmc/articles/PMC4266438/	TARE is recommended in case of any liver metastases (singular, multiple, etc.) from NET, when the palliation is needed	Low/C2
11.	NICE advice (SIR-spheres for treating inoperable HCC)	2016	https://www.nice.org.uk/advice/mib63/chapter/technology-overview	SIR-Spheres can be used to treat inoperable HCC. It may be an alternative or adjunct to TACE, drug-eluting bead TACE (DEB-TACE), or systemic drugs to control tumor size, extend life, reduce symptoms, or shrink tumors for resection or transplantation	NA
12.	NCCN clinical practice	2017	https://www.nccn.org/professionals/physician_gls/f_guidelines.asp	Might be an effective treatment option for patients with liver-limited, unresectable disease	NA

NA not available, *RE* radioembolization, *EANM* European Association of Nuclear Medicine, *HCC* hepatocellular carcinoma, *AASLD* American Association for the Study of Liver Diseases, *EASL-EORCT* European Association for the Study of the Liver-European Organisation for Research and Treatment of Cancer, *TACE* trans-arterial chemoembolization, *ESMO-ESDO* European Society of Medical Oncology-European Society of Digestive Oncology, *CEPO* Comitè de l'evolution des pratiques en oncologie, *NET* neuroendocrine tumors, *NICE* National Institute for Health and Care Excellence, *NCCN* National Cancer Comprehensive Network

Level/grade of evidence: Category 2A, there is uniform panel consensus, based on lower-level evidence including clinical experience, that the recommendation is appropriate; Grade B, moderate (further research is likely to have an important impact on our confidence in the estimate of effect and may change the estimate. Disposable: one high-quality study and several studies with some limitations); C2, low or scarce evidence grade microsphere treatment but also how to perform I-131 lipiodol treatment to liver tumors. Although it is mostly written on a purpose of procedure guideline, some informative explanations on the different features of the Y90 microspheres and how they may affect the microsphere selection on patient basis were also included. The strong aspects of this guideline are that it presents from an objective point of view all advantages and disadvantages of each microsphere type (resin and glass) and that this comparison is based on literature evidences. This guideline also has a special part which includes "issues to be further clarified" as listed at the end of the manuscript which mentioned some important points not assessed or studied at the time that it was written. The weak aspect of this guideline is that it is mostly a procedural guideline, without any extensive information with regard to clinical studies which show the impact of this therapeutic approach. The place of Y90 microsphere treatment in multidisciplinary therapy algorithm is also not very much mentioned.

The research reporting standards of RE of hepatic malignancies [4] are designed for reporting research and are not intended for clinical procedural notes for individual patients. It is written by a large group of authors who are dealing with research on RE for hepatic tumors. In this paper, it is advised to use the word "RE" for the procedure instead of "trans-arterial radionuclide therapy" or "selective internal radiation therapy" which may imply substantial technical jargon and marketing terminology. It is preferred to use the term "procedure" instead of "operation," and a procedure refers one treatment session. According to this report, it is impossible to strictly predefine a patient population to be offered RE due to intra- and interinstitutional variability. However, the reason why this therapy is chosen over alternative therapies and the intent of therapy should be stated in the research articles. In this guideline it is suggested to describe all therapies that were given to patients before RE, but the panel recognizes the controversy over the definition of a line of systemic therapy. The paper encourages to give in detail the dosimetric approach to create reproducibility between researchers in articles given the ongoing controversy over dosimetry. This guideline also mentions about some technical parameters to be provided for publication such as the median dose to treatment site and lungs along with the number of sessions required to achieve technical success. The guideline focuses on the difference of "technical success" from "technique effectiveness." It is clearly explained that technical success implies the dose delivery to all targeted area, while technique effectiveness is the clinical success for which follow-up data is needed. The guideline suggests the use of World Health Organization (WHO), Response Evaluation Criteria in Solid Tumors (RECIST) or European Association for the Study of Liver (EASL) criteria for response evaluation. Analyses of the results and how to design a RE research study are also among the topics that are mentioned in this guideline.

The guidelines from AASLD and EASL-EORCT cannot give final clinical indications for the employment of RE in patients with HCC [5, 6]. They suggest to use RE only in clinical trials, particularly in patients with advanced HCC.

Conversely, the guidelines from ESMO-ESDO [7], BC Cancer Agency, NICE, and NCCN recommend the use of RE in the following category of patients:

1. Those with prior TACE failure, excellent liver function, macrovascular invasion, and the absence of extra-liver disease (ESMO, NICE, NCCN)
2. With portal venous thrombosis (BC Cancer Agency), although it is relatively contraindicated in the NCCN guidelines

The current scenario is inhomogeneous across the different guidelines. According to the NICE recommendation, 11 studies are now available about the employment of selective internal radiation therapy for primary liver cancer. The majority of the studies are prospective ($n = 5$), nonrandomized ($n = 8$), and single center ($n = 6$). On the other hand, two multicenter randomized controlled trials are now available, but their final results are not conclusive (i.e., underpowered study or weak

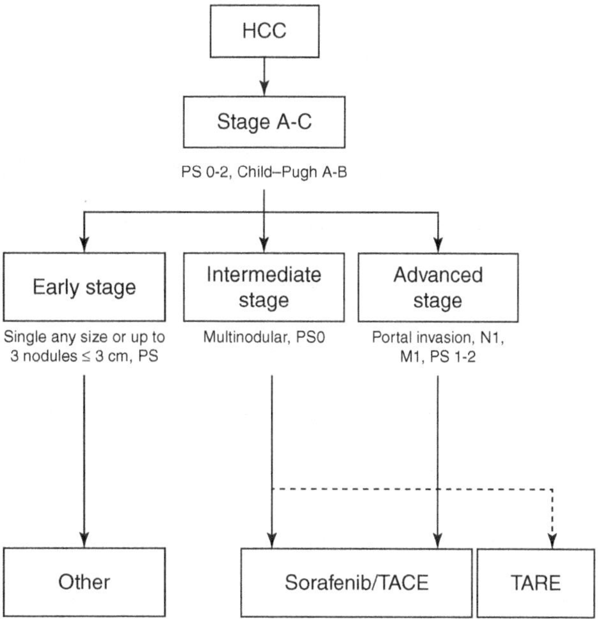

Fig. 16.1 A possible flowchart for the employment of RE in HCC

evidence). Therefore, considering the content of the abovementioned trials and the low level of evidence, the guidelines are not definitive for the employment of RE in patients with HCC. To date, on the basis of the available data, we can image a possible role of RE in HCC, in accordance with the below flowchart (Fig. 16.1).

References

1. Salem R, Thurston KG. Radioembolization with 90Yttrium microspheres: a state-of-the-art brachytherapy treatment for primary and secondary liver malignancies. Part 1: Technical and methodologic considerations. J Vasc Interv Radiol. 2006;17:1251–78.
2. Kennedy A, Nag S, Salem R, Murthy R, McEwan AJ, Nutting C, et al. Recommendations for radioembolization of hepatic malignancies using yttrium-90 microsphere brachytherapy: a consensus panel report from the radioembolization brachytherapy oncology consortium. Int J Radiat Oncol Biol Phys. 2007;68:13–23.
3. Giammarile F, Bodei L, Chiesa C, Flux G, Forrer F, Kraeber-Bodere F, et al. EANM procedure guideline for the treatment of liver cancer and liver metastases with intra-arterial radioactive compounds. Eur J Nucl Med Mol Imaging. 2011;38(7):1393–406. https://doi.org/10.1007/s00259-011-1812-2.
4. Salem R, Lewandowski RJ, Gates VL, Nutting CW, Murthy R, Rose SC, et al. Research reporting standards for radioembolization of hepatic malignancies. J Vasc Interv Radiol. 2011;22:265–78.
5. Bruix J, Sherman M. Management of hepatocellular carcinoma: an update. Hepatology. 2011;53:1020–2.
6. European Association For The Study Of The Liver; European Organisation For Research And Treatment Of Cancer. EASL-EORTC clinical practice guidelines: management of hepatocellular carcinoma. J Hepatol. 2012;56:908–43.
7. Verslype C, Rosmorduc O, Rougier P. Hepatocellular carcinoma: ESMO-ESDO clinical practice guidelines. Ann Oncol. 2012;23:vii41–8.
8. Boily G, Villeneuve J-P, Lacoursière L, Chaudhury P, Couture F, Ouellet J-F, et al. Transarterial embolization therapies for the treatment of hepatocellular carcinoma: CEPO review and clinical recommendations. HPB (Oxford). 2015;17:52–65.
9. Kennedy A, Bester L, Salem R, Sharma RA, Parks RW, Ruszniewski F. Role of hepatic intra-arterial therapies in metastatic neuroendocrine tumours (NET): guidelines from the NET-Liver-Metastases Consensus Conference. HPB (Oxford). 2015;17:29–37.

Part III

Neuroendocrine Tumors

17 Radiopharmaceuticals for Treatment of NETs

Mattia Asti, Michele Iori, Pier Cesare Capponi, and Sara Rubagotti

Abstract

Neuroendocrine tumours (NETs) are a group of unusual cancers which develop from cells of the diffuse endocrine system. They are found most commonly in lungs or gastrointestinal system, but they can also originate in other tissues such as pancreas, ovary and testes. A common feature of NETs is that they almost all overexpress somatostatin receptors. For this reason somatostatin receptors have been considered as a target for radiolabelled radiopharmaceuticals. These molecules are constituted by a peptide chain (i.e. a somatostatin-like structure), a partially or totally electron emitter radionuclide and a suitable bifunctional chelator able both to firmly complex the radionuclide as well as to be connected to the peptide chain by means of proper molecular spacers. Nowadays, the most used radiopharmaceuticals for treatments of NETs are [DOTA]^0-Tyr^3-octreotide (DOTATOC) and [DOTA^0]-Tyr^3-octreotate (DOTATATE) labelled with yttrium-90 and lutetium-177.

17.1 Introduction

Recently, a great interest in the therapeutic applications of radiolabelled analogues of biomolecules targeting specific tumours has been shown both in nuclear medicine research and in clinical practice [1]. Thanks to their smaller dimensions compared to other biological molecules, short-chain peptides have been extensively studied as they exhibit favourable pharmacological properties over antibodies or other bio-conjugates such as fast tissue penetration, rapid clearance, high target accessibility and low antigenicity [2]. Thanks to these facts, the feasibility of the imaging process and of the therapy of a large variety of tumours showing receptors specific for the peptide structures has been attested [3]. Nowadays, the most interesting results have been obtained with tumours overexpressing somatostatin receptors by *i.v.* injection of somatostatin derivatives labelled with positron or electron emitter radionuclide.

These radiopharmaceuticals rapidly accumulate in neoplastic tissues allowing the delivery of a high dose of radiation in the target and mainly sparing the surrounding healthy tissues. By this

M. Asti (✉) • M. Iori • P.C. Capponi • S. Rubagotti
Nuclear Medicine Unit, Oncology and Advanced Technologies Department, Azienda Unità Sanitaria Locale-IRCCS, Reggio Emilia, Italy
e-mail: mattia.asti@ausl.re.it

E. Bombardieri et al. (eds.), *Clinical Applications of Nuclear Medicine Targeted Therapy*,
https://doi.org/10.1007/978-3-319-63067-0_17

approach it is possible to combine both the diagnosis and the therapeutic process in the same molecule simply by exchanging the radionuclide employed for the labelling [4–6].

A peptide-based radiopharmaceutical for therapy is usually formed by a bio-conjugated molecules (i.e. a peptide chain), a suitable bifunctional chelator able both to firmly complex the radionuclide as well as to be connected to the peptide chain by means of proper molecular spacers and a partially or totally electron emitter radionuclide. The bio-conjugated molecules acts like a vector carrying the radioactive emission to a specific target. The targets are usually moieties overexpressed in tumour cells such as cell receptors.

In this chapter the theoretical aspects concerning the building of a radiopharmaceutical for peptide receptor radionuclide therapy (PRRT) as well as the practical aspects upon the preparation and the quality controls of these probes will be discussed.

17.2 The Vector and the Targets

17.2.1 Somatostatin and Its Analogues

Somatostatin (SST) or somatotropin release-inhibiting hormone (SRIH) is a cyclic neuropeptide whose biosynthesis mainly takes place at the hypothalamic level but also in the peripheral nervous system and in many other organs. SST is a molecule composed by 14 amino acids (SST-14) with a molecular weight of 1068 g/mol and can also be produced by the cleavage of its precursor the pro-somatostatin (SST-28) in which the 14 units are linked through the C-terminal to other 14 amino acids (Fig. 17.1). The two forms are synthesized in different amounts by different tissues: SST-14 producing cells are predominant in the pancreas, stomach, neuronal tissues as well as in the retina, peripheral nerves and enteric neurons; SST-28 producing cells are predominant in the intestinal mucosa and in the brain [7].

17.2.2 Physiological Activity

In addition to inhibiting the release of somatotropin, somatostatin exerts a large number of other inhibitory functions aimed to control the neuroendocrine system such as:

- Inhibition of dopamine, norepinephrine, thyroid-releasing hormone (TRH) and thyroid-stimulating hormone (TSH) excretion.
- Inhibition of somatotropin or growth hormone (GH) excretion. GH is responsible for body growth and cell metabolism regulation.
- Inhibition of prolactin release.
- Inhibition of gastrointestinal motility and secretions
- Inhibition of triiodothyronine (T3), thyroxine (T4) and calcitonin release
- Inhibition of insulin and glucagon secretion.

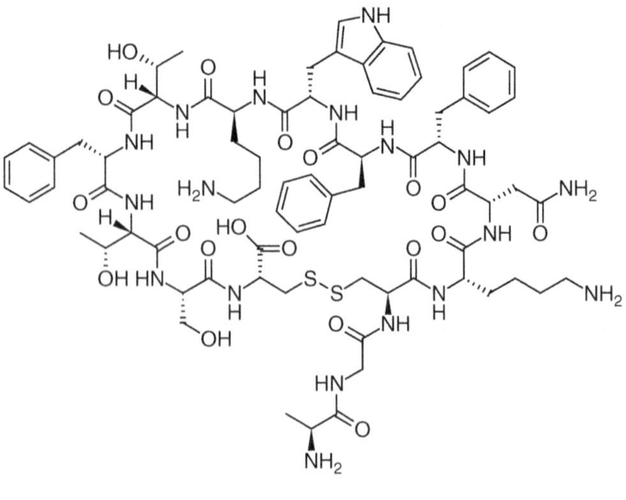

Fig. 17.1 Amino acid sequence of somatostatin-14 (source: Wikipedia)

- Inhibition of renin release (and consequently of angiotensin II and aldosterone, responsible for controlling the absorption of salts in the kidneys) and inhibition of antidiuretic hormone (ADH) that control the water reabsorption.
- Block of the release of growth factor IGF-1 (somatomedin) in the liver and of the epidermal growth (EGF) and the platelet-derived growth factor (PDGF)
- Vasoconstriction.
- Stimulation of phosphor-tyrosine-phosphatase or MAP kinase responsible for the regulation of cell proliferation.

17.2.3 Somatostatin Receptors

Somatostatin's multiple biological actions are mediated by the binding of the molecule to specific membrane receptors (SSTRs). Five somatostatin receptors subtypes have been identified and characterized (SSTR1-5). SSTRs are physiologically present in many tissues such as the intestine, brain, pituitary gland, endocrine and exocrine pancreas, thyroid, kidney and immune system cells, and both SST-14 and SST-28 exhibit great affinity for all five receptors subtypes [8]. SSTRs have been localized in a large variety of human tumours that originate from cells of the neuroendocrine system as well. This overexpression suggests that the receptor can exert a direct effect on the regulation of the tumour growth. However, the relative expression of the five receptor subtypes can sensibly vary among the different types of tumours, and, on the other hand, the same kind of tumour may express several different receptor subtypes. The most expressed receptor is definitely the SST2 subtype that proved to be predominant in the majority of neuroendocrine tumours such as pituitary adenomas (GH and TSH secreting), gastroenteropancreatic tumours (GEP), neuroendocrine lung tumours, pheochromocytomas and paragangliomas. Moreover, SSTR2 subtype is also expressed in the nervous system cancers such as blastomas of the bone marrow, meningiomas and neuroblastomas or even in non-neuroendocrine and non-neuronal tumours like breast cancers, small cell lung cancer, lymphomas, hepatocellular carcinomas and renal and gastric carcinomas although, in the latter, with a lower incidence and density. As already reported, there are a number of tumours that express other SSTR subtypes in addition or alternatively to SST2 receptors such as the subtypes SSTR1, SSTR3 and SSTR5. For instance, some pituitary adenomas and particularly GH-secreting adenomas express preferentially SST5 receptors, while many inactive adenomas express SST3 subtype. Prostatic tumours, instead, can express preferentially SST1 receptors. The same GEP, neuroendocrine lung and medullary thyroid tumours can frequently express different receptor subtypes as well [9]. In Fig. 17.2 a graphical representation of the five SST receptor subtypes is depicted.

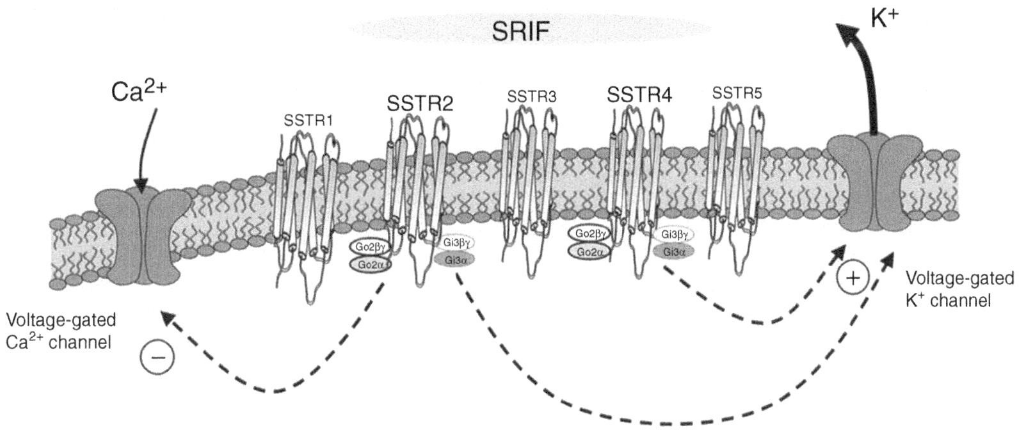

Fig. 17.2 Graphical representation of the five somatostatin receptor subtypes

17.2.4 Somatostatin Analogues

For the reasons expressed so far, somatostatin receptors appear to be a perfect target for selective deliver a radioactive dose to tumour tissues overexpressing this functionality.

Unfortunately somatostatin administered exogenously disappears quickly from the bloodstream (biological half-life 1–3 min) due to the action of peptidase enzymes present in many tissues and in the blood itself. In particular, the kidney seems to play a key role in SST metabolism and secretion. For this reason and for the fact that it has multiple effects on secretory systems as well, SST itself is not a suitable carrier to bring radioactivity to the cancer tissues [10].

Therefore, research turned to the study and synthesis of analogous peptides, with similar receptor affinities but with greater biological stability and consequently higher plasma half-life. Numerous synthetic peptides with high metabolic stability and receptor selectivity were realized starting from the amino acid chain of SST-14. The end result led to the recognition of the central segment Phe^{7}-Trp^{8}-Lys^{9}-Thr^{10} as responsible of the affinity to the receptors and thus of the biological activity.

Moreover, the use of particular expedients in the molecule design has allowed to obtain derivatives with an in vivo biological half-life of about 80 min, that is about 30-fold greater than the original somatostatin. In particular the synthesis strategy includes:

- The use of D-amino acids (D-phenylalanine and D-tryptophan) that are not recognized by the physiological peptidases.
- The prevailing use of lipophilic amino acids as the lipophilic peptides are seized by the liver and eliminated by biliary secretion, while the hydrophilic peptides are rapidly removed by renal excretion.
- The cyclization of the peptide using disulphide bridges, useful to limit his mobility and increase its biological activity.

Among the numerous analogues, a structure containing eight amino acids (named octreotide or Sandostatin) has proved to be the most effective for therapeutic purposes, and it was the first

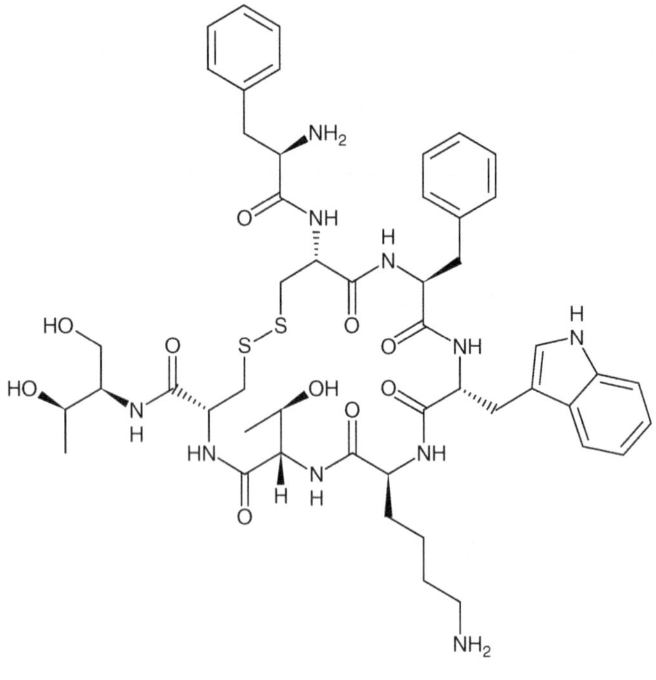

Fig. 17.3 Amino acid sequence of octreotide (source: Wikipedia)

peptide introduced in therapy [11]. In Fig. 17.3 the amino acid sequence of octreotide is shown.

Obviously, the differences on the structure with respect to the original sequence of the SST-14 lead to changes in the biological activity. In fact, by means of binding studies in cell lines infected with segments of DNA coding for the genes of the five somatostatin receptor subtypes turned out that octreotide maintains a high affinity for SSTR2 receptors and has an intermediate and moderate affinity, respectively, for SSTR3 and SSTR5 receptors, but it totally lost the affinity for the receptors SSTR1 and SSRT4. The structure was furtherly perfected by replacing some natural amino acids with peptide mimetic groups (e.g. 3(beta-naphtyl)alanine) and by replacing some chemical groups by others (i.e. –OH moiety with –COOH moiety). In any case, the predominant expression of the receptor subtype SST2 in human tumours of neuroendocrine origin lays the foundations for the clinical use of this peptide as a base vector for PRRT.

17.2.5 The Radionuclides

The great availability and variety of radionuclides have permitted to identify the better candidates to such kind of theranostic application, and, in the case of the labelling of peptide-based radiopharmaceuticals and in particular of somatostatin derivatives, it has reached the current peak using metal radioisotopes such as gallium-68, indium-111, yttrium-90 and lately lutetium-177.

Focusing on therapeutic applications, the latter two are the radionuclide of main choice.

Yttrium-90 is a pure β-emitter with a physical half-life of 64.1 h. The emitted electrons show an average energy of 935 keV, a maximum energy of 2284 keV and are able to penetrate surrounding tissue to up to 12 mm.

Lutetium-177 is a medium-energy β-emitter, with 6.73 days of physical half-time. The emitted electrons (78.6%) show a maximum β-energy of 498 keV and penetrate surrounding tissue up to 2 mm. Lutetium-177 also shows two additional γ-emissions (11% and 6.4%) of 210 and 113 keV, respectively [12]. Coupled to the proper carrier, it has been shown that both yttrium-90 and lutetium-177 are able to deliver the required dose for the treatment of extended tumour lesions or micrometastases, respectively [13, 14].

Unfortunately, it is chemically not possible to connect a metal radionuclide to a peptide structure without using a so-called bifunctional chelating group (BFC) intended as a chemical structure able both to firmly complex the metal core and also to be linked to the peptide chain through a stable covalent bond. The BFC have an influence on the SSTR affinity profile of the derivative and actually influences the biodistribution and pharmacokinetics of the future radiopharmaceutical.

17.2.6 The Bifunctional Chelators

Usually, BFC are molecules with an elevated number of coordinating group containing hard donor nitrogen or oxygen atoms (such as primary or secondary amines or carboxylates groups). Trivalent metal such as yttrium or lutetium require high coordinated scaffolds (usually eightfold or greater coordination) with preferred square-based antiprismatic geometries. An ancillary carboxylate group of the chelator is usually employed to form a covalent bond with the terminal amino group of the peptide sequence. Molecules of wide use are the open-chain chelators diethylenetriaminepentaacetic acid (DTPA), ethylenediaminetetraacetic acid (EDTA) and their derivatives, but numerous other aminopolycarboxylic chelators are used to label peptide-based molecules with the cited metallic radionuclides. In particular, DTPA and its derivatives show excellent in vivo stability and can be linked to the octreotide N-terminal portion through an amide bond with one carboxyl group. The compound [DTPA-D-Phe^1]-octreotide was actually the first peptide-based radiopharmaceutical approved by FDA, and it is widely used as SPECT radiotracer when labelled with indium-111 (Octreoscan). In Fig. 17.4 the chemical structure of DTPA and some examples of DTPA derivatives are shown, and in Fig. 17.5 the chemical structure of ^{111}In-[DTPA-D-Phe^1]-octreotide is depicted.

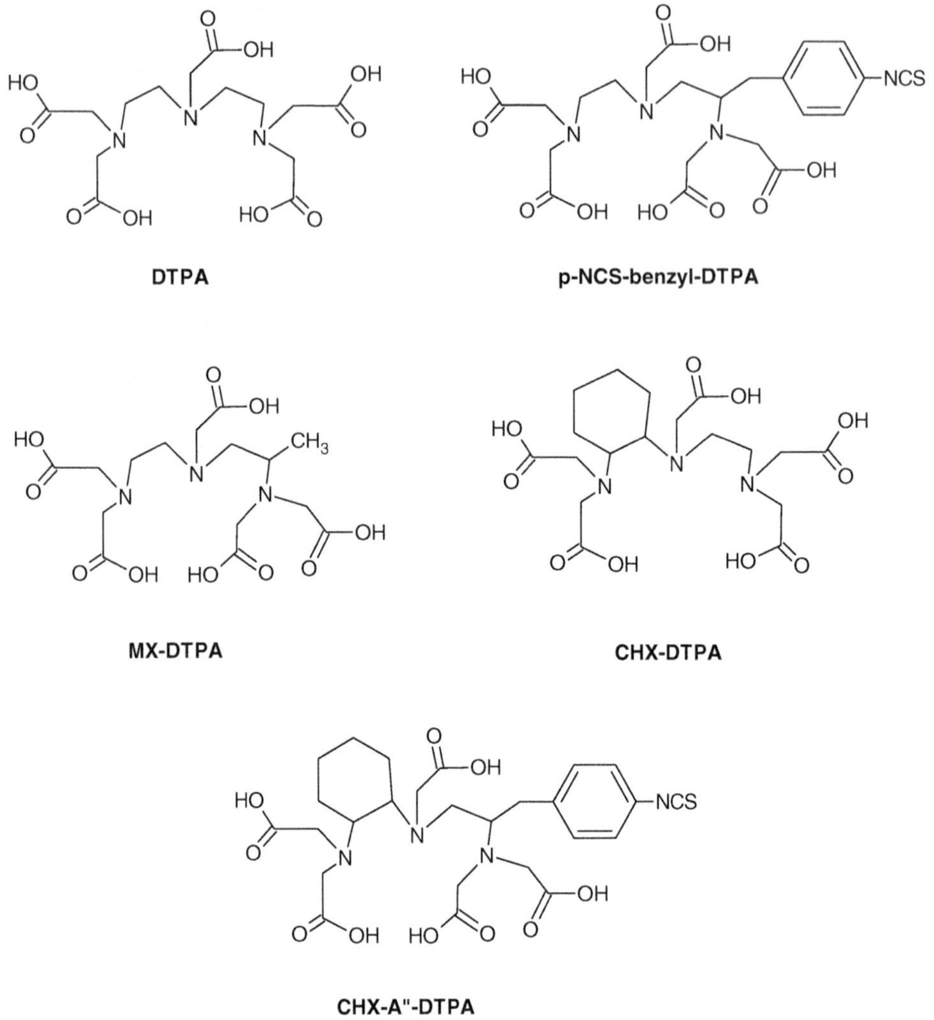

Fig. 17.4 Structures of DTPA and some derivatives

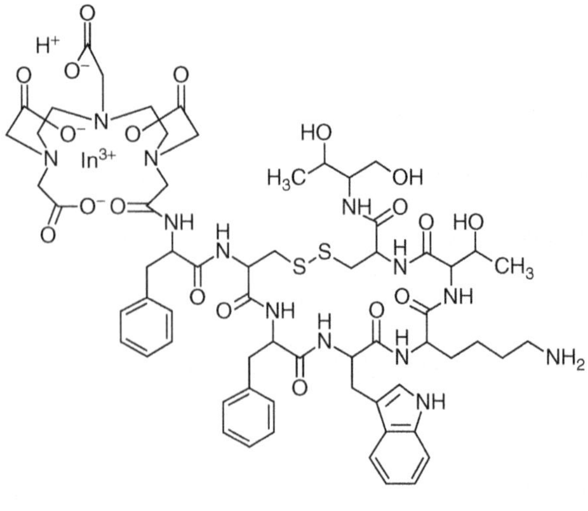

Fig. 17.5 Chemical structure of ^{111}In-[DTPA-D-Phe[1]]-octreotide (named Octreoscan)

Unfortunately, if DTPA derivatives have proved to be suitable for the coordination of metal radionuclides such as indium-111, the same assumption is not worth for radionuclides such as yttrium-90 or lutetium-177. In fact, the ^{90}Y-labelled DTPA-octreotide has been tried in preclinical trials with poor results because of the low in vivo stability. Actually, part of yttrium-90 was released from the chelator and was uptaken by bones causing excessive toxicity in the marrow [15].

Therefore, the introduction of new bifunctional chelators has been mandatory in order to use the metal radionuclides for therapeutic purpose. DTPA was mainly replaced with the cyclic 1,4,7,10-tetraazacyclododecane-1,4,7,10-tetraacetic acid (DOTA) and its derivatives. Nowadays, the structure of the theranostic vectors mainly implements the DOTA chelator connected to the receptor-binding motif (i.e. the Phe-D-Trp-Lys-Thr sequence in the case of somatostatin receptors) through a proper linker or through the amino-acidic chain of the original biological molecule properly modified for enhancing its stability to the proteases. DOTA is a very efficient bifunctional chelator able to form stable complexes with trivalent metal cations such as yttrium-90 and lutetium-177, the most used radionuclides for PRRT, as well as gallium-68, the most common radiometal used for positron emission tomography (PET) imaging. Further development on this field is based on the principle to create new connective moiety between the DOTA chelator and the peptide chain. For this reason a further carboxylate group has been added to the structure for obtaining DOTA derivatives such as DOTAGA or DOTASA, or a benzyl-NCS group was bond directly on one carbon atom of the chelator ring in order to obtain a derivative named p-NCS-Bz-DOTA. Both of these strategies achieve the purpose to maintain the eight coordinating sites of the chelator available for interacting with the metal core and hence guaranteeing a completion of the coordination geometry of yttrium and lutetium. In Fig. 17.6 the chemical structure of DOTA and some examples of DOTA derivatives are shown.

17.2.7 Final Structures

The first derivative, and probably still the most used in the clinical practice, is [DOTA]^0-Tyr^3-octreotide (DOTATOC) mainly labelled with gallium-68 and yttrium-90, but, more recently, many new somatostatin analogues have been developed [16]. These derivatives have an even

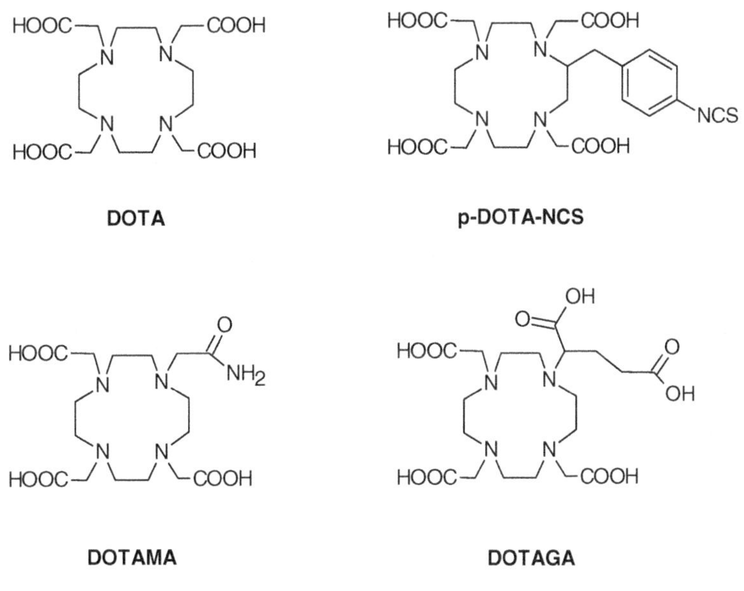

Fig. 17.6 Structures of DOTA chelator and some derivatives

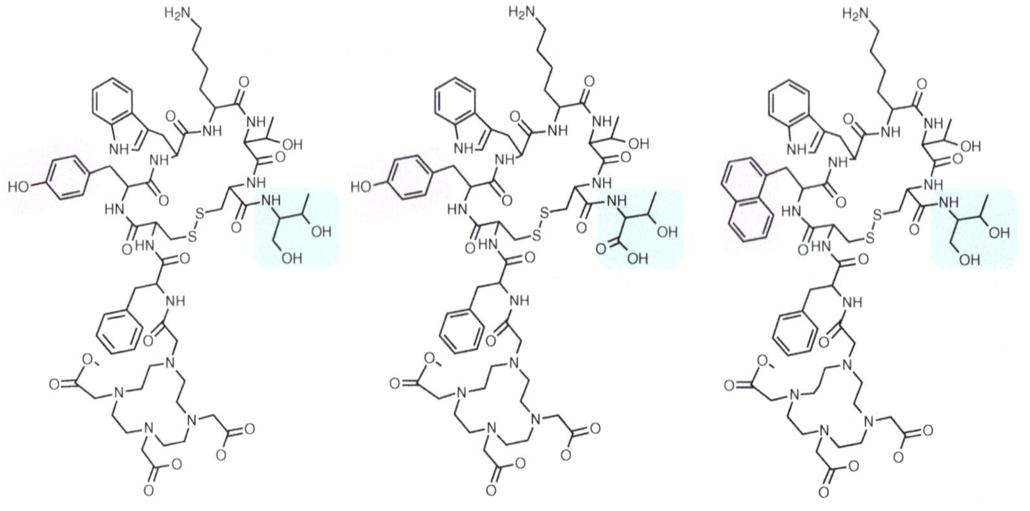

Fig. 17.7 Structures of DOTATOC, DOTATATE and DOTANOC somatostatin analogues

greater affinity for certain receptor subtypes compared to DOTATOC or have an affinity distribution more various between the different subtypes than DOTATOC itself. For instance, the [DOTA^0]-Tyr^3-octreotate (DOTATATE), a derivative where the threoninol residue at the C-terminal portion of the Tyr^3-octreotide was replaced by a threonine residue, showed even greater affinity for SSTR2 than DOTATOC but lower affinity for SSTR5. DOTATATE was mainly used labelled with the lutetium-177 and, as of recently, a multicentric, phase III, clinical study is leading towards marketing authorization of ^{177}Lu-DOTATATE as the first somatostatin analogue-based radiopharmaceutical (called LUTATHERA™) for the treatment of gastroenteropancreatic neuroendocrine tumours [17].

The derivatives [DOTA^0]-NaI^3-octreotide (DOTANOC), a molecule where the tyrosine residue of the original octreotide chain has been replaced with the peptide mimetic group 3(beta-naphtyl)alanine, is largely used in diagnostic PET labelled with gallium-68. DOTANOC has an affinity higher than DOTATOC for receptor subtypes SSTR3, SSTR4 and SSTR5. However, it has been shown that the therapeutic performances of DOTANOC when labelled with lutetium-177 are inferior to those with DOTATOC and DOTATATE due to the higher dose delivered to the healthy tissue in particular to the whole body, kidney and spleen [18, 19]. In Fig. 17.7 the structures of DOTATOC, DOTATATE and DOTANOC are represented.

As a matter of a fact, it has been shown the affinity profile to SST receptors in vitro cannot certainly predict by itself the effective behaviour of the radiopharmaceutical in vivo. For example, the derivatives [DOTA^0]-lanreotide although presenting a higher affinity for SSTR5 subtypes than DOTATOC showed a lower tumour uptake of about 10%. Moreover, it must be considered that also the different radionuclides influence the affinity of these compounds to the SST receptor; therefore the final considerations on the functionality of a molecule must always be carried out on the final drug in vivo [20].

17.3 Biodistribution and Pharmacokinetics

Biodistribution and pharmacokinetics of the DOTATOC derivative labelled with yttrium have been reported in an interesting preliminary study [21] In this study, as the pure β^- emitter yttrium-90 is not suitable for quantitative imaging, DOTATOC was labelled with the positron-emitting isotope yttrium-86 ($T_{1/2}$ = 14.74 h, 33% β+). ^{86}Y-DOTATOC is chemically identical to ^{90}Y-DOTATOC and can be considered the most appropriate agent to predict the pharmacokinetics and biodistribution of the therapeutic radiopharmaceutical.

The activity in blood was found to decrease to less than 10% within the first 3 h and to less than 1% within 13–15 h. The mean (range) cumulative activity excreted in the urine and expressed as % injected dose was 47.6% ID (40.3–54.8) 5 h post injection and 60.1% ID (53.2–67.0) 24 h post injection.

The distribution patterns of ^{86}Y-DOTATOC show rapid visualization of the kidneys. 4 h after injection, tracer accumulation in the liver, spleen, kidneys and tumour lesions exceeds background radioactivity. When ^{86}Y-DOTATOC biodistribution is compared to ^{111}In-DTPA-octreotide (Octreoscan), it is apparent that the kinetics in the organs are relatively similar, the similarity being most pronounced for the liver and least pronounced for the spleen. By contrast, the uptake kinetics of the metastases show marked differences, with much higher uptake and slower washout for ^{86}Y-DOTATOC. The effective dose estimated for ^{86}Y-DOTATOC was in the same order of magnitude of ^{111}In-Octreoscan, so that this tracer has no relevant disadvantage as far as the radiation burden for the patient is concerned. The highest tracer uptake in the kidneys, followed by the spleen, urinary bladder and liver, identifies these organs as critical during therapy with ^{90}Y-DOTATOC.

In contrast to yttrium-90, which is a pure β^--emitter, lutetium-177 is also a γ-emitter of low emission abundance. This characteristic enables both the imaging and therapy with the same compound labelled with this radionuclide and allows dosimetry during treatment as well. Schuchardt and co-workers [18] conducted a study with the aim to compare the pharmacokinetics and dosimetry of ^{177}Lu-DOTATATE, ^{177}Lu-DOTATOC and ^{177}Lu-DOTANOC.

Significant differences were found for the pharmacokinetics of the three compounds concerning the whole body, normal tissue, kidneys, and spleen. ^{177}Lu-DOTANOC performed in the worst way with a general slow washout in normal tissue, a higher persistence in the whole body (ca. 40% ID 20 h p.i. and 20% ID 70 h p.i.) and a higher uptake in the kidneys and spleen (ca. 3.2% ID 20 h p.i. and 1.7% ID 70 h p.i. for the kidneys and ca. 1.7% ID 20 h p.i. and 1.0% ID 70 h p.i. for the spleen, respectively) with respect to both DOTATOC and DOTATATE. DOTATOC was the compound that exhibited the best pharmacokinetics with a whole body persistence of ca. 20% ID 20 hours p.i. and 10% ID 70 h p.i., an uptake in the kidneys of ca. 1.7% ID 20 h p.i. and 1% ID 70 h p.i. and an uptake in the spleen of ca. 1% ID 20 h p.i. and 0.5% ID 70 h p.i.

All three peptides showed high specific uptake in somatostatin receptor-positive tumours, but, in contrast to the kinetics in normal organs, ^{177}Lu-DOTATATE revealed the highest uptake at 20 h p.i. (ca. 0.05 ID/ml) and at 70 h (ca. 0.03 ID/ml). DOTATOC exhibited the highest initial uptake followed by a faster decline than DOTATATE in the first 20 h (ca. 0.04 ID/ml 20 h p.i.) and then a comparable behaviour (0.03 ID/ml 70 h p.i.). Initial uptake of DOTATATE and DOTANOC were almost similar, but while the uptake of DOTATATE in the first 20 h, a fast and persistent decline was found for DOTANOC (ca. 0.02 ID/ml 20 h p.i. and 0.01 ID/ml 70 h p.i.).

However, all the difference in uptake and mean absorbed dose were not statistically significant.

17.4 Preparation of ^{90}Y- and ^{177}Lu-labelled Somatostatin Derivatives

The preparation of ^{90}Y- and ^{177}Lu-labelled somatostatin derivatives (namely, DOTATOC as a paradigmatic example of all the class of compounds) is still mainly performed using manual procedures although the radioactivity handled during the synthesis and fractioning of these radiopharmaceuticals can be up to 20 GBq for yttrium-90 and 40 GBq for lutetium-177, respectively. Radiation protection requirements related to manipulations of a

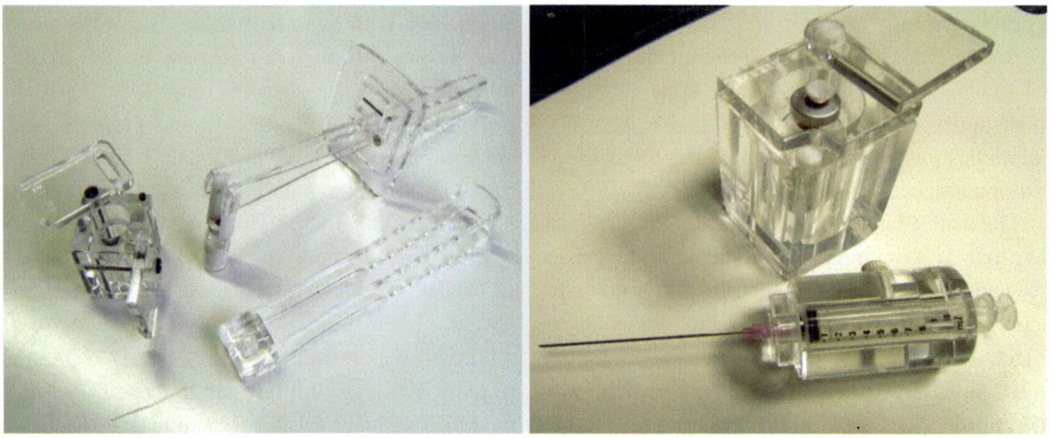

Fig. 17.8 PMMA shielding and tongues for the manual labelling of ^{90}Y- and ^{177}Lu-labelled somatostatin derivatives

large amount of electron emitter radionuclides have always been considered one of the main limitations of this practice. For this reason the use of dedicated poly(methyl methacrylate) (PMMA) tongues and shielding for syringes and vial during the manipulation has to be considered mandatory. In Fig. 17.8 an example of this protective device is shown. Moreover, any operations concerning the preparation should be carefully evaluated a priori and in the absence of radioactivity in order to exert the most advantageous movements to spare the dose exposure to the operator hands. In spite of these considerations, the hazard due to radiation exposure demands a strict rotation of operators involved in the process and limits the quantity of radioactivity that can be manipulated in a single therapeutic session.

In this section the practical operations needed to manually prepare ^{90}Y- and ^{177}Lu-labelled somatostatin analogues as well as the reagents and excipients necessary for a successful preparation will be deeply described. Moreover, alternative preparation methods by using a semiautomated synthesizer and a commercial automated synthesizer will be described and evaluated.

It is worth to highlight that as these kinds of preparations are not fully standardized, the method and substances described in the following paragraphs have to be considered as a general example.

17.4.1 Manual Preparation

Syntheses and fractionating are normally performed by carrying out the following procedure [22, 23]:

1. The delivery vial, containing the commercial $^{90}YCl_3$ or $^{177}LuCl_3$ solutions, is transferred to the proper reaction shielding. $^{90}YCl_3$ or $^{177}LuCl_3$ are usually dissolved in small volume (50–700 μL) of 0.04–0.05 M hydrochloric acid.
2. A syringe filled with the proper amount of a solution able to buffer the reaction to a pH ranging from 4.6 to 4.9 and with a volume of DOTA-peptide solution proportional to the delivered radioactivity was added to the radionuclide solution. Most utilized buffers are, for instance, 0.15 M sodium ascorbate or 2,5-dihydroxybenzoic acid solutions in a volume ranging between 1 and 2 mL. The amount of DOTA peptide depends on the specific activity of the radionuclide to be labelled as well as on the amount of metal contaminants in the original product and in the reagents used for the preparation. For this reason, it is difficult to give a general proportion, but in the right conditions a ratio of 13 ng peptide per MBq of yttrium-90 and 11 ng peptide per MBq of lutetium-177, respectively, can be achieved keeping the radiochemical purity (RCP) of the final product >97%.

3. The vial is then transferred to a heating block and heated for 20–30 min at 90 °C. At the end of the reaction, a small aliquot of activity (15–60 MBq) is withdrawn and usually diluted with 0.3 ml of 0.1 M HCl for assessing RCP.
4. The solution is transferred through a sterilizing filter to a final vial and diluted with the chosen amount of physiological solution by means of a manually assembled system consisting of tubes, valves and syringes. The final vial usually already contained a volume 1 mM DTPA solution proportional to the initial activity in order to complex any potentially unlabelled radionuclide [24, 25] as well as other stabilizers like as ascorbic/ascorbate solutions. These solutions decrease radiolysis phenomena enhancing stability of the products [26]. A representation of the manual dilution is depicted in Fig. 17.9.

When the manual approach is used, an average radiochemical yields (intended as the ratio between the starting radionuclide radioactivity and the radioactivity of the labelled product in the final vial) > 95% for both ^{90}Y- and ^{177}Lu-DOTA-peptide is normally obtained. This result is due to the fact that the reaction occurs directly inside the radioactivity delivery vial. This means that the radionuclide radioactivity is all employed in the labelling, and the only source of leakage may happen during transfer and dilution of the labelled precursor to the final vial through a sterile filter. The rare case where the RCY is below 95% is due to a defective transfer of the product caused by a leak in the manually assembled tubing system. The whole procedure takes normally about 120 min including preparation of tubing, labelling and quality controls of the final product. The manual method offers the chance to actively manage the labelling process, stopping or modifying the procedure if something goes in a wrong direction. This opportunity is limited by the main drawback of the method, namely, the high exposure of the operator's hands to radiations. The following handling steps have been identified as critical in terms of radiation exposure: (1) manual injection of buffer/ligand solution, (2) transfer of the original vial from the

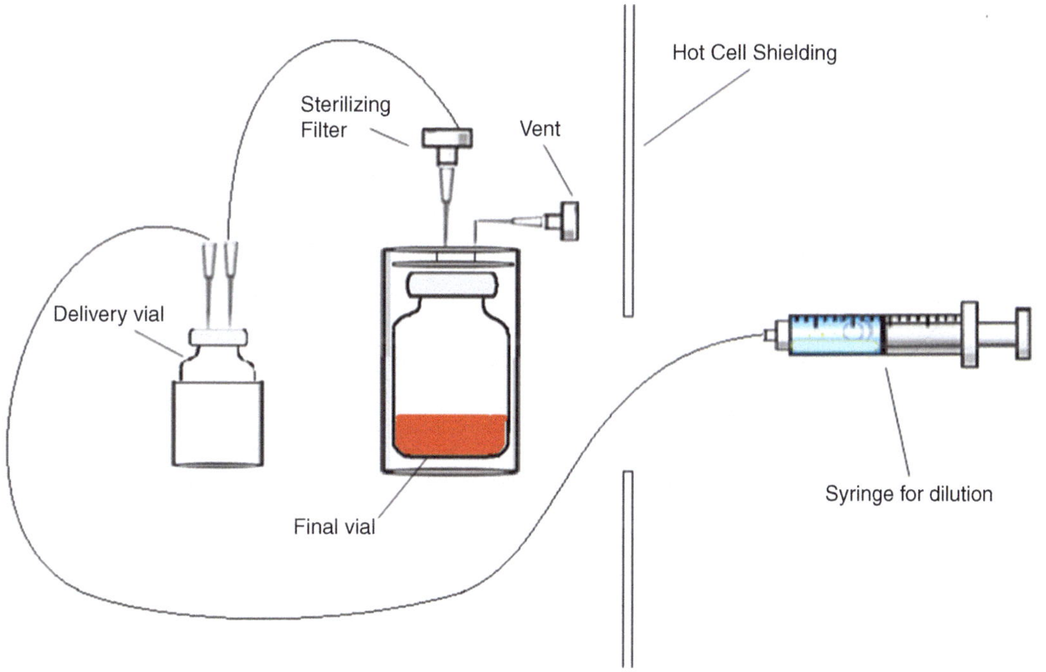

Fig. 17.9 Scheme of the manual assembled system for the filtration and dilution of ^{90}Y- and ^{177}Lu-labelled radiopharmaceuticals

delivering shielding to the heating block and (3) transfer from the heating block to the final shielding at the end of the warming, (4) insertion of the tubes for dilution and (5) removal of disposables (tubing and sterile filter) at the end of the process. In some of these steps, radioactivity is not shielded in a proper PMMA shielding, and the only protection for the operator was guaranteed by wearing anti-X 0.20 mmPb-equivalent gloves. In particular, dosimetry was especially high in ^{90}Y-labelled radiopharmaceutical preparations due to the high-energy β^--emissions of the radionuclide.

17.4.2 Semiautomated Preparation

In this approach, the radiolabelling was performed by using an ADD-2 (Amercare, Thame, UK), a prototype of a semi-automatic dose dispenser device modified for performing simple radiolabelling procedures avoiding the use of disposable cassettes [27]. The ADD-2 is an automatic device designed to transfer liquids from vials to syringes (Fig. 17.10a, b). These operations are carried out by a combination of movements performed by four-stepper motors which allow the ADD-2 to mimic manual operations. Two motors are dedicated to syringe movements: the first one pulls the shielded syringe from the loading position into the filling position. When the syringe operations are completed, the same motor pushes the shielded syringe out, allowing it to be unloaded by the operator. The second motor accurately moves the syringe plunger to perform the transfer of liquid from syringe to vials and vice versa. A third motor lifts the shielding containing the vial so that the syringe needle can accurately penetrate the centre of vial septum and reach to the required depth. When liquid needs to be withdrawn, a forth stepper motor performs a 180° inversion of the shielded syringe and shielded vial in order to minimize the residue remaining into the vial (Fig. 17.10c). The depth of needle penetration can be preset by the operator to ensure that nearly all of the liquid in vials can be extracted by the syringe.

Using these basic mechanical motions, the ADD-2 can fill a syringe from a vial with the required volume, and it can empty the syringe contents into multiple vials in as many aliquots as required. The ADD-2 can also add or empty liquid to or from a syringe that already contains liq-

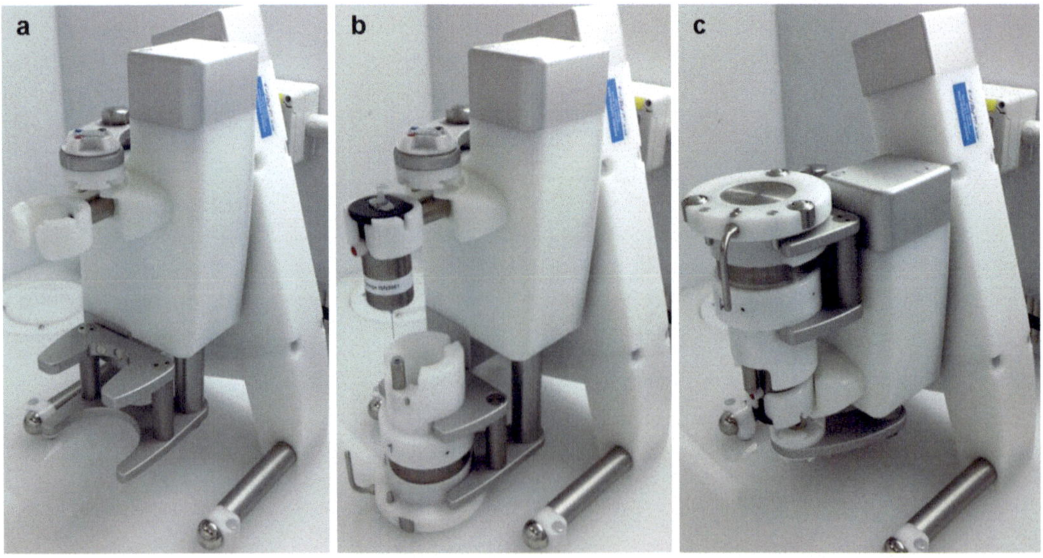

Fig. 17.10 Pictures of the automatic dispenser device (ADD) prototype. Base instrument asset (**a**). Instrument with syringe and vial shielding loaded (**b**). Instrument in the inverted position (**c**). Figure is reproduced from reference [27]

uid. The prototype used in this study has been modified in order to perform additional operations such as filtration or heating. These functions allow the system to carry out some relatively complex synthesis procedures.

The ADD-2 is controlled by a single board motion control system connected through specially designed stepper motor drivers to the stepper motors themselves. The position of the stepper motors is checked on every cycle by optical detectors which correct for any variations in the position. The stepper motors provide highly accurate positioning and enable the dispenser to achieve high accuracy in filling depending on the size of syringe used. The ADD-2 is preprogrammed to hold syringes from 1 ml up to 10 ml in size and for dispensing in vials from 2 ml up to 25 ml in size. During the operations, both syringes and vials are enclosed in a suitable 25 mm tungsten and plastic shielding in order to protect the operator's hands from radiation exposure (Fig. 17.11).

Vial shieldings are equipped with small metal rollerballs under the base and have a side handle that allow the operator to move the shielding along the work plane with minimal efforts. The operator is able to make the ADD-2 withdraw liquid from a vial with a syringe and deliver that liquid to other vials simply by replacing the first shielding in the work zone of the instrument with another shielding containing a different vial. A simple keypad allows the operator to input immediate commands to ADD-2 (namely, to fill, empty or add liquid to a syringe) or, alternatively, to program a sequence of movements in order to performed synthesis steps.

The synthesis path described above for the manual method can be performed by using ADD-2. Liquid transferring is achieved by using the syringes of suitable dimension depending on the step to be performed. A special filter holder and shielding can be supplied by the supplier for performing sterilizing filtration of the final solution (Fig. 17.12).

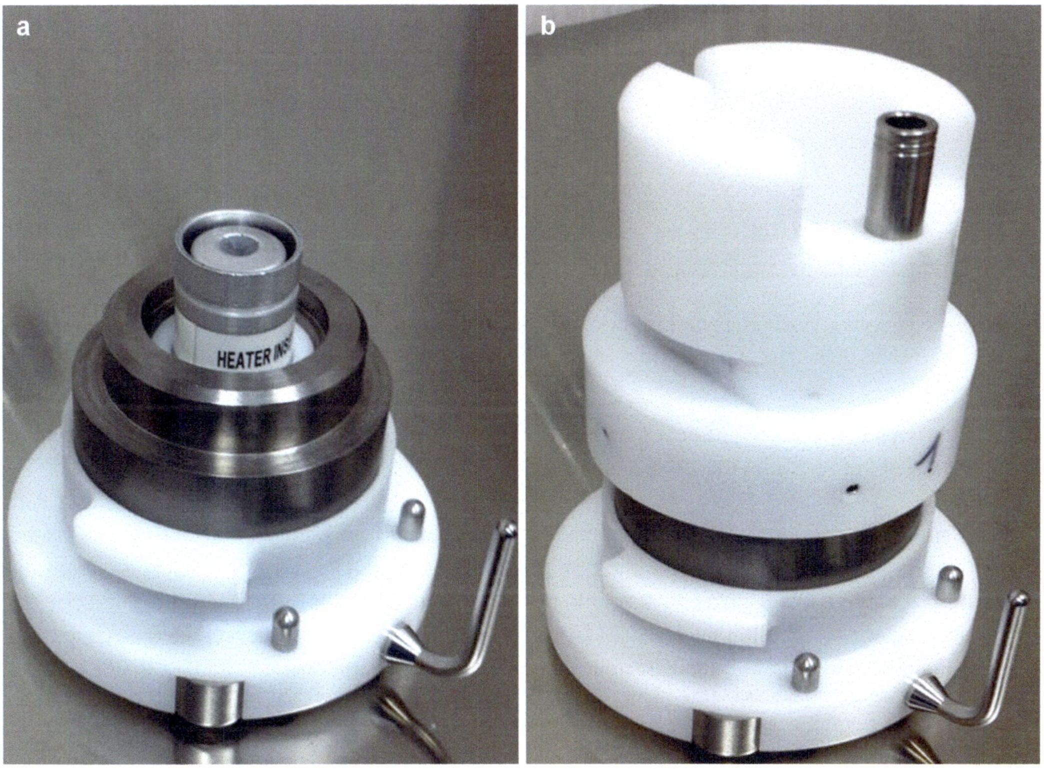

Fig. 17.11 Pictures of the reaction vial shielding. (**a**) open (**b**) closed with the proper shielding cover. Figure is reproduced from reference [27]

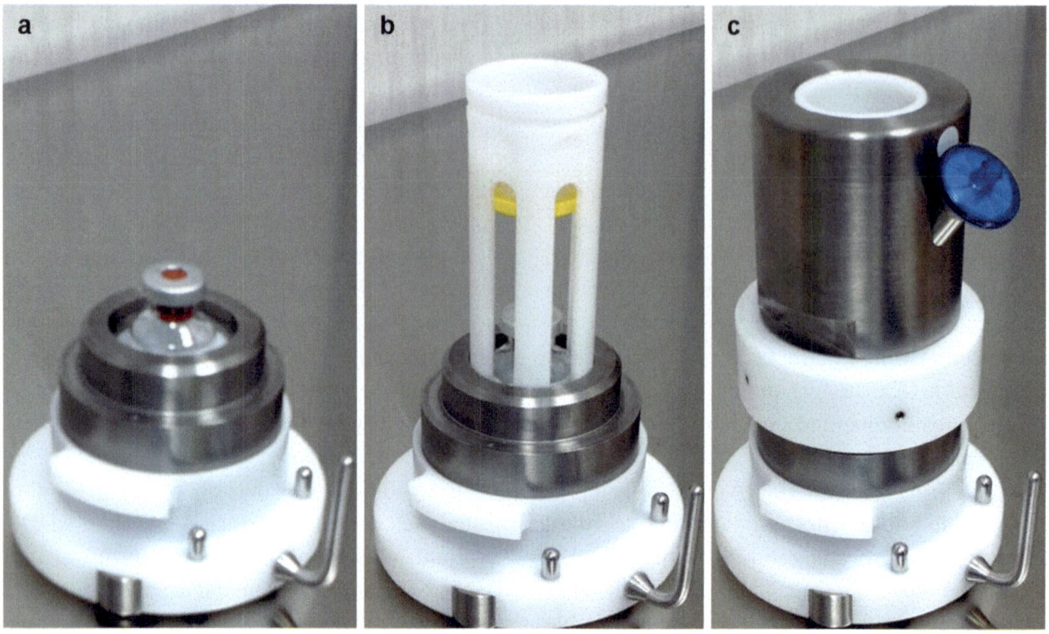

Fig. 17.12 Pictures of the final vial shielding with the sterilizing filter holder. (**a**) base situation (**b**) with filter holder placed (**c**) closed with the proper shielding cover. Figure is reproduced from reference [27]

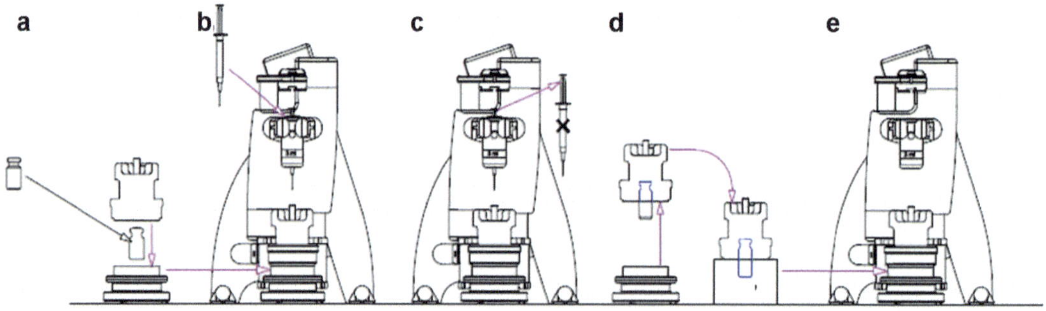

Fig. 17.13 Representation of operations performed with the ADD-2 semiautomated synthesizer. The picture is reproduced from reference [27]

Semi-automatic synthesis and doses fractionating are carried out by following these steps:

1. A 10 ml vial containing ^{90}Y/^{177}Lu chloride solutions is put in the suitable shielding and transferred in the ADD-2 carriage. A prefilled (sodium ascorbate solution and DOTATOC solution) 3 ml syringe is loaded into the ADD-2 syringe holder. Syringe solution is injected into the vial.
2. The vial, inside the suitable shielding, is removed from the ADD-2 carriage and heated for 30 min at 90 °C in a heating block. A schematic representation of these steps is shown in Fig. 17.13.
3. The vial is retransferred in the ADD-2 carriage, and an empty 1 ml syringe is loaded into the ADD-2 syringe holder. A small aliquot is drawn into the syringe. The operator manually unloads the shielded syringe and dilutes the contents in 0.2 ml of 0.1 M HCl for performing quality controls.
4. A 5 ml syringe with 3 ml of 0.9% NaCl solution is loaded into the ADD-2 syringe holder, and the liquid is dispensed in the vial containing the radiopharmaceutical preparation.

Using the same syringe, nearly all the radiopharmaceutical solution was withdrawn. A 25 ml vial with a sterilizing filter inside the suitable shielding was put in the ADD-2 carriage (Fig. 17.12). The radiopharmaceutical solution is filtered and dispensed from the syringe to 25 ml vial. A schematic representation of the dilution process is shown in Fig. 17.14. These operations (dilution, withdrawing, filtration) are repeated twice in order to minimize the residue remaining in the reaction vial, in the syringe and in the sterilizing filter.

5. The 25 ml vial containing ^{90}Y-/^{177}Lu-labelled preparation is measured in a dose calibrator.
6. A new syringe of suitable dimension is loaded in the ADD-2 syringe holder. The computed volume for having a single dose is withdrawn from the 25 ml dilution vial. The shielding containing the dilution vial is removed from the ADD-2 carriage, and a new shielded 25 ml vial was loaded. Dose is dispensed from the syringe to this vial and measured in the dose calibrator. These operations are repeated for every single dose.

Similar to the manual approach, the semiautomated methods (ADD-2 system) perform the labelling reaction directly in the delivery vial of the radionuclides. Transferring to and dilution of the radiopharmaceuticals to the final vial is carried out automatically by the system instead. The process takes ca. 60 min and assures a RCY around 90% for both yttrium-90 and lutetium-177 preparation with the greater loss due to radioactivity remaining in the delivery vial or small leaks during the transfer. These leaks can mainly occur after long periods of use of the instrument when the original symmetry and perfect overlap of the parts can be partially lost. In these cases, a growing laxity of the engine movement and an increase in the software communication failures can also be observed. These findings highlight the greatest drawback of the system, i.e. the need of frequent maintenance to maintain a high level of performance.

17.4.3 Fully Automated Preparation

The automated radiolabelling is described by using a ML eazy system (EZAG, Berlin). Modular-Lab eazy automatic synthesizer, disposable cassettes, hardware and reagent kits can be purchased from the supplier. The reagents kits for the labelling of ^{90}Y- or ^{177}Lu-DOTA peptides include vial 1 (50 ml of isotonic saline solution, 0.9% sodium chloride), vial 2 (50 ml of water for injection) and vial 3 (50 mg of ascorbic acid). The hardware kits are composed of 1 × 2 ml luer lock sterile syringe, 3 × 0.9 × 70 mm injection needle, 3 × 1.1 × 30 mm vent needle, 3 × 0.6 × 25 mm injection needle, 1× sterile empty 10 ml vial and 1× cation exchange CM cartridge.

The system uses a new technology working with a pressure distribution system instead of stopcocks or solenoid valves for liquid transfer. This internal and independent pressure system is set up inside the body of the synthesizer, while the disposable cassette is mounted on the top of the system simply clicking in the synthesis cassette (Fig. 17.15).

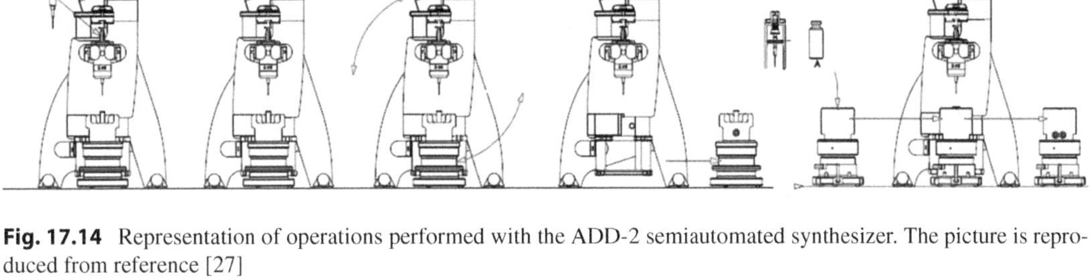

Fig. 17.14 Representation of operations performed with the ADD-2 semiautomated synthesizer. The picture is reproduced from reference [27]

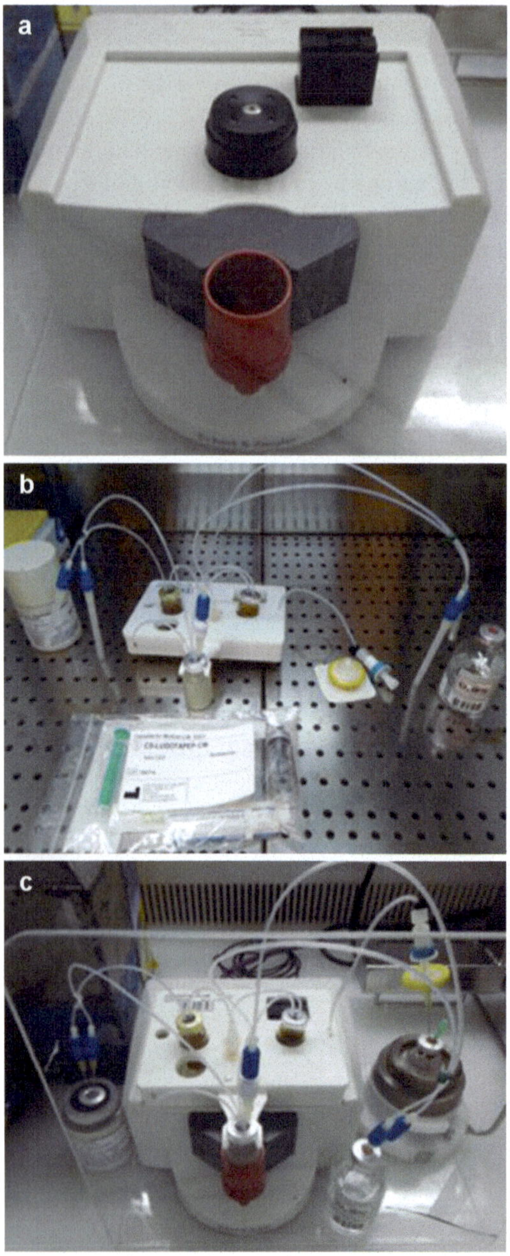

Fig. 17.15 Images of the ML eazy device (**a**), a disposable cassette (**b**) and disposable cassettes assembled onto the system (**c**)

All pressure connections are ensured automatically. After transferring all the required reagents in the proper vials, the cassette is subsequently mounted on the synthesizer. Vial containing the starting activity is connected to the synthesis cassette (delivery vial is kept in lead shielding throughout the whole process) in the last step prior to start the synthesis. The process works without external interaction as all steps are implemented in the synthesis template. Synthesis steps can be monitored via the HMI-scheme (Fig. 17.16). The Modular-Lab software is compliant with GMP standards (annex 11 for computerized systems), 21 CFR 210/211 cGMP, GAMP5 and 21 CFR part 11 regulations.

All consumables and reagents needed (excluding the precursors) are provided as part of the reagent kit. The light CM cartridge, the sterile filter and a needle are connected to the end of the product line of the cassettes, and the needle is inserted through the septum of a 25 ml vented vial. The reagents are prepared and filled as follows:

1. A 1.5 ml of water is withdrawn from vial 2 with a syringe and injected into vial 3 containing ascorbic acid. The vial was gently shaken to completely dissolve the substance.
2. A solution of the precursor proportional to the delivered radioactivity is added to vial 3.
3. The solution from vial 3 is withdrawn with a syringe and slowly injected into the dedicated vented vial of the cassette. Afterwards, the vent needle is discarded.

The cassette is assembled to the eazy system, and vial 1, containing isotonic solution, is connected to the cassette through the dedicated needles. The vial containing yttrium-90 or lutetium-177 chloride solutions is connected to the cassette by inserting the two dedicated needles. The software is started and the project corresponding to the synthesis is selected. After confirming the "preparation steps" displayed, the synthesis is started and moves towards the following steps: preheating of reaction vial (90 °C), transfer of buffer/precursor solution from buffer vial through delivery vial and then into the reaction vial, reaction time (about 30 min of heating), product transfer, purification and dilution into the product vial through CM and sterile filter. At the end of the synthesis, the cassette is automatically ejected, and aliquots for quality control are withdrawn directly from the final vial.

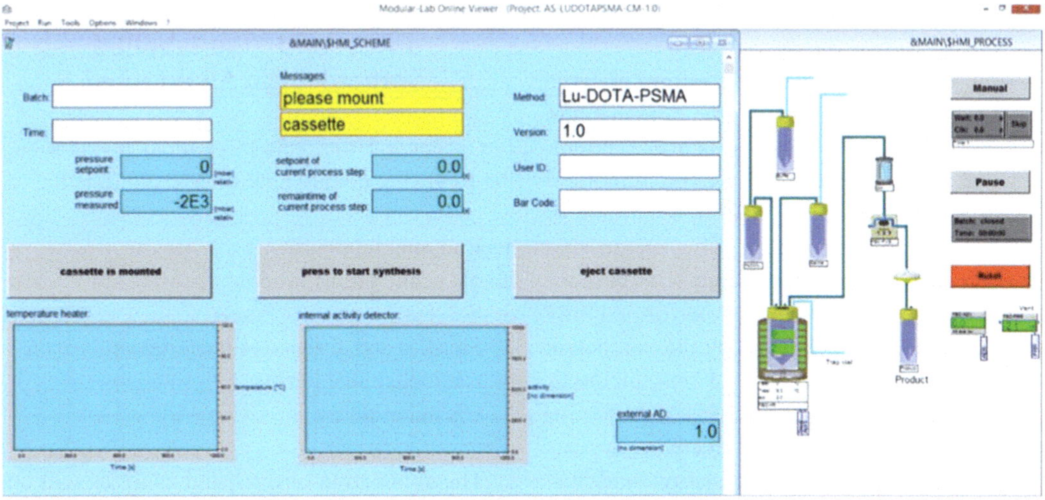

Fig. 17.16 Screenshot of ML eazy software interface. Synthesis steps, amount of radioactivity in the reactor and synthesis parameters are displayed during each synthesis run

The fully automated device described exhibits the advantage of a completely automated process where, after assembling of the disposable cassette and the reagents, the procedure is performed without any interference of the operator. Differently from the two precedent approaches, in this method the starting activity is transferred in a disposable reactor where the reaction takes place. The mixture is subsequently transferred to the final vial passing a CM cartridge. By using this approach, a RCY of around 83% for both ^{90}Y- and ^{177}Lu-DOTATOC is normally obtained. The lower RCY respect to the other two methods is mainly due to the fact that parts of radionuclide solution are not transferred to the reactor and, therefore, remain in the starting vial. Secondly, some radioactivity is lost in the reactor vial and in the CM cartridge during the transfer to the final vial.

In conclusion, the automated approach with the ML eazy synthesizer guarantees a decent RCY but a high reliability and reproducibility of the process. The operations are generally simpler, and no direct intervention of the operators is needed. The total time needed to prepare the system and perform the labelling is around 45–60 min.

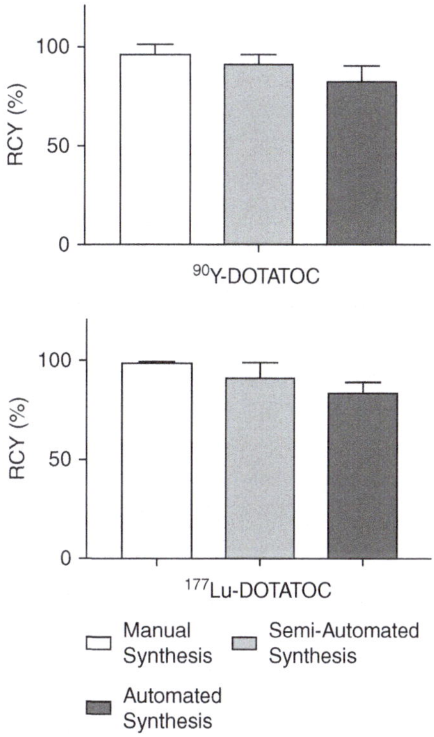

Fig. 17.17 Comparison of the performances of three different approaches preparing ^{90}Y- and ^{177}Lu-DOTATOC

A direct comparison of the performance of the three synthetic approaches in terms of RCY for the synthesis of ^{90}Y- and ^{177}Lu-DOTATOC is given in Fig. 17.17.

17.4.4 Quality Controls

In spite of a widespread utilization in large parts of the world, none of the somatostatin analogues labelled with therapeutic radionuclide has at the moment a marketing authorization or a dedicated monograph in a national or international pharmacopoeia. This means that these preparations are considered with purpose of clinical research and can be performed only under clinical trials approved by the competent authorities. This mean also that sets, methods, instrumentations and criteria of acceptance for quality controls are not described in the current radiopharmaceutical legislation and that the responsibility of their utilization is completely under the institution performing these preparations. A set of quality controls could actually be derived from general monographs on radiopharmaceutical preparations or monograph of similar radiotracer (e.g. monograph of ^{68}Ga-DOTATOC) in pharmacopoeia as well as from international/national guidelines, scientific publication or experience of the users [28–30]. To this purpose, a useful practical guidance on peptide receptor radionuclide therapy has been recently published together by the European Association of Nuclear Medicine (EANM), Society of Nuclear Medicine and Molecular Imaging (SNMMI) and International Atomic Energy Agency (IAEA) [31]. In this publication some suggestions on the parameters that have to be assessed and on the quality controls that have to be performed are given. However, the guidance is not specifically focused on quality controls.

In the following section, a brief analysis of the quality controls suggested by the European general monograph on radiopharmaceutical preparation will be given with the purpose to establish a base set of quality controls to be performed in a ^{90}Y- or ^{177}Lu-labelled somatostatin analogues preparation. Practical references to the analysis methods and practical advice on the manipulation of aliquots for quality controls will be given as well.

17.5 Which Quality Controls on ^{90}Y- and ^{177}Lu-labelled Somatostatin Analogues?

For a general radiopharmaceutical preparation, the following quality controls are suggested:

1. Radionuclidic purity
2. pH of the preparation
3. Solvent
4. Sterility and absence of bacterial endotoxins
5. Radiochemical purity
6. Chemical purity

The application of the listed analyses will be commented and contextualized for the preparation of a ^{90}Y- and ^{177}Lu-labelled somatostatin analogue, and criteria of acceptance will be given on the basis of scientific literature and international guidelines as well. In particular, the acceptance criteria are derived from the practical guidance published jointly by EANM, SNMMI and IAEA [31].

17.5.1 Radionuclidic Purity: Acceptance >99.99%

The radionuclidic purity is defined as the ratio between the activity of the base radionuclide and total activity of a radioactive compound. Radionuclidic impurities with half-lives of the order of several days constitute an unnecessary radiation burden for the patient. Long-lived radionuclides (half-life in the range of months to years) are problematic especially with respect to waste disposal at hospitals where a large number of treatments are conducted.

The main impurities in ^{90}Y- and ^{177}Lu-chloride solutions employed in the labelling of somatostatin analogues for therapeutic purpose are strontium-90 and lutetium-177 m, respectively. Yttrium-90 is produced by chemical high-purity separation from strontium-90, a fission product of uranium in nuclear reactors. For this reason, strontium-90 may be present in really low amount in the final yttrium-90 solutions [32, 33]. Lutetium-177 can be produced by irradiation of isotopically enriched lutetium-176 (direct way) and irradiation of ytterbium enriched with ytterbium-176 (indirect way) [34, 35].

The long-lived (160.5 days) isomer of ^{177}Lu is inevitably produced in the ^{176}Lu (n, γ)^{177m}Lu reaction during the direct production of lutetium-177, while a lutetium-177 preparation produced by the indirect route virtually does not contain this impurity.

To the purpose of quality controls, it is worth to notice that both the radionuclides used in the labelling of somatostatin analogues (i.e. yttrium-90 and lutetium-177) are supplied as commercial products with a marketing authorization or at least as good manufactured precursors.

This means that the radionuclidic purity is guaranteed by the supplier, and the amount of strontium-90 and lutetium-177 m is clearly indicated in the data sheet of the product. No further assessment is required to the final user if not checking these values on the datasheet. A structure owning the suitable instrumentations could also sometimes verify these data, but the procedure is not mandatory.

17.5.2 pH of the Preparation: Acceptance, 4.5–8.5

Although the pH of the final solution can be addressed by adding specific buffers (as described in the preparation paragraph) and the patient doses are normally injected after a large dilution in 0.9% NaCl solution, pH of the preparation should be assessed. The easiest way is by means of pH-indicator strips.

17.5.3 Solvents

This controls in not necessary in a ^{90}Y- and ^{177}Lu-labelled somatostatin analogue preparation whereas, as described before, only water solution are used.

17.5.4 Sterility and Absence of Bacterial Endotoxins: Acceptance, Sterility (<10 cfu/mL), Endotoxins (<175 EU/V)

Radiopharmaceuticals are administered by intravenous injection, and to avoid potential microorganism infection in the patients, it is essential that the preparations are sterile at the time of administration. However, since a sterility test takes 2 weeks and many radiopharmaceuticals have a really short half-life, it is normally not possible to do a prospective sterility test on most radiopharmaceuticals before injection. Moreover, the sterility tests are normally performed in laboratories not authorized to retain radioactive probes; hence, the radioactivity of samples taken for the sterility test has to be completely decayed before delivering them to the laboratories. In the case of ^{90}Y- and ^{177}Lu-labelled somatostatin analogue preparations, this latter consideration is critic. In fact, if the total amount of radioactivity handled and the volume needed for a sterility test are considered, it can be speculated that an aliquot of around 720 MBq has to be withdrawn for the test. Starting from this amount, around 64 days for yttrium-90 and 130 days for lutetium-177, respectively, are necessary to reach a radioactivity level deliverable outside an authorized facility. During these days the possibility of an external bacterial contamination is much more probable than an original contamination in the production process. For all these reasons, a standard sterility test is normally not suitable for assessing the sterility of a ^{90}Y- or ^{177}Lu-labelled radiopharmaceutical. However, this does not relieve these radiopharmaceuticals from the need to ensure their sterility. Confidence in the sterility of these products can be achieved by working in a clean environment and following a defined operating procedure which incorporates aseptic transfer techniques. This confidence can be endorsed by carrying out prospective procedure like media-fill tests.

Pyrogen (fever-inducing agent), principally known as bacterial endotoxin, is one of the most potent bacterial toxins. Its only source is Gram (−) bacteria (GNB), where endotoxin comprises about 75% of the GNB cell wall. Bacterial contamination (bioburden) in water and on surfaces normally contains GNB, so endotoxin is ubiquitous in nature. The most likely sources of endotoxins in PET radiopharmaceuticals are containers, tubing and non-sterile water and chemicals used in the preparation of the product [36, 37]. Nowadays, bacterial endotoxin level in radiopharmaceuticals preparation can be assessed by photometric tests. These tests require a highly processed reagent, a spectrophotometer, endotoxin-specific software and printout capability. In its most simplistic form, the simplest photometric system exists as a handheld unit employing a single-use, LAL cartridge that contains dried, pre-calibrated reagents. In the last years, an international-approved handheld system unit was introduced under the trade name of Endosafe PTS™ (Charles River Laboratories, Charleston, SC) [38]. The device requires about 15 min to analyse 4 × 25 mL amounts of sample. The simplicity and speed of this new automated system make it ideally suited for radiopharmaceutical preparation including ^{90}Y- and ^{177}Lu-labelled somatostatin analogues.

17.5.5 Radiochemical Purity (RCP): Acceptance, >98% by HPLC and/or >99% by TLC or SPE

Radiochemical purity is defined as the proportion of the total activity of a specific radionuclide in a specific chemical or biological form present in a preparation and is definitely the most important parameter in a radiopharmaceutical preparation. In the case of ^{90}Y- and ^{177}Lu-labelled somatostatin analogues, the potential impurities are due to unlabelled radionuclides (namely, free $^{90}Y^{3+}$ and $^{177}Lu^{3+}$), partially hydrolysed products (a mixture of ^{90}Y- and ^{177}Lu-oxide and hydroxide) and by-products due to radiolysis or oxidation phenomena. In particular, the first species are really dangerous for the patients because the free radionuclides accumulate in the bone giving an excessive radioactive dose with consequent toxicity to the bone marrow. For this reason it is of basilar importance that the RCP is as higher as possible.

RCP can be assessed mainly by three methods:

1. Solid-phase extraction (SPE) method: this method is based on the different interaction of the radiolabelled somatostatin analogues and the impurities (free $^{90}Y^{3+}$ and $^{177}Lu^{3+}$ and partially hydrolysed products) with a C-18 commercial cartridge (Waters, Milan) when eluted with different solvents. The method consists in the following steps:
   - Charging the C-18 cartridge properly conditioned (3 mL of MeOH followed by 3 ml of 1 M sodium acetate solution) with a small aliquot of the radiopharmaceutical solution.
   - Eluting the cartridge with 3 mL of a 1 M sodium acetate solution and collecting the fraction in a test tube A (in this fraction free $^{90}Y^{3+}$ and $^{177}Lu^{3+}$ and partially hydrolysed products if present are gathered).
   - Eluting the cartridge with 3 mL of MeOH and collecting the radiolabelled product in a test tube B.
   - Measuring both the tubes in a dose calibrator and computing the RCP as percentage of the ratio between the radioactivity measured in the fraction B and the sum of the radioactivity measured in both the fraction.

   The method is quite simple and cheap as no particular instrumentations is necessary, but, although suitable for assessing the RCP of these preparation, it is not really precise or reproducible as it mainly depends on the manual skill of the operator. The sequence of the steps of this method is represented in Fig. 17.18.
2. Radio-thin-layer chromatography (TLC): like all the chromatographic method, TLC is based on the different interaction of the radiolabelled products and impurities with a stationary phase (in this case proper TLC strips) and a mixture of eluents used to separate the analytes positioned on the strip. To run a thin-

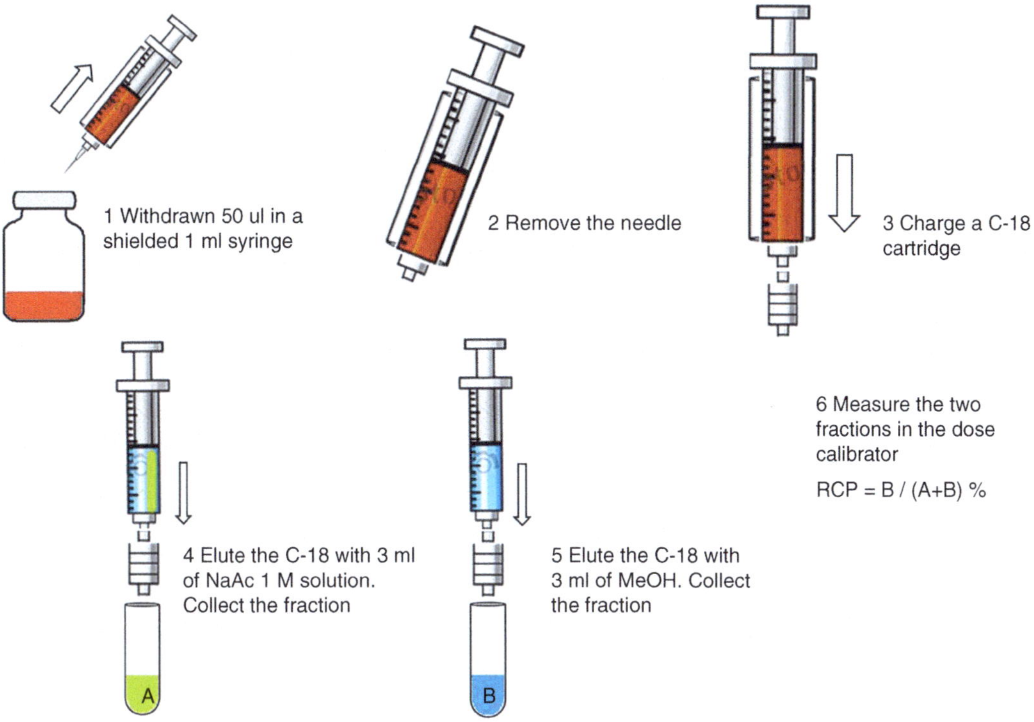

Fig. 17.18 Schematic representation of RCP assessment by SPE method

layer chromatography plate, the following procedure is carried out:

- Using a capillary, a small spot of radiopharmaceutical solution (around 5 μL) is applied to the strip, about 1.0 cm from the bottom edge. The solvent is allowed to completely evaporate off to prevent it from interfering with sample's interactions with the mobile phase in the next step.
- A small amount of an appropriate solvent (eluent) is poured into a glass beaker or any other suitable transparent container (separation chamber) to a depth of less than 0.5 cm. The container is closed with a cover glass or any other lid and is left for a few minutes to let the solvent vapours saturate the air in the chamber. (Failure to saturate the chamber will result in poor separation and non-reproducible results.)
- The TLC strip is then placed in the chamber so that the spot of the sample do not touch the surface of the eluent in the chamber and the lid is closed. The solvent moves up the plate by capillary action, meets the sample mixture and carries it up the plate (elutes the sample). The strip is removed from the chamber when the solvent front reaches 0.5 cm from the top edge of the stationary phase.
- The plate is visualized by a proper radio-TLC scanner and the radioactivity associated to any spot is computed. RCP is calculated as a percentage of the ratio between the radioactivity measured in the spot associated to ^{90}Y- or ^{177}Lu-somatostatin analogue and the sum of the radioactivity measured in all the spot on the strip. The position of a spot is indicated as the ratio between the distance travelled by the substance being considered and the total distance travelled by the mobile phase. This ratio is called the retention factor (R_f) and depends on the TLC strips and on the eluent used.

For the assessment of the RCP of ^{90}Y- or ^{177}Lu-somatostatin analogue, the following two systems are normally used [27, 39, 40]:

System 1: RP-18F plates (Merck, Whitehouse Station, NJ, USA) as stationary phase and 0.1 M sodium citrate/1 M HCl (97:3) solution as mobile phase. In this system the following R_f are obtained: ^{90}Y-/^{177}Lu-somatostatin analogue = 0.1; free radionuclides or hydrolysed products = 0.9.

System 2: ITLC-SG plates (Varian, Milan, Italy) as stationary phase and 1 M ammonium acetate/methanol (1:1) solution as mobile phase. In this system the following R_f are obtained: hydrolysed products = 0.0; free radionuclides = 0.4; and ^{90}Y-/^{177}Lu-somatostatin analogue = 0.9.

The distribution of the radioactive compounds when these two systems are employed for assessing the RCP of a ^{90}Y-DOTATOC preparation is shown in Fig. 17.19.

The method is simple and rapid but do not allow to discriminate the potential by-products due to radiolysis or oxidation that are not separated from the radiolabelled product. In Figs. 17.20 and 17.21, an example of TLC chromatograms of ^{177}Lu-DOTATOC preparations with RCP inside and outside criteria of acceptance is shown, respectively.

3. High-performance liquid chromatography (HPLC): the method uses the same principles of TLC, but the process is totally automatized and relies on pumps to pass a pressurized mixture of liquid eluent containing the sample mixture through a high-packed column filled with a solid adsorbent material. In the case of the quality control of ^{90}Y-/^{177}Lu-somatostatin analogue, the column normally used is a reverse phase C18 column (the exact specification depends on the HPLC instrumentation on use). After the separation, the analytes are detected by means of a radioactivity detector, and the signals proportional to the radioactivity in the fraction are processed by an internal validated software giving the final RCP of the

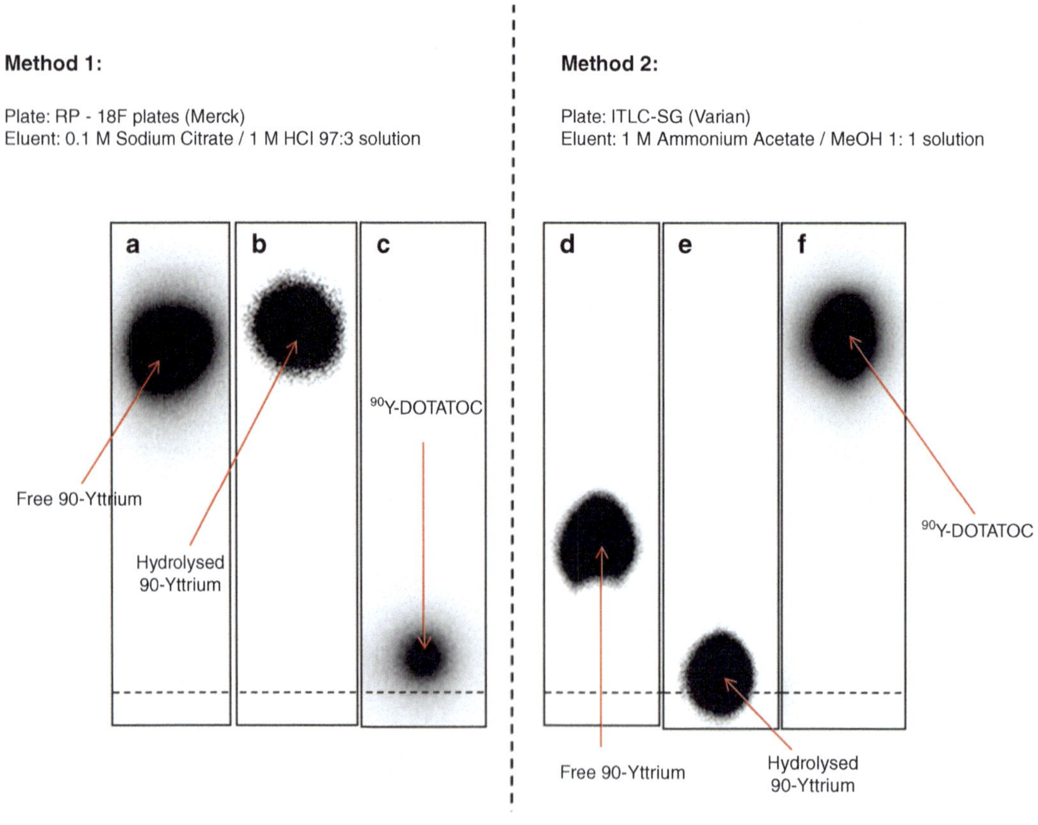

Fig. 17.19 Images of the radioactivity distribution when the RCP of a ^{90}Y-DOTATOC preparation is assessed by the two TLC methods. Figure is modified from reference [27]

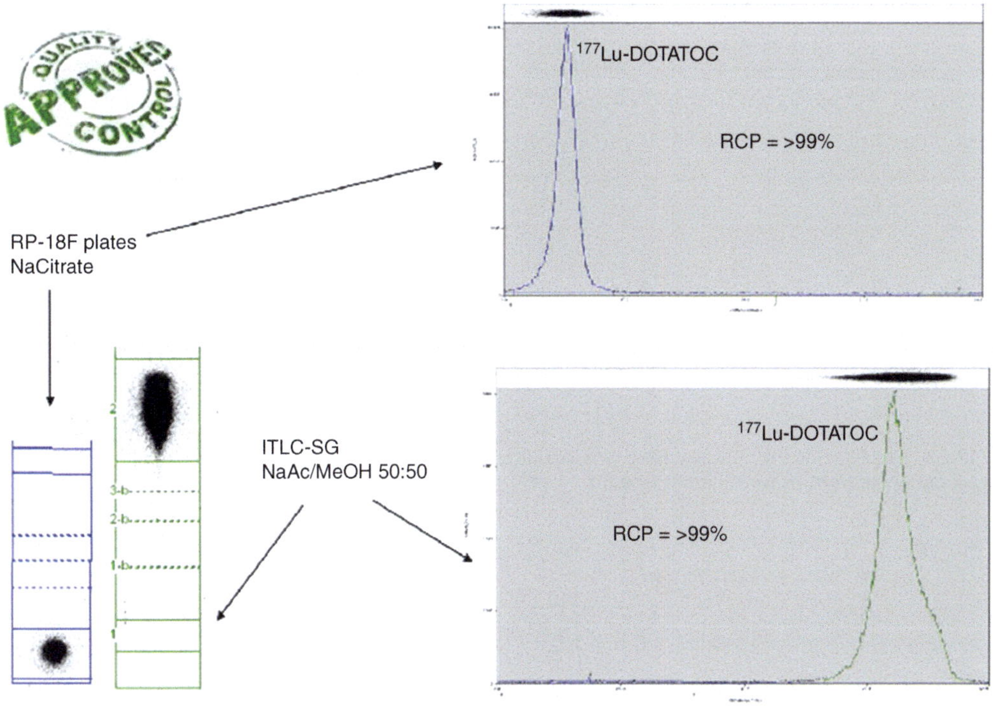

Fig. 17.20 TLC strips and the correspondent TLC chromatograms of a ^{177}Y-DOTATOC preparation with RCP inside the criteria of acceptance

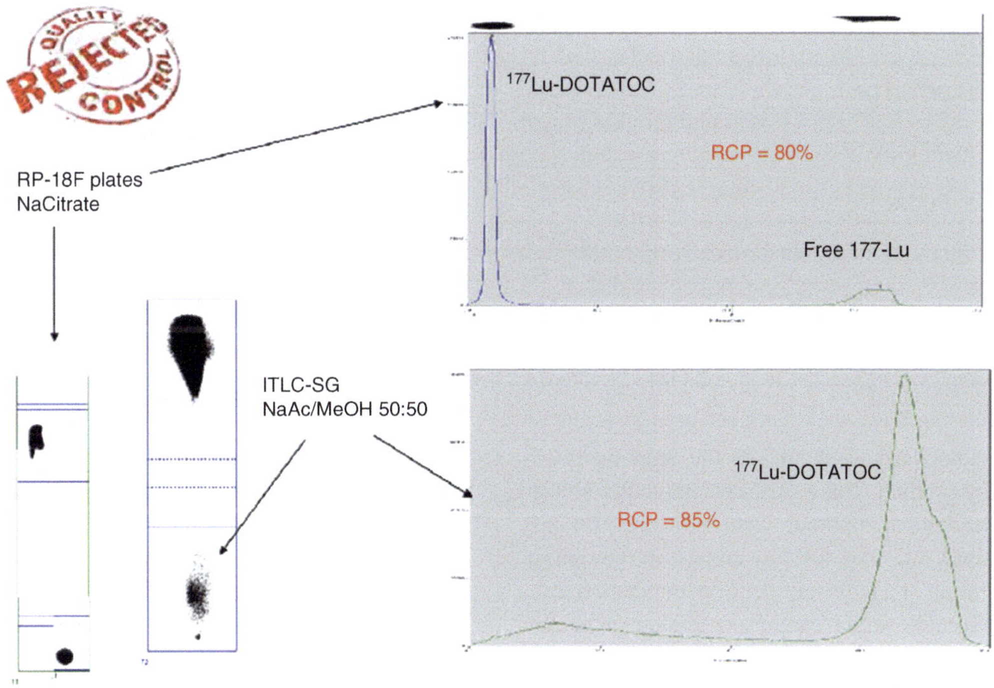

Fig. 17.21 TLC strips and the correspondent TLC chromatograms of a ^{177}Y-DOTATOC preparation with RCP outside the criteria of acceptance

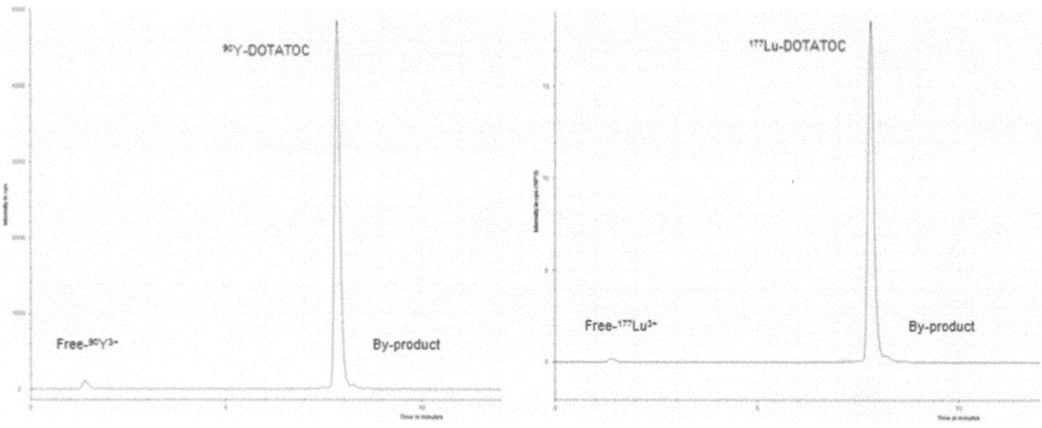

Fig. 17.22 Paradigmatic HPLC chromatograms (radiochemical detector) of ^{90}Y-DOTATOC and ^{177}Lu-DOTATOC preparations obtained by using example method 1

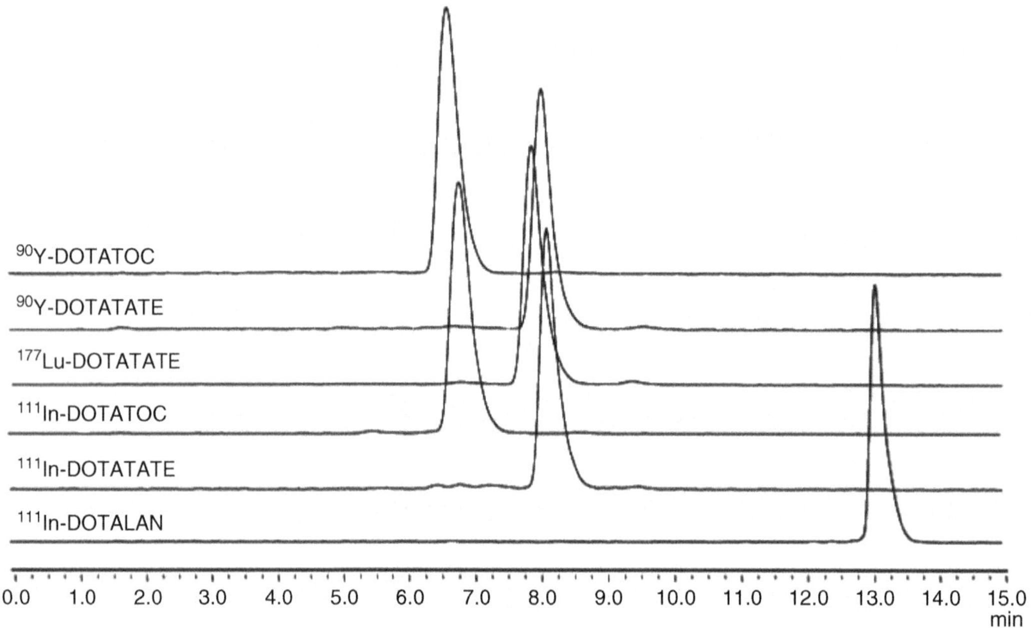

Fig. 17.23 Paradigmatic HPLC chromatograms (radiochemical detector) of radiolabelled somatostatin analogues obtained by using example method 2. Figure is reproduced from reference [41]

radiopharmaceutical and the amount of any by-product. Many different methods able to lead to an optimal separation are currently used, and they actually consist in the optimization of a large number of parameters such as eluent flow rate, eluent sort, change in the concentration of the eluents over time (gradient elution), column type, column temperature, volume of injection and many others. To the purpose of this chapter, some examples of HPLC methods commonly used and reported in scientific publications [41–43] are cited.

Example method 1: Column, Acclaim 120 C18 column (3 μm, 3 × 150 mm) (Thermo Scientific). Eluent flow rate: 0.6 ml/min Eluent A, 0.1% TFA water solution. Eluent B: acetonitrile; Gradient: 0–11 min 82% A, 11–16 min. 40% A , 11–20 min 16% A. At these conditions the following retention times (R_t) were found: unreacted radionuclides or hydrolysed product R_t = 1.3–1.4 min, ^{90}Y-/^{177}Lu-DOTATOC R_t = 7.7 min, by-products R_t = 8.2 min.

An example of HPLC chromatograms obtained by using this method is shown in Fig. 17.22.

Example method 2: Column, ACE 3 C18 (150 × 3 μm) column. Eluent flow rate: 0.5 ml/min Eluent A, acetonitrile. Eluent B: 0.1% TFA/water solution. Gradient: time, 0–1 min 20% A, 1–9 min 20–24% A, 9–11 min 24–60% A, 11–12 min 60% A, 12–12.1 min. 60–20% A and 12.1–15 min 20% A. At these conditions the following retention times (R_t) were found: unreacted radionuclides or hydrolysed product R_t = 1.3–1.4 min, ^{90}Y-/^{177}Lu-DOTATATE R_t = 8 min, by-products R_t = 9.2 min.

An example of HPLC chromatograms obtained by using this method is shown in Fig. 17.23.

HPLC is a really reliable and reproducible method because it is not operator-dependent. This analysis gives incontestable results as the software, if correctly calibrated, automatically computes the RCP and any change on the chromatograms or on the analysis is registered as well. HPLC has superior separation capability and precision than TLC as high-pressurized eluents and tightly packed specific columns are used. For this reason, the analysis is able to detect impurities due to radiolysis phenomena as well as free radionuclides or hydrolysed product. Finally, HPLC analysis is able to assess radiochemical purity and chemical purity of the radiopharmaceutical at the same time as described in the following paragraph. On the other hand, HPLC analysis involves expensive instrumentation, and the full exploitation of the potential of the technique requires trained operators.

17.5.6 Chemical Purity (CP): Acceptance, <250 μg of Somatostatin Analogue Per Patient

Chemical purity is defined as "the fraction of the total mass present in the stated chemical form". Due to the extremely low mass of the radiolabelled compounds, chemical purity itself cannot normally be determined, but the amount of some non-radioactive constituents, precursors or by-product may be determined. If significant levels of such chemical impurities are present, then it is possible that they may interfere in the labelling process. Some compounds may also be toxic for the patient. For that reason, all the reagents used in radiopharmaceutical formulations are normally of the highest purity that can be obtained.

In the case of ^{90}Y- and ^{177}Lu-somatostatin analogues, it is particularly important that the amount of unlabelled precursor in the final preparation is lower than 250 μg per patient, whereas somatostatin analogues have a great number of physiological effects as described in the first paragraph of this section. To this purpose, it is worth to notice that in these preparations the somatostatin analogue is always in large molar excess with respect to the radionuclide (ca. 2000-fold higher), and so the greater part of the precursor remains unlabelled. In spite of the fact that the operators should know the exact amount of precursor added to the preparation at the beginning of the reaction, the CP can be assessed by the same HPLC system and conditions described for the RCP but using a UV-visible detector connected in series with the radiochemical detector. UV detector is normally set at 220 nm and exploits the natural UV absorption of the many chromophores present on the peptide chain of the precursor. For the same reason explained for the unlabelled precursor, other molecules whose amount should be assessed are the by-products derived from the cleavage of the linker between the chelator and the peptide chain during the reaction (e.g. the TOC sequence derived from the cleavage of DOTATOC) and the by-product originated from the precursor oxidation [44]. An example of HPLC chromatogram of the substances employed in a ^{177}Lu-DOTATOC preparation is shown in Fig. 17.24.

Another aspect of the chemical purity regards the amount of metal cations in the commercial ^{90}Y- and ^{177}Lu-chloride solution. Some metal cations can strongly influence the completion of the labelling reaction by competing with the radionuclides in the complexation reaction [45]. For this

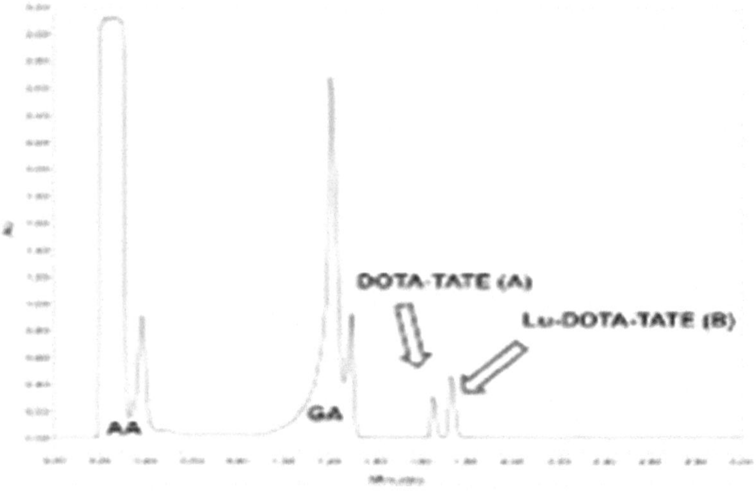

Fig. 17.24 Paradigmatic HPLC chromatograms (UV detector) of the standards for assessing the RC of a ^{177}Lu-DOTATATE preparation. Figure is reproduced from reference [44]

reason, the amount of metal cations and the limits of acceptance are usually indicated in the data sheet of the radionuclides and should be carefully assessed by the operator before starting the preparation.

Key Points

- Vector and targets: somatostatin and its analogues.
- Radionuclides for therapy: yttrium-90 and lutetium-177.
- The bifunctional chelator.
- Radiopharmaceuticals for therapy: biodistribution and pharmacokinetics.
- Preparation of yttrium-90- and lutetium-177-labelled somatostatin analogues.
- Quality controls: methods and instrumentation.
- Somatostatin receptors (in particular subtype 2) are overexpressed in many tumours and, in particular, in neuroendocrine ones. For the reason, somatostatin receptors appear to be a perfect target for selective deliver a radioactive dose to tumour tissues.
- Yttrium-90 and lutetium-177 are the most used radionuclide for peptide receptor radionuclide therapy. Yttrium-90 is a pure β-emitter with a physical half-life of 64.1 h. Lutetium-177 is a medium-energy β-emitter, with 6.73 days of physical half-time and also shows two additional γ-emissions of 210 and 113 keV.
- A bifunctional chelator (BFC) is a chemical structure able both to firmly complex the metal radionuclide core and also to be linked to the peptide chain through a stable covalent bond. Examples of the most used BFCs for therapeutic application are DOTA and its derivatives.
- Yttrium-90- and lutetium-177-labelled DOTATOC, DOTATATE and DOTANOC are the most used radiopharmaceuticals for the treatment of neuroendocrine tumour. They present comparable biodistribution and pharmacokinetics also if DOTATOC derivatives have a slightly more favourable behaviour.
- ^{90}Y- and ^{177}Lu-labelled somatostatin derivatives can be prepared in high yield and purity both by manual operations and by automatic procedures.
- None of the somatostatin analogues labelled with therapeutic radionuclide has at the moment a marketing authorization or a dedicated monograph in a national or international pharmacopoeia. This means that these preparations are considered with the purpose of clinical research and can be performed only under clinical trials approved by the competent authorities.

Acknowledgements The author thanks Coruzzi Chiara for the work on the raw material, the proofs for correction and for the bibliographic research.

References

1. Gudkov SV, Shilyagina NY, Vodeneev VA, et al. Targeted radionuclide therapy of human tumors. Int J Mol Sci. 2016;17:33.
2. De Jong M, Breeman WA, Kwekkeboom DJ, et al. Tumor imaging and therapy using radiolabeled somatostatin analogues. Acc Chem Res. 2009;42:873–80.
3. Ambrosini V, Fani M, Fanti S, et al. Radiopeptide imaging and therapy in Europe. J Nucl Med. 2011;52:42S–55S.
4. Gabriel M, Oberauer A, Dobrozemsky G, et al. 68Ga-DOTA-Tyr3 octreotide PET for assessing response to somatostatin-receptor-mediated radionuclide therapy. J Nucl Med. 2009;50:1427–34.
5. Kwekkeboom DJ, Krenning EP. Peptide receptor radionuclide therapy in the treatment of neuroendocrine tumors. Hematol Oncol Clin North Am. 2016;30:179–91.
6. Sabet A, Biersack HJ, Ezziddin S. Advances in peptide receptor radionuclide therapy. Semin Nucl Med. 2016;46:40–6.
7. Patel YC. General aspects of the biology and function of somatostatin. In: Somatostatin, Basic and clinical aspects of neuroscience, vol. 4. Berlin: Springer; 1992.
8. Patel YC. Somatostatin and its receptor family. Front Neuroendocrinol. 1999;20(3):157–98.
9. Reubi JC. Peptide receptors as molecular targets for cancer diagnosis and therapy. Endocr Rev. 2003;24(4):389–427.
10. Froidevaux S, Eberle AN. Somatostatin analogs and radiopeptides in cancer therapy. Biopolymers. 2002;66:161–83.
11. van der Lely AJ, de Herder WW, Krenning EP, et al. Octreoscan radioreceptor imaging. Endocrine. 2003;20(3):307–11.
12. Delacroix D, Guerre JP, Leblanc P, et al. Radionuclide and radiation protection data handbook 2nd edition (2002). Radiat Prot Dosim. 2002;98:9–168.
13. Barone R, Borson-Chazot F, Valkema R, et al. Patient-specific dosimetry in predicting renal toxicity with ^{90}Y-DOTATOC: relevance of kidney volume and dose rate in finding a dose–effect relationship. J Nucl Med. 2005;46:99S–106S.
14. Hind E, Zanotti-Fregonara P, Quinto MA, et al. Dose deposits from ^{90}Y, ^{177}Lu, ^{111}In, and ^{161}Tb in micrometastases of various sizes: implications for radiopharmaceutical therapy. J Nucl Med. 2016;57:759. https://doi.org/10.2967/jnumed.115.170423.
15. Smith-Jones PM, Stolz B, Albert R, et al. Synthesis and characterisation of [90Y]-Bz-DTPA-oct: a yttrium-90-labelled octreotide analogue for radiotherapy of somatostatin receptor-positive tumours. Nucl Med Biol. 1998;25(3):181–8.
16. Otte A, Jermann E, Behe M, et al. DOTATOC: a powerful new tool for receptor-mediated radionuclide therapy. Eur J Nucl Med. 1997;24(7):792–5.
17. Strosberg J, El-Haddad G, Wolin E, et al. Phase 3 trial of 177Lu-dotatate for midgut neuroendocrine tumors. N Engl J Med. 2017;376(2):125–35.
18. Schuchardt C, Kulkarni HR, Prasad V, et al. The bad berka dose protocol: comparative results of dosimetry in peptide receptor radionuclide therapy using 177Lu-DOTATATE, 177Lu-DOTANOC, and 177Lu-DOTATOC. In: Baum R, Rösch F, editors. Theranostics, gallium-68, and other radionuclides, Recent results in cancer research, vol. 194. Berlin: Springer; 2013.
19. Esser JP, Krenning EP, Teunissen JJ, et al. Comparison of [(177) Lu-OTA(0), Tyr(3)] octreotate and [(177) Lu-DOTA(0), Tyr(3)] octreotide: which peptide is preferable for PRRT? Eur J Nucl Med Mol Imaging. 2006;33:1346–51.
20. Antunes P, Ginj M, Zhang H, et al. Are radiogallium-labelled DOTA-conjugated somatostatin analogues superior to those labelled with other radiometals? Eur J Nucl Med Mol Imaging. 2007;34:982–93.
21. Förster GJ, Engelbach M, Brockmann J, et al. Preliminary data on biodistribution and dosimetry for therapy planning of somatostatin receptor positive tumours: comparison of 86Y-DOTATOC and 111In-DTPA-octreotide. Eur J Nucl Med. 2001;28(12):1743–50.
22. De Jong M, Bakker WH, Krenning EP, et al. Yttrium-90 and indium-111 labelling, receptor binding and biodistribution of [DOTA0,d-Phe1,Tyr3]octreotide, a promising somatostatin analogue for radionuclide therapy. Eur J Nucl Med. 1997;24:368–71.
23. Breeman WA, Chan HS, de Zanger RM, et al. Overview of development and formulation of 177Lu-DOTA-TATE for PRRT. Curr Radiopharm. 2016;9(1):8–18.
24. Breeman WA, van der Wansem K, Bernard BF, et al. The addition of DTPA to [177Lu-DOTA0,Tyr3] octreotate prior to administration reduces rat skeleton uptake of radioactivity. Eur J Nucl Med Mol Imaging. 2003;30(2):312–5.
25. Breeman WA, De Jong MT, De Blois E, et al. Reduction of skeletal accumulation of radioactivity by co-injection of DTPA in [^{90}Y-DOTA^{0},Tyr^{3}]octreotide solutions containing free $^{90}Y^{3+}$. Nucl Med Biol. 2004;31(6):821–4.
26. Scott PJ, Hockley BG, Kung HF, et al. Studies into radiolytic decomposition of fluorine-18 labeled radiopharmaceuticals for positron emission tomography. Appl Radiat Isot. 2009;67(1):88–94.
27. Asti M, Atti G, Iori M, et al. Semi-automated labelling and fractionation of yttrium-90 and lutetium-177 somatostatin analogues using disposable syringes and vials. Nucl Med Commun. 2012;33:1144–52.
28. European Directorate for the Quality of Medicines & Healthcare (EDQM). Gallium (68Ga) edotreotide injection. European Pharmacopoeia 7.6. 2013;2482:4847–48.
29. European Directorate for the Quality of Medicines & Healthcare (EDQM). Extemporaneous preparation of radiopharmaceutical preparations. Chapter 5.19.

In: European pharmacopoeia. 8th ed. Strasbourg: EDQM; 2016.
30. Elsinga P, Todde S, Penuelas I, et al. Guidance on current good radiopharmacy practice (cGRPP) for the small-scale preparation of radiopharmaceuticals. Eur J Nucl Med Mol Imaging. 2010;37:1049–62.
31. Zaknun JJ, Bodei L, Mueller-Brand J, et al. The joint IAEA, EANM, and SNMMI practical guidance on peptide receptor radionuclide therapy (PRRNT) in neuroendocrine tumours. Eur J Nucl Med Mol Imaging. 2013;40(5):800–16.
32. International Atomic Energy Agency. Therapeutic radionuclide generators: 90Sr/90Y and 188W/188Re generators, Technical Reports Series No. 470. Vienna: International Atomic Energy Agency; 2009.
33. Castillo AX, Pérez-Malo M, Isaac-Olivé K, et al. Production of large quantities of 90Y by ion-exchange chromatography using an organic resin and a chelating agent. Nucl Med Biol. 2010;37(8): 935–42.
34. Dash A, Pillai MR, Knapp FF Jr. Production of (177)Lu for targeted radionuclide therapy: available options. Nucl Med Mol Imaging. 2015;49(2): 85–107.
35. Tarasov VA, Andreev OI, Romanov EG, et al. Production of no-carrier added lutetium-177 by irradiation of enriched ytterbium-176. Curr Radiopharm. 2015;8(2):95–106.
36. Williams K. Endotoxins. 3rd ed. New York: Informa Healthcare; 2007. p. 27–90.
37. Cooper JF, Thoma LA. Screening extemporaneously compounded intraspinal injections with the bacterial endotoxins test. Am J Health Syst Pharm. 2002;59:2426–33.
38. Dragotakes SC, Cooper JF, Hubers D. A new system for the rapid detection of endotoxin in PET radiopharmaceuticals. (abstract). 2005. Society of Nuclear Medicine. Toronto.
39. Biasiotto G, Bertagna F, Zanella I, et al. Production and quality control of [(90)Y]DOTATOC for treatment of metastatic neuroendocrine tumors: results of 85 syntheses. Nucl Med Commun. 2013;34(3):265–70.
40. Kunikowska J, Królicki L, Dydejczyk AH, et al. Clinical results of radionuclide therapy of neuroendocrine tumours with 90Y-DOTATATE and tandem 90Y/177Lu-DOTATATE: which is a better therapy option? Eur J Nucl Med Mol Imaging. 2011;38(10):1788–97.
41. Petrik M, Knetsch PA, Knopp R, et al. Radiolabelling of peptides for PET, SPECT and therapeutic applications using a fully automated disposable cassette system. Nucl Med Commun. 2011;32:887–95.
42. Mukherjee A, Lohar S, Dash A, et al. Single vial kit formulation of DOTATATE for preparation of (177) Lu-labeled therapeutic radiopharmaceutical at hospital radiopharmacy. J Label Compd Radiopharm. 2015;58(4):166–72.
43. Taşdelen B, Ergun A, Büyükkaya F, et al. Rapid isocratic HPLC investigation of radiochemical purity for 90Y-DOTATATE. J Radioanal Nucl Chem. 2011;289(2):573–5.
44. Breeman WAP, Chan HS, de Blois E. Determination of peptide content and purity of DOTA-peptides by metal ion titration and UPLC: an alternative method to monitor quality of DOTA-peptides. J Radioanal Nucl Chem. 2004;302(2):825–30.
45. Asti M, Tegoni M, Farioli D, et al. Influence of cations on complexation yield of DOTATATE with yttrium and lutetium: a perspective study for enhancing the ^{90}Y and ^{177}Lu labeling conditions. Nucl Med Biol. 2012;39(4):509–17.

18 Paediatric Tumours of Neuroendocrine/Peripheral Neuroectodermal Origin

Roberto Luksch, Carlo Chiesa, Ettore Seregni, Carlo Morosi, Marta Podda, Davide Biasoni, Gemma Gatta, Lorenza Gandola, Paola Collini, Paolo Scanagatta, Giovanna Riccipetitoni, Nadia Puma, and Maria Rita Castellani

Abstract

The neoplasms arising from the neural crest-derived cells in the adrenal medulla or extra-adrenal paraganglia include peripheral neuroblastic tumours, pheochromocytoma and paraganglioma.

Peripheral neuroblastic tumours (neuroblastoma, ganglioneuroblastoma and ganglioneuroma) account for 7–10% of all tumours in childhood. In these tumours, the *MYCN* oncogene status, extension of the disease and age are the most relevant prognostic factors. The 5-year survival probability ranges from >95% for patients with nonmetastatic resectable tumour and absence of *MYCN* amplification to <20% for patients with metastatic disease and *MYCN*-amplified tumour.

R. Luksch (✉) • M. Podda • N. Puma
SC Pediatria Oncologica, Fondazione IRCCS Istituto Nazionale dei Tumori, Milan, Italy
e-mail: roberto.Luksch@istitutotumori.mi.it

C. Chiesa • M.R. Castellani
SC Medicina Nucleare, Fondazione IRCCS Istituto Nazionale dei Tumori, Milan, Italy

E. Seregni
SS Terapia Medico-Nucleare ed Endocrinologia, Fondazione IRCCS Istituto Nazionale dei Tumori, Milan, Italy

C. Morosi
SS Radiologia Paediatrica, Fondazione IRCCS Istituto Nazionale dei Tumori, Milan, Italy

D. Biasoni
SC Chirurgia Urologica, Fondazione IRCCS Istituto Nazionale dei Tumori, Milan, Italy

G. Gatta
SSD Epidemiologia Valutativa, Fondazione IRCCS Istituto Nazionale dei Tumori, Milan, Italy

L. Gandola
SS Radioterapia Paediatrica, Fondazione IRCCS Istituto Nazionale dei Tumori, Milan, Italy

P. Collini
SS Patologia dei tessuti molli e dell'osso e diagnostica generale e dell'età evolutiva, Fondazione IRCCS Istituto Nazionale dei Tumori, Milan, Italy

P. Scanagatta
SC Chirurgia Toracica, Fondazione IRCCS Istituto Nazionale dei Tumori, Milan, Italy

G. Riccipetitoni
Dip. Chirurgia Paediatrica, Ospedale dei Bambini V. Buzzi, ASST Fatebenefratelli Sacco, Milan, Italy

E. Bombardieri et al. (eds.), *Clinical Applications of Nuclear Medicine Targeted Therapy*,
https://doi.org/10.1007/978-3-319-63067-0_18

Pheochromocytoma and paraganglioma are very rare. Functioning tumours are associated with symptoms related to catecholamine secretion, whereas nonfunctioning tumours present with symptoms related to tumour mass effect, or present incidentally. These tumours are generally benign, but a small percentage of them are high-grade malignancies requiring multimodality therapies. Ninety percent of the cases are sporadic, while 10% are familial, such as those that occur as part of the multiple endocrine neoplasia syndromes.

18.1 Introduction

Neuroendocrine tumours comprise different neoplasms arising from the endocrine glands or neuroendocrine tissues. The focus of this chapter are tumours arising from the neural crest-derived cells in the adrenal medulla or extra-adrenal paraganglia: peripheral neuroblastic tumours (including neuroblastoma, ganglioneuroblastoma and ganglioneuroma), pheochromocytoma and paraganglioma. In the present chapter, we review the current approach to the diagnosis, staging and management of patients. Peripheral neuroblastic tumours (PNTs) account for 7–10% of all tumours in children, while pheochromocytoma and paraganglioma are very rare. Due to the rarity of these tumours, we believe that the best treatment is provided at tertiary care centres with multidisciplinary teams specialized in the management of these tumours.

18.2 Neuroblastoma and Other Peripheral Neuroblastic Tumours

Neuroblastoma and other peripheral neuroblastic tumours (PNTs) are a family of tumours of the sympathetic nervous system derived from the primitive neural crest. In fact, the term PNTs encompasses the histologic variants neuroblastoma, ganglioneuroblastoma (with two variants: nodular and intermixed) and ganglioneuroma. Neuroblastoma is the most common and clinically relevant variant and, together with the very uncommon nodular ganglioneuroblastoma, is considered malignant in nature, as they tend to progress to death in the absence of treatment. By contrast, intermixed ganglioneuroblastoma and ganglioneuroma are composed of mature cells and are therefore considered benign and curable by surgery alone.

18.2.1 Epidemiology and Risk Factors

PNTs are very rare but are the most frequent solid tumours in children in pre-scholar age, accounting for around 8% of all tumours in childhood. Ninety-five percent of all PNET occur in children under 5 years of age, and the median age at diagnosis is about 19 months. The occurrence of PNTs is unusual in adolescents and adults [1]. These tumours are slightly more frequent in boys than girls [2]. In Europe according to the RARECAREnet project (period of diagnosis 2000–2007), the annual incidence rate was six cases per million in children 0–14 years old [3]. The rarity of neuroblastoma and other PNTs is a challenge for the feasibility of epidemiological studies, but data from recent literature suggest that certain types of exposure are more common in neuroblastoma patients [4]. Several studies have provided evidence of an increasing risk of disease with alcohol use during pregnancy, with odds ratios (OR) ranging between 1.2 and 12.0 [4–6]. A significant risk was identified for nonvolatile and volatile hydrocarbons (OR: 1.5), specifically diesel fuels, lacquer thinner and turpentine [6]. Two studies showed a strong association between the use of oral contraceptives or other sex hormones in early pregnancy, and a positive significant association was also found with the administration of codeine during pregnancy or lactation (OR: 3.4) [7, 8].

18.2.2 Pathology

PNTs derive from neuroectodermal embryonic cells [9]. These tumours show two main components, neuroblastic cells and Schwannian cells, in various proportions. PNTs are assigned to one of four categories:

1. Neuroblastoma (Schwannian stroma-poor). Neuroblastomas are defined as neuroblastic Schwannian stroma-poor. By definition, the proportion of tumour tissue with stroma-rich histology should not exceed 50%.
2. Ganglioneuroblastoma, intermixed (Schwannian stroma-rich). This is a tumour in which well-defined microscopic nests of neuroblastic cells are intermixed, or randomly distributed, in a ganglioneuromatous component. The nests are made up of neuroblastic cells in various stages of differentiation in a background of abundant neuropil.
3. Ganglioneuroblastoma, nodular (composite Schwannian stroma-rich/stroma-dominant/stroma-poor). This tumour is characterized by the presence of one or more microscopic nodule(s) of stroma-poor neuroblastoma in a background of stroma-rich or stroma-dominant component.
4. Ganglioneuroma (Schwannian stroma-dominant). This tumour consists of a predominant Schwannian stromal component with completely differentiated ganglion cells ("mature ganglioneuroma") or incompletely differentiated ganglion cells ("maturing ganglioneuroma").

The International Neuroblastoma Pathology Classification (INPC) distinguishes different categories of neuroblastoma and defines the prognostic impact of each category. For neuroblastoma and ganglioneuroblastoma nodular, age and two microscopic features—mitosis-karyorrhexis index (MKI) and grade of differentiation—have to be taken into account (Table 18.1) [9–11].

Table 18.1 Prognostic groups according to the International Neuroblastoma Pathology Classification (INPC) [9–11]

Ganglioncuroma mature: favourable histology	
Ganglioneuroma maturing: favourable histology Neuroblastoma: favourable histology	
	<18 months: neuroblastoma poorly differentiated or differentiating with low MKI (<2%) or intermediate MKI (>2% and <4%)
	Between 18 months and 5 years: neuroblastoma differentiating with low MKI
Neuroblastoma: unfavourable histology	<18 months: neuroblastoma undifferentiated Neuroblastomas with high MKI (>4%)
	Between 18 months and 5 years: neuroblastoma undifferentiated or poorly differentiated, any MKI Neuroblastoma differentiating with intermediate or high MKI
	>5 years: neuroblastoma, all histotypes
Ganglioneuroblastoma: favourable histology	Ganglioneuroblastoma with nodule(s) of neuroblastoma with favourable histology
Ganglioneuroblastoma: unfavourable histology	Ganglioneuroblastoma with nodule(s) of neuroblastoma with unfavourable histology

18.2.3 Biological Features

Neuroblastoma cells display several genomic and chromosomal abnormalities, and the modern technologies have revealed a complex picture of chromosomal abnormalities in both localized and metastatic tumours. The first molecular marker strongly associated with a poor prognosis was *MYCN* gene amplification. *MYCN* is a member of the *MYC* proto-oncogene family, which encodes transcription factors that regulate the expression of approximately 15% of all human genes, and its overexpression markedly impacts cell behaviour [12]. *MYCN* amplification plays a crucial role in the aggressiveness of the tumour, and several studies have shown that *MYCN* amplification promotes tumour growth and tumour progression. *MYCN* is found to be amplified in at least 20% of neuroblastomas, with a greater prevalence in patients with metastatic disease at onset [12]. A significant correlation between *MYCN* amplification and poor prognosis has been demonstrated in patients with localized tumours, and patients with disseminated tumour showing *MYCN* amplification have more rapid progression than those who do not have *MYCN* amplification [12, 13]. The discovery of structural (or segmental) chromosomal abnormalities in neuroblastoma is very important because, apart from *MYCN*, other aberrations have been found to be associated with a poor prognosis: chromosome 1p deletion, chromosome 17q gain and chromosome 11q loss. Chromosome 11q loss is less frequent than other aberrations but is very important and has been included in the new international staging and risk stratification of neuroblastoma as a negative predictive factor in patients under 18 months of age with localized or metastatic tumours (see below in the following paragraph) [14–18].

A group of genes that are mostly involved in PNTs belong to the TRK gene family that encode for tyrosine kinases. These kinases regulate cell growth, differentiation and programmed cell death of neurons in both the central and peripheral nervous systems [19]. TRKA is the receptor for nerve growth factor (NGF), and its expression may be involved in the regulation of cell differentiation and in the induction of programmed cell death of neural crest cells of sympathoadrenal lineage. Tumour cells expressing TRKA undergo cell differentiation in the presence of NGF, and their presence in the tumour is associated with a favourable patient's outcome, while its expression is almost completely downregulated in tumours with *MYCN* amplification [19, 20]. *ALK*, the anaplastic lymphoma kinase gene, is a fused gene between nucleophosmin and a tyrosine kinase region in the t(2;5)(p23;q35) chromosome translocation. When inappropriately activated, *ALK* acts as an oncogene and triggers signalling cascades of different metabolic pathways. Recently, the *ALK* gene has been identified as the first neuroblastoma-predisposing gene [21, 22]. In neuroblastoma cells, *ALK* becomes activated by point mutations in the tyrosine kinase domain and is overexpressed in advanced neuroblastoma and in Schwannian stroma-poor tumours [21–25]. These alterations are present in 10–14% of neuroblastomas.The importance of *ALK* determination in neuroblastoma is due to the recent availability for clinical use of small molecule inhibitors that could target the *ALK*-activated receptor [24].

18.2.4 Clinical Presentation

About 70% of PNTs originate in the retroperitoneum (in adrenal glands or paravertebral ganglia) and present as an abdominal mass with symptoms of compression of the abdominal viscera. When PNTs originate in the posterior mediastinal ganglia (20% of cases), they cause frequently respiratory symptoms. In about 5% of cases, PNTs originate in the neck, causing the presence of a palpable laterocervical mass, and the symptoms of the Bernard-Horner syndrome are evident when the cranial proportion of the mediastinum is also involved. A 5% of cases of PNTs arises in the pelvis, causing sphincteral impairment [26, 27]. When a paravertebral tumour infiltrates the spinal canal through the intervertebral foramina (about 7% of cases), the signs and symptoms of spinal epidural compression are present [28, 29]. In cases of nonmetastatic disease, usually the outcome is favourable, but the majority of them develop definitive neurologic and orthopaedic sequelae. For this reason, an early diagnosis and a rapid therapy are crucial to avoid permanent damages [28, 29]. In 1–2% of cases, PNTs present with paraneoplastic syndromes. Opsoclonus-myoclonus-ataxia is a paraneoplastic pattern consequent to the production of anti-cerebellar autoantibodies [30]. As in the case of spinal compression, most of these patients survive but are at risk of developing psychomotor sequelae and intellectual deficits [30]. Rarely, a vasoactive intestinal peptide (VIP) syndrome is present at onset causing profuse watery diarrhoea as the result of a

VIP production by the tumour [31]. In 50% of patients with neuroblastoma, metastatic dissemination at onset is present. The cortical bone and the bone marrow are the most frequently involved sites. Patients with metastatic disease present often with systemic symptoms (fever, pain, weight loss, periorbital ecchymoses) [26, 27].

18.2.5 Diagnostic Criteria

For diagnosis and staging, the following examinations are required, as indicated by the International Neuroblastoma Staging System (INSS) [26, 27, 32]:

- CT or MR of the site of the primary tumour, to evaluate the extension of the primary disease.
- Histological evaluation of the primary tumour or of one of the sites of metastases if present.
- Bone marrow aspirate and biopsy at two different sites, to evaluate whether bone marrow infiltration is present; immunocytochemical detection or RT-PCR/FISH techniques to detect bone marrow infiltration may be performed but are considered investigative [33].
- Metaiodobenzylguanidine (I-MIBG) scintigraphy, to evaluate the site of the primary tumour and to detect metastatic sites, both in the skeleton and in the soft tissues. Nowadays, in the ongoing international trials of high-risk neuroblastoma, an MIBG scan score has been introduced for the evaluation of response [34].
- Levels of urinary catecholamine metabolites (homovanillic and vanillylmandelic acids).
- Additional evaluations are ferritin level, serum LDH and neuron-specific enolase (NSE).

18.2.6 Staging and Prognosis

The staging system used in the past two decades, called International Neuroblastoma Staging System (INSS), was based on the surgeon's judgement of resectability at the time of diagnosis [32], while in 2009 the International Neuroblastoma Risk Group (INRG) classification system was developed (Table 18.2) [18].

Table 18.2 Image-defined risk factors (IDRFs) in neuroblastic tumours [35]

Ipsilateral tumour extension within two body compartments	
Neck	Tumour encasing carotid and/or vertebral artery and/or internal jugular vein
	Tumour extending to the base of the skull
	Tumour compressing the trachea
Cervicothoracic junction	Tumour encasing brachial plexus roots
	Tumour encasing subclavian vessels and/or vertebral and/or carotid artery
	Tumour compressing the trachea
Thorax	Tumour encasing the aorta and/or major branches
	Tumour compressing the trachea and/or principal bronchi
	Lower mediastinal tumour, infiltrating the costovertebral junction between T9 and T12
Thoraco-abdominal	Tumour encasing the aorta and/or the vena cava
Abdomen/pelvis	Tumour infiltrating the porta hepatis and/or the hepatoduodenal ligament
	Tumour encasing branches of the superior mesenteric artery and the mesentery root
	Tumour encasing the origin of celiac axis and/or of the superior mesenteric artery
	Tumour invading one or both renal pedicles
	Tumour encasing the aorta and/or the vena cava
	Tumour encasing the iliac vessels
	Pelvic tumour across the sciatic nerve
	Intraspinal tumour extension whatever the location provided that more than one-third of the spinal canal in the axial plane is invaded and/or the perimedullary leptomeningeal spaces are not visible and/or the spinal cord signal is abnormal
	Infiltration of adjacent organs/structures: pericardium, diaphragm, kidney, liver, duodeno-pancreatic block and mesentery
Conditions to be recorded, but not considered IDRFs	Multifocal primary tumours; pleural effusion, with or without malignant cells; ascites, with or without malignant cells

This system defines reproducible risk groups more homogeneously, and radiological criteria at diagnosis based on the relation of the tumour to the adjacent structures and vasculature have been adopted as image-defined risk factors (IDRFs) potentially associated with surgery-related complications [17, 18, 35, 36]. These IDRFs are the basis for the new International Neuroblastoma Risk Group Staging System (INRGSS) that is nowadays universally accepted (Table 18.3) [17]. Several international groups developed models of risk stratification to facilitate the delivery of risk-adapted treatments, and various biological features have been added to the clinical characteristics [17, 37, 38]. Nowadays the most important prognostic factors include age, stage and *MYCN* amplification. Additional prognostic markers, such as histopathological classification, tumour ploidy and chromosomal anomalies including 11q aberration, have been integrated in the International Neuroblastoma Risk Group Consensus Pretreatment Classification Scheme, in order to establish a consensus approach to pretreatment risk stratification (Table 18.4) [17].

Table 18.3 International Neuroblastoma Risk Group Staging System (INRGSS) [18]

Stage	Characteristics
Stage L1	Radiological risk factors absent: localized tumour not involving vital structures as defined by the list of image-defined risk factors, and confined to one body compartment
Stage L2	Locoregional tumour with presence of one or more image-defined risk factors
Stage M	Distant metastatic disease (except stage MS)
Stage MS	Metastatic disease in children younger than 18 months with metastases confined to the skin, liver and/or bone marrow (bone marrow involvement should be limited to <10% of total nucleated cells on smears or biopsy)

Table 18.4 International Neuroblastoma Risk Group consensus pretreatment classification scheme [17]

INRG stage	Age (months)	Historical category	Grade of tumour differentiation	*MYCN*	11q aberration	Ploidy	Pretreatment risk group
L1/L2		GN maturing; GN intermixed					A Very low
L1		Any, except GN maturing or GNB intermixed		NA[a]			B Very low
				Amp[b]			K High
L2	<18	Any, except GN maturing or GNB intermixed		NA	No		D Low
					Yes		G Intermediate
	>18	GNB nodular; neuroblastoma	Differentiating	NA	No		E Low
					Yes		H Intermediate
			Poorly differentiated or undifferentiated	NA			
				Amp			N High
M	<18			NA		Hyperdiploid	F Low
	<12			NA		Diploid	I Intermediate
	12 to <18				NA	Diploid	J Intermediate
	<18			Amp			O High
	≥18						P High
MS	<18			NA	No		C Very low
					Yes		Q High
				Amp			R High

[a]NA = *MYCN* not amplified
[b]Amp = *MYCN* amplified

In infants, the prognosis is very good, while it is somewhat unfavourable in older children. Five-year survival in patients diagnosed between 2000 and 2007 declined from 87% 1 year after diagnosis to 70% at 3 years [39]. Five-year survival for patients with neuroblastoma and ganglioneuroblastoma was lowest in adolescents and adults: 48% and 40%, in 15-/24-year-old patients and 25-/64-year-old patients, respectively [3, 40–43]. The clinical course of neuroblastoma in adults seems only modestly influenced by therapy, the outcome being poorer at all stages [40].

18.2.7 Treatment Modalities

The therapeutic modalities include surgery, chemotherapy, radiotherapy and biotherapy based on the use of vitamin A derivatives and immunotherapy, while observation-only is undertaken only in few patients [14, 26, 27]. The different treatment modalities can be combined basing on prognostic factors and the consequent risk-group assignment [17].

Surgery plays an important role as diagnostic and therapeutic tool. In patients with nonmetastatic disease, surgery may achieve complete tumour excision, and in this case, it may be the only treatment. In other cases, when the features of the tumour and the image-defined risk factors indicate that surgical resection is not feasible without risk, surgery is limited to providing enough tumour tissue to make the histological diagnosis and to carry out biologic studies. In these cases, pre-surgical chemotherapy should be administered in order to shrink the tumour and enable safe tumour resection [18, 44–47]. Since neuroblastoma has an elevated tropism for lymphatic vessels, surgical tumour resection should include exploration of locoregional lymph nodes. In the case of spinal canal invasion through intervertebral foramina, laminotomy is indicated only in the presence of rapidly progressive neurological symptoms, as chemotherapy can rapidly reduce the volume of the tumour and relieve compression [28, 48, 49]. In case of metastatic disease at onset, surgery has a role for the diagnosis to assess histology and biologic studies, preferably with the biopsy of the primary tumour, while has a controversial role as therapeutic tool [50–52]. However, given the high incidence of local relapses, the current indication in the ongoing trials is the resection of the primary tumour after induction chemotherapy that in the majority of cases permits a shrinking of the primary tumour [50–52].

Chemotherapy is the pivotal treatment modality for patients with metastatic or locally advanced disease. Different drugs have proved effective in the last four decades, and are nowadays commonly used in the first-line treatments, usually as combination chemotherapy including different combinations of vincristine, cyclophosphamide, *cis*-platin, doxorubicin, epipodophyllotoxins (VP16, VP26) and melphalan [53]. Subsequent studies have proved the activity and efficacy of other drugs (ifosfamide, carboplatin, topotecan, irinotecan and taxol) [26, 27, 54, 55]. Owing to the poor results yielded by previous modalities in metastatic patients, a number of trials including "consolidation" therapy with high-dose chemotherapy and autologous bone marrow or peripheral blood stem cell rescue were designed in the hope of increasing the rates of responders and long-term survivors. The use of high doses increased both response rates and the number of long-term survivors [56–59].

Radiotherapy is an important tool, since neuroblastoma is a radiosensitive tumour. Effective doses are in the range of 15–32 Gy, and external beam radiotherapy is being continuously refined as risk factors that limit its use in low-risk patients are identified [60–63]. New technologies, such as intensity-modulated photon techniques (IMRT or VMAT) and proton therapy could nowadays offer the possibility to optimize tumour volume coverage, thus minimizing the risk of toxic effects on vital surrounding organs [64, 65]. In the current protocols, irradiation of the primary tumour bed is commonly undertaken after surgery in patients with locally advanced disease + unfavourable biology and/or histopathology *or in patients with* metastatic disease. External beam radiation therapy is often used on symptomatic lesions in the palliative care setting [66]. Another important radiotherapeutic approach is radio-metabolic therapy with I-131, which is carried by means of benzylguanidine (I-131 MIBG). Radio-metabolic treatments for PNTs are described in another dedicated chapter.

Biotherapy consisting of the use of differentiative therapy with vitamin A derivatives and with immunotherapy has been demonstrated efficacious in the context of minimal residual disease. The efficacy of the use of 13-*cis*-retinoic acid as maintenance phase after intensive treatments for high-risk patients was demonstrated by the Children's Oncology Group trial conducted between 1991 and 1996 [59]. In a subsequent trial of the same group, immunotherapy with an anti-disialoganglioside-2(anti-GD2) monoclonal antibody plus cytokines was added to 13-*cis*-retinoic acid during the maintenance phase, in a randomized fashion (13-*cis*-retinoic acid alone vs. 13-*cis*-retinoic acid and anti-GD2 + GM-CSF/IL2). The addiction of immunotherapy is translated into a significant improvement of both 3-year and long-term survival [67]. This was the best clinical result obtained in a randomized study in high-risk patients, and the maintenance with 13-*cis*-retinoic acid + anti-GD2 and GM-CSF/IL2 is considered up to now the standard in the United States. The ongoing SIOPEN study for high-risk patients evaluates in a randomized fashion the use of ch.14.18 anti-GD2 monoclonal antibody with/without IL2, and the anti-GD2 monoclonal antibody is given in long-term infusion with the objective to reduce the side effects of this treatment.

18.2.8 Risk-Based Treatments

Very low- and low-risk disease—(nearly one-third of all subjects newly diagnosed PNT). Ganglioneuroma and ganglioneuroblastoma intermixed are tumours that do not possess malignant potential and thus require only surgical resection followed by observation [26, 27, 68]. The prognosis in these cases is very good. According to the SIOP Europe Neuroblastoma (SIOPEN) recommendations, this group includes patients with a single *MYCN* gene copy number and L1 stage, or L2 stage + age younger than 18 months, or Ms stage + age younger than 12 months.

Surgical resection of the primary tumour is the only treatment required for L1 stage patients, while a few courses of low-dose chemotherapy are considered sufficient for the majority of L2 stage patients in preparation for surgery. Some studies have supported this policy, with overall survival (OS) rates around 99% for stage 1 and 95% for stage 2 were reported [47, 69, 70]. The German Neuroblastoma Group studied infants with localized neuroblastoma without *MYCN* amplification. These patients received chemotherapy only in the event of life-threatening symptoms, while in the other cases the tumour was either resected or kept under observation. Of the group of 93 patients with partially resected tumours, spontaneous regression was seen in 44. OS at 3 years was 99%, and EFS was 94% [71]. For patients with stage Ms disease, both the Children's Oncology Group and SIOP Europe Neuroblastoma studies found an OS rate close to 100% among infants with normal *MYCN* gene and minimal mild chemotherapy treatment, or observation for those without life-threatening symptoms [72, 73].

Intermediate-risk disease—(10–15% of newly diagnosed patients). This category includes L1 stage patients with amplified *MYCN* gene; L2 stage patients older than 18 months with normal *MYCN* gene copy number, including patients with symptomatic epidural compression; and stage M patients 1 year old or younger with normal *MYCN* gene copy number.

For L1 stage patients with amplified *MYCN* gene (very rare cases), the limited data available are not yet sufficient to define the amount and intensity of treatment, and we know that 3-year EFS does not exceed 60% with surgery alone [69, 74]. At the moment, the SIOPEN guidelines suggest four to six courses of standard chemotherapy for these patients. Patients with L2 stage older than 18 months with normal *MYCN* gene copy number, when treated with four to six courses of standard-dose chemotherapy and surgery, have 5-year OS around 85%, with significantly better results in younger patients (age 12–18 months) and those with favourable histology [75–79]. The effectiveness of administering 21–30 Gy radiotherapy to an incompletely resected tumour in this setting is under investigation.

High-risk disease—(approximately 40% of all newly diagnosed). This category includes patients over 1 year of age with disseminated disease (the large majority of cases), L2 stage patients with amplified *MYCN* and Ms stage patients with amplified *MYCN*.

The treatment of these patients remains one of the greatest challenges in paediatric oncology, as such cases account for most of the mortality associated with this malignancy. Although the current 5-year OS rate remains no greater than 35%, much progress has been made since the 10% OS rate reported in the 1970s [26, 27, 80, 81]. This improvement has been achieved through intensification of induction therapy plus the use of myeloablative chemotherapy as consolidation treatment and biologic treatment of minimal residual disease (MRD). In fact, given that neuroblastoma is sensitive to chemotherapy, intensive multi-agent induction regimens have been employed to induce rapid and massive reduction of the tumour burden. The results of several studies have supported the efficacy of this strategy, as greater response rates have been obtained by increasing dose intensity, particularly of platinum compounds [26, 27, 82]. The aim of consolidation treatment with high-dose chemotherapy is to eliminate the tumour cells remaining from the previous phase [55–59, 83–86]. After the favourable results with the introduction of a maintenance phase including vitamin A derivatives and immunotherapy as above described [59, 67], the ongoing SIOPEN study for high-risk patients is evaluating the use of ch.14.18 anti-GD2 with/without IL2, anti-GD2 is given by means of long-term infusion, in order to reduce the side effects of this treatment.

18.2.9 Therapeutic Perspectives for the Future

During the last decade, tremendous advances have been made in clarifying the genetic features of PNTs. This enabled the prognosis of the individual patient to be better defined [37, 87]. A fuller understanding of tumour biology could also significantly improve patient management both on diagnosis and on relapse [37] and may enable us to identify the molecular aberrations and the cellular networks leading to tumour initiation and progression in each individual patient. Furthermore, access to an increasing number of actionable drugs now offers the possibility to develop new clinical trials with adaptive designs based on the presence of selective tumour characteristics. Different therapeutic agents are under investigation, including those targeting *MYCN* [88], or aurora kinases [89, 90], or RTKs and PI3K [91, 92], histone deacetylases (HDACS) [93] and *ALK* [94, 95]. *ALK*-targeted therapy seems to play an important role in patients with tumours with activating mutations in *ALK* that are observed in 8–10% of neuroblastoma, and de novo or acquired resistance to the *ALK* inhibitors is present in some cases [94], a phenomenon which will necessitate new strategies [25]. Considerable evidence suggests that neuroblastoma is a potentially immunogenic tumour and that it may elicit responses on the part of either adaptive or innate immunity [14]. Among adoptive immunotherapies, the use of anti-disialoganglioside-2 (GD2) has yielded the most notable clinical results as described above, and preclinical studies and early clinical trials have shown the potential role of adoptive for GD2 [67, 96]. The refinement of biotechnology has enabled new generation of anti-GD2 chimeric antigen receptors (CARs) T-cells to be produced, with a view to obtaining the best possible immune recognition and durable immune responses [96–99].

18.2.10 Follow-Up and Sequelae

The relapse of PNTs usually occurs within 2 years after the end of treatment in patients with metastatic disease or within 2 years after surgery in the case of localized disease [26, 27]. However, relapses occurring more than 5 years after the end of treatment are not exceptional, which means that patients need fairly long follow-up. Furthermore, since the very intensive treatment administered to patients with metastatic disease carries the risk of a number of late toxic complications, a long-term follow-up programme for those patients has to be planned. Any signs or symptoms indicative of relapse should be evaluated by means of physical examination, urinary catecholamine assay, complete blood count and imaging at the site of the primary tumour. It is currently recommended that patients be assessed every 3 months for the first year, every 4 months in the second year and every 6 months thereafter up to the fifth post-treatment year. As relapse in patients with stage 4 disease usually involves metastatic sites, MIBG scan and bone marrow evaluation should be performed every 6 months in the first 2 years of follow-up [26, 27].

As described above, the treatment is tailored according to risk classification, and high-risk patients receive very intensive treatment [17]. Data from the Childhood Cancer Survivor Study showed that survivors have a higher rate of mortality (standardized mortality ratio of 5.6) and of further malignant neoplasms (7% cumulative incidence at 30 years) than the US population of the same age and sex and suffer a greater number of chronic health conditions. The most frequently reported long-term sequelae are endocrine deficits, mainly hypothyroidism, growth hormone deficiency/diminished growth and gonadal damage [100–105].

The risk of developing second malignancies in high-risk patients is well known [106]. The risk of second malignancies is even higher when an excess of epipodophyllotoxins and high-dose alkylants has been used. Indeed, in patients who had undergone high-dose chemotherapy with stem cell rescue, 15-year cumulative incidence of second malignancies exceeds 10%, without evidence of a plateau at 15 years [106, 107].

18.3 Pheochromocytoma and Paraganglioma

These tumours arise from neural crest-derived neuroendocrine cells in the adrenal medulla or extra-adrenal paraganglia. Pheochromocytoma (PHEO) is the term used to describe a chromaffin tumour arising from the adrenal medulla, whereas paraganglioma (PARAGL) is an extra-adrenal tumour that arises from both sympathetic and parasympathetic paraganglia located outside the cerebrospinal axis [108].

18.3.1 Epidemiology

PHEO and PARAGL are very rare tumours and represent <7% of tumours that arise from the sympathetic nervous system. Together, they have an estimated incidence of 0.3 cases/million/year [109]. Only 10–20% of cases are identified during childhood, the majority being PHE. In childhood, the diagnosis is done at an average age of 11 years, with a slight predominance in boys [109–112].

18.3.2 Biological Characteristics

These tumours show differences in biological characteristics, malignant potential and clinical presentation, depending on site and secretive characteristics. PHEO is a tumour arising in the adrenal gland and is composed of cells secreting catecholamines and their metabolites (dopamine/3-methoxytyramine, norepinephrine/3-methoxytyramine and epinephrine/metanephrine) [108, 113]. PARAGL is an extra-adrenal tumour and can arise anywhere from the base of the skull to the pelvis, most commonly in the abdomen, near the renal vessels or from the organ of Zuckerkandl, an adrenal structure consisting of chromaffin tissue located around the origin of the inferior mesenteric artery. PARAGL can be secretory or nonsecretory [108, 114]. The vast majority of head and neck PARAGL are nonsecretory, whereas those at intra-abdominal localization are usually secretory.

PHEO often occur as sporadic tumours (90% of cases) but can also develop as part of a hereditary tumour syndrome including VHL disease, MEN2A, MEN2B, NF1, the familial PGL syndromes (PGL1-4) and rarely the TSC [113–115]. VHL disease is responsible for the majority of cases in childhood followed by the familial PARAGL syndromes and MEN2 [110, 114, 115]. Hereditary tumours often occur multifocally and, in the case of PHE, bilaterally. *SDHB* is the suspected gene responsible for aggressive disease in children [110, 113–116].

Areas of ganglioneuroblastoma, ganglioneuroma or carcinoma are sometimes admixed, in which case the term composite pheochromocytoma or composite paraganglioma is used [117, 118].

18.3.3 Clinical Characteristics

PHEO and PARAGL can present clinically with signs correlated to catecholamine hypersecretion. In 80% of cases, PHEO is accompanied by hypertension, and the classic triad headache + palpitations + diaphoresis can be present; other frequent signs/symptoms are pallor, orthostatic hypotension, syncope, tremor and anxiety [110, 113, 119]. Symptoms in nonsecreting tumours can be related to the tumour mass effect (e.g. pain) and can also be nonspecific such as gastrointestinal symptoms, weight loss, low-grade fever and behavioural problems. The diagnosis can also be an incidental radiographic finding or because of the screening for an associated hereditary tumour syndrome [108, 119, 120].

PHEO and PARAGL in childhood are malignant in a % ranging from 12 to 65, depending on the case series reported [108, 110, 121]. Malignancy is established by identification of metastases where paraganglia are absent (bones, liver, lungs) or when secondary lymph nodes infiltration is present [117, 121, 122]. The risk of malignant transformation is greater for secreting PARAGL, and the highest risk for malignancy and death is in *SDHB*-related sympathetic PARAGL [114, 121, 123].

The prognosis of children diagnosed with PHEO or PARAGL is generally good. Five- and 10-year survival rates are 98%, and 20-year survival rate is 84% [108, 113, 120]. However, PHEO and PARAGL have unpredictable behaviour. In fact, children are at risk for the development of metachronous delayed presentation of metastatic disease at several years after the diagnosis. Children with metastatic disease demonstrate usually an indolent clinical course, with average overall survival >6 years after the diagnosis of metastatic disease.

18.3.4 Diagnosis

The initial biochemical test when a secreting PHEO or PARAGL is suspected is the assessment of plasma and urine metanephrines (metanephrines and normetanephrines) [108, 119, 124]. Additionally, chromogranin A (a secretory protein present in the soluble matrix of chromaffin granules) is an effective tumour marker that may correlate with tumour size and malignant potential [125, 126].

Once the diagnosis of a secretory tumour is made, radiographic studies are undertaken to identify the location of the tumour [118, 119, 127]. Abdominal US, followed by CT or MRI of the abdomen and pelvis, should be done initially. If these examinations are negative, radiological evaluation of the neck and chest is necessary. Functional testing with ^{123}I-labelled metaiodobenzylguanidine scintigraphy is highly specific, can reveal tumours not detected with cross-sectional imaging and could identify other sites of disease [128]. Other nuclear imaging modalities evaluated for these tumours are SST receptor scintigraphy using ^{111}In-DTPA-pentetreotide (octreotide), [^{18}F] fluoro-dihydroxyphenylalanine PET, [^{18}F]-fluorodopamine PET or FDG-PET [129–131]. [^{18}F]FDG-PET seems superior in the evaluation of cases with *SDHB* mutation carriers [131].

There is no clinical staging system for malignant PHEO or PARAGL.

18.3.5 Treatment

Surgery has a pivotal role in the treatment of chromaffin tumours. The surgical procedure for PHEO is adrenalectomy. In the setting of bilateral tumours or PHEO arising within a hereditary tumour syndrome, cortical-sparing procedures should be considered [132–134]. The surgical approach to PARAGL depends upon the location of the tumour [119, 135]. Medical treatment in functional PHEO or PARAGL should be initiated in preparation for surgery in order to minimize the complications that may arise from acute secretion of catecholamines during induction of anaesthesia and manipulation of the tumour (i.e. alfa-blockers or alfa-blockers + beta-blockers) [113, 118, 136, 137]. Intravenous antihypertensive medications and vasopressors (sodium nitroprusside, beta-blockers, antiarrhythmics) would be necessary for intraoperative use. Postoperatively, the patient should be monitored to avoid hypotension and hypoglycaemia [136, 137].

Patients with unresectable tumours or metastases can have excellent palliation of symptoms related to catecholamine hypersecretion through the use of the same medications employed for preoperative blockade. Radiation therapy can be used in cases of unresectable PARAGL. Treatment modalities for advanced malignant PHEO or PARAGL include also ^{131}I-MIBG and other radiolabelled compounds, chemotherapy and targeted therapies, among which sunitinib showed promise [122–124, 138]. Chemotherapy permits to obtain partial or complete remission in around 50% of cases and include cyclophosphamide-based or dacarbazine-based regimens combined with vincristine (CVD) or doxorubicin (CVDD or CDD) [12, 81, 127, 134].

18.3.6 Follow-Up

As described above, children with PHEO and PARAGL have unpredictable behaviour and are at risk for the development of metachronous tumours at several years after the diagnosis. Children who underwent gland-sparing procedures for multicentric adrenal lesions are also at risk for recurrence of the primary tumour [139, 140].

The patients at higher risk of relapse or appearance of metachronous metastases are those with PARAGL or a known *SDHB* mutation. For these reasons, a follow-up on regular basis and at long-term is necessary, with biochemical screening and intermittent imaging studies [117–119].

Genetic testing is recommended for all children who present with these tumours, whether or not there is a positive family history [118], and specific recommendations have been made to help the clinician prioritize genetic testing [108, 119].

Acknowledgements The authors want to thank for their support the Associazione Bianca Garavaglia ONLUS, Busto Arsizio (Varese) and the Associazione UNA-Milano, Milan, Italy.

References

1. Gatta G, Ferrari A, Stiller CA, Pastore G, Bisogno G, Trama A, et al. Embryonal cancers in Europe. Eur J Cancer. 2012;48:1425–33.
2. Spix C, Pastore G, Sankila R, Stiller CA, Steliarova-Foucher E. Neuroblastoma incidence and survival in European children (1978-1997): report from the automated childhood cancer information system project. Eur J Cancer. 2006;42:2081–91.
3. RARECAREnet project. Available at http://www.rarecarenet.eu/rarecarenet/.
4. Heck JE, Ritz B, Hung RJ, Hashibe M, Boffetta P. The epidemiology of neuroblastoma: a review. Paediatr Perinat Epidemiol. 2009;23:125–43.
5. Schuz J, Kaletsch U, Meinert R, Kaatsch P, Spix C, Michaelis J. Risk factors for neuroblastoma at different stages of disease. Results from a population-based case-control study in Germany. J Clin Epidemiol. 2001;54:702–9.
6. De Roos AJ, Olshan AF, Teschke K, Poole C, Savitz DA, Blatt J, et al. Parental occupational exposures to chemicals and incidence of neuroblastoma in offspring. Am J Epidemiol. 2001;154:106–14.
7. Michalek AM, Buck GM, Nasca PC, Freedman AN, Baptiste MS, Mahoney MC. Gravid health status, medication use, and risk of neuroblastoma. Am J Epidemiol. 1996;143:996–1001.
8. Cook MN, Olshan AF, Guess HA, Savitz DA, Poole C, Blatt J, et al. Maternal medication use and neuroblastoma in offspring. Am J Epidemiol. 2004;159:721–31.
9. Shimada H, Ambros IM, Dehner LP, Hata J, Joshi VV, Roald B, et al. The international neuroblastoma pathology classification (the Shimada system). Cancer. 1999;86:364–728.
10. Umehara S, Nakagawa A, Matthay KK, Lukens JN, Seeger RC, Stram DO, et al. Histopathology defines prognostic subsets of ganglioneuroblastoma, nodular. Cancer. 2000;89(5):1150–61.
11. Teshiba R, Kawano S, Wang LL, He L, Naranjo A, London WB, et al. Age-dependent prognostic effect by mitosis-karyorrhexis index in neuroblastoma: a report from the Children's Oncology Group. Pediatr Dev Pathol. 2014;17(6):441–9.
12. Schwab M, Alitalo K, Klempnauer KH, Varmus HE, Bishop JM, Gilbert F, et al. Amplified DNA with limited homology to myc cellular oncogene is shared by human neuroblastoma cell lines and a neuroblastoma tumour. Nature. 1983;305:245–8.
13. Tonini GP, Boni L, Pession A, Rogers D, Iolascon A, Basso G, et al. MYCN oncogene amplification in neuroblastoma is associated with worse prognosis, except in stage 4s: the Italian experience with 295 children. J Clin Oncol. 1997;15:85–93.
14. Cheung NK, Dyer MA. Neuroblastoma: developmental biology, cancer genomics and immunotherapy. Nat Rev Cancer. 2013;13(6):397–411.
15. Ambros PF, Ambros IM, Brodeur GM, Haber M, Khan J, Nakagawara A, et al. International consensus for neuroblastoma molecular diagnostics: report from the International Neuroblastoma Risk Group (INRG) Biology Committee. Br J Cancer. 2009;100(9):1471–82.
16. Bagatell R, Beck-Popovic M, London WB, Zhang Y, Pearson AD, Matthay KK, et al. Significance of

MYCN amplification in international neuroblastoma staging system stage 1 and 2 neuroblastoma: a report from the International Neuroblastoma Risk Group database. J Clin Oncol. 2009;27(3):365–70.
17. Cohn SL, Pearson AD, London WB, Monclair T, Ambros PF, Brodeur GM, et al. The International Neuroblastoma Risk Group (INRG) classification system: an INRG task force report. J Clin Oncol. 2009;27(2):289–97.
18. Monclair T, Brodeur GM, Ambros PF, Brisse HJ, Cecchetto G, Holmes K. The International Neuroblastoma Risk Group (INRG) staging system: an INRG task force report. J Clin Oncol. 2009;27(2):298–303.
19. Brodeur GM, Minturn JE, Ho R, Simpson AM, Iyer R, Varela CR, et al. Trk receptor expression and inhibition in neuroblastomas. Clin Cancer Res. 2009;15(10):3244–50.
20. Scaruffi P, Cusano R, Dagnino M, Tonini GP. Detection of DNA polymorphisms and point mutations of high-affinity nerve growth factor receptor (TrkA) in human neuroblastoma. Int J Oncol. 1999;14(5):935–8.
21. Longo L, Panza E, Schena F, Seri M, Devoto M, Romeo G, et al. Genetic predisposition to familial neuroblastoma: identification of two novel genomic regions at 2p and 12p. Hum Hered. 2007;63(3-4):205–11.
22. Mossé YP, Laudenslager M, Longo L, Cole KA, Wood A, Attiyeh EF, et al. Identification of ALK as a major familial neuroblastoma predisposition gene. Nature. 2008;455(7215):930–5.
23. Passoni L, Longo L, Collini P, Coluccia AM, Bozzi F, Podda M, et al. Mutation-independent anaplastic lymphoma kinase overexpression in poor prognosis neuroblastoma patients. Cancer Res. 2009;69(18):7338–46.
24. Mossé YP, Lim MS, Voss SD, Wilner K, Ruffner K, Laliberte J, et al. Safety and activity of crizotinib for paediatric patients with refractory solid tumours or anaplastic large-cell lymphoma: a Children's Oncology Group phase 1 consortium study. Lancet Oncol. 2013;14(6):472–80.
25. Bresler SC, Weiser DA, Huwe PJ, Park JH, Krytska K, Ryles H, et al. ALK mutations confer differential oncogenic activation and sensitivity to ALK inhibition therapy in neuroblastoma. Cancer Cell. 2014;26(5):682–94.
26. Brodeur GM, Hogarty MD, Bagatell R, Mossé YP, Maris JM. Neuroblastoma. In: Pizzo DA, editor. Principles and practice of paediatric oncology. 7th ed. Philadelphia: Wolters Kluwer; 2016. p. 772–97.
27. Luksch R, Castellani MR, Collini P, De Bernardi B, Conte M, Gambini C, Gandola L, Garaventa A, Biasoni D, Podda M, Sementa AR, Gatta G, Tonini GP. Neuroblastoma (Peripheral neuroblastic tumours). Crit Rev Oncol Hematol. 2016 Nov;107:163–81.
28. De Bernardi B, Quaglietta L, Haupt R, Castellano A, Tirtei E, Luksch R, et al. Neuroblastoma with symptomatic epidural compression in the infant: the AIEOP experience. Pediatr Blood Cancer. 2014;61:1369–75.
29. Angelini P, Plantaz D, De Bernardi B, Passagia JG, Rubie H, Pastore G. Late sequelae of symptomatic epidural compression in children with localized neuroblastoma. Pediatr Blood Cancer. 2011;57:473–80.
30. Krug P, Schleiermacher G, Michon J, Valteau-Couanet D, Brisse H, Peuchmaur M, et al. Opsoclonus-myoclonus in children associated or not with neuroblastoma. Eur J Paediatr Neurol. 2010;14(5):400–9.
31. Han W, Wang HM. Refractory diarrhea: a paraneoplastic syndrome of neuroblastoma. World J Gastroenterol. 2015;21:7929–32.
32. Brodeur GM, Pritchard J, Berthold F, Carlsen NL, Castel V, Castelberry RP, et al. Revisions of the international criteria for neuroblastoma diagnosis, staging, and response to treatment. J Clin Oncol. 1993;11:1466–77.
33. Viprey VF, Lastowska MA, Corrias MV, Swerts K, Jackson MS, Burchill SA. Minimal disease monitoring by QRT-PCR: guidelines for identification and systematic validation of molecular markers prior to evaluation in prospective clinical trials. J Pathol. 2008;216(2):245–52.
34. Matthay KK, Shulkin B, Ladenstein R, Michon J, Giammarile F, Lewington V, et al. Criteria for evaluation of disease extent by (123) I-metaiodobenzylguanidine scans in neuroblastoma: a report for the International Neuroblastoma Risk Group (INRG) task force. Br J Cancer. 2010;102(9):1319–26.
35. Cecchetto G, Mosseri V, De Bernardi B, Helardot P, Monclair T, Costa E, et al. Surgical risk factors in primary surgery for localized neuroblastoma: the LNESG1 study of the European International Society of Paediatric Oncology Neuroblastoma Group. J Clin Oncol. 2005;23(33):8483–9.
36. Brisse HJ, McCarville MB, Granata C, Krug KB, Wootton-Gorges SL, Kanegawa K, et al. Guidelines for imaging and staging of neuroblastic tumors: consensus report from the International Neuroblastoma Risk Group project. Radiology. 2011;261(1):243–57.
37. Pinto NR, Applebaum MA, Volchenboum SL, Matthay KK, London WB, Ambros PF, et al. Advances in risk classification and treatment strategies for neuroblastoma. J Clin Oncol. 2015;33:3008–17.
38. Maris JM. Recent advances in neuroblastoma. N Engl J Med. 2010;362(23):2202–11.
39. Gatta G, Botta L, Rossi S, Aareleid T, Bielska-Lasota M, Clavel J, et al. Childhood cancer survival in Europe 1999-2007: results of EUROCARE-5 – a population-based study. Lancet Oncol. 2014;15:35–47.
40. Sorrentino S, Gigliotti AR, Sementa AR, Morsellino V, Conte M, Erminio G, et al. Neuroblastoma in the adult: the Italian experience with 21 patients. J Pediatr Hematol Oncol. 2014;36:499–505.
41. Conte M, Parodi S, De Bernardi B, Milanaccio C, Mazzocco K, Angelini P, et al. Neuroblastoma

in adolescents: the Italian experience. Cancer. 2006;106(6):1409–17.

42. Podda MG, Luksch R, Polastri D, Gandola L, Piva L, Collini P, et al. Neuroblastoma in patients over 12 years old: a 20-year experience at the Istituto Nazionale Tumori of Milan. Tumori. 2010;96(5):684–9.
43. Mossé YP, Deyell RJ, Berthold F, Nagakawara A, Ambros PF, Monclair T, et al. Neuroblastoma in older children, adolescents and young adults: a report from the International Neuroblastoma Risk Group project. Pediatr Blood Cancer. 2014;61(4):627–35.
44. Monclair T, Mosseri V, Cecchetto G, De Bernardi B, Michon J, Holmes K. Influence of image-defined risk factors on the outcome of patients with localised neuroblastoma. A report from the LNESG1 study of the European International Society of Paediatric Oncology Neuroblastoma Group. Pediatr Blood Cancer. 2015;62(9):1536–42.
45. Gunther P, Holland-Cunz S, Schupp CJ, Stockklausner C, Hinz U, Schenk JP. Significance of image-defined risk factors for surgical complications in patients with abdominal neuroblastoma. Eur J Pediatr Surg. 2011;21:314–7.
46. Lim II, Goldman DA, Farber BA, Murphy JM, Abramson SJ, Basu E, et al. Image-defined risk factors for nephrectomy in patients undergoing neuroblastoma resection. J Pediatr Surg. 2016;51:975. https://doi.org/10.1016/j.jpedsurg.2016.02.069.
47. Strother DR, London WB, Schmidt ML, Brodeur GM, Shimada H, Thorner P, et al. Outcome after surgery alone or with restricted use of chemotherapy for patients with low-risk neuroblastoma: results of Children's Oncology Group study P9641. J Clin Oncol. 2012;30(15):1842–8.
48. Plantaz D, Hartmann O, Kalifa C, Sainte-Rose C, Passagia JG, Lemerle J. Dumbbell neuroblastoma. Experience at the Gustave Roussy Institute in 38 cases treated from 1982 to 1987. Arch Fr Pediatr. 1991;48(8):529–33. Review. French. Erratum in: Arch Fr Pediatr 1991;48(10):742.
49. De Bernardi B, Balwierz W, Bejent J, Cohn SL, Garrè ML, Iehara T, et al. Epidural compression in neuroblastoma: diagnostic and therapeutic aspects. Cancer Lett. 2005;228:283–99.
50. Simon T, Häberle B, Hero B, von Schweinitz D, Berthold F. Role of surgery in the treatment of patients with stage 4 neuroblastoma age 18 months or older at diagnosis. J Clin Oncol. 2013;31(6):752–8.
51. La Quaglia MP, Kushner BH, Su W, Heller G, Kramer K, Abramson S, et al. The impact of gross total resection on local control and survival in high-risk neuroblastoma. J Pediatr Surg. 2004;39(3):412–7.
52. Yeung F, Chung PH, Tam PK, Wong KK. Is complete resection of high-risk stage IV neuroblastoma associated with better survival? J Pediatr Surg. 2015;50(12):2107–11.
53. Carli M, Green AA, Hayes FA, et al. International criteria for diagnosis, staging and response to treatment in patients with neuroblastoma. A review. In: Raybaud E, Clément R, editors. Peadiatric oncology. Amsterdam: Excerpta Medica; 1982. p. 141–50.
54. De Kraker J, Pritchard J, Hartmann O, Ninane J. Single-agent ifosfamide inpatient with recurrent neuroblastoma. Pediatr Hematol Oncol. 1987;4:101–4.
55. Philip T, Ghalie R, Pinkerton R. A phase II study of cis-platin and VP16 in neuroblastoma. J Clin Oncol. 1987;5:941–50.
56. Pritchard J, Cotterill SJ, Germond SM, Imeson J, de Kraker J, Jones DR. High dose melphalan in the treatment of advanced neuroblastoma: results of a randomised trial (ENSG-1) by the European Neuroblastoma Study Group. Pediatr Blood Cancer. 2005;44:348–57.
57. Dini G, Lanino E, Garaventa A, Rogers D, Dallorso S, Viscoli C, et al. Myeloablative therapy and unpurged autologous bone marrow transplantation for poor-prognosis neuroblastoma: report of 34 cases. J Clin Oncol. 1991;9(6):962–9.
58. Luksch R, Podda M, Gandola L, Polastri D, Piva L, Castellani R, et al. Stage 4 neuroblastoma: sequential hemi-body irradiation or high-dose chemotherapy plus autologous haemopoietic stem cell transplantation to consolidate primary treatment. Br J Cancer. 2005;92(11):1984–8.
59. Matthay KK, Reynolds CP, Seeger RC, Shimada H, Adkins ES, Haas-Kogan D, et al. Long-term results for children with high-risk neuroblastoma treated on a randomized trial of myeloablative therapy followed by 13-cis-retinoic acid: a Children's Oncology Group study. J Clin Oncol. 2009;27(7):1007–13.
60. Haas-Kogan DA, Swift PS, Selch M, Haase GM, Seeger RC, Gerbing RB, et al. Impact of radiotherapy for high-risk neuroblastoma: a Children's Cancer Group study. Int J Radiat Oncol Biol Phys. 2003;56(1):28–39.
61. Gatcombe HG, Marcus RB Jr, Katzenstein HM, Tighiouart M, Esiashvili N. Excellent local control from radiation therapy for high-risk neuroblastoma. Int J Radiat Oncol Biol Phys. 2009;74(5):1549–54.
62. Laprie A, Michon J, Hartmann O, Munzer C, Leclair MD, Coze C, et al. High-dose chemotherapy followed by locoregional irradiation improves the outcome of patients with international neuroblastoma staging system stage II and III neuroblastoma with MYCN amplification. Cancer. 2004;101(5):1081–9.
63. Gaze MN, Boterberg T, Dieckmann K, Hörmann M, Gains JE, Sullivan KP, et al. Results of a quality assurance review of external beam radiation therapy in the International Society of Paediatric Oncology (Europe) Neuroblastoma Group's high-risk neuroblastoma trial: a SIOPEN study. Int J Radiat Oncol Biol Phys. 2013;85(1):170–4.
64. Hill-Kayser C, Tochner Z, Both S, Lustig R, Reilly A, Balamuth N, et al. Proton versus photon radiation therapy for patients with high-risk neuroblastoma: the need for a customized approach. Pediatr Blood Cancer. 2013;60:1606–11.
65. Hattangadi JA, Rombi B, Yock TI, Broussard G, Friedmann AM, Huang M, et al. Proton radiotherapy for high-risk paediatric neuroblastoma: early outcomes and dose comparison. Int J Radiat Oncol Biol Phys. 2012;83(3):1015–22.

66. Caussa L, Hijal T, Michon J, Helfre S. Role of palliative radiotherapy in the management of metastatic paediatric neuroblastoma: a retrospective single-institution study. Int J Radiat Oncol Biol Phys. 2011;79:214–9.
67. Yu AL, Gilman AL, Ozkaynak MF, London WB, Kreissman SG, Chen HX, et al. Anti-GD2 antibody with GM-CSF, interleukin-2, and isotretinoin for neuroblastoma. N Engl J Med. 2010;363(14):1324–34.
68. De Bernardi B, Gambini C, Haupt R, Granata C, Rizzo A, Conte M, et al. Retrospective study of childhood ganglioneuroma. J Clin Oncol. 2008;26:1710–6.
69. De Bernardi B, Mosseri V, Rubie H, Castel V, Foot A, Ladenstein R, et al. Treatment of localised resectable neuroblastoma. Results of the LNESG1 study by the SIOP Europe Neuroblastoma Group. Br J Cancer. 2008;99:1027–33.
70. Rubie H, De Bernardi B, Gerrard M, Canete A, Ladenstein R, Couturier J, et al. Excellent outcome with reduced treatment in infants with nonmetastatic and unresectable neuroblastoma without MYCN amplification: results of the prospective INES 99.1. J Clin Oncol. 2011;29(4):449–55.
71. Hero B, Simon T, Spitz R, Ernestus K, Gnekow AK, Scheel-Walter HG, et al. Localized infant neuroblastoma often show spontaneous regression: results of the prospective trials NB95-S and NB97. J Clin Oncol. 2008;26:1504–10.
72. Suarez D, Shuster JJ, Vassal G, et al. Treatment of stage IV-S neuroblastoma: a study of 34 cases treated between 1972-1987. Med Pediatr Oncol. 1991;19:473–7.
73. De Bernardi B, Gerrard M, Boni L, Rubie H, Canete A, Di Cataldo A, et al. Excellent outcome with reduced treatment for infants with disseminated neuroblastoma without MYCN gene amplification. J Clin Oncol. 2009;27(7):1034–40.
74. Perez CA, Matthay KK, Atkinson JB, Seeger RC, Shimada H, Haase GM, et al. Biologic variables in the outcome of stages I and II neuroblastoma treated with surgery as primary therapy: a Children's Cancer Group study. J Clin Oncol. 2000;18(1):18–26.
75. Kohler JA, Rubie H, Castel V, Beiske K, Holmes K, Gambini C, et al. Treatment of children over the age of one year with unresectable localised neuroblastoma without MYCN amplification: results of the SIOPEN study. Eur J Cancer. 2013;49(17):3671–9.
76. Modak S, Kushner BH, LaQuaglia MP, Kramer K, Cheung NK. Management and outcome of stage 3 neuroblastoma. Eur J Cancer. 2009;45(1):90–8.
77. Baker DL, Schmidt ML, Cohn SL, Maris JM, London WB, Buxton A, et al. Outcome after reduced chemotherapy for intermediate-risk neuroblastoma. N Engl J Med. 2010;363(14):1313–23.
78. De Bernardi B, Pianca C, Pistamiglio P, Veneselli E, Viscardi E, Pession A, et al. Neuroblastoma with symptomatic spinal cord compression at diagnosis: treatment and results with 76 cases. J Clin Oncol. 2001;19:183–90.
79. Plantaz D, Rubie H, Michon J, Mechinaud F, Coze C, Chastagner P, et al. The treatment of neuroblastoma with intraspinal extension with chemotherapy followed by surgical removal of residual disease, a prospective study of 42 children. Results of the NBL 90 study of the French Society of Paediatric Oncology. Cancer. 1996;78:311–9.
80. Wilson LMK, Draper GJ. Neuroblastoma, its natural history and prognosis: a study of 487 cases. BMJ. 1974;3:301–7.
81. Zucker JM. Retrospective study of 462 neuroblastomas treated between 1950 and 1970. Maandschr Kindergeneeskd. 1974;42:369–85.
82. Pearson AD, Pinkerton CR, Lewis IJ, Imeson J, Ellershaw C, Machin D, et al. High-dose rapid and standard induction chemotherapy for patients aged over 1 year with stage 4 neuroblastoma: a randomised trial. Lancet Oncol. 2008;9(3):247–56.
83. Ladenstein R, Pötschger U, Pearson ADJ, Brock P, Luksch R, Castel V, et al. Busulfan and melphalan versus carboplatin, etoposide, and melphalan as high-dose chemotherapy for high-risk neuroblastoma (HRNBL1/SIOPEN): an international, randomised, multi-arm, open-label, phase 3 trial. Lancet Oncol. 2017;18(4):500–14.
84. Ladenstein R, Philip T, Lasset C, Hartmann O, Zucker JM, Pinkerton R, et al. Multivariate analysis of risk factors in stage 4 neuroblastoma patients over the age of one year treated with megatherapy and stem-cell transplantation: a report from the European Bone Marrow Transplantation Solid Tumor Registry. J Clin Oncol. 1998;16:953–65.
85. Haupt R, Garaventa A, Gambini C, Parodi S, Cangemi G, Casale F, et al. Improved survival of children with neuroblastoma between 1979 and 2005: a report of the Italian Neuroblastoma Registry. J Clin Oncol. 2010;28:2331–8.
86. Yalçin B, Kremer LC, van Dalen EC. High-dose chemotherapy and autologous haematopoietic stem cell rescue for children with high-risk neuroblastoma. Cochrane Database Syst Rev. 2015;5:(10):CD006301.
87. Bosse KR, Maris JM. Advances in the transational genomics of neuroblastoma: from improving risk stratification and revealing novel biology to identifying actionable genomic alterations. Cancer. 2016;122:20–33.
88. Kiessling MK, Curioni-Fontecedro A, Samaras P, Lang S, Scharl M, Aguzzi A, et al. Targeting the mTOR complex by everolimus in NRAS mutant neuroblastoma. PLoS One. 2016;11(1):e0147682.
89. Gustafson WC, Meyerowitz JG, Nekritz EA, Chen J, Benes C, Charron E, et al. Drugging MYCN through an allosteric transition in Aurora kinase A. Cancer Cell. 2014;26(3):414–27.
90. Ramani P, Nash R, Rogers CA. Aurora kinase A is superior to Ki67 as a prognostic indicator of survival in neuroblastoma. Histopathology. 2015;66(3):370–9.
91. Smith JR, Moreno L, Heaton SP, Chesler L, Pearson AD, Garrett MD. Novel pharmacodynamic biomarkers for MYCN protein and PI3K/AKT/mTOR pathway signaling in children with neuroblastoma. Mol Oncol. 2016;10(4):538–52.

92. Minturn JE, Evans AE, Villablanca JG, Yanik GA, Park JR, Shusterman S, et al. Phase I trial of lestaurtinib for children with refractory neuroblastoma: a new approaches to neuroblastoma therapy consortium study. Cancer Chemother Pharmacol. 2011;68(4):1057–65.
93. Rettig I, Koeneke E, Trippel F, Mueller WC, Burhenne J, Kopp-Schneider A, et al. Selective inhibition of HDAC8 decreases neuroblastoma growth in vitro and in vivo and enhances retinoic acid-mediated differentiation. Cell Death Dis. 2015;6:e1657.
94. Schleiermacher G, Javanmardi N, Bernard V, Leroy Q, Cappo J, Rio Frio T, et al. Emergence of new ALK mutations at relapse of neuroblastoma. J Clin Oncol. 2014;32(25):2727–34.
95. Li T, LoRusso P, Maitland ML, Ou SH, Bahceci E, Ball HA, et al. First-in-human, open-label dose-escalation and dose-expansion study of the safety, pharmacokinetics, and antitumor effects of an oral ALK inhibitor ASP3026 in patients with advanced solid tumors. J Hematol Oncol. 2016;9:23.
96. Louis CU, Savoldo B, Dotti G, Pule M, Yvon E, Myers GD, et al. Antitumor activity and long-term fate of chimeric antigen receptor-positive T cells in patients with neuroblastoma. Blood. 2011;118(23):6050–6.
97. Sun J, Huye LE, Lapteva N, Mamonkin M, Hiregange M, Ballard B, et al. Early transduction produces highly functional chimeric antigen receptor-modified virus-specific T-cells with central memory markers: a Production Assistant for Cell Therapy (PACT) translational application. J Immunother Cancer. 2015;3:5.
98. Gargett T, Brown MP. Different cytokine and stimulation conditions influence the expansion and immune phenotype of third-generation chimeric antigen receptor T cells specific for tumor antigen GD2. Cytotherapy. 2015;17(4):487–95.
99. Louis CU, Shohet JM. Neuroblastoma: molecular pathogenesis and therapy. Annu Rev Med. 2015;66:49–63.
100. Laverdière C, Liu Q, Yasui Y, Nathan PC, Gurney JG, Stovall M, et al. Long-term outcomes in survivors of neuroblastoma: a report from the Childhood Cancer Survivor Study. J Natl Cancer Inst. 2009;101(16):1131–40.
101. Perwein T, Lackner H, Sovinz P, Benesch M, Schmidt S, Schwinger W, et al. Survival and late effects in children with stage 4 neuroblastoma. Pediatr Blood Cancer. 2011;57:629–35.
102. Hobbie WL, Moshang T, Carlson CA, Goldmuntz E, Sacks N, Goldfarb SB, et al. Late effects in survivors of tandem peripheral blood stem cell transplant for high-risk neuroblastoma. Pediatr Blood Cancer. 2008;51:679–83.
103. van Santen HM, de Kraker J, Vulsma T. Endocrine late effects from multi-modality treatment of neuroblastoma. Eur J Cancer. 2005;41:1767–74.
104. Flandin I, Hartmann O, Michon J, Pinkerton R, Coze C, Stephan JL, et al. Impact of TBI on late effects in children treated by megatherapy for stage IV neuroblastoma. A study of the French Society of Paediatric Oncology. Int J Radiat Oncol Biol Phys. 2006;64(5):1424–31.
105. Gurney JG, Tersak JM, Ness KK, Landier W, Matthay KK, Schmidt ML, Children's Oncology Group. Hearing loss, quality of life, and academic problems in long-term neuroblastoma survivors: a report from the Children's Oncology Group. Pediatrics. 2007;120:e1229–36.
106. Martin A, Schneiderman J, Helenowski IB, Morgan E, Dilley K, Danner-Koptik K, et al. Secondary malignant neoplasms after high-dose chemotherapy and autologous stem cell rescue for high-risk neuroblastoma. Pediatr Blood Cancer. 2014;61:1350–6.
107. Moreno L, Vaidya S, Pinkerton R, Lewis IJ, Imeson J, Machin D, et al. Long-term follow-up of children with high-risk neuroblastoma: the ENSG5 trial experience. Pediatr Blood Cancer. 2013;60:1135–40.
108. Gunawardane PT, Grossman A. Phaeochromocytoma and paraganglioma. In: Hypertension: from basic research to clinical practice, Advances in experimental medicine and biology, vol. 956. Cham: Springer; 2016. p. 239.
109. Goodman MT, Gurney JG, Smith MA, et al. Sympathetic nervous system tumors. In: Ries LAG, Smith MA, Gurney JG, et al., editors. Cancer incidence and survival among children and adolescents: United States SEER Program 1975–1995, NIH publication no. 99-4649. Bethesda: National Cancer Institute; 1999. p. 65–72.
110. Barontini M, Levin G, Sanso G. Characteristics of pheochromocytoma in a 4- to 20-year-old population. Ann N Y Acad Sci. 2006;1073:30–7.
111. Beltsevich DG, Kuznetsov NS, Kazaryan AM, et al. Pheochromocytoma surgery: epidemiologic peculiarities in children. World J Surg. 2004;28(6):592–6.
112. Ross JH. Pheochromocytoma. Special considerations in children. Urol Clin North Am. 2000;27(3):393–402.
113. Waguespack S, Ying AK. Pheochromocytoma and multiple endocrine neoplasia syndromes. In: Sperling MA, editor. Paediatric endocrinology. 4th ed. Philadelphia: Elsevier Saunders; 2014. p. 533–68.
114. Fishbein L, Leshchiner I, Walter V, Danilova L, Robertson AG, Johnson AR, Cancer Genome Atlas Research Network, et al. Comprehensive molecular characterization of pheochromocytoma and paraganglioma. Cancer Cell. 2017;31(2):181–93.
115. Bausch B, Schiavi F, Ni Y, Welander J, Patocs A, Ngeow J, European-American-Asian Pheochromocytoma-Paraganglioma Registry Study Group, et al. Clinical characterization of the pheochromocytoma and paraganglioma susceptibility genes SDHA, TMEM127, MAX, and SDHAF2 for gene-informed prevention. JAMA Oncol. 2017;3:1204. https://doi.org/10.1001/jamaoncol.2017.0223.

116. Neumann HP, Bausch B, McWhinney SR, et al. Germ-line mutations in nonsyndromic pheochromocytoma. N Engl J Med. 2002;346(19):1459–66.
117. Tischler AS. Pheochromocytoma and extra-adrenal paraganglioma: updates. Arch Pathol Lab Med. 2008;132(8):1272–84.
118. Armstrong R, Sridhar M, Greenhalgh KL, et al. Phaeochromocytoma in children. Arch Dis Child. 2008;93(10):899–904.
119. Waguespack SG, Rich T, Grubbs E, et al. A current review of the etiology, diagnosis, and treatment of paediatric pheochromocytoma and paraganglioma. J Clin Endocrinol Metab. 2010;95(5):2023–37.
120. Pham TH, Moir C, Thompson GB, et al. Pheochromocytoma and paraganglioma in children: a review of medical and surgical management at a tertiary care center. Pediatrics. 2006;118(3):1109–17.
121. King KS, Prodanov T, Kantorovich V, et al. Metastatic pheochromocytoma/paraganglioma related to primary tumor development in childhood or adolescence: significant link to SDHB mutations. J Clin Oncol. 2011;29(31):4137–42.
122. Jimenez C, Rohren E, Habra MA, et al. Current and future treatments for malignant pheochromocytoma and sympathetic paraganglioma. Curr Oncol Rep. 2013;15(4):356–71.
123. Eisenhofer G, Bornstein SR, Brouwers FM, et al. Malignant pheochromocytoma: current status and initiatives for future progress. Endocr Relat Cancer. 2004;11(3):423–36.
124. Berruti A, Baudin E, Gelderblom H, et al. Adrenal cancer: ESMO clinical practice guidelines for diagnosis, treatment and follow-up. Ann Oncol. 2012;23(Suppl 7):vii131–8.
125. Bilek R, Safarik L, Ciprova V, et al. Chromogranin A, a member of neuroendocrine secretory proteins as a selective marker for laboratory diagnosis of pheochromocytoma. Physiol Res. 2008;57(Suppl 1):S171–9.
126. Grossrubatscher E, Dalino P, Vignati F, et al. The role of chromogranin A in the management of patients with phaeochromocytoma. Clin Endocrinol. 2006;65(3):287–93.
127. Pacak K, Eisenhofer G, Ahlman H, et al. Pheochromocytoma: recommendations for clinical practice from the First International Symposium, October 2005. Nat Clin Pract Endocrinol Metab. 2007;3(2):92–102.
128. Jacobson AF, Deng H, Lombard J, et al. ^{123}I-metaiodobenzylguanidine scintigraphy for the detection of neuroblastoma and pheochromocytoma: results of a meta-analysis. J Clin Endocrinol Metab. 2010;95(6):2596–606.
129. Timmers HJ, Taieb D, Pacak K. Current and future anatomical and functional imaging approaches to pheochromocytoma and paraganglioma. Horm Metab Res. 2012;44(5):367–72.
130. Chang CA, Pattison DA, Tothill RW, Kong G, Akhurst TJ, Hicks RJ, et al. (68)Ga-DOTATATE and (18)F-FDG PET/CT in paraganglioma and pheochromocytoma: utility, patterns and heterogeneity. Cancer Imaging. 2016;16(1):22.
131. Timmers HJ, Chen CC, Carrasquillo JA, et al. Staging and functional characterization of pheochromocytoma and paraganglioma by 18F-fluorodeoxyglucose (18F-FDG) positron emission tomography. J Natl Cancer Inst. 2012;104(9):700–8.
132. Ludwig AD, Feig DI, Brandt ML, et al. Recent advances in the diagnosis and treatment of pheochromocytoma in children. Am J Surg. 2007;194(6):792–6. discussion 796–797
133. Mannelli M, Dralle H, Lenders JW. Perioperative management of pheochromocytoma/paraganglioma: is there a state of the art? Horm Metab Res. 2012;44(5):373–8.
134. PDQ Adult Treatment Editorial Board. Pheochromocytoma and Paraganglioma Treatment (PDQ®): Patient Version. PDQ Cancer Information Summaries [Internet]. Bethesda: National Cancer Institute (US). 2002–2016 Jul 19.
135. Walz MK, Alesina PF, Wenger FA, et al. Posterior retroperitoneoscopic adrenalectomy—results of 560 procedures in 520 patients. Surgery. 2006;140(6):943–8. discussion 948–950
136. Pacak K. Preoperative management of the pheochromocytoma patient. J Clin Endocrinol Metab. 2007;92(11):4069–79.
137. Groeben H, Nottebaum BJ, Alesina PF, Traut A, Neumann HP, et al. Perioperative α-receptor blockade in phaeochromocytoma surgery: an observational case series. Br J Anaesth. 2017;118(2):182–9.
138. Ayala-Ramirez M, Chougnet CN, Habra MA, et al. Treatment with sunitinib for patients with progressive metastatic pheochromocytomas and sympathetic paragangliomas. J Clin Endocrinol Metab. 2012;97(11):4040–50.
139. Grubbs EG, Rich TA, Ng C, et al. Long-term outcomes of surgical treatment for hereditary pheochromocytoma. J Am Coll Surg. 2013;216(2):280–9.
140. Amar L, Lussey-Lepoutre C, Lenders JW, Djadi-Prat J, Plouin PF, Steichen O. Management of endocrine disease: recurrence or new tumors after complete resection of pheochromocytomas and paragangliomas: a systematic review and meta-analysis. Eur J Endocrinol. 2016;175(4):135–45.

19 Treatment with ^{131}I-mIBG (Metaiodobenzylguanidine): Indications, Procedures, and Results

Maria Rita Castellani, Antonio Scarale, Alice Lorenzoni, Marco Maccauro, Julia Balaguer Guill, and Roberto Luksch

Abstract

Since the 80s, treatment with ^{131}I-metaiodobenzylguanidine (mIBG) has been introduced in the management of neuroendocrine tumors (NET). In several chromaffin tumors (neuroblastoma, pheochromocytoma, paraganglioma), but also medullary thyroid carcinoma and carcinoids, the efficacy and the possible role of ^{131}I-mIBG treatment along disease course have been extensively investigated.

In children with high-risk refractory or recurrent neuroblastoma, the results of ^{131}I-mIBG treatment have been improved by combinations with chemotherapy, radiosensitizers, and autologous stem cell support. Consequently, this treatment has been progressively incorporated into the more important multicenter trials.

For adult pheochromocytoma and paraganglioma, ^{131}I-mIBG therapy is currently the most efficient nonsurgical therapeutic modality for inoperable or metastatic disease. In low-growing but symptomatic tumors, the powerful palliation of hormone-related secretory symptoms should also be considered when judging treatment benefit.

For other various NET types, with a wide range variability of mIBG-avid lesions, the role of this treatment is progressively decreasing by the emergence of peptide receptor radionuclide (PRRT).

M.R. Castellani (✉) • A. Scarale • A. Lorenzoni
M. Maccauro
Nuclear Medicine Unit,
Fondazione IRCCS Istituto Nazionale Tumori,
Milan, Italy
e-mail: rita.castellani@istitutotumori.mi.it;
scarale.antonio@hotmail.it;
alice.lorenzoni@istitutotumori.mi.it;
marco.maccauro@istitutotumori.mi.it

J. Balaguer Guill
Pediatric Oncology Unit, Hospital Universitario y Politecnico La Fe, Valencia, Spain
e-mail: balaguer_jul@gva.es; julbagui@yahoo.es

R. Luksch
Pediatric Oncology Unit, Fondazione IRCCS Istituto Nazionale Tumori, Milan, Italy
e-mail: roberto.luksch@istitutotumori.mi.it

E. Bombardieri et al. (eds.), *Clinical Applications of Nuclear Medicine Targeted Therapy*,
https://doi.org/10.1007/978-3-319-63067-0_19

Nevertheless in carcinoid tumors, ^{131}I-MIBG remains a valid alternative radionuclide option for patients with renal impairment.

In this article, the most important practical aspects of ^{131}I-MIBG therapy are listed and discussed.

19.1 Background

The use of labeled mIBG for diagnosis and therapy has a long history. Early studies in the 1970s identified a number of guanethidine derivates, including metaiodobenzylguanidine (mIBG).

Metaiodobenzylguanidine is an aralkylguanidine resulting from the combination of the benzyl group of bretylium and the adrenergic neuron blocker guanidine. Due to its molecular analogy with norepinephrine, MIBG binds to the norepinephrine transporter [1] and is taken up by the adrenal chromaffin cells and presynaptic terminals. Nevertheless, mIBG uptake is inhibited by norepinephrine, in a competitive manner [2].

19.1.1 mIBG Uptake

MIBG enters neuroendocrine cells by two pathways: the former specific, defined as Uptake-1 and the latter nonspecific, called Uptake-2.

The Uptake-1 is an active, ATP-dependent, saturable uptake process [3, 4], dependent on co-transported substrates, leading to the specific concentration of the molecule within the cells.

With the Uptake-2, a small portion of the tracer is passively brought into cells by nonspecific mechanism which is energy-independent and unsaturable and results in low-level norepinephrine accumulation in most tissues [5].

Cell line works have shown that in normal adrenomedullary tissue or in pheochromocytoma tumors, mIBG is transported and accumulated in the secretory granules via vesicular monoamine transporters [6], but in the evenience of a paucity of the neurosecretory granules, i.e., in neuroblastoma cells lines, the storage is predominantly extravesicular, and mIBG may remain in the cytoplasm and mitochondria [7–9].

MIBG uptake shows a strong correlation with norepinephrine transporter expression levels [10].

Several pharmaceuticals can inhibit the norepinephrine transporter and consequently have to be withheld before mIBG imaging or therapy (see chapter 10.2.3 "Patient Preparation") [11].

19.1.2 mIBG Radiolabeled for Imaging and Therapy

In 1979 Donald Wieland introduced mIBG radiolabeled with iodine I-131 for imaging of adrenal medulla. Early studies in the 1970s and 1980s demonstrated the effectiveness of this radiopharmaceutical as imaging agent in the neuroendocrine tumors [12] and in neuroblastoma [13].

In 1984 the first experience with ^{131}I-mIBG for therapeutic use was described in patients with pheochromocytoma (PHEO) [14]. In the same period, the first reports appeared on the use of this radiopharmaceutical in patients with neuroblastoma [15] and neuroendocrine carcinomas [16].

Since that time all over the world, many patients have been investigated for imaging (^{123}I/^{131}I-mIBG) or treated with ^{131}I-MIBG.

Radiolabeled mIBG is an exemplar of theranostics, as it is used for imaging, and when labeled with I-131, or the treatment of mIBG-avid neuroendocrine tumors.

So far, despite the introduction of positron emission tomography (PET) into daily practice, ^{123}I-mIBG imaging, particularly if performed with SPECT/TC modality, is a diagnostic and prognostic cornerstone in neuroblastoma patients enrolled in multicentric therapeutic protocols, providing an essential contribution to staging the disease and evaluating its response to treatment [17, 18].

In other neuroendocrine tumors, ^{123}I-mIBG is routinely studied with the aim to select patients who are possible candidates for radionuclide therapy with ^{131}I-mIBG.

19.1.3 Pharmacokinetics: Administration Modalities and Cytotoxic Effect of ^{131}I-MIBG Therapy

After intravenous administration, MIBG shows a rapid clearance from the blood pool, with 10% or less remaining in the blood few hours after injection. This data is consistent with the idea that the cytotoxic effect of ^{131}I-MIBG is due to local radioactivity rather than a general blood radioactivity.

^{131}I-MIBG is taken up quickly into the tumor cells compared to the normal tissues, with an early peak 6 h after administration [19].

An important component of the rapid clearance is the enzymatic deiodination of mIBG. The percentage of free ^{131}I -I increases to more than 10% at the end of the infusion and is quickly cleared through the urine [20].

In order to limit the early ^{131}I-mIBG loss due to deiodination, ^{131}I-mIBG infusion should be fast, not more than an hour, even in the event of very high activities injected. During the first 4 h post-infusion ^{131}I-MIBG, the elimination half-life is about 10 h, slightly faster in children than in adults [21].

In urinary excretions over 4–5 days, 75–90% of the radioactivity is in the form of undegraded ^{131}I-MIBG; small amounts of various metabolites, including ^{131}I-iodide, comprise the remainder [22].

Low concentrations of MIBG are not cytotoxic. Unlabeled MIBG up to concentrations of 10 μM has no direct effect on the cells [23]. However, small concentrations of radiolabeled MIBG are highly cytotoxic, due to the direct effect on tissues by beta radiation. The cytotoxic effect of ^{131}I-MIBG appears relatively fast, with tumor growth significantly inhibited for several days following administration [24].

Repeated administrations don't reduce the ^{131}I-MIBG uptake on tumor accumulation. Even if the greatest therapeutic effect occurs after the first cycle of therapy, further responses are frequently observed in the subsequent treatment courses [25].

19.1.4 Factors Modulating Therapeutic mIBG Uptake and Patient Selection

There are several evidences that the grade of malignancy is an important tumor characteristic affecting the imaging sensitivity and the therapeutic efficacy of radioiodinated mIBG: between the several subsubtypes of neuroendocrine tumors, high-grade/poorly differentiated carcinomas have a lower MIBG uptake capacity than well-differentiated carcinomas [26].

Moreover, during the course of disease, in the same patient, the genetic layout can change by selecting the growth of poorly differentiated subtypes influencing mIBG response to treatment.

Recently, some authors reported that patients who underwent mIBG therapy for relapsed or refractory neuroblastoma showed different outcomes: patients with prior relapse had higher rates of progressive disease and lower 2-year overall survival than patients treated for refractory disease. This report confirms that the biological characteristics of the tumor may play a role in disease responsiveness or being a surrogate for unfavorable prognosis [27].

During the last years, some preclinical and clinical studies have been performed with the aim to identify genetic, biological, or chemotherapy agents able to increase the intracellular mIBG uptake.

As human norepinephrine transporter (hNET) seems to be a critical step in the treatment of MIBG-concentrating tumors, in 1991 in a preclinical study, it has been demonstrated the increased MIBG uptake in rat hepatoma cells induced by retroviral transfection of the hNET gene. However, the retention of MIBG was brief; therefore, the absorbed dose of radiation in vivo was not expected to be therapeutically effective [28].

Moreover, experimental studies with human neuroblastoma cell lines showed that a pretreatment with cisplatin and doxorubicin is able to significantly intensify MIBG uptake in the tumor cells by acting on norepinephrine transporter gene and subsequent norepinephrine receptor expression during and after chemotherapy [29, 30].

Experimental study with topotecan, another chemotherapeutic agent used in treatment of neuroblastoma, showed that a combined topotecan-mIBG treatment produced a significant inhibition of the tumor cell growth, as both agents impaired DNA repair mechanism in the tumor cells. These studies were the basis of recent phase I/II studies [5, 31–33].

More recently, vincristine and irinotecan have been employed as systemic radiation sensitizers of ^{131}I-mIBG in a phase I/II study for advance neuroblastoma [34].

19.2 Planning for an ^{131}I-MIBG Therapy

^{131}I-MIBG therapy needs a multidisciplinary team that includes oncologists, pediatricians, oncology/pediatric nurses, nuclear medicine physicians, and medical physicist experienced in therapeutic nuclear medicine. All the procedures, in particular referred to hospitalization and radioprotection rules, informed consent from the patient or parent, and treatment scheduling has to be continuously reviewed and formally approved. Education of the patient and family should include appropriate radiation safety instructions during hospitalization period and after patient discharge.

mIBG therapy needs the patient's admission in a dedicated shielded room, where the radiopharmaceutical is administered, and all potentially contaminated biological materials, patient's dose rates, and personnel radiation exposures are all the time monitored until the patient's hospital discharge. According to Italy radioprotection recommendations, patients are discharged when the dose rate measured was below 40 μSv/h at 1 m with safety instructions delivered for the patient and parents.

19.2.1 Patient Selection

There are no uniform guidelines for selecting or excluding patients to be treated.

In general, ideal candidates to ^{131}I-mIBG are those patients with progressing or symptomatic disease with evidence of disease uptake on imaging mIBG scan. Furthermore, in pheochromocytomas/paragangliomas (PHEO/PGL), ^{131}I -mIBG therapy can be considered in the presence of a stable disease, in order to reduce the catecholamine-related symptoms [35].

Finally, in neuroblastoma ^{131}I-mIBG therapy is so far included into several therapeutic protocols, within a specific step of the treatment planning (see chapter 19.3.2 "Neuroblastoma").

Nevertheless, there are not uniform criteria for the identification of the uptake entity valued as "adequate" for selecting the patient. Dosimetric estimate of tumor-absorbed dose allows the maximization of the administered activities [36] but in most cases is not feasible due to several clinical reasons: not measurable lesions, fast disease evolution, and patient accessibility.

A good compromise is to perform a whole-body dosimetry after the ^{131}I-mIBG administration of a high activity, empirically determined on the basis of the body weight: The result is employed to calculate the activity to administer during the second treatment, in order to raise a whole-body cumulative dose of 4 Gy [37] (see Sect. 19.3.2). Other methods are based on subjective (visual) criteria or a semiquantitative measurement of uptake (lesion/background ratio >2) [38].

In most cases, all the clinical or radiological lesions should have been seen by imaging. Anyway, some neuroendocrine tumors with multiple lesions can be treated even in the presence of a relatively small number of sites of mIBG uptakes, if there is the clinical evidence of the absence of progression of the cold sites of disease.

Patients candidates for ^{131}I-MIBG therapy should have a reasonable performance status (Karnofsky >60) and a life expectancy of at least 3 months, unless they have intractable bone pain.

Reasonable hematopoietic parameters (WBC >3000/μL, platelets >100 K/μL) are required prior to ^{131}I-MIBG therapy, especially when stem cells are not available [11].

There are no limitation to treat patients previously nephrectomized, i.e., for a large adrenal tumor, anyway the residual kidney function have to be acceptable. Patients with nephrotic syndrome may develop to bronchiolitis obliterans organizing pneumonia or acute distress respiratory distress syndrome [38].

19.2.2 Therapy Modalities

Even for the long-lasting experience, there is no standardized practice in terms of choosing the activities for a single therapeutic treatment, ranging from low (<200 mCi) to intermediate (≥200 mCi) to high doses (>500 mCi). The administered activity, respectively, sometimes was fixed, based on empirical evidence of limited toxicity, sometimes adjusted to body weight, or sometimes progressively escalating as in phase II trials [39].

Some investigators have calculated activities to deliver by performing a dosimetry study, with the aim to administer a dose less than 2–4 Gy to blood or whole body, calculated using prior imaging. Generally, whole-body doses up to 2 Gy can be administered without bone marrow support [36, 37].

At the same time, the frequency of retreatment was variable, tailored from few weeks to >6 months intervals on the basis of tumor growth rate or by considering an adequate marrow recovery from toxicity, in particular if high activities are administered [35, 40–44].

Regarding the parameter of assessing treatment response, a wide range of evaluation methods has been reported. Sometimes the disease was evaluated by functional (mIBG or PET) imaging, sometimes based on the radiological (CT or MR) imaging. Moreover, the response rate has been evaluated at few months or at more longtime intervals.

In general, response rate was determined using size measurement criteria, in most cases WHO criteria, but in PHEO/PGL hormone-secreting tumors with elevated catecholamine levels, also biochemical parameters were also used to gauge response. In some studies, both the degree of the objective tumor response and the hormonal response have been evaluated [35, 45].

High vs low activities, tumor grow rate, response rate, and marrow toxicity were the principal factors affecting the total therapy time, the overall number of retreatments (1 to >10 cycles), and the cumulative activities reached [35].

A brief overview of the most significant experiences is resumed and discussed in chapter 19.3 "Clinical Experience."

19.2.3 Patient Preparation

From several years, it is well known the list of the drugs surely or potentially interfering with the uptake and/or retention of mIBG, particularly certain antihypertensives, such as labetalol, tricyclic antidepressants, and some sympathomimetics. Doubtful is the interference of some calcium-channel blockers, such as nifedipine.

However in patients with pheochromocytomas, it is not always permitted to stop the antihypertensive medications. Therefore, when possible, these drugs are substituted with phenoxybenzamine and atenolol, plus eventually nifedipine, in order to maintain the control of blood pressure. The detailed list of drugs that may interfere, including the length of their withdrawal before mIBG administration, can be consulted in published EANM procedure guidelines for ^{131}I-mIBG therapy [11].

Thyroid blockade is necessary to prevent hypothyroidism due to the thyroid uptake of free radioactive iodide dissociating from the mIBG molecule.

A variety of regimens using potassium iodide (KI), saturated solution of potassium iodide (SSKI), or Lugol's solution is available. Thyroid blockade usually starts 1 day prior to administration of the ^{131}I-MIBG. The length of blockade is linked to the therapeutic ^{131}I-mIBG schedule, in particular by considering the administered activity, the extension and intensity of uptake, and the biological half-life, and can range from 7 to 30 days.

If the patient is candidate to high-activity therapeutic regimen of ^{131}I-mIBG (see chapter 19.3 "Neuroblastoma"), harvest of peripheral blood stem cells (PBSC) is recommended in order to manage the blood marrow toxicity [46].

Harvest should be performed following stimulation with filgrastim (G-CSF, granulocyte-colony-stimulating factor) which is widely used for peripheral blood stem cell (PBSC) mobilization.

Harvest may be scheduled either after the last chemotherapy cycle or out of steady-state mobilization.

The aim is to obtain a total CD34 harvest of at least 3 × 10^6/kg cells. The stem cells are to be returned after ^{131}I-mIBG therapy, after an interval time of 7–15 days, depending on the length of the radionuclide retention [47].

19.2.4 Supportive Care

Antiemetic therapy should be given according to the clinical condition and institutional procedures.

To minimize the radiation dose to the bladder, oral and/or parenteral hydration is recommended. In small children, urinary catheterization is often performed to minimize bladder dose and avoid contamination.

^{131}I-mIBG is administered by pump i.v. through a plastic indwelling catheter or central line. A variety of infusion times has been suggested. In any cases, when high specific mIBG activity is given, the radiopharmaceutical infusion should be shortened to a maximum of 1 h.

Since patients, in particular PHEO/PGL, may develop a hypertensive response, during the administration it is recommended to monitor vital signs, in order to eventually control the cardiovascular side effects.

19.3 Clinical Experience of ^{131}I-mIBG Therapy in Neuroendocrine Tumors

Among the neuroendocrine tumors, ^{131}I-mIBG therapy has been more extensively studied in neuroblastoma, pheochromocytomas, paragangliomas, medullary thyroid carcinoma, and carcinoid tumors.

19.3.1 Pheochromocytomas and Paragangliomas

Pheochromocytomas and paragangliomas are rare neuroendocrine neoplasms arising from chromaffin cells of the adrenal medulla or the sympathetic nervous system. The intra-adrenal tumors are referred as pheochromocytoma (PHEO). If they occur outside of the adrenal, in the extra-adrenal sympathetic tissue, or of the parasympathetic tissue, they are referred as paraganglioma. Intra-adrenal pheochromocytomas are more frequent than extra-adrenal or parasympathetic paragangliomas.

PHEO secrete catecholamines in most of the cases, and consequently, patients present with hypertension and other symptoms of adrenergic excess. In some instances, however, they are nonfunctional, and presentation is related to mass effect or incidental findings.

About 75% of PHEO/PGL are sporadic, but some are familiar and related to several genetic defects with typical presentations, often associated with an increased incidence of malignant and/or extra-adrenal disease [48–50].

Paragangliomas are present in about 30% of patients lower than 20 years old, demonstrate multicentricity in 15–24% of cases, and secrete catecholamines only in case of sympathetic origin [35].

Although most PHEO/PGL are benign, 36% of extra-adrenal PGL are malignant.

Because of lack of robust morphological and histological criteria, it is difficult to differentiate benign from malignant tumors. Consequently, the malignancy can only be determined by the presence of distant metastases, which occur in

3–13% of cases. The most common sites of metastatic disease are the lymph nodes, bone, liver, and lung. The 5-year survival rate depends on the location of metastases; patients with lung and liver metastases have the worst survival, while bone metastases are associated with a more favorable survival. Patients with malignant disease typically have an overall 5-year survival of less than 50%. Nonetheless, some metastatic patients may exhibit a more indolent course and may live >20 years with limited therapy [51].

The unpredictable nature of this disease suggests that in the absence of early prognostic indicators, the effectiveness of therapy in patients with long survival cannot easily be assessed. Similarly, this unpredictable aspect can cause delays in initiation of therapeutic applications in patients with rapidly progressing disease [35].

Urinary fractionated or plasma-free metanephrines are the most sensitive laboratory tests to confirm the diagnosis of PHEO/PGL, which have sensitivities of more than 95% [45].

The diagnostic and functional imaging modalities most often used for staging include CT and MRI, ^{123}I-MIBG, ^{18}F-fluorodopamine, ^{111}In-pentetreotide scintigraphy, and several PET-tracers: ^{18}F-FDG-PET, ^{18}F- DOPA, the precursor of dopamine and the catecholamines, and different forms of ^{68}Ga-DOTA-conjugated peptides, expression of somatostatin receptors (SSTR) [52, 53]. The comparison between imaging functional tracers revealed findings showing association with radionuclide imaging, genetic features, and clinical outcome [54], which has been considered in the recent European guidelines [55].

Main treatment for malignant pheochromocytomas/paragangliomas includes surgery, ^{131}I-mIBG therapy, chemotherapy, and external beam radiotherapy. ^{131}I-MIBG therapy has been utilized for the treatment of malignant pheochromocytoma since the second half of the 1980s in many centers across the world.

At Michigan University in 1984, Sisson's group first reported the initial experience of ^{131}I-mIBG therapy in malignant pheochromocytoma [56].

The first international comprehensive report on indications and results of ^{131}I-MIBG therapy was illustrated in the international workshop held in Rome in 1991 [57]. In the cumulative experience of seven institutions, which reported the results obtained in a total of 106 patients, ^{131}I-mIBG resulted able to induce major responses (RC + RP > 50%) in 15/85(18%) of the cases and 47% of stabilizations, sometimes very long-lasting (52–72 months) [35].

In 1997, Loh et al. reviewed in a meta-analysis the studies performed in 23 institutions from 1983 to 1997 [58]. On the 116 patients treated, the mean activity/course was 158 mCi, with a range of 96–300 mCi. Cumulative activity administered ranged from 96 to 2322 mCi with a mean for patient of 490 mCi and 3.3 retreatments, with a maximum of 11 courses. Of the 116 patients, 4% had an objective CR, 26% had PR, 57% showed no change, and 13% progressed. ^{131}I-mIBG induced a symptomatic improvement of symptoms related to catecholamine excess in 76% of 96 cases. Five patients achieved complete antitumor and hormonal response lasted between 16 and 58 months. Moreover, the authors found that responders had a longer overall survival than non-responders. Specifically, 33% of responders survived for 22 months, while 45% of non-responders died in 13 months.

Even if these studies were not fully comparable because mIBG therapy was performed in small group of patients with a wide range of activities, modalities, patient's selection criteria, and different response evaluations, it was clear that in PHEO/ PGL, ^{131}I-mIBG therapy undoubtedly resulted to be an effective treatment modality. In fact, it proved to be able to induce a significant tumor response, to produce long-term stabilization of disease in several cases and to significantly reduce catecholamine-related symptoms in almost all patients.

After initial experiences, methodology of ^{131}I-mIBG treatment progressively evolved in two clinical directions: palliation of symptoms and reduction of tumor mass. In the former, the studies have been carried out administering relatively low activities (median < 200 mCi) with long intervals between each cycle. In the latter, intermediate (200–500 mCi) or high activities (12–18 mCi/kg) were administered with short intervals between each retreatment.

In Table 19.1 are summarized some of the most important experiences performed between 1991 and 2010. Only in six studies the number of patients studied reached 20 cases [39, 59, 63, 64, 66, 69].

The reported administered activity varied widely for single treatment, ranging from 2.6 to 43.8 GBq (90–1622 mCi), but the criteria of activity choice are well described only by the San Francisco group [39], which performed a phase I/II dose-escalation trial with the aim to determine the tolerance limits and the activity-related effectiveness of treatment [39]. It is important to notice that the activity per kilogram to be administered in adults without incurring the need of bone marrow transplantation is still to be defined. During the Rome Symposium, it emerged that the well-tolerated activity per kilogram for children corresponded to a significantly lower average activity for adults: thus adults received 1/3–1/5 whole-body dose than children. In his phase II study, Gonias reported that successful peripheral blood stem cell (PBSC) harvest was required for patients that received more than 12 mCi/kg or in cases of administered activity equal or higher than 500 mCi.

Apart from the experience of this group, a standard administration criterion is not yet established, in particular due to the lack of a systematic comparison of regimens using low, mild, or high doses of ^{131}I-mIBG.

Each center continued to use mIBG treatment with different modalities with results that are not well comparable. So, the debate about the optimal activity and schedule is still ongoing.

Table 19.1 ^{131}I-mIBG: summary of cumulative experience in pheochromocytoma/paraganglioma

	Year	Number	Single activity (mCi)	Cumulative activity (mCi)	Objective PR or CR-PR response rate	Duration of response (years)
Shapiro [59]	1991	28	97–301 (mean 181)	Mean 479 (111–916)	7%	Less than 1
Mukherjee [60]	2001	15	Mean 268	274–1754	40%	NA
Rose [61]	2003	12	528–1184 mean 1095	529–2313	83%	0.5–8.4 Median 3.6
Bomanji [62]	2003	6	300–1469 Mean 414	300–1469	83%	0.75–5.1
Safford [63]	1003	33	96–714 Mean 391	70–1223 (mean 549)	67%	NA
Buscombe [44]	2005	3	90–142	37–703	33%	1.5
Sisson [64]	2006	21	137–349	329–1254 median 588	30%	1–21
Fitzgerald [65]	2006	30	762–1622 Mean 1140		67%	NA
Gedik [66]	2008	19	100–700 (median 200)	183–2200 (median 800)	47%	0.66–5
Navalkissoor [67]	2009	4	Mean 218	400–1450	50%	0.66–3.33
Shilkrut [68]	2009	10	Mean 200	137–829	80%	0.5–3.9
Gonias [39]	2009	50	6–19 mCi/kg (492–1160) or 500 mCi, if no stem cells	492–3919	64%	NA
Castellani [69][a]	2010	12 16	124–149 (median 149) 200–350 (median 268)	149–1800 (median 1065) 249–1546 (median 651)	33 25	Median 1.9 y Median 3 y

[a]Two groups of patients: low vs intermediate activity

Response rate does not significantly differ if a patient is treated with low or intermediate activities. Nevertheless, Milan experience demonstrated that the increased activity shortened time to achieve a significant response (7 versus 19 months) and, consequently, reduced the number of retreatment and the cumulative activity with only a modest increase in toxicity. Moreover, as significant scintigraphic responses have been observed even after the first treatment, the speed of response in Group 2 showed prognostic information [69].

The duration of response ranges from few months to 8, 4 [61], or 21 years [64]. These results are in accordance with the large variability of evolution of these tumors: sometimes very aggressive, but often with a long-lasting slow evolution, even in case of visceral metastases. In the presence of an indolent disease course, the impact and the real efficacy of each treatment, not only of ^{131}I -mIBG, in terms of overall survival, or stabilization of disease, are questionable [64]. For this reason, in many cases, ^{131}I-mIBG therapy should be performed only with the aim to reduce symptoms or in the presence of a clear progression of disease.

In conclusion, although ^{131}I-mIBG has proved to be the most efficient nonsurgical therapeutic modality in PHEO/PLG, more than 25 years later, and after hundreds of patients treated, there is still a significant interest about the therapeutic impact of ^{131}I-mIBG, but there isn't still a general consensus on procedures and guidelines.

19.3.2 Neuroblastoma

Neuroblastoma is an embryonal malignancy arising from the sympathetic nervous system, which is the most frequent extracranial solid tumor in childhood. About 90% of neuroblastoma occurs before 5 years of age. Infants younger than 12 months of age, even with metastatic disease, have a favorable outcome with chemotherapy and surgery. Despite substantial progress in the understanding of the disease and aggressive treatment regimens, the prognosis of children older than 18 months of age remains poor. Patients who present metastatic disease and do not achieve a complete response to induction therapy have a less than 35% of 3-year event-free survival rate [18, 70, 71]. The 5-year overall survival of patients with stage 4 neuroblastoma is only 50% [72]. Consequently, improved therapeutic strategies including mIBG-targeted therapy are probably necessary.

From 1984 ^{131}I-mIBG therapy has been extensively employed in neuroblastoma. In a systematic review of ^{131}I-mIBG therapy, Wilson et al. analyzed 1121 patients treated with ^{131}I-mIBG in the time period from 1987 until 2012 [39].

From the late 1980s, in the vast majority of the studies, ^{131}I-mIBG was used as single agent (monotherapy) in patients with a poor prognosis, in particular those with recurrent/refractory disease, as a palliative treatment. While most studies have been designed to administer repeated therapeutic doses of ^{131}I-mIBG, several authors have used single doses.

In most of the old studies, mIBG doses have been based on fixed activity [73–79] or by considering different class of body weight [82, 84] or based on mCi/body weight, or with an escalation activity, one of the earliest phase 1 dose-escalation trials with increasing ^{131}I-mIBG activities ranging from 50 to 220 mCi [77]. In two cases, the activity has been administered by considering both body weight and dosimetry WB dose estimation [80, 83], as so far it is carried out in currently neuroblastoma international therapy protocols.

Fixed doses usually consisted of repeated treatments of 100–200 mCi, with cumulative activities up to 600–1000 mCi and several cycles of retreatments (Table 19.2a, b).

These monotherapy pilot trials are not comparable in term of results, due to their large variability in terms of patients studied, most of them with an extensive prior treatment. Consequently, these studies showed a wide range of tumor response, with very rare CR, and overall response (CR + PR) ranging between 2 and 59% [39].

Nevertheless, these studies demonstrated that ^{131}I-MIBG could be performed safely with repeated treatments in patients with advanced disease who had failed conventional therapy and gave relevant information regarding the side effects, in particular the hematologic toxicity.

Table 19.2 Neuroblastoma: ^{131}I-mIBG therapy modalities and hyperbaric oxygen therapy

(a) Monotherapy-fixed doses

Author	Year	Number of patients	Number of cycles	Modality
Hoefnagel [73]	1987	16	1	40–200 mCi
Treuner [74]	1988	27	1–6	35–448 mCi (mean 135 mCi)
Troncone [75]	1991	11	1–4	70–260 mCi
Lumbroso [76]	1991	26	1–5	30–108 mCi (mean 70 mCi)
Hutchinson [77]	1992	14	1–3	Fixed/escalated 50–220 mCi (median154 mCi)
Voute [78]	1995	36 + 27 with HBO	1–4	200–100 mCi + HBO
Castellani [79]	2000	22	1–6	244–388 mCi

(b) Monotherapy weight-based activity

Study	Year	Number of patients	Number of cycles	Modality	Total activity related to WB dose
Schwabe [80]	1987	11	1–6	2 cycles 10 mCi/kg tandem	WB dose: 2 Gy
Klingebiel [81]	1991	47	1–6	1.6–16.2 mCi/kg	//
Claudiani [82]	1991	42	1–6	70–150 mCi (depending by class of weight)	//
Lashford [83]	1992	25	1	65–327 mCi	WB dose: 1–2.5 Gy
Garaventa [84]	1999	43	1–5	70–200 mCi (depending by class of weight	//
Kang [85]	2003	17	1–3	First administration 8 mCi/kg; second mean 245 mCi; third mean 116 mCi	

Table 19.3 Neuroblastoma: ^{131}I-mIBG therapy escalating-dose studies alone or in association with stem cell support (PBSC) or with high-dose chemotherapy plus autologous stem cell transplant (ASCT)

Author	Year	N patients	Modality	Association with HD CHEMO + ASCT	PBSC
Matthay [40]	1998	30	2.6–18 mCi/kg	No	Yes
Miano [86]	2001	17	4–11 mCi/kg	Yes	Yes
Howard [25]	2005	28	3–19 mCi/kg	No	No[a]
Matthay [87]	2007	164	12–18 mCi/kg	No	Yes
Matthay [88]	2009	21	22–50 mCi/kg[b]	No	Yes
Matthay [89]	2012	15	12–21 mCi/kg[c]	No	Yes
Klingebiel [90]	1998	11	15.67 mCi/kg	Yes	Yes
Yanik [91]	2002	12	12 mCi/kg	Yes	Yes
Matthay [92]	2006	22	12 mCi/kg[c]	Yes	Yes
Yanik [93]	2015	42	12 mCi/kg	Yes	Yes

[a]Platelets transfusions; weight-based phase I dose escalation
[b]Two infusions tandem therapy
[c]No carrier added

In the same period, phase I dose-escalation trials started in Europe and North America with the aim to determine the most appropriate I^{131}I-mIBG treatment dose as monotherapy or in combination therapies with autologous stem cell transplantation. In these studies, the activity has been administered by escalating doses of mCi/kg (Table 19.3).

In 1998, Matthay reported the results of their phase I dose-escalation trial with ^{131}I-mIBG doses escalated from 2.6 to −18 mCi/kg. This study demonstrated that doses above 12 mCi/kg cause significant hematologic toxicity and require preharvesting of stem cells. Consequently, 12 mCi/kg is the maximal tolerated mIBG dose that does not require bone marrow rescue [40].

In 2007, Matthay treated with ^{131}I-mIBG as monotherapy 148 patients with progressive, refractory, or relapsed high-risk mIBG-avid neuroblastoma. Patients with stem cells available received 18mCi/kg of ^{131}I-mIBG, whereas 16 patients without available stem cells received 12 mCi/kg. The overall CR plus PR rate to ^{131}I-mIBG therapy was 36%. Patients aged 12 years or older showed a 55% response rate compared to a 40% response rate in those less than 12 years old. Hematologic toxicity occurred in 33% of patients requiring autologous hematopoietic stem cell support. Hepatic, pulmonary, and infectious toxicities were observed in 5%, 4%, and 11%, respectively [87].

Another study that experimented very high pro kilo activities, by administering median individual doses of 35.8 mCi/kg in one to four sessions, found as expected an improvement of response rate and median overall survival of 12 months, but myelosuppression required platelet support in about 80% of the cases [25].

Matthay administered a total 22–51 mCi/kg in two sequential doses delivered over 14 days (tandem scheme) with an OS of 48% at 18 months [88].

To maximize the therapeutic effect of ^{131}I-mIBG, some groups combined ^{131}I-mIBG therapy with high-dose chemotherapy, in particular in conjunction with carboplatin, etoposide, and melphalan (CEM) followed by stem cell rescue [92, 93]. The NANT consortium trial [95, 96] studies demonstrated that the addiction of ^{131}I-mIBG to the conditioning therapy had a tolerable toxicity and did not affect the post-transplant hematologic recovery. Moreover, 27% of patients achieved a CR or PR, and patients who had a PR to induction therapy had a mild better 3-year EFS and OS than non-responders to previous therapy EFS 38% vs 20% and OS 75% vs 62%, respectively.

More recently, several clinical and preclinical studies have investigated the possibility to improve the mIBG uptake and efficacy administering ^{131}I-mIBG therapy in conjunction with those agents able to enhance the norepinephrine transporter (NET) expression.

A pretreatment with corticosteroids, gamma interferon, retinoic acid, cisplatin, and doxorubicin is able to increase NET expression, as well as radiosensitizers such as vorinostat, irinotecan, or topotecan, the hyperbaric oxygen, gene therapy, or ionizing radiation from external beam radiation [5].

Recently, in some experimental studies, cisplatin, topotecan, vincristine, and irinotecan have been combined with ^{131}I-mIBG in order to improve mIBG tumor uptake [34, 37, 46, 94]. Even if these drugs have independent tumor activity against neuroblastoma, they are been administered in very small doses, in order to act only as radiosensitizers and don't overlap ^{131}I-mIBG toxicity.

One study experimented a single mIBG treatment (200 mCi) in combination with cisplatin and cyclophosphamide with or without etoposide and vincristine [94]. In another phase I/II study, low doses of vincristine and irinotecan have been administered in conjunction with myeloablative doses of ^{131}I-mIBG in 32 patients with refractory neuroblastoma [34]. Myelosuppression and diarrhea were the most common toxicities.

Finally, topotecan has been experimented in a small pilot study consisting of dosimetry-based high-dose ^{131}I-mIBG [37]. This study consists of two ^{131}I-mIBG cycles administered with topotecan between an interval time of 2 weeks (Tandem scheme). In the first treatment, 12 mCi/kg are given and then the dosimetry study starts. Based on this dosimetry estimation, in the second treatment, the remnant mIBG activity is administered in order to rich a total WB dose of 4 Gy. So far, this very promising therapy scheme is applied in several European hospitals as "palliative treatment," and only a multicentric European study phase II/III trial will start in the so-called very high-risk neuroblastoma patients.

The last therapeutic goal of ^{131}I-mIBG is its use as a first-line therapy in mIBG-avid tumors.

The rationale of giving ^{131}I-mIBG before chemotherapy is to utilize at the best the radiotherapeutic effect of radionuclide therapy in order to reduce the tumor mass but at the same time avoid the unfavorable effects of previous chemotherapy: uptake reduction due to the response, selection of de-differentiated cell lines not mIBG avid, and the negative effects on bone marrow supply.

Nevertheless, only limited data are available on its use as up-front therapy in presurgical patients.

In 1994, ^{131}I-mIBG was able to induce a response rate greater than 70% in 31 children with inoperable neuroblastoma. Side effects were significantly lower than after conventional therapy [95].

In a more recent study, the Dutch group used ^{131}I-mIBG as induction therapy in 41 evaluable patients with newly diagnosed stage IV neuroblastoma. Therapy planning consisted of two ^{131}I-mIBG treatments, followed by surgery or by both neo-adjuvant chemotherapy and surgery. Each cycle was administered with a fixed dose of 200 mCi and 100 mCi at an interval time of 4–6 weeks. If objective responses were obtained, the patients proceeded to surgery; if not, they were switched to chemotherapy until surgery. After surgery, patients underwent myeloablative chemotherapy +ASCT and subsequent consolidation therapy, independent of the preoperative therapeutic regimen. The ^{131}I-mIBG induction obtained an objective response rate of 66%, higher than values observed in induction chemotherapy regimens currently employed in high-risk trials [96].

More recently, Dutch group reported the results of a similar up-front ^{131}I-mIBG therapy study, performed in 32 consecutive newly diagnosed stage 4 NBL patients. Twenty-one patients with high mIBG uptake level in both the primary tumor and known metastases and not in poor clinical conditions underwent two ^{131}I-mIBG courses, fixed doses 200 mCi and 150 mCi, respectively. Subsequently all patients, including 11 patients excluded from ^{131}I-mIBG induction, followed the standard high-risk arm of the German Pediatric Oncology Group (GPOH) 2004 [97]. Patients RR post-^{131}I-mIBG was 38% and post-MAT + ASCT was 71%. Overall, the patients in the ^{131}I-mIBG group had a better RR and survival than patients in the chemotherapy group, but probably due to selection bias (more sick patients). In any case, radionuclide induction didn't significantly delayed interval between chemo courses and resulted feasible, in particular with respect to harvest stem cells and to hematological reconstitution post-ASCT, and the toxicity acceptable.

19.3.3 Medullary Thyroid Carcinoma

Medullary thyroid carcinoma (MTC) is a rare neuroendocrine tumor originating from the parafollicular C cells which releases calcitonin, carcinoembryonic antigen (CEA), and occasionally other substances.

MTC appear in sporadic and familiar form. A germline mutation of the RET proto-oncogene is present in 20–30% of cases and occurs in three different hereditary forms: familial MTC, multiple endocrine neoplasia (MEN) 2A, and MEN 2B syndrome. Prognosis of MTC is largely related to tumor extension at disease onset. Surgery remains the most effective therapy for potential cure.

So far, the experience of ^{131}I-mIBG therapy is very limited, due in part to the low incidence of this tumor, in part because only one third of the cases presents lesions with an intensity of mIBG uptake so high to be favorably considered for radionuclide treatment [98]. Moreover, often the lesions present a variable ability to take up the tracer; consequently, the presence of "cold" metastasis limits the global efficacy of this treatment.

The indication of ^{131}I-mIBG therapy remains the palliation of inoperable metastatic disease or of the hormone-related symptoms.

The overall response rate is near 30%, in most case minor responses, but in few patients unresponsive to any other established treatments, ^{131}I-mIBG therapy showed a surprising long-lasting stabilization of the disease (more than 10 years). In some cases, the efficacy is limited to decrease the hormone-related symptoms, similar as in pheochromocytoma [99].

19.3.4 Carcinoid Tumors

Malignant carcinoid tumors are in most cases small tumors, slow growing, and associated with an overall 5-year survival rate of 67%. About 75% of carcinoids developed in abdominal sites, in particular the ileum, and frequently metastasized to the liver. The remnant 25% developed in the bronchopulmonary system [100].

Most carcinoid tumors present secretory granules releasing active hormones, in particular serotonin. In many cases, the diagnosis is suspected by appearance of the hormone-releasing symptoms, in particular flushing and diarrhea, overall defined as carcinoid syndrome, and confirmed by measurements of serum serotonin or its urinary metabolite, 5-hydroxyindoleacetic acid.

Carcinoids express high concentrations of somatostatin receptors, but frequently the intracellular secretory granules contain a NET system that facilitates the uptake of mIBG. In any cases, only a small fraction of carcinoids is mIBG avid. The mIBG diagnostic sensitivity is near 60% in tumors of midgut origin, but tumors of the foregut, including those of bronchial origin, show a very low ability of uptake. Tumor uptake of MIBG is less frequently present than respective uptake of somatostatin analog [101, 102].

The worldwide cumulative experience with ^{131}I-mIBG therapy in carcinoid tumors has been consistent. ^{131}I-mIBG treatment resulted mainly efficacy to attenuate symptoms related to carcinoid syndrome. On about 350 cases reported, ^{131}I-mIBG treatment has been able to induce a significant long-lasting symptomatic response in 50–75% of the cases, while the median objective response rate, in most cases limited to stabilization of disease, was near to 20% [103, 104].

On the last years, the relevance of ^{131}I-mIBG treatment has substantially decreased due to the success of peptide receptor radionuclide therapy (PRRT) in gastro-entero-pancreatic neuroendocrine tumors, which induces higher morphologic response rates than mIBG therapy [105, 106].

However, mIBG, if taken up, can be considered a safe and effective treatment for carcinoid patients able to reduce tumor-related symptoms and to arrest tumor progression, prolonging survival [104]. In some particular cases, with lesions presenting uptake of both diagnostic MIBG and somatostatin analog receptor imaging, the combination of mIBG therapy and PRRT can be performed according to dosimetric considerations [107].

Finally, mIBG may be considered a good alternative to PRRT in patients with kidney disease, as it is lacking of significant renal irradiation.

19.4 Brief Summary of Indications of ^{131}I-mIBG Therapy in Neuroendocrine Tumors

Clinical experiences suggest the following considerations.

An important precondition to consider is an adequate uptake of all growing lesions based on a pre-therapy imaging.

In adults with neuroendocrine tumors, ^{131}I-mIBG therapy is indicated:

- In all cases who are not suitable candidates for local treatment with surgery, external beam radiotherapy, intra-arterial radioembolization, and peptide receptor radiotherapy (PPRT).
- In some slow-growing tumors, such as pheochromocytomas or carcinoid tumors, the main indication to therapy is reduction of hormone-related symptoms.
- In patients with progressing or symptomatic disease, the main indication to therapy is to arrest the tumor progression and to induce a reduction of tumor mass.
- In multi-metastatic patients, the indication to therapy is mainly palliative, with the aim to induce a stabilization of disease and a reduction of symptoms related.
- In some pheochromocytomas and paragangliomas with a locoregional extended tumor, not suitable for surgical resection, ^{131}I-mIBG therapy can be performed with the aim to reduce the tumor mass in order to be surgically removed.
- In mIBG-avid carcinoid tumors that are indicated in the presence of renal impairment.

In children with neuroblastoma, ^{131}I-mIBG therapy is indicated:

- As palliative therapy in advance/recurrent disease
- As a part of therapy planning in high-risk neuroblastoma, i.e., as post-induction consolidation
- As a frontline therapy in dedicated trials of therapy
- As myeloablative treatment in very high-risk, recurred, or advanced disease and sometimes in conjunction with radiosensitizers

19.5 Potential Toxicity and Late Side Effects of ^{131}I-mIBG Therapy

Several of the most side effects of ^{131}I-mIBG therapy have been previously discussed.

The earliest toxicity is pharmacologic, occurring within the first hours and days after the infusion, and consists of nausea and emesis due to radiation gastritis. Transient tachycardia and hypertension occur in less than 10% of the patients [108].

Hematopoietic toxicity consists of myelosuppression with anemia, thrombocytopenia, neutropenia, and lymphopenia. Usually it appears 2–4 weeks after infusion but the nadir occurs 2–3 weeks later, and the recovery can be very slow after4–6 weeks. In children treated with ^{131}I-mIBG, the degree of the hematopoietic toxicity has been recognized to be activity/weight related. As previously discussed, an activity greater than 12 mCi/kg (444 MBq/kg) needs as a precaution the stem cell rescue PBSC. In adults hematopoietic toxicity is not activity/weight related but due to several clinic conditions: disease extent, in particular bone metastases, age, previous chemotherapy, or extended fields of external beam radiotherapy [69]. Usually in adults, myelosuppression is limited to thrombocytopenia and lymphopenia and is of mild degree, but the completed recovery can occur even 2–3 months later.

Despite prophylaxis with potassium iodide, hypothyroidism is a late radiation-induced effect related to ^{131}I uptake by thyroid due to free radioactive iodide present in the product or dissociating from the mIBG molecule. This side effect has an incidence of 7–12% and may occur several months after therapy [109].

Late radiation-induced toxicities include the development of secondary malignancies. In particular, acute myelogenous leukemia and myelodysplastic syndrome were reported both in adults and children in about 3% of patients [69, 108, 110]. Nevertheless, in children treated with a chemotherapy multimodality therapy, it is difficult to distinguish the risk of developing secondary malignances derived from ^{131}I-mIBG radiation effects and the risk derived from the alkylator-based chemotherapies [108].

Other nonematologic grades 3–4 are rare when ^{131}I-mIBG is used as monotherapy, but may rise when radionuclide therapy is combined with myeloablative chemotherapy.

In a recent study, a transient asymptomatic elevation of transaminases has been referred in less than 10% of children treated with high pro kilo activities [111].

Key Points

- Since the 1980s, ^{131}I-mIBG therapy is delivered in patients with neuroendocrine tumors.
- The main clinical experience has been developed in children with high-risk recurrent/refractory neuroblastoma with mIBG-avid disease. As a consequence of both bad prognosis of this tumor and the discrete efficacy of ^{131}I-mIBG therapy, this radionuclide treatment has been extensively investigated with several modalities and regimens, as monotherapy or in combination therapies and in frontline therapy.
- So far, in high-risk neuroblastoma, ^{131}I-mIBG therapy is progressively incorporated in the most important international trials of therapy.
- In other neuroendocrine tumors, in particular malignant pheochromocytoma and paraganglioma, ^{131}I-mIBG therapy has been mainly employed as palliative treatment, in any case able to induce long-lasting objective tumor and symptomatic (hormonal) responses.
- Due to relevant myelotoxicity, special attention is necessary regarding the administered activities, interval between retreatments, and the opportunity to manage myelosuppression with blood transfusions or infusions of autologous stem cell for rescue.

Acknowledgments The authors are grateful to Emilio Bombardieri, MD, Scientific Director of Humanitas Gavazzeni Hospital, Bergamo (Italy), for his help and support in preparing this manuscript.

References

1. Wieland DM, Brown LE, Tobes MC, et al. Imaging the primate adrenal-medulla with [I-123] and [I-131] metalodobenzylguanidine: concise communication. J Nucl Med. 1981;22:358–64.

2. Iavarone A, Lasorella A, Servidei T, Riccardi R, Troncone L, Mastrangelo R. Biology of metaiodobenzylguanidine interactions with human neuroblastoma cells. J Nucl Biol Med. 1991;35:186–90.
3. Bönisch H, Brüss M. The norepinephrine transporter in physiology and disease. Handb Exp Pharmacol. 2006;175:485–524.
4. Iversen LL. The uptake of noradrenaline by the isolated perfused rat heart. Br J Pharmacol Chemother. 1963;21:523–37.
5. Streby KA, Shah N, Ranalli MA, Kunkler A, Cripe TP. Nothing but NET: a review of norepinephrine transporter expression and efficacy of 131I-mIBG therapy. Pediatr Blood Cancer. 2015;62:5–11. https://doi.org/10.1002/pbc.25200.
6. Kolby L, Bernhardt P, Levin-Jakobsen AM, et al. Uptake of meta-iodobenzylguanidine in neuroendocrine tumours is mediated by vesicular monoamine transporters. Br J Cancer. 2003;89:1383–8.
7. Smets LA, Janssen M, Rutgers M, et al. Pharmacokinetics and intracellular-distribution of the tumor-targeted radiopharmaceutical M-iodobenzylguanidine in SK-N-SH neuroblastoma and PC-12 pheochromocytoma cells. Int J Cancer. 1991;48:609–15.
8. Lashford LS, Hancock JP, Kemshead JT. Metaiodobenzylguanidine (metaiodobenzylguanidine) uptake and storage in the human neuroblastoma cell-line SK-N-BE(2C). Int J Cancer. 1991;47:105–9.
9. Gaze MN, Huxham IM, Mairs RJ, Barrett A. Intracellular localization of metaiodobenzyl guanidine in human neuroblastoma cells by electron spectroscopic imaging. Int J Cancer. 1991;47(6):875–80.
10. Carlin S, Mairs RJ, McCluskey AG, Tweddle DA, Sprigg A, Estlin C, Board J, et al. Development of a real-time polymerase chain reaction assay for prediction of the uptake of meta-[(131)I]iodobenzylguanidine by neuroblastoma tumors. Clin Cancer Res. 2003;9:3338–44.
11. Giammarile F, Chiti A, Lassmann M, Brans B, Flux G, EANM. EANM procedure guidelines for 131I-metaiodobenzylguanidine (131I-mIBG) therapy. Eur J Nucl Med Mol Imaging. 2008;35:1039–47.
12. McEwan AJ, Shapiro B, Sisson JC, Beierwaltes WH, Ackery DM. Radio-iodobenzylguanidine for the scintigraphic location and therapy of adrenergic tumors. Semin Nucl Med. 1985;15:132–53.
13. Treuner J, Feine U, Niethammer D, et al. Scintigraphic imaging of neuroblastoma with [131-I] iodobenzylguanidine. Lancet. 1984;1:333–4.
14. Sisson JC, Shapiro B, Beierwaltes WH. Scintigraphy with I-131 MIBG as an aid to the treatment of pheochromocytomas in patients with the MEN-2 syndromes. Henry Ford Hosp Med J. 1984;32:254–61.
15. Treuner J, Klingebiel T, Feine U, Buck J, Bruchelt G, et al. Clinical experiences in the treatment of neuroblastoma with ^{131}I-metaiodobenzylguanidine. Pediatr Hematol Oncol. 1986;3:205–16.
16. Hoefnagel CA, den Hartog Jager FC, van Gennip AH, Marcuse HR, Taal BG. Diagnosis and treatment of a carcinoid tumor using Iodine-131 meta-iodobenzylguanidine. Clin Nucl Med. 1986;11:150–2.
17. Park JR, Bagatell R, Cohn SL, Pearson AD, et al. Revisions to the international neuroblastoma response criteria: a consensus statement from the National Cancer Institute clinical trials planning meeting. J Clin Oncol. 2017;35(22):2580–7.
18. Lewington V, Lambert B, Poetschger U, Bar Sever Z, Giammarile F, McEwan AJB, Castellani R, et al. 123I-mIBG scintigraphy in neuroblastoma: development of a SIOPEN semi-quantitative reporting, method by an international panel. Eur J Nucl Med Mol Imaging. 2017;44:234–41.
19. Hickeson MP, Charron M, Maris JM, Brophy P, Kang TI, Zhuang H, Khan J, Nevrotski T. Biodistribution of post-therapeutic versus diagnostic ^{131}I-MIBG scans in children with neuroblastoma. Pediatr Blood Cancer. 2004;42:268–74.
20. Ehninger G, Klingebiel T, Kumbier I, Schuler U, Feine U, Treuner J, Waller HD. Stability and pharmacokinetics of m-[131I]iodobenzylguanidine in patients. Cancer Res. 1987;47(22):6147–9.
21. Wafelman AR, Nortier YL, Rosing H, Maessen HJ, Taal BG, Hoefnagel CA, Maes RA, Beijnen JH. Renal excretion of meta-iodobenzylguanidine after therapeutic doses in cancer patients and its relation to dose and creatinine clearance. Nucl Med Commun. 1995;16:767–72.
22. Mangner TJ, Tobes MC, Wieland DW, et al. Metabolism of iodine-131 metaiodobenzylguanidine in patients with metastatic pheochromocytoma. J Nucl Med. 1986;27:37–44.
23. Bruchelt G, Girgert R, Buck J, Wolburg H, Niethammer D, Treuner J. Cytotoxic effects of w-[^{131}I]-and m-[^{125}I]Iodobenzylguanidine on the human neuroblastoma cell lines SK-N-SH and SK-N-LO[1]. Cancer Res. 1988;48:2993–7.
24. Rutgers M, Buitenhuis CK, van der Valk MA, Hoefnagel CA, Voute PA, Smets LA. [(131)I] and [(125)I] metaiodobenzylguanidine therapy in macroscopic and microscopic tumors: a comparative study in SK-N-SH human neuroblastoma and PC12 rat pheochromocytoma xenografts. Int J Cancer. 2000;90:312–25.
25. Howard JP, Maris JM, Kersun LS, Huberty JP, Cheng SC, Hawkins RA, Matthay KK. Tumor response and toxicity with multiple infusions of high dose ^{131}I-MIBG for refractory neuroblastoma. Pediatr Blood Cancer. 2005;44:232–9.
26. Vöö S, Bucerius J, Mottaghy FM. I-131-MIBG therapies. Methods. 2011;55:238–45.
27. Zhou MJ, Dorala MY, DuBoisa SG, Villablancab JG, Yanikc GA, Matthay KK. Different outcomes for relapsed vs. refractory neuroblastoma after therapy with 131I-metaiodobenzylguanidine (131I-MIBG). Eur J Cancer. 2015;51(16):2465–72.

28. Altmann A, Kissel M, Zitzmann S, Kubler W, Mahmut M, Peschke P, Haberkorn U. Increased MIBG uptake after transfer of the human norepinephrine transporter gene in rat hepatoma. J Nucl Med. 2003;44(6):973–80.
29. Armour A, Cunningham SH, Gaze MN, Wheldon TE, Mairs RJ. The effect of cisplatin pretreatment on the accumulation of MIBG by neuroblastoma cells in vitro. Br J Cancer. 1997;75(4):470–6.
30. Meco D, Lasorella A, Riccardi A, Servidei T, Mastrangelo R, Riccardi R. Influence of cisplatin and doxorubicin on 125I-meta-iodobenzylguanidine uptake in human neuroblastoma cell lines. Eur J Cancer. 1999;35(8):1227–34.
31. McCluskey AG, Boyd M, Ross SC, Cosimo E, Clark AM, Angerson WJ, Gaze MN, Mairs RJ. [131I]meta-iodobenzylguanidine and topotecan combination treatment of tumors expressing the noradrenaline transporter. Clin Cancer Res. 2005;11(21):7929–37.
32. McCluskey AG, Boyd M, Gaze MN, Mairs RJ. [131I]MIBG and topotecan: a rationale for combination therapy for neuroblastoma. Cancer Lett. 2005;228(1–2):221–7.
33. McCluskey AG, Mairs RJ, Tesson M, et al. Inhibition of poly(ADP-ribose) polymerase enhances the toxicity of 131I-metaiodobenzylguanidine/topotecan combination therapy to cells and xenografts that express the noradrenaline transporter. J Nucl Med. 2012;53(7):1146–54.
34. DuBois SG, Allen S, Bent M, Hilton JF, Hollinger F, Hawkins R, Courtier J, Mosse YP, Matthay KK. Phase I/II study of 131I-MIBG with vincristine and 5 days of irinotecan for advanced neuroblastoma. Br J Cancer. 2015;112:644–9.
35. Castellani MR, Aktolun C, Buzzoni R, Seregni E, Chiesa C, Maccauro M, Aliberti GL, Vellani C, Lorenzoni A, Bombardieri E. Iodine-131 metaiodobenzylguanidine (I-131 MIBG) diagnosis and therapy of pheochromocytoma and paraganglioma: current problems, critical issues and presentation of a sample case. Q J Nucl Med Mol Imaging. 2013;57(2):146–52.
36. Chiesa C, Castellani R, Mira M, Lorenzoni A, Flux GD. Dosimetry in 131I-MIBG therapy: moving toward personalized medicine. Q J Nucl Med Mol Imaging. 2013;57:161–70.
37. Gaze MN, Chang YC, Flux GD, Mairs RJ, Saran FH, Meller ST. Feasibility of dosimetry-based high-dose 131I-meta-iodobenzylguanidine with topotecan as a radiosensitizer in children with metastatic neuroblastoma. Cancer Biother Radiopharm. 2005;20(2):195–9.
38. Gonias S, Goldsby R, Matthay KK, et al. Phase II study of highdose I-131 metaiodobenzylguanidine therapy for patients with metastatic pheochromocytoma and paraganglioma. J Clin Oncol. 2009;27:4162–8.
39. Wilson JS, Gains JE, Moroz V, Wheatley K, Gaze MN. A systematic review of 131I-meta iodobenzylguanidine molecular radiotherapy for neuroblastoma. Eur J Cancer. 2014;50(4):801–15.
40. Matthay KK, DeSantes K, Hasegawa B, et al. Phase I dose escalation of I-131-metaiodobenzylguanidine with autologous bone marrow support in refractory neuroblastoma. J Clin Oncol. 1998;16:229–36.
41. Averbuch SD, Steakley CS, Young RC, et al. Malignant pheochromocytoma: effective treatment with a combination of cyclophosphamide, vincristine, and dacarbazine. Ann Intern Med. 1988;109:267–73.
42. Goncalves E, Ninane J, Wese FX, et al. Familial pheochromocytoma: successful treatment with I-131 MIBG. Med Pediatr Oncol. 1990;18:126–30.
43. Bomanji J, Britton KE, Ur E, Hawkins L, Grossman AB, Besser GM. Treatment of malignant pheochromocytoma, paraganglioma and carcinoid-tumors with I-131 metaiodobenzylguanidine. Nucl Med Commun. 1993;14:856–61.
44. Buscombe JR, Cwikla JB, Caplin ME, Hilson AJW. Long-term effi cacy of low activity meta-[I-131]iodobenzylguanidine therapy in patients with disseminated neuroendocrine tumours depends on initial response. Nucl Med Commun. 2005;26:969–76.
45. Carrasquillo JA, Chen CC. 131 I-MIBG therapy. In: Strauss HW, et al., editors. Nuclear oncology: pathophysiology and clinical applications. New York: Springer; 2013. p. 691–714.
46. DuBois SG, Matthay KK. 131I-metaiodobenzylguanidine therapy in children with advanced neuroblastoma. Q J Nucl Med Mol Imaging. 2013;57(1):53–65.
47. Lisenko K, Baertsch MA, Meiser R, Pavel P, Bruckner T, Kriegsmann M, Schmitt A, Witzens-Harig M, Ho AD, Hillengass J, Wuchter P. Comparison of biosimilar filgrastim, originator filgrastim, and lenograstim for autologous stem cell mobilization in patients with multiple myeloma. Transfusion. 2017;57(10):2359–65.
48. Neumann HPH, Bausch B, McWhinney SR, et al. Germ-line mutations in nonsyndromic pheochromocytoma. N Engl J Med. 2002;346:1459–66.
49. Amar L, Bertherat J, Baudin E, et al. Genetic testing in pheochromocytoma or functional paraganglioma. J Clin Oncol. 2005;23:8812–8.
50. Zarnegar R, Kebebew E, Duh QY, Clark OH. Malignant pheochromocytoma. Surg Oncol Clin N Am. 2006;15:555.
51. Tischler AS, Kimura N, McNicol AM. Pathology of pheochromocytoma and extra-adrenal paraganglioma. In: Pacak K, Eisenhofer G, editors. Pheochromocytoma. Oxford: Blackwell; 2006. p. 557–70.
52. Timmers HJ, Chen CC, Carrasquillo JA, Whatley M, Ling A, Havekes B, et al. Comparison of 18F-fluoro-L-DOPA, 18F-fluoro-deoxyglucose, and 18F-fluorodopamine PET and 123I-MIBG scintigraphy in the localization of pheochromocytoma and paraganglioma. J Clin Endocrinol Metab. 2009;94:4757–67.

53. Kauhanen S, Seppanen M, Ovaska J, Minn H, Bergman J, Korsoff P, et al. The clinical value of [18F]fluoro-dihydroxyphenylalanine positron emission tomography in primary diagnosis, staging, and restaging of neuroendocrine tumors. Endocr Relat Cancer. 2009;16:255–65.
54. Rufini V, Treglia G, Castaldi P, Perotti G, Calcagni ML, Corsello SM, et al. Comparison of 123I-MIBG SPECT-CT and 18F-DOPA PET-CT in the evaluation of patients with known or suspected recurrent paraganglioma. Nucl Med Commun. 2011;32:575–82.
55. Taïeb D, Timmers HJ, Hindié E, Guillet BA, Neumann HP, Walz MK, European Association of Nuclear Medicine, et al. EANM 2012 guidelines for radionuclide imaging of phaeochromocytoma and paraganglioma. Eur J Nucl Med Mol Imaging. 2012;39:1977–95.
56. Sisson JC, Shapiro B, Beierwaltes WH, Glowniak JV, Nakajo M, Mangner TJ, et al. Radiopharmaceutical treatment of malignant pheochromocytoma. J Nucl Med. 1984;25:197–206.
57. The role of [131I]Metaiodobenzylguanidine in the treatment of neural crest tumors. Proceedings of an international workshop. Rome, Italy, September 6–7, 1991. J Nucl Biol Med. 1991;35:177–363.
58. Loh KC, Fitzgerald PA, Matthay KK, et al. The treatment of malignant metaiodobenzylguanidine (I-131-MIBG): a comprehensive review of 116 reported patients. J Endocrinol Investig. 1997;20:648–58.
59. Shapiro B, Sisson IC, Wieland DM, et al. Radiopharmaceutical therapy of malignant pheochromocytoma with I-131 metaiodobenzylguanidine: results from ten years of experience. J Nucl Biol Med. 1991;35:269–76.
60. Mukherjee JJ, Kaltsas GA, Islam N, Plowman PN, Foley R, Hikmat J, et al. Treatment of metastatic carcinoid tumours, phaeochromocytoma, paraganglioma and medullary carcinoma of the thyroid with (131)I-meta-iodobenzylguanidine [(131)I-mIBG]. Clin Endocrinol. 2001;55:47–60.
61. Rose B, Matthay KK, Price D, et al. High-dose I-131-metaiodobenzylguanidine therapy for 12 patients with malignant pheochromocytoma. Cancer. 2003;98:239–48.
62. Bomanji JB, Wong W, Gaze MN, Cassoni A, Waddington W, Solano J, Ell PJ. Treatment of neuroendocrine tumours in adults with 131I-MIBG therapy. Clin Oncol (R Coll Radiol). 2003;15(4):193–8.
63. Safford SD, Coleman E, Gockerman JP, et al. Iodine-131 metaiodobenzylguanidine is an effective treatment for malignant pheochromocytoma and paraganglioma. Surgery. 2003;134:956–62.
64. Sisson JC, Shulkin BL, Esfandiari NH. Courses of malignant pheochromocytoma: implications for therapy. Ann N Y Acad Sci. 2006;1073:505–11.
65. Fitzgerald PA, Goldsby RE, Huberty JP, Price DC, Hawknis RA, Veatch JJ, et al. Malignant pheochromocytomas an paragangliomas. A phase II study of therapy with high-dose ^{131}I-Metaiodobenzylguanidine (^{131}I-MIBG). Ann N Y Acad Sci. 2006;1073:465–90.
66. Gedik GK, Hoefnagel CA, Bais E, et al. (131) I-MIBG therapy in metastatic phaeochromocytoma and paraganglioma. Eur J Nucl Med Mol Imaging. 2008;35:725–33.
67. Navalkissoor S, Alhashimi DM, Quigley AM, Caplin ME, Buscombe JR. Efficacy of using a standard activity of ^{131}I-MIBG therapy in patients with disseminated neuroendocrine tumours. Eur J Nucl Med Mol Imaging. 2009;37(5):904–12.
68. Shilkrut M, Bar-Deroma R, Bar-Sela G, Berninger A, Kuten A. Low-dose iodine-131 metaiodobenzylguanidine therapy for patients with malignant pheochromocytoma and paraganglioma. Am J Clin Oncol. 2009;33(1):79–82.
69. Castellani MR, Seghezzi S, Chiesa C, et al. I-131-MIBG treatment of pheochromocytoma: low versus intermediate activity regimens of therapy. Q J Nucl Med Mol Imaging. 2010;54:100–13.
70. Matthay KK, Villablanca JG, Seeger RC, Stram DO, Harris RE, Ramsay NK, Swift P, Shimada H, Black CT, Brodeur GM, Gerbing RB, Reynolds CP. Treatment of high-risk neuroblastoma with intensive chemotherapy, radiotherapy, autologous bone marrow transplantation, and 13-cis-retinoic acid. Children's cancer group. N Engl J Med. 1999;341:1165–73.
71. Ladenstein R, Philip T, Lasset C, Hartmann O, Garaventa A, Pinkerton R, Michon J, et al. Multivariate analysis of risk factors in stage 4 neuroblastoma patients over the age of one year treated with megatherapy and stem-cell transplantation: a report from the European bone marrow transplantation solid tumor registry. J Clin Oncol. 1998;16:953–65.
72. Pinto NR, Applebaum MA, Volchenboum SL, et al. Advances in risk classification and treatment strategies for neuroblastoma. J Clin Oncol. 2015;33:3008–17.
73. Hoefnagel CA, Voute PA, De KJ, Marcuse HR, Hoefnagel CA, Voute PA, et al. Radionuclide diagnosis and therapy of neural crest tumors using iodine-131 metaiodobenzylguanidine. J Nucl Med. 1987;28(3):308–14.
74. Treuner J, Gerein V, Klingebiel T, Schwabe D, Feine U, Happ J, et al. MIBG-treatment in neuroblastoma; experiences of the Tubingen/Frankfurt group. Prog Clin Biol Res. 1988;271:669–78.
75. Troncone L, Rufini V, Riccardi R, Lasorella A, Mastrangelo R, Troncone L, et al. The use of [131I] metaiodobenzylguanidine in the treatment of neuroblastoma after conventional therapy. J Nucl Biol Med. 1991;35(4):232–6.
76. Lumbroso J, Hartmann O, Schlumberger M, Lumbroso J, Hartmann O, Schlumberger M. Therapeutic use of [131I]metaiodobenzylguanidine in neuroblastoma: a phase II study in 26 patients. "Societe Francaise d'Oncologie Pediatrique" and

nuclear medicine co-investigators. J Nucl Biol Med. 1991;35(4):220–3.
77. Hutchinson RJ, Sisson JC, Shapiro B, Miser JS, Normole D, Shulkin BL, et al. 131-I-metaiodobenzylguanidine treatment in patients with refractory advanced neuroblastoma. Am J Clin Oncol. 1992;15(3):226–32.
78. Voute PA, van der Kleij AJ, De KJ, Hoefnagel CA, Tiel-van-Buul MM, Van GH. Clinical experience with radiation enhancement by hyperbaric oxygen in children with recurrent neuroblastoma stage IV. Eur J Cancer. 1995;31A:596–600.
79. Castellani MR, Rottoli L, Maffioli L, Massimino M, Gasparini M, Buraggi GL, et al. Experience with palliative [131I]metaiodobenzylguanidine therapy in advanced neuroblastoma. J Nucl Biol Med. 1991;35(4):241–3.
80. Schwabe D, Sahm S, Gerein V, Happ J, Kropp-von RH, Maul F, et al. 131-Metaiodobenzylguanedine therapy of neuroblastoma in childhood. Eur J Pediatr. 1987;146(3):246–50.
81. Klingebiel T, Berthold F, Treuner J, Schwabe D, Fischer M, Feine U, et al. Metaiodobenzylguanidine (mIBG) in treatment of 47 patients with neuroblastoma: results of the German neuroblastoma trial. Med Pediatr Oncol. 1991;19(2):84–8.
82. Claudiani F, Garaventa A, Bertolazzi L, Villavecchia GP, Cabria M, Scopinaro G, et al. [131I]metaiodobenzylguanidine therapy in advanced neuroblastoma. J Nucl Biol Med. 1991;35(4):224–7.
83. Lashford LS, Lewis IJ, Fielding SL, Flower MA, Meller S, Kemshead JT, et al. Phase I/II study of iodine 131 metaiodobenzylguanidine in chemoresistant neuroblastoma: a United Kingdom Children's cancer study group investigation. J Clin Oncol. 1992;10(12):1889–96.
84. Garaventa A, Bellagamba O, Lo Piccolo MS, Milanaccio C, Lanino E, Bertolazzi L, et al. 131I-metaiodobenzylguanidine (131IMIBG) therapy for residual neuroblastoma: a mono-institutional experience with 43 patients. Br J Cancer. 1999;81(8):1378–84.
85. Kang TI, Brophy P, Hickeson M, Heyman S, Evans AE, Charron M, et al. Targeted radiotherapy with submyeloablative doses of 131I-MIBG is effective for disease palliation in highly refractory neuroblastoma. J Pediatr Hematol Oncol. 2003;25(10):769–73.
86. Miano M, Garaventa A, Pizzitola MR, Piccolo MS, Dallorso S, Villavecchia GP, et al. Megatherapy combining 131I metaiodobenzylguanidine and high-dose chemotherapy with haematopoietic progenitor cell rescue for neuroblastoma. Bone Marrow Transplant. 2001;27(6):571–4.
87. Matthay KK, Yanik G, Messina J, Quach A, Huberty J, Cheng SC, et al. Phase II study on the effect of disease sites, age, and prior therapy on response to iodine-131-metaiodobenzylguanidine therapy in refractory neuroblastoma. J Clin Oncol. 2007;25(9):1054–60.
88. Matthay KK, Quach A, Huberty J, Franc BL, Hawkins RA, Jackson H, et al. Iodine-131-metaiodobenzylguanidine double infusion with autologous stem-cell rescue for neuroblastoma: a new approaches to neuroblastoma therapy phase I study. J Clin Oncol. 2009;27(7):1020–5.
89. Matthay KK, Weiss B, Villablanca JG, Maris JM, Yanik GA, Dubois SG, et al. Dose escalation study of no-carrier-added 131Imetaiodobenzylguanidine for relapsed or refractory neuroblastoma: new approaches to neuroblastoma therapy consortium trial. J Nucl Med. 2012;2012:1155–63.
90. Klingebiel T, Bader P, Bares R, et al. Treatment of neuroblastoma stage 4 with 131I-meta-iodobenzylguanidine, high dose chemo therapy and immunotherapy. A pilot study. Eur J Cancer. 1998;34:1398–402.
91. Yanik GA, Levine JE, Matthay KK, Sisson JC, Shulkin BL, Shapiro B, et al. Pilot study of iodine-131-metaiodobenzylguanidine in combination with myeloablative chemotherapy and autologous stem-cell support for the treatment of neuroblastoma. J Clin Oncol. 2002;20(8):2142–9.
92. Matthay KK, Tan JC, Villablanca JG, et al. Phase 1 dose escalation of iodine-131-metaiodobenzylguanidine with myeloablative chemotherapy and autologous stem-cell transplantation in refractory neuroblastoma: a new approaches to neuroblastoma therapy consortium study. J Clin Oncol. 2006;24:500–6.
93. Yanik GA, Villablanca J, Maris JM, et al. 131I-metaiodobenzylguanidine with intensive chemotherapy and autologous stem cell transplantation for high-risk neuroblastoma. A new approaches to neuroblastoma therapy (NANT) phase II study. Biol Blood Marrow Transplant. 2015;21:673–81.
94. Mastrangelo R, Tornesello A, Lasorella A, et al. Optimal use of the 131-I- metaiodobenzylguanidine and cisplatin combination in advanced neuroblastoma. J Neurooncol. 1997;31:153–8.
95. Hoefnagel CA, DeKraker J, Valdes-Olmos RA, et al. 131I-MIBG as a first line treatment in high-risk neuroblastoma patients. Nucl Med Commun. 1994;15:712–7.
96. de Kraker J, Hoefnagel KA, Verschuur AC, van Eck B, van Santen HM, Caron HN. Iodine-131-metaiodobenzylguanidine as initial induction therapy in stage 4 neuroblastoma patients over 1 year of age. Eur J Cancer. 2008;44(4):551–6.
97. Kraal KCJM, Bleeker GM, van Eck-Smit BLF, van Eijkelenburg NKA, Berthold F, van Noesel MM, Caron HN, Tytgat GAM. Feasibility, toxicity and response of upfront metaiodobenzylguanidine therapy therapy followed by German pediatric oncology group neuroblastoma 2004 protocol in newly diagnosed stage 4 neuroblastoma patients. Eur J Cancer. 2017;76:188–96.

98. Castellani MR, Alessi A, Savelli G, Bombardieri E. The role of radionuclide therapy in medullary thyroid cancer. Tumori. 2003;89(5):560–2.
99. Castellani MR, Seregni E, Maccauro M, Chiesa C, Aliberti G, Orunesu E, Bombardieri E. MIBG for diagnosis and therapy of medullary thyroid carcinoma: is there still a role? Q J Nucl Med Mol Imaging. 2008;52(4):430–40.
100. Sisson JC, Yanik GA. Theranostics: evolution of the radiopharmaceutical meta-iodobenzylguanidine in endocrine tumors. Semin Nucl Med. 2012;42:171–84.
101. Zuetenhorst JM, Hoefnagel CA, Bott H, et al. Evaluation of 111 in-pentetreotide,131 I-MIBG and bone scintigraphy in the detection and clinical management of bone metastases in carcinoid disease. Nucl Med Commun. 2002;23:735–41.
102. Ezziddin S, Logvinski T, Yong-Hing C, et al. Factors predicting tracer uptake in somatostatin receptor and MIBG scintigraphy of metastatic gastroenteropancreatic neuroendocrine tumors. J Nucl Med. 2006;47:223–33.
103. Grünwald F, Ezziddin S. 131I-Metaiodobenzylguanidine therapy of neuroblastoma and other neuroendocrine tumors. Semin Nucl Med. 2010;40:153–63.
104. Taal BG, Hoefnagel CA, Valdes Olmos RA, et al. Palliative effect of metaiodobenzylguanidine in metastatic carcinoid tumors. J Clin Oncol. 1996;14:1829–38.
105. Forrer F, Waldherr C, Maecke HR, et al. Targeted radionuclide therapy with 90Y-DOTATOC in patients with neuroendocrine tumors. Anticancer Res. 2006;26:703–7.
106. Kwekkeboom DJ, de Herder WW, Kam BL, et al. Treatment with the radiolabeled somatostatin analog [177 Lu-DOTA 0, Tyr3]octreotate: toxicity, efficacy, and survival. J Clin Oncol. 2008;26:2124–30.
107. Madsen MT, Bushnell DL, Juweid ME, et al. Potential increased tumor dose delivery with combined 131I-MIBG and 90Y-DOTATOC treatment in neuroendocrine tumors: a theoretic model. J Nucl Med. 2006;47:660–7.
108. Parisi MT, Eslamy H, Park JR, Shulkin BL, Yanik GA. 131I-Metaiodobenzylguanidine theranostics in neuroblastoma: historical perspectives; practical applications. Semin Nucl Med. 2016;46:184–202.
109. vanSanten HM, DeKraker J, vanEck BL, et al. High incidence of thyroid dysfunction despite prophylaxis with potassium iodide during 131I-metaiodobenzylguanidine treatment in children with neuroblastoma. Cancer. 2002;94:2081–9.
110. Weiss B, Vora A, Huberty J, et al. Secondary myelodysplastic syndrome and leukemia following 131I-metaiodobenzylguanidine therapy for relapsed neuroblastoma. J Pediatr Hematol Oncol. 2003;25:543–7.
111. Quach A, Ji L, Mishra V, et al. Thyroid and hepatic function after high- dose 131I-metaiodobenzylguanidine(131I-MIBG) therapy for neuroblastoma. Pediatr Blood Cancer. 2011;56:191–201.

Dosimetry for ^{131}I mIBG Therapy

20

Carlo Chiesa and Glenn Flux

Abstract

In ^{131}I-mIBG of paediatric neuroblastoma, the first dosimetric method introduced was whole-body dosimetry by Lashford et al. (J Clin Oncol 10(12):1889–96, 1992). This aims to prevent haematological toxicity. Despite its simplicity and level of approximation, this method is the basis for a forthcoming European multicentre trial, in which the activity of a second administration is planned according to the whole-body absorbed dose delivered in the first. Lesion dosimetry has also been performed, though in a small number of centres. The limited number of lesion dosimetry studies derives from the challenge of high activity quantitative imaging of I-131, incurring gamma camera saturation in peri-therapy imaging, and the need for children to remain steady during sequential camera scans. The major goal now is to establish absorbed dose-effect correlation studies, which will provide a fundamental basis for individualised treatment planning. Thanks to the improvement of methods for internal dosimetry and radiobiology over the last two decades and the increasing availability of quantitative ^{124}I PET imaging, in the near future, we could have a more systematic basis for standardisation and individualisation of mIBG therapy.

20.1 Goal of Dosimetry in mIBG Treatments

The general goal of dosimetry is to optimise the treatment, i.e. choose the optimal administered activity capable of maximising efficacy whilst keeping toxicity low. Advances in mIBG therapy have mainly stemmed from development for the treatment of paediatric neuroblastoma, since the international experience of ^{131}I-MIBG therapy in phaeochromocytoma and paragangliomas is

C. Chiesa (✉)
Nuclear Medicine, Fondazione IRCCS Istituto Nazionale Tumori, Milan, Italy
e-mail: Carlo.Chiesa@istitutotumori.mi.it

G. Flux
Joint Department of Physics, Royal Marsden Hospital and Institute of Cancer Research, Sutton, UK

E. Bombardieri et al. (eds.), *Clinical Applications of Nuclear Medicine Targeted Therapy*,
https://doi.org/10.1007/978-3-319-63067-0_20

still limited [1]. Treatment of young children can present challenges to data acquisition for dosimetric methodology in centres without sufficient experience. Pretreatment dosimetry has been rarely performed. Whole-body dosimetry can be obtained without blood sampling or imaging but simply external counts of the child lying on the bed in the therapy unit [2, 3]. This simplified methodology aims to prevent toxicity in the subsequent administration and from this point of view is safety-orientated. However, it also allows the maximisation of further administered activities, in compliance with the generally accepted 2 Gy whole-body absorbed dose limit. From this point of view, it could also be considered an efficacy-orientated method. No information about lesion absorbed dose is deducible with this methodology. This is a major limitation, since high activity administration to a child should be justified by a predicted therapeutic lesion absorbed dose.

20.2 The Practical Implementation of Dosimetry in mIBG Treatments

20.2.1 Whole-Body Dosimetry

In practical terms, the implementation of whole-body dosimetry is simpler than lesion dosimetry, particularly if the patient is young. The use of ^{123}I mIBG for pretreatment dosimetry is reported in the literature [4]. However, the uncertainty in the prediction of the time activity curve for the long-lived ^{131}I-mIBG using the short-lived ^{123}I mIBG (12.3 h half-life) may be large [5]. For whole-body dosimetry, the best prediction of therapeutic time activity curve is given by a previous peri-therapeutic study, with an uncertainty range of −30% + 20% on the whole-body absorbed dose [6].

The simplest and reliable method to monitor the activity burden remaining in a patient following an administration of ^{131}I mIBG is by a counter from a distance. Care must be taken to ensure that the distance between the patient and the detector is reproduced for each reading. A convenient approach is to monitor the counts from the patient using a Geiger counter placed at least 2 m from the patient. A setup for this approach, using a ceiling-mounted counter that enables the patient to lie down in a reproducible position, has been described by Chittenden et al. [7].

A spectroscopic NaI probe can be used as well (thyroid uptake probe) with the drawback that it cannot be fixed to the ceiling and the need of larger distance (3–4 m) to include the whole body in the conical field of view defined by the collimator. According to our experience, a 10 mm lead shield is mandatory for peri-therapy 3″ × 3″ NaI counting to avoid saturation from dead time.

Portable counters, such as those ordinarily used to monitor the patient external exposure rate at patient release, can be used peri-therapeutically, provided that the patient-detector distance may be reproducible and that the duration of the measurement could be integrated over a time to reduce statistical fluctuations.

The steps required to perform accurate whole-body dosimetry using this method are as follows:

1. *Background readings.* A first background rate reading BKG_0 [cps] should be acquired prior to administration.
2. *Patient-counter geometry.* When using a ceiling-mounted counter, for each reading patients should lie in the same position. Particular care should be taken with young patients to ensure that they are in the same position on the bed for each measurement and the bed should not be moved with respect to the counter between readings. In the case of using a handheld counter, it is essential to ensure that the patient-counter geometry is reproduced as accurately as possible.
3. *First measurement.* The first patient reading should be acquired immediately following administration and before the first void to obtain the baseline to which further measurements will be calibrated. Ideally, both anterior

and posterior scans should be acquired to obtain a geometric mean of the count rate or of the exposure rate (depending on the instrument display) C_0.

$$C_0 = \sqrt{(C_{0\mathrm{ANT}} - \mathrm{BKG}_0)\times(C_{0\mathrm{POST}} - \mathrm{BKG}_0)}$$

4. *Second measurement.* The second reading C_1 should be acquired immediately after the first void to determine the level of administered activity that is immediately excreted.
5. *Subsequent readings.* These should be taken ideally at least every 2 h for the first 24 h, and every 4–6 h thereafter, subject to the patient being awake and in accordance with (2) above. This will generally require the omission of readings taken at night. Patients must void before each reading. Practically a minimum of three counts in the first day and two counts in the following days (early morning and late evening) result in acceptable clearance curves. The last count should be taken at more than about 66 h from administration.

$$C_\mathrm{j} = \sqrt{(C_{\mathrm{jANT}} - \mathrm{BKG_j})\times(C_{\mathrm{jPOST}} - \mathrm{BKG_j})}$$

6. *Activity-time curve (TACT).* Decay phases may be determined from the activity-time curve, starting from C_1 but excluding C_0, which is used for quantification purpose only (Fig. 20.1). The minimal approach suggested is a bi-exponential fit although many phases may be determined in some treatments.
7. *Cumulated activity.* Integration of the curve to determine the cumulated activity, $\tilde{A}$ in MBq h, and the residence time τ in hours can be calculated from consideration of sequential decay phases.
8. *Calculate absorbed dose.* The whole-body absorbed dose may then be calculated using the standard MIRD equation:

$$D = \tilde{A}\times S_{WB\leftarrow WB}$$

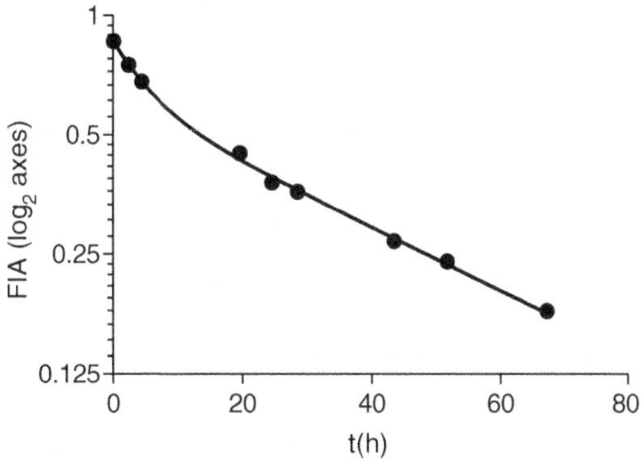

Fig. 20.1 An example of whole-body clearance curve obtained with a Geiger mounted on the ceiling. *FIA* is the Fraction of Injected Activity

20.2.2 Lesion Dosimetry

Lesion dosimetry requires a sequence of images. This may be more demanding on children than on adults. Due to the heterogeneity of uptake in larger lesions, SPECT dosimetry is recommended. A series of 3–4 scans is advisable. The last scan should be acquired at least at day 3 after administration (72 h). To acquire such a series of acquisitions, the possibility of performing scans in narcosis may be considered, as younger patients may be treated in narcosis with external beams.

An additional problem is that peri-therapeutic scans are heavily affected by the saturation problem deriving from the dead time of the detector. The easiest solution is to wait for sufficient clearance, typically for 2 days. This however prolongs the sequence in the second week. An ideal solution is to develop or purchase a SPECT dead time correction method [8]. This allows the first scan to be acquired at an earlier time (for instance, 24 h). Images should be corrected for scatter with a triple energy window and for attenuation. The partial volume effect is particularly pronounced with imaging of small volumes in systems of low spatial resolution with high-energy collimators.

20.3 Feasibility in Routine Practice

Whole-body dosimetry during hospitalisation is a common procedure. Tricks to convince a child to remain still on a bed for 1 min can be used, turning the procedure into a game (e.g. saying "Let's play the mummy" or "I challenge you to be steady for 1 min"). For very young children, the presence of parents or grandparents, required anyway, can help during the counting procedure.

The feasibility of lesion dosimetry is less studied. Our experience confirms that four planar whole-body scintigrams on babies as young as 3 years old, assisted by their mother, hand in hand, without narcosis may be obtained.

20.4 Short Review

Internal dosimetry offers the potential to play an important role in the harmonisation and optimisation of a standard methodological framework for mIBG therapy. The acquisition of a series of gamma camera scintigrams for dosimetry in paediatric neuroblastoma can however be demanding for children. For this reason, and to improve accuracy, the whole-body dosimetry method using an external counter was introduced as a surrogate for bone marrow dosimetry, which is the activity-limiting criteria for administration. This method is intended as a basis for the European protocol VERITAS under the auspices of SIOPEN following a protocol developed whereby two mIBG therapeutic administrations are administered within a 15-day interval. Whole-body dosimetry from the first cycle is then used as a basis to calculate the activity for the second, in order to reach a total of 4 Gy to the whole body [9].

The predictive power of such dosimetric methodology on haematological toxicity is powerful, but its reliability is limited by bone marrow infiltration and pretreatment with chemotherapy. These factors bias the relationship between red marrow dosimetry and toxicity.

With regard to dose efficacy of tumours, a single dose-response correlation has been published [10, 11]. The intrinsic feature of neuroblastoma lesions presents a challenge for assessing dosimetry-related responses as they frequently comprise large tumours with heterogeneous uptake, leading to non-uniformity of absorbed dose distributions. In many other cases, lesions are infiltrative in the bone marrow, and their volume cannot be accurately measured. An interesting case report [12] casts a renewed light after 20 years [13] on the potential to determine the non-uniformity of uptake, adopting ^{124}I-mIBG PET/MR for phaeochromocytoma dosimetry. The lack of absorbed dose-effect relationships in lesions may be considered the result of an absence of clinical trials and the paucity of data on tumour dosimetry.

20.4.1 Dosimetry to Prevent Toxicity

20.4.1.1 Peculiarities of Methodology Implemented for ^{131}I mIBG Dosimetry

Red marrow dosimetry for agents without active or passive bone or red marrow uptake, including radioiodine, ^{131}I mIBG and ^{131}I MoAbs, relies on a series of blood samples and of whole-body counts [14]. mIBG exhibits a fast blood clearance. The direct beta irradiation from the blood to bone marrow is less important in ^{131}I mIBG than in ^{131}I NaI [15]. In addition, the potential difficulty of obtaining blood samples from children led many researchers after Sisson et al. [2] towards the use of whole-body counting only and to consider the whole-body absorbed dose as a surrogate for red marrow absorbed dose evaluation. This methodology, which is easy to implement both pre- and peri-therapeutically, has proven to be effective.

20.4.1.2 Dosimetry and Haematological Toxicity

The first dosimetric evaluation of ^{131}I mIBG dosimetry, and to date the only absorbed dose escalation study performed, was undertaken by the United Kingdom Children's Cancer Study Group (UKCCSG) in 1991 (Fielding et al. [3]). Twenty five children suffering from neuroblastoma were studied in 6 centres. Absorbed doses for organs were studied pre-therapeutically with a static scintigram at a minimum of 5 time points up to 72 h p.i., with a later scan also acquired. Therapeutic activity was chosen on a dosimetric basis, escalating from 1.0 Gy to 2.5 Gy, rather than on injected activity. The two distributions of red marrow and whole-body absorbed dose per unit activity fairly but not exactly overlap, with the majority of patients receiving less than 0.39 Gy/GBq. Differences between the two values in each patient reached 30%. The blood absorbed dose was markedly lower. A discrepancy between the predicted and peri-therapeutically verified whole- body absorbed dose was observed in 10/26 treatments, with the absorbed dose at therapy being lower than that predicted in 9/10 cases by up to 32%. This was attributed to the different specific activity of the two dosimetry sessions. A dose-effect correlation is reported by Lashford et al. [16]). Bone marrow toxicity increased with whole-body absorbed dose, with 80% of patients developing grade 3 or 4 thrombocytopenia at a prescribed whole-body radiation dose of 2.5 Gy.

The correlation of bone marrow toxicity with activity or absorbed dose was investigated by Matthay et al. in two consecutive studies in pretreated neuroblastoma patients. The first phase I study [10] determined that with an activity-limiting cut-off of 444 MBq/kg (12 mCi/kg), bone marrow rescue was not required. Dose-limiting haematological toxicity, requiring bone marrow reinfusion, was reached at 555 MBq/kg (15 mCi/kg). Prolonged thrombocytopenia was common.

In the second study [11] on 42 patients with the same range of activity per kg, it was found that the whole-body absorbed dose correlated with activity/kg with a Spearman analysis (r = 0.59, $p < 0.0001$). However, in a figure of that paper, it is evident that in some individual cases, the actual whole-body absorbed dose is twice than that predicted by a weight-based activity administration. This correlation therefore cannot justify the avoidance of individualised dosimetry.

A two-interval normal tissue complication probability (NTCP) for haematological toxicity of grades 3 and 4 resulted in 24/24 toxicity cases (NTCP = 100%) above 555 MBq/kg (15 mCi/kg), with an NTCP = 50% below that value. The value of 555 MBq/kg corresponded in that paper to a 2.5 Gy whole-body absorbed dose, confirming that above 2.5 Gy all patients experience toxicity, whilst below that value probability and individual radiosensitivity play a major role. No stem cell reinfusion was required below that cut-off value, whilst 11/24 reinfusions were necessary above that value ($p < 0.001$). Neutrophil (N) and platelet (PLT) values at nadir correlated both with administered MBq/kg and with whole-body dose, independently measured. The Spearman correlation factors were $r = -0.44$ (N) and r = −0.37 (PLT) for MBq/kg, whilst values for the whole-body absorbed dose were better ($r = -0.56$, $r = -0.40$). The need for stem cell reinfusion also correlated with whole-body absorbed dose, which had a median value of 3.2 Gy (range [1.8–6.5] Gy) for the 11/24 patients that required reinfusion, whilst it was 2.2 [0.6–5.4] Gy in patients without the need of PBSCS ($p = 0.03$).

Whole-body absorbed dose-toxicity correlations were also the focus of a study by Buckley et al. [6], which demonstrated a statistically significant correlation between the whole-body absorbed dose and neutropenia, whereas no correlation was found between the administered activity and toxicity. The whole-body absorbed dose of patients with grade 1 neutropenia was 0.90 ± 0.12 Gy, whilst for those with grade 4 toxicity, it was 1.63 ± 0.4 Gy ($p = 0.05$). It was found that the administration of previous or concomitant chemotherapy resulted in lower PLT and WBC nadir values with respect to ^{131}I mIBG treatments alone. Moreover, PLT and neutrophil nadir occurred significantly earlier in the presence of concomitant therapy. Buckley et al. also showed that dosimetry performed during the previous treatment is the most accurate and precise predictor of the whole-body absorbed dose.

20.4.1.3 Liver Dosimetry

If stem cell support is available, the 2 Gy limit for haematological toxicity can be overcome. Activity per kg higher than 555 MBq/kg (15 mCi/kg) can be repeatedly administered. This brings into question the issue of the next organ at risk which is the liver. Liver dosimetry requires sequential imaging, as is the case for tumour dosimetry. Fielding et al. [3] reported the mean absorbed doses to the liver to be 0.9 Gy/GBq but with a maximum of 2.0 Gy/GBq. Koral et al. [17] compared liver dosimetry in pre- and peri-therapeutic dosimetry, demonstrating a statistically significant reduction in the absorbed dose delivered to the liver at therapy of a factor 1.28 with respect to the tracer study. This phenomenon was ascribed to an initial indication of hepatocyte toxicity. The median liver absorbed dose agreed closely with the Fielding study at 0.8 Gy/GBq, with a range of [0.5–1.1] Gy/GBq.

A patient with the upper extreme value of 1 Gy/GBq administered twice with 15 GBq (400 mCi) would reach a total of 30 Gy to the liver, the irradiation limit adopted in external beam radiotherapy for a 5% of risk of radioinduced disease in 5 years. Such direct comparison to the external beam absorbed dose limits however is not correct, since the role of different dose rate is neglected. The lower dose rate with ^{131}I-mIBG compared to external beam radiation therapy (EBRT), i.e. the dilution of the irradiation in a longer time, could mitigate the damage, for the same absorbed dose. In more rigorous terms, it could be considered that the Biologically Effective Dose (BED) from 30 Gy, delivered at 2 Gy/day with external beam radiotherapy, with a value of $\alpha/\beta = 2.5$ Gy for the liver, is given by:

$$BED_{\mathrm{EBRT}} = D\left[1 + d/(\alpha/\beta)\right] = 30\,\mathrm{Gy}\left[1 + 2/2.5\right] = 54\,\mathrm{Gy}$$

For mIBG irradiation, a different formula should be used for BED. If the liver clearance curve was mono-exponential, with generally adopted $T^{REP} = 2.5$ h, this gives:

$$BED = D + \frac{1}{\alpha/\beta} \frac{T_{1/2}^{REP}}{T_{1/2}^{REP} + T_{1/2}^{EFF}} D^2$$

Radioiodine is long-lived isotope. According to in vivo measurements, it may be assumed that T^{EFF} is larger than 50 h, so that

$$BED_{\mathrm{mIBG}} < 48\,\mathrm{Gy}$$

Therefore the same absorbed dose of 30 Gy delivered with a single mIBG administration is less toxic to the liver than EBRT. In case of two mIBG administrations delivering an absorbed dose of 15 Gy each, the total BED_{mIBG} is even lower, i.e. < 39 $\mathrm{Gy_{BED}}$.

Consider moreover that the liver is the second tissue, after the bone marrow, capable of regeneration within about 3 months.

These two factors (that BED is lower for I-131 mIBG therapy than for EBRT and regeneration of liver) could explain the fact that liver toxicity has not been reported after repeated mIBG treatment. Consider however that the interval between treatments is usually of some months. The proposed treatment algorithm in the VERITAS project (two high activity administrations 2 weeks apart) poses a new scenario. Liver dosimetry and follow-up would be very interesting in this protocol.

20.4.2 Dosimetry to Investigate Efficacy

A wide range of lesion absorbed doses per unit activity have been reported [18]. The use of ^{123}I mIBG pre-therapy lesion dosimetry was studied by Tristam et al. [19]. Sudbrock et al. [20] used daily whole-body scans commencing the day following therapeutic administration and developed a dead time correction method to compensate for the count losses due to camera saturation. Delpon et al. [21] and Chiesa et al. [22] stated that any dead time correction method for whole-body images requires a step and shoot modality for whole-body acquisition, since the degree of saturation is dependent on the level of activity seen by the detector, which varies continuously in continuous WB scanning and therefore cannot be corrected using this modality.

To avoid the dead time problem for SPECT imaging, Buckley et al. [23] took the first scan when the remaining activity was less than 1.5 GBq, as deduced from whole-body counting. This was usually at least 48 h following administration. Matthay et al. [11] developed a simple method to simultaneously correct for attenuation and dead time on planar static images, using an ^{131}I point source within the field of view. They were able to demonstrate a Spearman correlation between the tumour absorbed dose and volume reduction. Their tumour control probability (TCP) histogram indicated that in absorbed dose ranges of [0–17] Gy, [17–70] Gy and [70–300] Gy, the response probability was, respectively, 33%, 44% and 100%.

20.5 Future Perspectives

The difficulties of ^{131}I imaging have led to consideration of dosimetry based on ^{124}I mIBG PET imaging as indicated over 20 years ago by Fielding et al. [3]. Further dosimetric ^{124}I mIBG

PET studies are likely with the advent of hybrid PET-MRI systems [12]. The most recent paper about ^{124}I mIBG PET dosimetry found a marked difference between usual S factors derived by the Cristy-Eckerman phantom, presently used in OLINDA 1.1, and those derived using a more refined virtual phantom developed by the Florida University and National Cancer Institute [24]. Four PET/CT were taken up to 115 h post injection. The 10-year-old female, 29 kg weight, was then treated without considering the predicted dosimetry, with an activity of 666 MBq/kg (18 mCi/kg), with an administration of ^{131}I-mIBG of 19.3 GBq (522 mCi). The predicted absorbed dose to the spleen, lungs, thyroid, liver, heart wall and salivary glands were, respectively, 16, 21, 23, 34, 36 and 98 Gy. Note that lung and liver dose of 21 Gy and 34 Gy are above the tolerance limit adopted in EBRT (but remember the BED argument presented above for liver dosimetry). In conclusion, the trend towards high ^{131}I mIBG activity administrations can potentially result in high absorbed doses delivered to normal organs, even after a single injection. This demands the development of a reliable pretreatment dosimetry.

Key Points

- 131-I mIBG therapy is mainly delivered to children affected by neuroblastoma. This remarks the importance of optimising the treatment using a quantitative approach.
- A very simple and accessible methodology has been developed and tested on several cases. This consists of a series of whole-body counts without the need of imaging, using either a Geiger counter fixed to the ceiling above the bed in the therapy unit, or thyroid uptake probe, or portable counters. The whole-body dose correlates with haematological toxicity. A safety limit of 2 Gy is generally accepted if stem cells are not available. The dosimetric study performed during the first treatment allows to maximise the activity for the subsequent treatments.
- Imaging-based dosimetry has been rarely performed for the challenge of having a child steady. It is however feasible and is the root to real optimisation of the treatment (balance between whole-body and lesion absorbed dose). Liver dosimetry might be important in high activity approach repeated within a short interval.
- 124-I mIBG PET is a promising option to plan the treatment.

References

1. Castellani MR, Seghezzi S, Chiesa C, Aliberti GL, Maccauro M, Seregni E, et al. ^{131}I-MIBG treatment of pheochromocytoma: low versus intermediate activity regimens of therapy. Q J Nucl Med Mol Imaging. 2010;54(1):100–13.
2. Sisson JC, Hutchinson RJ, Carey JE, Shapiro B, Johnson JW, Mallette SA, Wieland DM. Toxicity from treatment of neuro-blastoma with 131I-meta-Iodobenzylguanidine. Eur J Nucl Med. 1988; 14(7-8):337–40.
3. Fielding SL, FLower MA, Ackery D, Kemshead JT, Lashford LS, Lewis I. Dosimetry of iodine 131 metaiodobenzylguanidine for treatment of resistant neuroblastoma: results of a UK study. Eur J Nucl Med. 1991;18:308–16.
4. Monsieurs M, Brans B, Bacher K, Dierckx R, Thierens H. Patient dosimetry for I-131-MIBG therapy for neuroendocrine tumours based on I-123-MIBG scans. Eur J Nucl Med Mol Imaging. 2002;29(12):1581–7.
5. Flux GD, Guy MJ, Beddows R, Pryor M, Flower MA. Estimation and implications of random errors in whole-body dosimetry for targeted radionuclide therapy. Phys Med Biol. 2002;47(17):3211–23.
6. Buckley SE, Chittenden SC, Saran FH, Meller ST, Flux GD. Whole-body dosimetry for individualized treatment planning of 131I-mIBG radionuclide therapy for neuroblastoma. J Nucl Med. 2009;50(9):1518–24.
7. Chittenden S, Pratt B, Pomeroy K, Black P, Long C, Smith N, Buckley SE, Saran F, Flux GD. Optimization of equipment and methodology for whole-body activity retention measurements in children undergoing targeted radionuclide therapy. Cancer Biother Radiopharm. 2007;22(2):247–53.
8. Dewaraja YK, Ljungberg M, Green AJ, Zanzonico PB, Frey EC, SNMMI MIRD Committee, Bolch WE, Brill AB, Dunphy M, Fisher DR, Howell RW, Meredith RF, Sgouros G, Wessels BW. MIRD pamphlet no. 24: guidelines for quantitative 131I SPECT in dosimetry applications. J Nucl Med. 2013;54(12):2182–8.
9. Gaze MN, Chang YC, Flux GD, Mairs RJ, Saran FH, Meller ST. Feasibility of dosimetry-based high-dose131i-meta-Iodobenzylguanidine with topotecan as a radiosensitizer in children with metastatic neuroblastoma. Cancer Biother Radiopharm. 2005;20(2):195–9.

10. Matthay KK, DeSantes K, Hasegawa B, Huberty J, Hattner RS, Ablin A, et al. Phase I dose escalation of 131I-metaiodobenzylguanidine with autologous bone marrow support in refractory neuroblastoma. J Clin Oncol. 1998;16(1):229–36.
11. Matthay KK, Panina C, Huberty J, Price D, Glidden DV, Tang HR, et al. Correlation of tumor and whole-body dosimetry with tumor response and toxicity in refractory neuroblastoma treated with (131)I-MIBG. J Nucl Med. 2001;42(11):1713–21.
12. Hartung-Knemeyer V, Rosenbaum-Krumme S, Buchbender C, Poppel T, Brandau W, Jentzen W, et al. Malignant pheochromocytoma imaging with [^{124}I]mIBG PET/MR. J Clin Endocrinol Metab. 2012;97(11):3833–4.
13. Ott RJ, Tait D, Flower MA, Babich JW, Lambrecht RM. Treatment planning for ^{131}I mIBG radiotherapy of neural crest tumors using ^{124}I-mIBG positron emission tomography. Br J Radiol. 1992;65:787–91.
14. Hindorf C, Glatting G, Chiesa C, Lindèn O, Flux G. EANM dosimetry committee guidelines for bone marrow and whole-body dosimetry. Eur J Nucl Med Mol Imaging. 2010;37(6):1238–5.
15. Chiesa C, Castellani R, Mira M, Lorenzoni A, Flux GD. Dosimetry in 131I-MIBG therapy: moving toward personalized medice. Q J Nucl Med Mol Imaging. 2013;57:161–70.
16. Lashford LS, Lewis IJ, Fielding SL, Flower MA, Meller S, Kemshead JT, Ackery D. Phase I/II study of iodine 131 metaiodobenzylguanidine in chemoresistant neuroblastoma: a United Kingdom Children's Cancer Study Group investigation. J Clin Oncol. 1992;10(12):1889–96.
17. Koral KF, Huberty JP, Frame B, Matthay KK, Maris JM, Regan D, et al. Hepatic absorbed radiation dosimetry during 131I metaiodobenzylguanidine (MIBG) therapy for refractory neuroblastoma. Eur J Nucl Med Mol Imaging. 2008;35:2105–12.
18. Flux GD, Chittenden SJ, Saran F, Gaze MN. Clinical applications of dosimetry for mIBG therapy. Q J Nucl Med Mol Imaging. 2011;55:116–25.
19. Tristam M, Alaamer AS, Fleming JS, Lewington VJ, Zivanovic MA. Iodine-131-metaiodobenzylguanidine dosimetry in cancer therapy: risk versus benefit. J Nucl Med. 1996;37(6):1058–63.
20. Sudbrock F, Schmidt M, Simon T, Eschner W, Berthold F, Schica H. Dosimetry for ^{131}I mIBG therapies in metastatic neuroblastoma, phaeochromocytoma and paraganglioma. Eur J Nucl Med Mol Imaging. 2010;37:1279–90.
21. Delpon G, Ferrer L, Lisbona A, Bardies M. Correction of count losses due to deadtime on a DST-XLi (SMVi-GE) camera during dosimetric studies in patients injected with iodine-131. Phys Med Biol. 2002;47:N79–90.
22. Chiesa C, Negri A, Albertini C, Azzeroni R, Setti E, Mainardi L, Aliberti G, Seregni E, Bombardieri E. A practical dead time correction method in planar activity quantification for dosimetry during radionuclide therapy. Q J Nucl Med Mol Imaging. 2009;53(6):658–70.
23. Buckley SE, Saran FH, Gaze MN, Chittenden S, Partridge M, Lancaster D, Pearson A, Flux GD. Dosimetry for fractionated ^{131}I-mIBG therapies in patients with primary resistant high-risk neuroblastoma: preliminary results. Cancer Biother Radiopharm. 2007;22(1):105–12.
24. Huang S, Bolch WE, Lee C, Brocklin H, Pampaloni M, Hawkins R, Sznewajs A, DuBois S, Matthay K, Seo Y. Patient-specific dosimetry using pretherapy [^{124}I]m-iodobenzylguanidine ([^{124}I]mIBG) dynamic PET/CT imaging before [^{131}I]mIBG targeted radionuclide therapy for neuroblastoma. Mol Imaging Biol. 2015;17:284–94.

Medical Treatment of Gastroenteropancreatic (GEP) Neuroendocrine Tumors

21

Carlo Carnaghi and Valeria Smiroldo

Abstract

Neuroendocrine tumors (NETs) are a heterogeneous group of neoplasms that arise from the diffuse endocrine system present in various organs. These tumors are classified as functioning and nonfunctioning due to the presence of a specific syndrome determined by the production of some peptides and, due to the low incidence, they are considered rare. This landscape is going to change due to the steadily rising prevalence and incidence as reported by a recent SEER database analysis. The first aim of the treatment of patients with diagnosis of NETs is to cure, and this goal could be achieved by surgery. If patients are not suitable for surgery with curative intent, a medical management for symptom and disease is required. Somatostatin analogues are the backbone of the treatment of symptoms; a few years later after their introduction in clinical practice, the antiproliferative effects were demonstrated by two clinical trials. Significant clinical activity was also achieved with two different oral target therapies: everolimus (mTOR inhibitor) and sunitinib (multi-targeted receptor tyrosine kinase inhibitor). Chemotherapy maintains a significat role for the most aggressive variants such as neuroendocrine cancers (NECs). At last, the peptide receptor radiotherapy is an innovative therapeutic approach for somatostatin receptor-positive inoperable and metastatic NETs.

21.1 Introduction

Neuroendocrine tumors (NETs) are an heterogeneous group of malignancies that sometimes produce peptides that cause characteristic hormonal syndromes. NETs can be clinically symptomatic (functioning) or silent (nonfunctioning); both types frequently synthesize more than one peptide,

C. Carnaghi (✉) • V. Smiroldo
Oncology and Hematology Unit, Humanitas Cancer Center, Istituto Clinico Humanitas, Rozzano, Italy
e-mail: carlo.carnaghi@cancercenter.humanitas.it

E. Bombardieri et al. (eds.), *Clinical Applications of Nuclear Medicine Targeted Therapy*,
https://doi.org/10.1007/978-3-319-63067-0_21

although often these are not associated with specific syndromes. In the last years, the incidence and prevalence of NETs are increasing [1]. The primary treatment goal for patients with NETs is curative, with symptom control and the limitation of tumor progression as secondary goals. Surgery is the only possible curative approach and it represents the traditional first-line therapy. However, as most patients with NETs are diagnosed once metastases have occurred, curative surgery is generally not possible. Patients therefore require chronic postoperative medical management with the aim of relieving symptoms and improving tumor growth and survival. Descriptions of the most common treatment options for metastatic GEP-NETs will be described. Treatment options and recommendations depend on several factors, including the type and stage of neuroendocrine tumor, possible side effects, and the patient's preferences and overall health.

Unfortunately, the limited number of clinical randomized trials and the lack of sequence trials didn't allow to draw a clear therapeutic algorithm.

21.2 Somatostatin Analogues in Gastroenteropancreatic Neuroendocrine Tumors

Octreotide was the first biologically somatostatin analogue (SSA) that has been synthesized; it binds with high, low, and moderate affinity to SSTR2, SSTR3, and SSTR5, respectively [2]. Long-acting formulation of octreotide (octreotide LAR) was approved in 1995; it is a depot preparation administered by monthly intramuscular injection. The pharmacokinetics show an initial peak within 1 h of administration and a second release reaching a plateau between days 14 and 42. Steady-state serum concentrations are reached after three injections [3]. *Lanreotide* is another different somatostatin analogue with a similar receptors binding profile. The original sustained-release formulation (lanreotide SR) was later followed by lanreotide Autogel [4]. After administration, lanreotide peptide monomers are slowly released over a period of 1 month.

Somatostatin analogues have long been indicated for symptom relief associated with GEP-NET, and their clinical use has contributed to improved patient survival. The benefits related to somatostatin analogues (SSAs) were shown in three phase III randomized trials (Table 21.1). Gastrointestinal-related complaints are the most frequently reported side effects; these are related to disruption of GEP hormone signaling and reduced secretion of digestive enzymes. Altered secretion of cholecystokinin can lead to abnormalities in the biliary system and development of biliary sediment/sludge, microlithiasis, or gallstones [5].

The phase III trial (PROMID), a multicenter, randomized, double-blind, placebo-controlled trial, was the first large trial to confirm the antitumor effect of octreotide LAR in a randomized setting. In 85 treatment-naïve patients with well-differentiated metastatic GEP-NET of the midgut, functional and nonfunctional, median time to tumor progression in the octreotide LAR and

Table 21.1 Published phase III trials with SSAs

Study	N of pts.	Tumor origin	Treatment	Primary endpoint	Prior therapy	Results (mo)	HR, *p*-value
PROMID [6]	85	G1 metastatic GEP-NET of the midgut	Octreotide LAR vs placebo	TTP	No	14.3 vs 6	HR 0.34; 95% CI 0.20–0.59; *P* 0.000072
RADIANT-2 [13]	429	NETs	EVE 10 mg/day + octreotide LAR vs placebo + octreotide LAR	PFS	Yes	16.4 vs 11.3	HR 0.77; 95% CI 0.59–1.00; *P* 0.026
CLARINET [8]	204	G1-G2, nonfunctional NETs	Lanreotide Autogel vs placebo	PFS	Yes	NR vs 18	HR 0.47; 95% CI 0.30–0.73; *P* < 0.001

mo months, *TTP* time to progression, *GEP* gastroenteropancreatic, *GI* gastrointestinal, *BSC* best supportive care, *SSAs* somatostatin analogues, *PFS* progression-free survival, *NR* not reached placebo groups was 14.3 and 6 months, respectively (HR 0.34; CI 0.20–0.59; P = 0.000072) [6]. Authors concluded that due to the low number of observed deaths, the survival analysis was not confirmatory, and the extent of tumor burden is a predictor for shorter survival. Overall survival was similar in patients receiving octreotide LAR or placebo treatment [7]. The Lanreotide Antiproliferative Response in Patients with GEP-NET (CLARINET) trial is a randomized, double-blind, placebo-controlled, multinational study of the somatostatin analogue lanreotide in patients with advanced, well-differentiated, or moderately differentiated, nonfunctioning, somatostatin receptor-positive neuroendocrine tumors. Patients were randomly assigned to receive lanreotide Autogel Depot at a dose of 120 mg or placebo once every 28 days for 96 weeks. The primary endpoint of progression-free survival (PFS) was met, lanreotide Autogel was superior to placebo in prolonging PFS, and median PFS was not reached with lanreotide Autogel vs 18 months with placebo (HR 0.47; 95% CI 0.30–0.73; $P < 0.001$). After 2 years of treatment, estimated rates of PFS were 65.1 and 33.0% in the lanreotide Autogel and placebo groups, respectively [8].

Pasireotide is a next-generation, multi-receptor-targeted somatostatin analogue with high affinity for SSTR1, SSTR2, SSTR3, and SSTR5. Binding affinity to SSTR5 is 39-fold higher than octreotide [9]. Pasireotide long-acting formulation (pasireotide LAR) is administered by monthly intramuscular injection. It has a similar safety profile as that of first-generation SSAs, except for a higher frequency and degree of hyperglycemia [10].

A phase III multicenter, randomized, double-blind clinical trial evaluated pasireotide LAR (160 mg) vs increased dose of octreotide LAR (40 mg) in patients with metastatic GEP-NETs with carcinoid symptoms failing at standard dose of octreotide LAR (30 mg). Pasireotide LAR and octreotide LAR showed similar effects on symptom control, and the trial was earlt stopped due to the higher toxicity profile of pasireotide. This trial was not designed for evaluating survival data, but in the analysis, pasireotide LAR was associated with a longer PFS compared with octreotide LAR; these data warrant further investigation into the role of pasireotide LAR in the treatment of GEP-NETs [11].

21.3 Targeted Therapies

Everolimus is a serine-threonine kinase inhibitor of mammalian target of rapamycin (mTOR) downstreamer of the PI3K/AKT pathway. Everolimus binds to an intracellular protein, FKBP-12, resulting in an inhibitory complex formation with mTOR complex 1 (mTORC1) and thus inhibition of mTOR kinase activity. Everolimus efficacy was investigated in four trials (Table 21.2).

Table 21.2 Published trials with everolimus

Study	Phase	N of pts.	Tumor origin	Treatment	Primary endpoint	Results	HR, p-value
RADIANT-1 [12]	II	160	pNETs	EVE 10 mg/day	ORR	8.7%	–
RADIANT-2 [13]	III	429	NETs	EVE 10 mg/day + octreotide LAR vs placebo + octreotide LAR	PFS	16.4 vs 11.3 mo	HR 0.77; 95% CI 0.59–1.00; P 0.026
RADIANT-3 [14]	III	410	pNETs, G1-G2	EVE 10 mg/day or placebo + BSC (±SSAs)	PFS	11 vs 4.6 mo	HR 0.35; 95% CI 0.27–0.45; $P < 0.001$
RADIANT-4 [15]	III	205	G1 nonfunctional NETs of the lung or GI	EVE 10 mg/day or placebo	PFS	11.0 vs 3.9 mo	HR 0.48; 95% CI 0.35–0.67; $P < 0.00001$

GI gastrointestinal, *BSC* best supportive care, *SSAs* somatostatin analogues, *PFS* progression-free survival, *ORR* objective response rate, *EVE* everolimus, *mo* months

RADIANT-1 is a multinational, single-arm phase II trial that evaluated everolimus 10 mg/day in patients with *advanced pNETs* refractory to cytotoxic chemotherapy. Patients who were previously on SSAs were continued on this regimen. This trial demonstrated an 8.7% objective response rate, and 84.7% of patients had at least stable disease. Median PFS was 9.7 months in patients receiving everolimus alone and 16.7 for everolimus and octreotide treatment. Median overall survival was 24.9 months in the everolimus group and had not yet been reached at the time of publication in the everolimus plus octreotide group [12].

The RADIANT-2 trial is a multicenter, randomized, placebo-controlled phase III trial looking at the role of adding everolimus 10 mg/day or placebo to octreotide LAR 30 mg every 28 days in patients with *advanced NETs and carcinoid syndrome*. Median PFS was 16.4 months in the everolimus group compared with 11.3 months in the placebo group. Although this trial demonstrated that treatment with everolimus was associated with a reduced risk of progression of 23%, the hazard ratio (0.77; $p = 0.026$) fell short of achieving statistical significance based on the prespecified cutoff value ($p = 0.0246$) [13].

RADIANT-3 is a multicenter, double-blind, randomized phase III trial that evaluated everolimus in patients with unresectable or *metastatic low- or intermediate-grade pNETs* progressing to prior chemotherapy or other systemic treatments. Patients received either everolimus 10 mg/day or placebo in addition to best supportive care, including SSAs in 40% of cases. PFS was 11 months for the everolimus group versus 4.6 months in the placebo group, with a hazard ratio for disease progression or death with everolimus of 0.35 ($p < 0.001$); no significant difference was documented in overall survival between the two treatment arms of the RADIANT-3 trial, since the trial design allowed crossover at disease progression [14].

RADIANT-4 is a randomized, double-blind, placebo-controlled, phase III trial that evaluated the PFS in patients with *advanced, progressive, well-differentiated, nonfunctional neuroendocrine tumors of the lung or gastrointestinal origin* treated with everolimus 10 mg/day or placebo. At central review analysis, everolimus-treated patients showed a prolonged median PFS, as compared with those receiving placebo (11.0 vs 3.9 months; HR 0.48; 95% CI 0.35–0.67; $p < 0.00001$); similar results were observed at investigator assessment (14.0 vs 5.5 months; HR 0.39; 95% CI 0.28–0.54; $p < 0.00001$). This benefit in PFS was achieved in all subgroup analyses. The first pre-planned interim OS analysis suggested that everolimus might be associated with a reduction in the risk of death (HR 0.64; 95% CI 0.40–1.05; $p = 0.037$, whereas the boundary for statistical significance was 0.0002) compared with placebo [15].

Sunitinib malate is a multitargeted tyrosine kinase inhibitor, whose targets include vascular endothelial growth factor receptors (VEGFRs) and stem cell factor receptor (c-KIT). A phase III (SUN-1111), randomized, double-blind, placebo-controlled trial was conducted to assess the efficacy and safety of continuous daily administration of sunitinib 37.5 mg/day in patients with advanced pancreatic neuroendocrine tumors. The study was discontinued early after the observation of serious adverse events and deaths in the placebo group as well as a difference in progression-free survival favoring sunitinib. Median progression-free survival was 11.4 months in the sunitinib group as compared with 5.5 months in the placebo group (hazard ratio for progression or death, 0.42; 95% confidence interval [CI], 0.26–0.66; $P < 0.001$) [16].

In 2016, the updated progression-free survival and the final overall survival of SUN-1111 were published. Five years after study closure, median OS was 38.6 months for sunitinib and 29.1 months for placebo (HR 0.73; 95% CI 0.50–1.06; $P = 0.094$), with 69% of placebo patients having crossed over to sunitinib; median PFS was 12.6 months for sunitinib and 5.8 months for placebo (HR 0.32; 95% CI 0.18–0.55; $P = 0.000015$). The authors conclude for the doubling of PFS with sunitinib compared with placebo [17].

Cabozantinib (XL-184) is a potent inhibitor of MET, VEGFR2/KDR, RET, and other receptor tyrosine kinases, such as KIT, AXL, and

FLT3. In an open-label phase II trial, cabozantinib demonstrated clinical activity in patients with advanced carcinoid and well or moderately differentiated pNET. Patients received cabozantinib 60 mg daily in 28-day cycles. A somatostatin analogue was allowed if the dose was stable for 2 months. There was no limit to prior therapy. The primary objective was to evaluate the overall response rate. Partial responses were observed in 15% of each cohort treated with cabozantinib, and stable disease was the best response in about two-thirds of patients. Median progression-free survival was 21.8 months (95% CI 8.5–32.0). Adverse events were consistent with those reported with the use of cabozantinib in other diseases. Grade 3/4 toxicity included hypertension in 13% of patients, hypophosphatemia in 11%, diarrhea in 10%, lymphopenia in 7%, thrombocytopenia in 5%, fatigue in 5%, and increased lipase or amylase in 8%. At present, a confirmation of cabozantinib activity in a randomized phase III trial in carcinoid tumors and pNETs is in development [18].

21.4 The Role of Chemotherapy in Advanced and Metastatic GEP-NETs

The majority of well-differentiated GEP-NETs have an indolent behavior, but in patients who develop clear tumor progression, systemic chemotherapy may be useful. Cytotoxic chemotherapy has been tested in GEP-NETs since the 1980s, but treatment recommendations are controversial in many instances.

Streptozotocin (STZ) was the most studied chemotherapy agents in NETs. The efficacy of STZ alone or in combination with 5FU and doxorubicin is documented by several small nonrandomized trials.

A recent systematic review and meta-analysis try to evaluate the role of "standard" combination of STZ and 5FU comparing its activity with the other available chemotherapy regimens. The results do not show any significant differences in terms of overall response rate, progression-free survival, and overall survival [19–24].

Other drugs that showed efficacy in NETs are dacarbazine, cisplatin, capecitabine, etoposide, carboplatin, temozolomide, and irinotecan, but due to the lack of data, also ENETS, NANETS, and NCCN guidelines do not give any clear suggestion about the ideal schedules and specific indication [25–27].

Differently to NETs, chemotherapy is the standard treatment for metastatic poorly differentiated neuroendocrine carcinoma (NEC) in which it represents the only therapeutic option. The standard combination is cisplatin and etoposide or irinotecan. Although these neoplasms are more chemosensitive than NETs (ORR about 55%), the prognosis is extremely poor [28].

21.5 Treatment Selection and Sequences

Considering the long median survival, documented in patients with diagnosis of locally advanced and metastatic NETs, one of the aims of treatment is the continuum of care that could be achieved by the individualization of the best therapy sequence. Comparing the different available guidelines, we could find some suggestions about the selection for first, second, and further lines of treatment, but the ideal sequence and how one therapy could influence the subsequent treatment outcomes are unknown. If we take, for example, NETs of the midgut, the favorable toxicity profile of somatostatin analogues makes them a good first choice for many patients [6, 8], but beyond first-line, physicians and patients often face decisions regarding where to proceed next, and for some patients with liver-dominant disease, liver-directed therapies are still an option. For others, everolimus is a systemic option, and then lutetium dotatate will be an option based on approval of the drug. Knowing how to choose among these three treatments is going to be a challenge. It's even more complicated for pancreatic NETs. Beyond somatostatin analogues, we have several strategies: everolimus, sunitinib, cytotoxic chemotherapy, liver-directed therapy, and peptide receptor radiotherapy. The use of everolimus or sunitinib is supported by randomized data, and their use is appropriate in this setting [14, 17]. Although no large, randomized trials have yet been completed with streptozocin- or temozolomide-based regimens, these are clearly active in pancreatic NETs and are associated with higher tumor response rates than somatostatin analogues or the biological agents. Cytotoxic therapies may also be an upfront treatment for highly symptomatic patients when tumor shrinkage rather than disease stabilization is the primary objective [19–24]. Moreover concomitant diseases of the patient and the different toxicity profiles could help clinicians to personalize treatment strategy. Combination therapies may be feasible, and effective but randomized trials are clearly needed to assess the safety and the efficacy of these regimens when compared with single-agent therapy.

At present, the landscape of therapeutic options for patients with poorly differentiated neuroendocrine carcinomas (NECs) is still lacking. For metastatic NECs the combination of cisplatin/etoposide is considered a standard option offering high rate of tumor response, but at the same time, short-lasting duration of response and high toxicity are reported [28].

There are a number of trials taking place looking at immunotherapy. If these agents work anywhere in the neuroendocrine field, they are more likely to work in poorly differentiated or high-grade tumors given the high mutational burden of these cancers.

In conclusion, there is a lack of real standard approaches and therapeutic sequences for metastatic GEP-NETs and NECs, and the appropriate selection and sequencing of treatments currently depend on clinical judgment.

Due to the complexity and heterogeneity of NETs, every treatment choice should take place in the setting of a multidisciplinary neuroendocrine tumor board.

To date research efforts are focused on translational studies in order to better select the patients who could benefit from different treatment options. Furthermore clinical trials comparing one agent to another would be beneficial in order to find the best treatment strategy.

References

1. Dasari A, Shen C, Halperin D, et al. JAMA Oncol. 2017;3(10):1335–42.
2. Hofland LJ, Lamberts SW. The pathophysiological consequences of somatostatin receptor internalization and resistance. Endocr Rev. 2003;24(1):28–47.
3. Lancranjan I, Bruns C, Grass P, et al. Sandostatin LAR: pharmacokinetics, pharmacodynamics, efficacy, and tolerability in acromegalic patients. Metabolism. 1995;44(Supplement 1):18–2.
4. Pouget E, Fay N, Dujardin E, et al. Elucidation of the self-assembly pathway of lanreotide octapeptide into beta-sheet nanotubes: role of two stable intermediates. J Am Chem Soc. 2010;132(12):4230–41.
5. Bornschein J, Drozdov I, Malfertheiner P. Octreotide LAR: safety and tolerability issues. Expert Opin Drug Saf. 2009;8(6):755–68.
6. Rinke A, Müller HH, Schade-Brittinger C, et al. Placebo-controlled, double-blind, prospective, randomized study on the effect of octreotide LAR in the control of tumor growth in patients with metastatic neuroendocrine midgut tumors: a report from the PROMID Study Group. J Clin Oncol. 2009;27(28):4656–63.
7. Rinke A, Wittenberg M, Schade-Brittinger C, et al. Placebo-controlled, double-blind, prospective, randomized study on the effect of octreotide LAR in the control of tumor growth in patients with metastatic neuroendocrine midgut tumors (PROMID): results of long-term survival. Neuroendocrinology. 2017;104(1):26–32.
8. Caplin ME, Pavel M, Ćwikła JB, et al. Lanreotide in metastatic enteropancreatic neuroendocrine tumors. N Engl J Med. 2014;371(3):224–33.
9. Schmid HA. Pasireotide (SOM230): development, mechanism of action and potential applications. Mol Cell Endocrinol. 2008;286(1–2):69–74.
10. Colao A, Auriemma RS, Pivonello R, et al. Medical consequences of acromegaly: what are the effects of biochemical control? Rev Endocr Metab Disord. 2008;9(1):21–31.
11. Wolin EM, Jarzab B, Eriksson B, et al. Phase III study of pasireotide long-acting release in patients with metastatic neuroendocrine tumors and carcinoid symptoms refractory to available somatostatin analogues. Drug Des Devel Ther. 2015;9:5075–86.
12. Yao J, Lombard-Bohas C, Baudin E, et al. Daily oral everolimus activity in patients with metastatic pancreatic neuroendocrine tumors after failure of cytotoxic chemotherapy: a phase II trial. J Clin Oncol. 2010;28(1):69–76.
13. Pavel ME, Hainsworth JD, Baudin E, et al. Everolimus plus octreotide long-acting repeatable for the treatment of advanced neuroendocrine tumours associated with carcinoid syndrome (RADIANT-2): a randomised, placebo-controlled, phase 3 study. Lancet. 2011;378(9808):2005–12.

14. Yao JC, Shah MH, Ito T, et al. Everolimus for advanced pancreatic neuroendocrine tumors. N Engl J Med. 2011;364(6):514–23.
15. Yao JC, Fazio N, Singh S, et al. Everolimus for the treatment of advanced, non-functional neuroendocrine tumours of the lung or gastrointestinal tract (RADIANT-4): a randomised, placebo-controlled, phase 3 study. Lancet. 2016;387(10022):968–77.
16. Raymond E, Dahan L, Raoul JL, et al. Sunitinib malate for the treatment of pancreatic neuroendocrine tumors. N Engl J Med. 2011;364(6):501–13.
17. Faivre S, Niccoli P, Castellano D, et al. Sunitinib in pancreatic neuroendocrine tumors: updated progression-free survival and final overall survival from a phase III randomized study. Ann Oncol. 2016;28(2):339–43.
18. Chan JA, Faris JE, Murphy JE, et al. Phase II trial of cabozantinib in patients with carcinoid and pancreatic neuroendocrine tumors (pNET). J Clin Oncol. 2017;35. (Suppl 4S; abstract 228).
19. Engstrom PF, Lavin PT, Moertel CG, et al. Streptozocin plus fluorouracil versus doxorubicin therapy for metastatic carcinoid tumor. J Clin Oncol. 1984;2(11):1255–9.
20. Moertel CG, Hanley JA. Combination chemotherapy trials in metastatic carcinoid tumor and the malignant carcinoid syndrome. Cancer Clin Trials. 1979;2(4, Winter):327–34.
21. Moertel CG, Hanley JA, Johnson LA. Streptozocin alone compared with streptozocin plus fluorouracil in the treatment of advanced islet-cell carcinoma. N Engl J Med. 1980;303(21):1189–94.
22. Moertel CG, Lefkopoulo M, Lipsitz S, et al. Streptozocin-doxorubicin, streptozocin-fluorouracil or chlorozotocin in the treatment of advanced islet-cell carcinoma. N Engl J Med. 1992;326(8):519–23.
23. Sun W, Lipsitz S, Catalano P, et al. Phase II/III study of doxorubicin with fluorouracil compared with streptozocin with fluorouracil or dacarbazine in the treatment of advanced carcinoid tumors: Eastern Cooperative Oncology Group Study E1281. J Clin Oncol. 2005;23(22):4897–904.
24. Meyer T, Qian W, Caplin ME, et al. Capecitabine and streptozocin +/- cisplatin in advanced gastroenteropancreatic neuroendocrine tumours. Eur J Cancer. 2014;50(5):902–11.
25. Garcia-Carbonero R, Sorbye H, Baudin E, et al. ENETS consensus guidelines for high-grade gastroenteropancreatic neuroendocrine tumors and neuroendocrine carcinomas. Neuroendocrinology. 2016;103(2):186–94.
26. Kunz PL, Reidy-Lagunes D, Lowell BA, et al. Consensus guidelines for the management and treatment of neuroendocrine tumors. Pancreas. 2013;42(4):557–77.
27. NCCN guidelines, version 2.2017 by the National Comprehensive Cancer Network.
28. Mitry E, Baudin E, Ducreaux M, et al. Treatment of poorly differentiated neuroendocrine tumours with etoposide and cisplatin. Br J Cancer. 1999;81:1351–5.

PRRT with Radiolabeled Peptides: Indications, Procedures, and Results

22

Ettore Seregni and Alice Lorenzoni

Abstract

Peptide receptor radionuclide therapy (PRRT) is an effective and usually well-tolerated treatment for unresectable or metastatic neuroendocrine tumors expressing somatostatin receptors. The two radiopharmaceuticals most commonly used for PRRT are 90Y-DOTATOC and 177Lu-DOTATATE which have been demonstrated to provide effective tumor response and symptom relief and have positive impact on survival. Chronic side effects on the kidneys and bone marrow are generally mild. Future perspectives include combinations with innovative therapeutic agents or the use of alpha-emitting radionuclide to improve PRRT efficacy.

22.1 Introduction

In patients with inoperable metastasized neuroendocrine tumors (NETs), therapeutic options are limited. Peptide receptor radionuclide therapy (PRRT) can be an effective strategy to treat these patients. The majority of NETs, in fact, express somatostatin-type receptors (SSTR), mainly subtypes 2 and 5, and these receptors can be targeted by radiolabeled somatostatin analogues (SSAs). NETs are a group of heterogeneous neoplasm that arise in the diffuse neuroendocrine system, present in almost all organs in the human body [1]. Most of NETs originate in the gastroenteropancreatic (GEP) and bronchopulmonary tract, and their incidence and prevalence have been increasing over the past decades, probably as a consequence of improvement of imaging methods [2]. The particular characteristic of NETs relies in the fact that are composed of specialized cells having the ability to produce, store, and secrete bioactive amines and peptide hormones. NETs are broadly classified into two categories termed functional NETs or nonfunctional NETs according to whether these tumors give rise to a clinical syndrome [3]. Functional NETs may be discovered when they are in the distinctive early stage, but they are often misdiagnosed on account of nonspecific and unpredictable symptoms. By contrast NETs with no symptoms or just local symptoms are not frequently identified until they have progressed to an advanced state, by which

E. Seregni (✉) • A. Lorenzoni
Nuclear Medicine, Fondazione IRCCS Istituto Nazionale Tumori, Milan, Italy
e-mail: ettore.seregni@istitutotumori.mi.it

E. Bombardieri et al. (eds.), *Clinical Applications of Nuclear Medicine Targeted Therapy*,
https://doi.org/10.1007/978-3-319-63067-0_22

time metastasis has already occurred [4]. Surgery is the only curative treatment for localized tumor. However, almost 50% of patients have metastatic disease at diagnosis, thus requiring systemic therapies. Targeted agents, such as SSAs (octreotide and lanreotide) and, recently, everolimus and sunitinib, demonstrated therapeutic efficacy in these patients [5]. From the early 1990s, PRRT has shown significant promise for treatment of advanced, low- to intermediate-grade NETs. However, for many years clinical evidence of antineoplastic efficacy of PRRT was poor deriving only from limited, nonrandomized, and I–II phase studies [6]. Very recently the randomized phase III NETTER-1 trial [7] unequivocally demonstrated the efficacy of PRRT in patients with metastatic and progressive NETs.

In this chapter we summarize from a practical point of view the role and the clinical indications of PRRT in patients with advanced NETs.

22.2 Radiopharmaceuticals

Several radiolabeled SSAs have been proposed for PRRT, and they are different in terms of radionuclide, somatostatin analogue, and chelator. DOTA is the most used chelator agent due to its high affinity for radiometals such as Yttrium-90 and Lutetium-177. Both [Tyr3]-octreotide (TOC) and [Tyr3]-octreotate (TATE) are well-experimented somatostatin analogues in clinical trials. The somatostatin analogue TATE differs from TOC only in that the C-terminal threoninol is replaced with threonine, resulting in a higher affinity for the somatostatin-receptor subtype 2 [8].

There are evident differences in physical properties between Yttrium-90 and Lutetium-177 (Table 22.1). The half-life of Lutetium-177 is 6.7 days versus 2.7 days for Yttrium-90. Furthermore, the tissue penetration range of Yttrium-90 is about 12 mm in contrast of 2 mm of Lutetium-177. This longer tissue penetration of Yttrium-90 could be beneficial in larger tumors with a heterogeneous receptor expression. By contrast, the shorter tissue penetration of Lutetium-177 makes this radionuclide probably more suitable to treat also smaller tumors [9]. Besides β-emission, Lutetium-177 also emits y-rays that can be used for imaging in the days after therapy. Therefore, these images can be used to verify the targeted delivery of the radiopharmaceutical and to calculate absorbed dose in organs/tissues and SSTR-positive tumors.

^{90}Y-DOTATOC and ^{177}Lu-DOTATATE have been extensively evaluated in the last two decades. No "ad hoc" study is available to demonstrate the superiority of one radiopharmaceutical in respect to another one. However, ^{90}Y-DOTATOC seems to display more side effects, and, for this reason, ^{177}Lu-DOTATATE is, at the moment, the first choice for treating patients with NETs. Furthermore, considering the results of NETTER-1 trial is reasonable that ^{177}Lu-DOTATATE will be registered in the near future and it will become the "standard" radiopharmaceutical for PRRT.

22.3 Pathologies and Tumor Characteristics

PRRT has been demonstrated of clinical efficacy in patients affected by NETs with high SSTR expression and, particularly, in patients affected by metastatic GEP and bronchial NETs. The grade of cell dedifferentiation represents a relevant tumor feature that is to be considered in selecting patients for PRRT. Patients with high-grade NETs have generally high aggressive poor-prognosis tumors with a clinical evolution that is not influenced by PRRT. By contrast low- or

Table 22.1 Physical characteristics of radionuclides for PRRT

Radionuclide	Emission	Max energy (MeV)	Penetration range (mm)	Half-life (days)
^{111}In	Auger/gamma	0.61	0.5	2.8
^{177}Lu	Beta/gamma	0.49	2	6.68
^{90}Y	Beta	2.27	11	2.67

intermediate- grade NETs have often an indolent course that can be successfully controlled by PRRT.

22.4 Patient Selection

22.4.1 Inclusion Criteria

SSTR expression in neoplastic lesions must be confirmed by molecular imaging, and only patients with high uptake of radiolabeled SSAs can be selected for PRRT. A qualitative index of radiolabeled SSA uptake, i.e., the "Krenning score," obtained from ^{111}In-pentetreotide scintigraphy (Octreoscan) can be adapted to select patients [10]. Patients with three- to four-grade uptakes (tumor uptake equal or greater than that of the spleen or kidneys) have higher possibilities to respond to PRRT. In recent years ^{68}Ga-DOTATOC PET/CT scan has been replacing scintigraphy, and it has been demonstrated that a maximum standard uptake (SUV) of >16 predicts response with good accuracy [11].

The success of PRRT is also influenced by the site of primary tumor and tumor burden. Different studies have demonstrated that pancreatic NETs have higher response rates even than other NETs even if they can relapse earlier [12–14]. Patients with high tumor load and with massive liver involvement have lower chance to respond to PRRT [15].

22.4.2 Exclusion Criteria

Patients with poor performance status (e.g., Karnofsky score <60) are not "ideal" candidates for PRRT even if unexpected and favorable responses are not rare in these clinically advanced patients.

Exclusion criteria are also renal function (creatinine levels >1.7–2.0 mg/dL or a creatinine clearance <50 mL/min), bone marrow (hemoglobin level <8 g/dL, white cell count <2000/mm^3, platelet count <75,000/mm^3), and liver (total bilirubin level of more than three times the upper limit of the normal range, serum albumin <3.0 g/dL) impairment.

Table 22.2 Treatment regimen

Radiopharmaceutical	Administered activity
^{90}Y-DOTATOC/TATE	2.8–3.7 GBq
^{177}Lu-DOTATOC/TATE	5.5–7.4 GBq
Combination ^{90}Y/^{177}Lu peptides	^{90}Y: 2.5–5.0 GBq ^{177}Lu: 5.5–7.4 GBq

22.5 Modality of Administration

^{90}Y/ ^{177}Lu-DOTATOC or ^{177}Lu-DOTATATE radiopharmaceuticals are systemically delivered in fractioned sequential cycles (generally four to six) every 4–12 weeks. Activities are generally ranging from 2.8–3.7 GBq (80–100 mCi) for ^{90}Y-labeled SSAs and 5.5–7.4 GBq (150–200 mCi) for ^{177}Lu-labeled SSAs, respectively (Table 22.2). Radiolabeled compound are infused over a period of 30 min, and to reduce renal toxicity, an intravenous amino acid solution (lysine and/or arginine) is administrated concomitantly for 4–8 h, starting 30 min to 2 h before the infusion of the radiopharmaceutical. These positive-charged amino acids are able to inhibit in a competitive manner the radiopeptide resorption in the nephron proximal tubuli. Different amino acid solutions have been proposed, and this point is still a matter of debate. In the NETTER-1 trial, investigators use commercial amino acid formulations (Aminosyn II 10% [21.0 g of lysine and 20.4 g of arginine in 2 L of solution] or VAMIN-18 [18 g of lysine and 22.6 g of arginine in 2 L of solution]) [7] which can cause nausea and vomiting when infused at high rates. These effects are almost never seen with the use of an infusion of 25 g of lysine and 25 g of arginine, as proposed by several institutional protocols.

22.6 Side Effects

In general, PRRT is well tolerated.

22.6.1 Acute Side Effects

Acute side effects are nausea and vomiting and in the majority of case are attributable to amino acid infusion (see above) [14]. These effects are often self-limiting or can be treated with antiemetics. The use of arginine reduces the rates and the severity of these events. Other common adverse events include fatigue or asthenia, abdominal pain, and diarrhea. However, in the majority of patients (>95%), these effects are of mild entity (WHO toxicity grade 1 or 2). A severe but rare complication (incidence around 1% of cases) is a carcinoid crisis related to a massive release of biologically active amine or peptides [16]. This crisis develops shortly after infusion and, in any cases, within 24–48 h after the first radiopharmaceutical administration and requires proper clinical management. Another subacute adverse event is increased hair loss. This unexplained, transitory, and mild (grade 1) side effect is observed in about one half of patients treated with ^{177}Lu-DOTATATE [12]. Myelosuppression due to irradiation of the bone marrow can occur after 4–6 weeks from infusion and is usually mild and reversible. Severe grade 3–4 hematological toxicities have been reported in about 13% and 4% of patients treated with ^{90}Y-DOTATOC and ^{177}Lu-DOTATATE, respectively [12–13, 17, 18]. Most susceptible to radiation-induced damage are platelets, followed by white blood cells (WBC) and red cell progenitors. Considering WBC, several studies have demonstrated that severe lymphopenia is not a rare event. However, its clinical impact seems to be minimal since opportunistic infections are not reported in patients treated with PRRT.

22.6.2 Chronic Side Effects

Kidneys and bone marrow are the dose-limiting organs, so long-term side effects can include renal failure and serious hematological adverse events such as myelodysplastic syndrome (MDS) and acute leukemia (AL). MDS is described in 1–2% and AL in <1% of patients [17]. It is to be noted, however, that different factors related either to antineoplastic treatments (previous chemo- or radiotherapy) or tumor evolution (bone marrow involvement) can affect the development of MDS, and, in some cases, it is quite impossible to relate the MDS to PRRT.

As described, the co-administration of positively charged amino acids is useful to partially reduce (up to 40%) the high radiation dose to kidneys [19, 20, 21]. However, despite the adsorbed dose, severe renal toxicities (grade 3–4) occur in less than 2% of patients [17]. Similar to hematological side effects, renal damage is observed more frequently after therapy with ^{90}Y-labeled SSAs than with ^{177}Lu-labeled radiopharmaceuticals. At regard, it has been observed a median decline in creatinine clearance of 7% per year in patients treated with ^{90}Y-DOTATOC with respect to 4% in those treated with ^{177}Lu-DOTATATE. Preexisting risk factors such as poorly controlled diabetes or hypertension seems to be correlated with more persistent renal damage [22].

22.7 Clinical Results: PRRT Efficacy in GEP-NETs

22.7.1 ^{90}Y-DOTATOC

^{90}Y-DOTATOC was evaluated in several phase I and phase II PRRT trials. Many factors make it virtually impossible to compare these studies. In fact, heterogeneity is reported either in patient selection and characteristics (e.g., tumor types, performance status, previous therapies) or in PRRT protocols (e.g., cycle doses, administered cumulative dose) and different criteria for tumor response assessment. Overall, the objective response rates (ORR) reported across studies of ^{90}Y-DOTATOC range from 4 to 33% with median progression-free survival (PFS) varying from 17 to 29 months and median overall survival (OS) from 22 to 37 months [22].

22.7.2 ^{177}Lu-DOTATATE

^{177}Lu-DOTATATE is currently the most widely used radiopeptide for PRRT. In several studies, this radiopharmaceutical has demonstrated similar efficacy as compared with ^{90}Y-DOTATOC while having a more favorable toxicity profile, particularly in terms of hematological and renal toxicity. In a recent meta-analysis [23] which considered

473 NET patients submitted to ^{177}Lu-DOTATATE, ORR varied from 18 to 44%, with an average disease control rate of about 80%. Furthermore, PFS in patients with advanced and progressive NETs is about 36 months. Also quality of life (QoL) improves significantly after ^{177}Lu-DOTATATE therapy. At regard, in a study of 265 NET patients, QoL improved in about 40% of patients and symptomatology up to 70% of patients [24]. Starting from these results derived from nonrandomized studies and obtained in heterogeneous patient populations of GEP-NETs, a randomized prospective phase 3 trial (NETTER-1) was designed in order to unequivocally demonstrate the efficacy of ^{177}Lu-DOTATATE therapy [7]. This trial investigated ^{177}Lu-DOTATATE versus high-dose octreotide LAR (60 mg/month) in 229 patients with advanced, somatostatin-receptor-positive midgut NETs who had progressed on standard dose of octreotide LAR. The primary endpoint of the study was PFS determination by RECIST criteria. After a median follow-up of 14 months, ^{177}Lu-DOTATATE therapy resulted in a 79% reduction in the risk of progression or death compared with high-dose octreotide. The median PFS was not reached in the PRRT arm while was 8.4 months in the control arm. The rate of PFS, evaluated after 20 months of follow-up, was 65% in ^{177}Lu-DOTATATE group and 10% in the control group. Furthermore, ORR was remarkably high in PRRT patients (18 vs. 3%), and these figures are of relevance considering that response rates above 5% have not been observed with other systemic therapies approved in the same patient population. Although longer follow-up is needed to draw definitive conclusions on the influence of lutetium on OS, interim analysis strongly suggests an improvement of OS in the PRRT arm. In any case, however, the results of the prospective and randomized NETTER-1 trial validate the results obtained by numerous early-phase studies (Table 22.3).

Table 22.3 Efficacy of PRRT

Radiopharmaceutical	Overall response rate (ORR)	Survival results
90Y-DOTATOC	4–33%	PFS: 17–29 months OS: 22–37 months
177Lu-DOTATATE	18–44%	PFS: 33–40 months 79% reduction in risk of progression or death (NETTER 1 study)
Combination or treatment tandem ^{90}Y/^{177}Lu peptides[a]	42–47%	OS is significantly longer in patients treated with the combination reduction in the risk of progression or death of 36%

[a]References: Seregni E et al. Eur J Nucl Med Mol Imaging. 2014;41:223–30; Villard L et al. J Clin Oncol. 2012;30(10):1100–6; Kunikowska J et al. Eur J Nucl Med Mol Imaging. 2011;38(10):1788–97

22.8 PRRT Efficacy in Bronchial NETs

Results of PRRT in patients with bronchial NETs (B-NETs) are encouraging, and they seem similar to those observed in GEP-NETs even if there are no any perspective phase III trial specific for patients with B-NETs. Therefore, for these tumors, results are commonly extrapolated from more general studies. For example, in a mono-institutional retrospective study [25], a median OS of about 60 months, with a median PFS of 28 months, was observed in 114 advanced stage B-NET patients treated with ^{90}Y-DOTATOC or ^{177}Lu-DOTATATE. In only ^{177}Lu-DOTATATE-treated patients, ORR and stable disease were 15% and 47%, respectively. It is important to note, however, that in respect to GEP-NETs, B-NETs express relatively low SSTR2, and therefore, it must be critically considered for a correct selection of patients suitable for PRRT.

22.9 Perspectives and Conclusions

Different strategies are now under evaluation in order to improve the clinical efficacy of PRRT or to expand its clinical indications. Regarding the latter aspect, preoperative PRRT with ^{177}Lu-DOTATATE is proposed as neoadjuvant therapy for downstaging inoperable locally advanced pancreatic NETs. Preliminary results seem to indicate that this approach is potentially effective. Association of different radionuclides, combination of PRRT with antineoplastic agents, selection of alternative isotopes, and targeting agents or administration routes are all new fields of investigation.

Several groups tried to improve the results by using two different radionuclides or combining PRRT with chemotherapy. Studies have shown that the combination of ^{177}Lu- and ^{90}Y-labeled SSAs might be more effective than PRRT with Lutetium-177 or Yttrium-90 alone. The rationale for this approach is the relatively short path length of the medium-energy β-emission of Lutetium-177 and the longer path length of the high energy of β-emission of Yttrium-90, which may have a maximal impact on small and large tumors, respectively. Preliminary studies indicate that the combination of PRRT with radiosensitizing chemotherapy (capecitabine- and temozolomide-based regimens) seems to improve clinical efficacy of PRRT with acceptable toxicities. Furthermore, the synergist combination with innovative and very promising drugs such as DNA repair and immune checkpoint inhibitors could be investigated considering the PRRT-induced DNA damage and antitumor immune response, respectively. A different promising new technique is the use of alpha-emitting radiolabeled SSAs. Alpha-emitting radionuclides such as ^{213}Bi have a very short tissue penetration range (about 50–100 μm) and a high linear energy (LET) with the consequence that they can induce more DNA damage to the target tissue with a marked irradiation reduction of no-target healthy tissue. At regard, however, only one pilot study in seven patients has been up to now published [26]. Finally, a new strategy to increase the tumor dose is the use of radiolabeled SSTR antagonists. Even if these compounds are not internalized into tumor cells, they can deliver higher doses to the target when compared with the canonical somatostatin analogues. This effect could be explained by their higher affinity for SSTR and lower dissociation rate in respect to agonist. A recent pilot study in four patients showed a 1.7–10.6 times higher tumor dose using the antagonist 177Lu-DOTA-JR11 compared to 177Lu-DOTATATE [27].

In conclusion, different approaches are now under evaluation to improve PRRT, but, in any case, with the recent publication of the impressive results of the NETTER-1 trial, it may be expected that the use of this therapy will increase in the coming years.

References

1. Cives M, Strosberg J. An update on gastroenteropancreatic neuroendocrine tumors. Oncology (Williston Park). 2014;28(9):749–56, 758.
2. Yao JC, Hassan M, Phan A, et al. One hundred years after "carcinoid": epidemiology of and prognostic factors for neuroendocrine tumors in 35,825 cases in the United States. J Clin Oncol. 2008;26(18):3063–72.
3. Kaltsas GA, Besser GM, Grossman AB. The diagnosis and medical management of advanced neuroendocrine tumors. Endocr Rev. 2004;25:458–511.
4. Kulke MH, Benson AB 3rd, Bergsland E, et al. Neuroendocrine tumors. J Natl Compr Canc Netw. 2012;10:724–64.
5. Castellano D, Grande E, Valle J, Capdevila J, Reidy-Lagunes D, O'Connor JM, Raymond E. Expert consensus for the management of advanced or metastatic pancreatic neuroendocrine and carcinoid tumors. Cancer Chemother Pharmacol. 2015;75(6):1099–114.
6. van der Zwan WA, Bodei L, Mueller-Brand J, et al. GEPNETs update: radionuclide therapy in neuroendocrine tumors. Eur J Endocrinol. 2015;172(1):R1–8.
7. Strosberg J, El-Haddad G, Wolin E, NETTER-1 Trial Investigators, et al. Phase 3 trial of (177)lu-dotatate for midgut neuroendocrine tumors. N Engl J Med. 2017;376(2):125–35.
8. Reubi JC, Schar JC, Waser B, et al. Affinity profiles for human somatostatin receptor subtypes SST1-SST5 of somatostatin radiotracers selected for scintigraphic and radiotherapeutic use. Eur J Nucl Med. 2000;27:273–82.
9. Volkert WA, Hoffman TJ. Thrapeutic radiopharmaceuticals. Chem Rev. 1999;99:2269–92.
10. Krenning EP, Kwekkeboom DJ, Bakker WH, et al. Somatostatin receptor scintigraphy with [^{111}In-DTPA-D-Phe1]- and [^{123}I-Tyr3]-octreotide: the Rotterdam experience with more than 1000 patients. Eur J Nucl Med. 1993;20:716–31.
11. Kratochwil C, Stefanova M, Mavriopoulou E, et al. SUV of [68Ga]DOTATOC-PET/CT predicts response probability of PRRT in neuroendocrine tumors. Mol Imaging Biol. 2015;17(3):313–8.
12. Kwekkeboom DJ, de Herder WW, Kam BL, et al. Treatment with the radiolabeled somatostatin analog [177 Lu-DOTA 0, Tyr3]octreotate: toxicity, efficacy, and survival. J Clin Oncol. 2008;26:2124–30.
13. Imhof A, Brunner P, Marincek N, et al. Response, survival, and long-termtoxicity after therapy with the radiolabeled somatostatin analogue [90Y-DOTA]-TOC in metastasized neuroendocrine cancers. J Clin Oncol. 2011;29:2416–23.

14. Sansovini M, Severi S, Ambrosetti A, et al. Treatment with the radiolabelled somatostatin analog Lu-DOTATATE for advanced pancreatic neuroendocrine tumors. Neuroendocrinology. 2013;97:347–54.
15. Kwekkeboom DJ, Teunissen JJ, Bakker WH, et al. Radiolabeled somatostatin analog [177Lu DOTA0,Tyr3]octreotate in patients with endocrine gastroenteropancreatic tumors. J Clin Oncol. 2005;23(12):2754–62.
16. De Keizer B, van Aken MO, Feelders RA, et al. Hormonal crises following receptor radionuclide therapy with the radiolabeled somatostatin analogue [177Lu-DOTA0,Tyr3]octreotate. Eur J Nucl Med Mol Imaging. 2008;35:749e55.
17. Bodei L, Kidd M, Paganelli G, et al. Long-term tolerability of PRRT in 807 patients with neuroendocrine tumours: the value and limitations of clinical factors. Eur J Nucl Med Mol Imaging. 2015;42:5e19.
18. Gupta SK, Singla S, Bal C. Renal and hematological toxicity in patients of neuroendocrine tumors after peptide receptor radionuclide therapy with 177Lu-DOTATATE. Cancer Biother Radiopharm. 2012;27:593.
19. Rolleman EJ, Valkema R, de Jong M, et al. Safe and effective inhibition of renal uptake of radiolabelled octreotide by a combination of lysine and arginine. Eur J Nucl Med Mol Imaging. 2003;30:9.
20. Jamar F, Barone R, Mathieu I, et al. (86Y-DOTA0)-D-Phe1-Tyr3-octreotide (SMT487)ea phase 1 clinical study: pharmacokinetics,biodistribution and renal protective effect of different regimens of amino acid co-infusion. Eur J Nucl Med Mol Imaging. 2003;30:510.
21. Bodei L, Cremonesi M, Ferrari M, et al. Long-term evaluation of renal toxicity after peptide receptor radionuclide therapy with 90Y-DOTATOC and 177Lu-DOTATATE: the role of associated risk factors. Eur J Nucl Med Mol Imaging. 2008;35:1847.
22. Brabander T, Teunissen JJ, Van Eijck CH, et al. Peptide receptor radionuclide therapy of neuroendocrine tumours. Best Pract Res Clin Endocrinol Metab. 2016;30(1):103–14.
23. Kim SJ, Pak K, Koo PJ, Kwak JJ, Chang S. The efficacy of (177)Lu-labelled peptide receptor radionuclide therapy in patients with neuroendocrine tumours: a meta-analysis. Eur J Nucl Med Mol Imaging. 2015;42(13):1964–70.
24. Khan S, Krenning EP, van Essen M, et al. Quality of life in 265 patients with gastroenteropancreatic or bronchial neuroendocrine tumors treated with [177Lu-DOTA0,Tyr3]octreotate. J Nucl Med. 2011;52(9):1361–8.
25. Mariniello A, Bodei L, Tinelli C, et al. Long-term results of PRRT in advanced bronchopulmonary carcinoid. Eur J Nucl Med Mol Imaging. 2016;43(3):441–52.
26. Kratochwil C, Giesel FL, Bruchertseifer F, et al. 213Bi-DOTATOC receptor-targeted alpha-radionuclide therapy induces remission in neuroendocrine tumours refractory to beta radiation: a first-in-human experience. Eur J Nucl Med Mol Imaging. 2014;41:2106.
27. Wild D, Fani M, Fischer R, et al. Comparison of somatostatin receptor agonist and antagonist for peptide receptor radionuclide therapy: a pilot study. J Nucl Med. 2014;55(8):1248–52.

23 Dosimetry in PRRT

Marta Cremonesi, Mahila Ferrari, and Francesca Botta

Abstract

Peptide receptor radionuclide therapy (PRRT) with ^{90}Y- and ^{177}Lu-radiolabelled peptides represents a promising option for patients with somatostatin receptor-expressing tumours. Several clinical trials have proven its efficacy and a general profile of low toxicity. Although in a minority of patients, severe events of kidney toxicity have occurred, so the kidneys represent the organ at risk, especially for ^{90}Y-peptides, followed by red marrow, as also haematological toxicity, rarely at high grade, may occur in both ^{90}Y- and ^{177}Lu-PRRT. The results of some studies have shown important dose-effect correlations, especially for renal damage, showing the possibility not only to avoid unwanted effects when absorbed dose prescriptions are respected but also to optimise therapy. However, due to the large variability of biokinetics among patients, individual dosimetry is necessary for tailored PRRT.

The following chapter summarises the methods for PRRT dosimetry and the major dosimetric and radiobiological results present in the literature, highlighting correlations and challenging perspectives. Possible approaches for simplified dosimetry are also described.

23.1 Goal of Dosimetry in PRRT

Many clinical trials have proven the efficacy of peptide receptor radionuclide therapy (PRRT) with ^{90}Y- and ^{177}Lu-radiolabelled peptides for the treatment of patients affected by inoperable tumours expressing somatostatin receptors, such as the neuroendocrine tumours (NET) [1–3]. Despite the collateral effects are generally mild, possible radiation-induced renal damage and large inter-patient variability in biodistribution and tumour uptake denote the need of accurate dosimetry for safe therapy planning.

Recent improvements in dosimetry methods in PRRT have provided promising results and correlations that represent challenging perspectives for optimised approaches and radiobiological models [4–18].

M. Cremonesi (✉) • M. Ferrari • F. Botta
Istituto Europeo di Oncologia, Milan, Italy
e-mail: marta.cremonesi@ieo.it

E. Bombardieri et al. (eds.), *Clinical Applications of Nuclear Medicine Targeted Therapy*,
https://doi.org/10.1007/978-3-319-63067-0_23

The clinical results available today indicate ^{177}Lu-PRRT as more tolerated with very rare cases of renal toxicity as compared with ^{90}Y-PRRT, at least with the commonly applied therapy schemes. Therefore, at a first glance, dosimetry seems especially important to ascertain safety in ^{90}Y-PRRT. However, the role of dosimetry is of most importance even in ^{177}Lu-PRRT, as efficacy, beyond safety, can be pursued. In fact, the traditional fixed activity of four cycles of 7.4 GBq of ^{177}Lu-DOTATATE has been proven to be quite harmless [2, 19], but some dose-based protocols with prescription of kidney dose limits have shown that optimisation is possible. Up to eight cycles of 7.4 GBq of ^{177}Lu-DOTATATE could be administered in some patients, within renal prescriptions, thus doubling the irradiation of target lesions [13]. The economic implications of dosimetry, which can prevent side effects and increase efficacy, consist in the sparing of cures for toxicity and the benefit of improved responses [20, 21].

23.2 The Practical Implementation of Dosimetry in PRRT

The dosimetry methods to be used for ^{90}Y- and ^{177}Lu-PRRT, typically administering ^{90}Y-DOTATOC or ^{177}Lu-DOTATATE, have to be considered separately, due to the different physical characteristics of the two radioisotopes.

23.2.1 ^{90}Y-PRRT

^{90}Y is an almost pure beta emitter radionuclide—besides a very low abundance of positron emission (branching ratio, 32×10^{-6}). The physical half-life of ^{90}Y (64.1 h) is compatible with the peptide kinetics, and the high energy of β-particles (E_{max} = 2.28 MeV) allows crossfire effect, with killing properties in a certain volume around the uptaking neoplastic cells. Unfortunately, the lack of γ emission makes imaging difficult with this isotope.

Some authors apply very sophisticated processing to planar and SPECT Bremsstrahlung images, after correction for attenuation, scatter and detector response, either based on Monte Carlo simulations or obtained by new generation equipment (SPECT/CT). However, this remains a technique of niche [22–24]. Other authors have considered the possibility to obtain ^{90}Y-PET images, thanks to the (low) β+ emission [24], following the experience of liver radioembolisation [25–27]. In any case, PET image statistics in PRRT remains poor, besides the few highly uptaking organs (kidneys, spleen, bladder), and more than one bed is necessary to have acquired the districts of interest.

Alternatively to ^{90}Y-imaging, the most practical method is to use the same peptide for therapy labelled with ^{111}In (e.g. ^{111}In-DOTATOC). The very similar chemical characteristics of ^{111}In and ^{90}Y and physical half-life (67.4 vs. 64.1 h) reasonably allow to assume a comparable behaviour in vivo of ^{111}In- and ^{90}Y-derivatives [28]. A diagnostic activity of ^{111}In (e.g. 185 MBq) can provide serial planar and SPECT images over 3–4 days.

Importantly, it is to remind that when dosimetry is performed out of therapy, renal protection has to be administered also for dosimetry.

Other proposed—but not ideal—options involve ^{86}Y-peptides, ^{111}In-octreotide and ^{68}Ga-peptides.

The same compound labelled with ^{86}Y (^{86}Y-DOTATOC) totally preserves the chemical nature of ^{90}Y-derivatives and offers PET resolution. Conversely, limitations are related to its short physical half-life (14.7 h) as compared to the peptide kinetics, complex image quantification, cost and poor availability [28].

^{111}In-octreotide and ^{68}Ga-peptides are not suitable for dosimetry. ^{111}In-octreotide is not suitable simply because different peptides have different biokinetics. In particular, the biokinetics of ^{111}In-octreotide and ^{111}In-DOTATOC are not comparable, even though some authors claim its use for a "practical" dosimetry [4, 29]. ^{68}Ga-peptides is not suitable because of the extremely short half-time of ^{68}Ga (68 min) as compared to peptide kinetics [28].

23.2.2 ^{177}Lu-PRRT

In comparison with ^{90}Y, the β-particles of ^{177}Lu (E_{max} = 0.5 MeV) induce less crossfire effect but release higher energy in smaller tissues, and the γ-rays of ^{177}Lu 113 (6%) and 208 (11%) keV are suitable for imaging and dosimetry. Most often dosimetry is evaluated during a cycle of PRRT, with typical activities administered of 3.7–7.4 GBq.

23.2.3 Dosimetry Methods

The details of dosimetry formalism are not the aim of this paragraph and can be found elsewhere [29–31]. It is just important to recall the essential dose calculation, which can be summarised by the following equation (MIRD method):

$$D_{target} = \sum_{s} \tilde{A}_s S_{t\leftarrow s} = A_0 \sum_{s} \alpha_s S_{t\leftarrow s}$$

where $\tilde{A}_s$ is the time-integrated activity (or total number of nuclear transformations) of the source tissue s, i.e. the integral of the time-activity curves); $S_{t\leftarrow s}$ is the Snyder factor for each source s to a target t, representing the mean absorbed dose rate to target tissue per unit nuclear transformation present in source tissue; and α_s is the time-integrated activity coefficient, i.e. the cumulative number of nuclear transformations occurring in source tissue per unit administered activity A_0 [30].

In summary, for dosimetry purposes, time-activity curves have to be generated for all the source organs, and from these, the time-integrated activity coefficients can be derived, e.g. by fitting methods [32, 33].

Despite the differences between radionuclides, a complete dosimetry study of both ^{90}Y- and ^{177}Lu-PRRT would require:

1. Serial blood samples for the estimate of red marrow absorbed dose
2. Complete urine collection to determine the rate of excretion and, consequently, the urinary bladder absorbed dose, while faeces collection is not requested—being the activity mainly excreted via the kidneys
3. At least five serial planar and/or SPECT images for the estimate of the absorbed dose to the normal organs and tumours

Concerning imaging, dosimetry can be based on three methods [12, 31, 33–35]:

1. A 2D protocol, using whole-body (WB) planar images, with the advantage of having under control the activity in the total body and, therefore, allowing to derive the time-integrated activity coefficients for all the organs and the remainder of the body. On the other hand, information about the 3D distribution of the activity is not available, and quantitative estimation of tumour dose is often prevented due to the overlap of uptaking tissues.
2. A hybrid protocol, using sequential WB planar images (2D) to derive the trend of time variation of the activity in source tissues, and one or two SPECT (better SPECT/CT) images (3D) to quantify the activity in the sources.
3. A pure 3D protocol, with serial SPECT (or SPECT/CT) images, with the advantage to have the 3D activity (and dose) distribution, but with the limit to have only a partial region of the body imaged, or the need to acquire 2 SPECT beds at each time to include all the volumes of interest.

Finally, two possible quantification strategies are to be distinguished. The first is the absolute calibration, which is not always easy to derive and presumes careful phantom studies, leading to the association of the counts inside appropriate phantom inserts with the calibrated activity filling those inserts. The second is the relative calibration, setting the total counts of the region/volume under examination equal to the total activity administered or the activity restricted to a certain volume (e.g. total counts of the first WB equal to 100% of the injected activity or to 100% of the activity subtracted by the activity eliminated in the first urine collection).

The different steps required for a practical dosimetry study in ^{90}Y-PRRT (with ^{111}In) and ^{177}Lu-PRRT are schematically summarised in Tables 23.1 and 23.2, respectively [28]. Details about timing and equipment settings are reported. In both

Table 23.1 Data collection for dosimetry in 90Y-PRRT with ^{111}In-peptides

	Item	Aim	Equipment	Settings	Timing	Is it possible to simplify?
Pharmacokinetics	Blood	To derive red marrow time-activity curve based on the same activity concentration in blood and in RM	γ-Counter	^{111}In energy peaks (e.g. 173 ± 10% and 243 ± 10% keV)	Blood sampling (e.g. 1 mL) typically at 20–30 min, 1, 4, 6, 10–16, 24, 48 h (if possible also 64 h) p.i.	Avoidable if RM dosimetry is based on imaging
	Urine	To derive the activity cumulatively eliminated in the urine vs. time	γ-Counter	^{111}In energy peaks (e.g. 173 ± 10% and 243 ± 10% keV)	Complete urine collection with time intervals up to 0–1, 1–3, 3–6, 6–16, 16–24, 24–40, 40–48 and if possible 48–64 h p.i.	Avoidable with quantitative imaging; up to the first image acquisition time in case of relative calibration
Anatomy	CT scan	To evaluate actual organ and possibly tumour masses	CT scanner		Close to the date of therapy	No
Metabolic data	WB transmission	To allow attenuation correction of WB	γ-Camera and flood source (^{57}Co) or CT scanner	Energy peak of ^{57}Co	Before administration	Avoidable if information from CT available (scout)
				Low CT settings	Before or after administration (scout)	
	WB scintigraphy	To derive time-activity curves of source organs (TB, spleen, kidneys, liver, testes and tumours), typically with two-exponential fitting Methods: (1) 2D planar (WB), (2) hybrid (WB + SPECT), (3) 3D (SPECT)	γ-Camera for WB protocols, γ-camera and CT or SPECT/CT for hybrid or 3D protocols	^{111}In energy peaks and scatter windows (e.g. 173 ± 10% and 243 ± 10% keV; scatter, 140 ± 10% keV)	At least five acquisitions, typically at 1, 3–4, 16–24, 40–48, 64–72 h p.i.	Reducible to three acquisitions for mono-exponential fitting, e.g. 1, 24, 48 h p.i. for relative calibration; 24, 48, 64 h p.i. With quantitative imaging
	SPECT (SPECT-CT)			^{111}In energy peaks and scatter windows (e.g. 173 ± 10% and 243 ± 10% keV; scatter, 140 ± 10% keV) possibly low CT for SPECT attenuation correction	If possible, at least one to two acquisitions at 24–48 h (at the level of the kidneys) for hybrid protocols; the same timing as for WB for pure 3D protocols	Avoidable if planar dosimetry is accepted

p.i. = postinjection, *RB* = remainder of the body, *RM* = red marrow, *TB* = total body, *WB* = whole body

Table 23.2 Data collection for dosimetry in ^{177}Lu-PRRT

	Item	Aim	Equipment	Settings	Timing	Is it possible to simplify?
Pharmacokinetics	Blood	To derive red marrow time-activity curve based on the same activity concentration in blood and in RM	γ-Counter	^{177}Lu energy peak 208 keV (±10%)	Blood sampling (e.g. 1 mL) typically at 20–30 min, 1, 4, 6, 10–16, 24, 48, 64 h (if possible 90 h) p.i.	Avoidable if RM dosimetry is based on imaging
	Urine	To derive the activity cumulatively eliminated in the urine vs. time	γ-Counter	^{177}Lu energy peak 208 keV (±10%)	Complete urine collection with time intervals up to 0–1, 1–3, 3–6, 6–16, 16–24, 24–40, 40–48 h (if possible 48–64 h) p.i.	Avoidable with quantitative imaging; up to the first image acquisition time in case of relative calibration
Anatomy	CT scan	To evaluate actual organ and possibly tumour masses	CT scanner	15% at 208 keV 4% at 189 keV + 4% at 229 keV	Close to the date of therapy	No
Metabolic data	WB transmission	To allow attenuation correction of WB	γ-Camera and flood source (^{57}Co) or CT scanner	Energy peak of ^{57}Co	Before administration	Avoidable if information from CT available (scout)
				Low CT settings	Before or after administration (scout)	
	WB scintigraphy	To derive time-activity curves of source organs (TB, spleen, kidneys, liver, testes and tumours), typically with two-exponential fitting Methods: (1) 2D planar (WB), (2) hybrid (WB + SPECT), (3) 3D (SPECT)	γ-Camera for WB protocols, γ-camera and CT or SPECT/CT for hybrid or 3D protocols	^{177}Lu energy peak and scatter windows (e.g. 208 ± 8%; scatter, 189 ± 4% and 229 ± 4% keV)	At least five acquisitions, typically at 1, 3–4, 24, 48, 64 or 90 and, if possible, 160 h p.i. Alternatively at 1, 24, 64, 90, 160 h p.i.	Reducible to three acquisitions for mono-exponential fitting, e.g. 1, 24, 64 h p.i. for relative calibration; 24, 48, 90 h p.i. With quantitative imaging
	SPECT (SPECT-CT)			^{177}Lu energy peak and scatter windows (e.g. 208 ± 8%; scatter, 189 ± 4% and 229 ± 4% keV) Possibly low CT for SPECT attenuation correction	If possible, at least one to two acquisitions at 24–48 h (at the level of the kidneys) for hybrid protocols; the same timing as for WB for pure 3D protocols	Avoidable if planar dosimetry is accepted

p.i. = postinjection, *RB* = remainder of the body, *RM* = red marrow, *TB* = total body, *WB* = whole body cases, PRRT is divided into multiple cycles, and dosimetry can be done in a forward-looking setting with a diagnostic activity (e.g. 185 MBq of ^{111}In-peptide or 740 MBq of ^{177}Lu-peptide), provided to use renal protection as in therapy, or, more practically, during the first cycle of PRRT, always with renal protection. In case of ^{90}Y-PRRT, 185 MBq of ^{111}In can be added to the therapeutic activity of ^{90}Y, and in case of ^{177}Lu-PRRT, the therapeutic activity is directly used for dosimetry. Assuming reproducible biokinetics, the activity in the subsequent cycles can be tuned based on the dosimetry results.

23.3 Feasibility of Dosimetry in the Routine

The application of a complete dosimetric study might seem quite complicated to non-trained or not- in-the-field personnel. Conversely, the experience from collaborative hospital divisions shows that once dosimetry has been applied, there is a very interesting exchange of information among scientists of different backgrounds that enriches not only work but, especially, patient care. Of note is that dosimetry for PRRT does not require any special patient preparation (besides renal protection), and this is a further advantage.

The dosimetric results from different patients and centres have shown wide inter-patient variations as well as frequent intra-patient differences on tumour uptake, leading to the need to assess individual dosimetry in the routine. On the other hand, the possibility to optimise therapy is extremely important. In many patients, tolerability has not been fully exploited, while higher tumour irradiation might notably increase the 30–35% response typically reported to date as clinical success of PRRT.

To be highlighted is also the possibility to simplify dosimetry for routine use, at the expense of a relatively lower accuracy. An abridged methodology (see Tables 23.1 and 23.2) could:

1. Avoid blood withdrawals and base red marrow dosimetry on imaging, e.g. considering the uptake of the lumbar vertebrae (this is because red marrow absorbed dose has not been shown to correspond to haematological toxicity [36, 37]).
2. Avoid urine collection if quantitative imaging is applied, and use the retention curve from imaging to elaborate the excretion curve for the urinary bladder.
3. Reduce from five or more to three acquisitions, and accept a mono-exponential trend in place of a bi-exponential, provided acquisitions are performed at sufficiently late time points [32].

23.4 Short Review on Dosimetry

The promising results of PRRT in terms of response rates and longer survival as compared to patients not receiving PRRT have diffused its application in most recent years ([38], van Essen [1–3, 19, 39]). As a natural consequence, this has stimulated the improvement of dosimetry, in terms of accuracy and methodologies for practical request. Numerous papers dealing with dosimetry have been published, reporting dose estimates, comparisons of 2D and 3D methods, dose-effect correlations and dosimetry-based PRRT optimization. This paragraph provides a short review of these issues.

23.4.1 Y- and Lu-PRRT Absorbed Doses

^{90}Y-DOTATOC and ^{177}Lu-DOTATATE are the most used radiopeptides. They have in common a rapid pharmacokinetics, with very fast blood clearance and urinary elimination that ensures a low irradiation of the whole body, and the highest absorbed doses to the spleen, kidneys, urinary bladder and liver. The kidneys are the organs at risk, followed by the red marrow, although no significant uptake in bone or red marrow is generally observed. After the first experimental administrations of ^{90}Y-DOTATOC with cases of serious nephropathy, the administration of radiopeptides has been performed always with the infusion of renal protective agents (essentially, amino acids), which are able to reduce at least of 30% the kidney uptake [40]. In spite of this, the kidneys remain the dose-limiting organs.

The graphs reported in Figs. 23.1 and 23.2 for ^{90}Y-DOTATOC and ^{177}Lu-DOTATATE, respectively, collect the absorbed dose values to the major target organs (spleen; kidneys; urinary bladder; liver; total body; red marrow) and tumours available in the literature.

An immediate observation emerging is the wide variability in normal organs and even

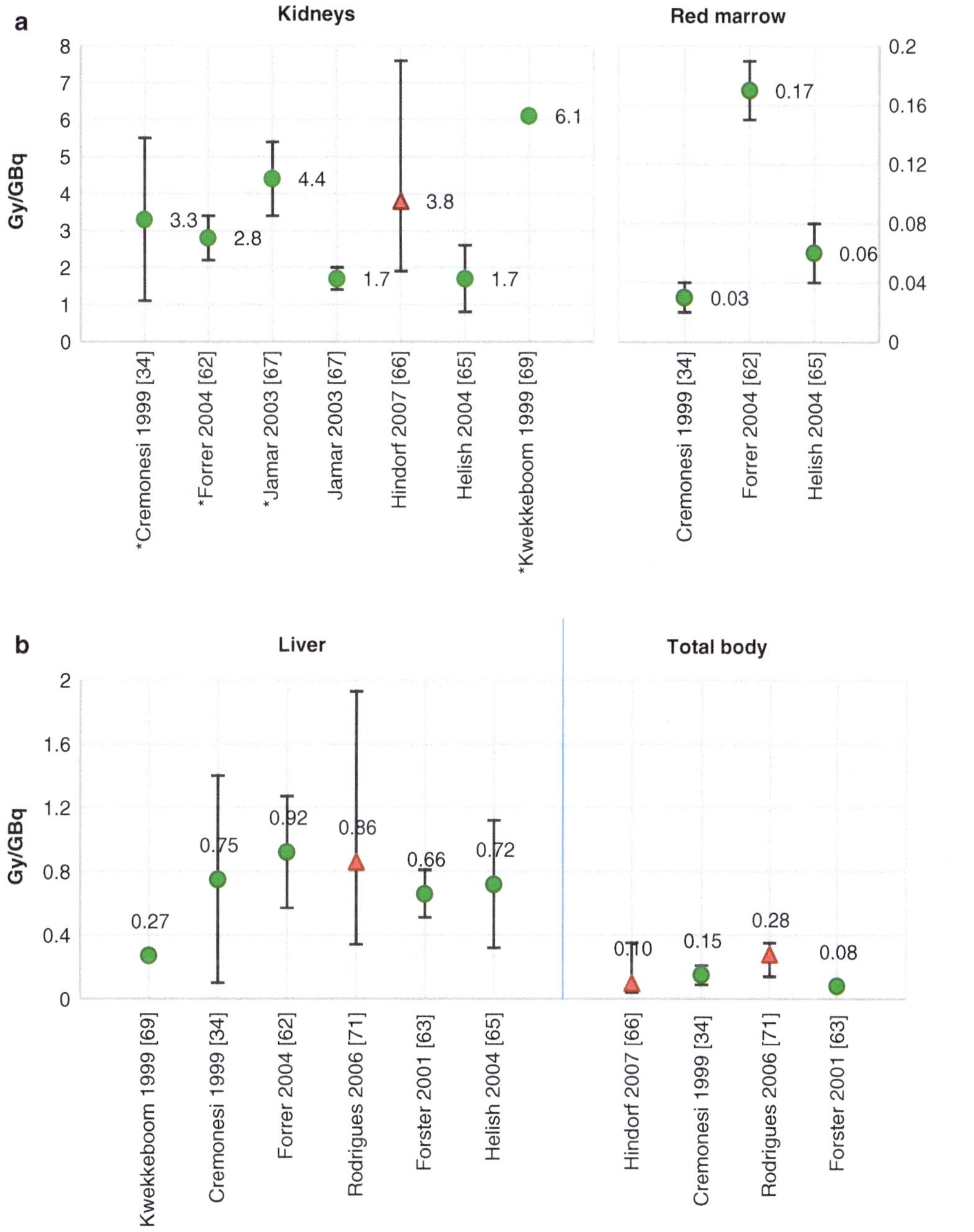

Fig. 23.1 Absorbed doses per unit activity (Gy/GBq) of ^{90}Y-DOTATOC in kidneys and red marrow (**a**), liver and total body (**b**), spleen and urinary bladder (**c**), and tumour (**d**). Circles and corresponding error bars represent mean values and standard deviations; triangles and corresponding error bars represent median values and ranges of variability. For the kidneys, the values with the asterisk next to the first author indicate that values refer to therapy without renal protection

c

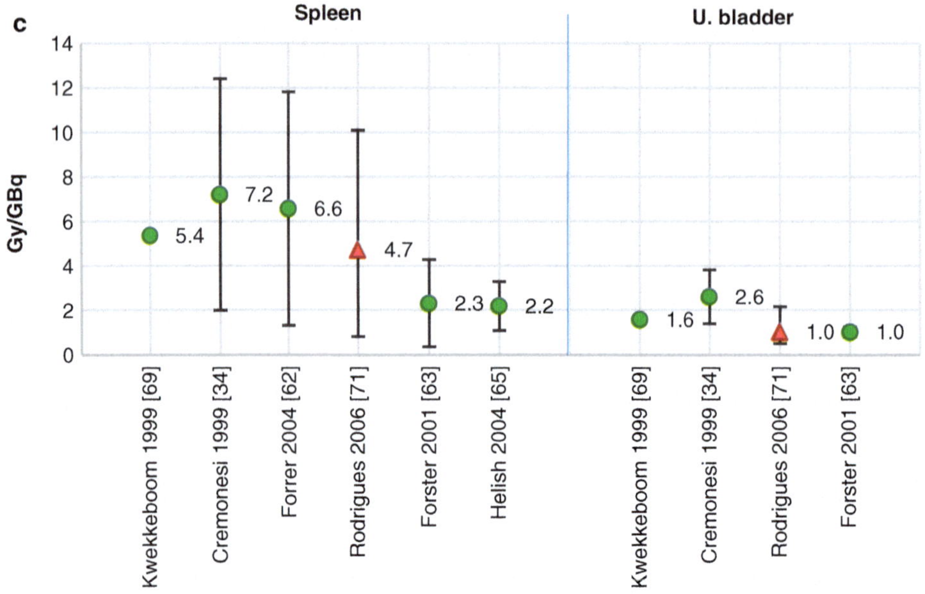

d

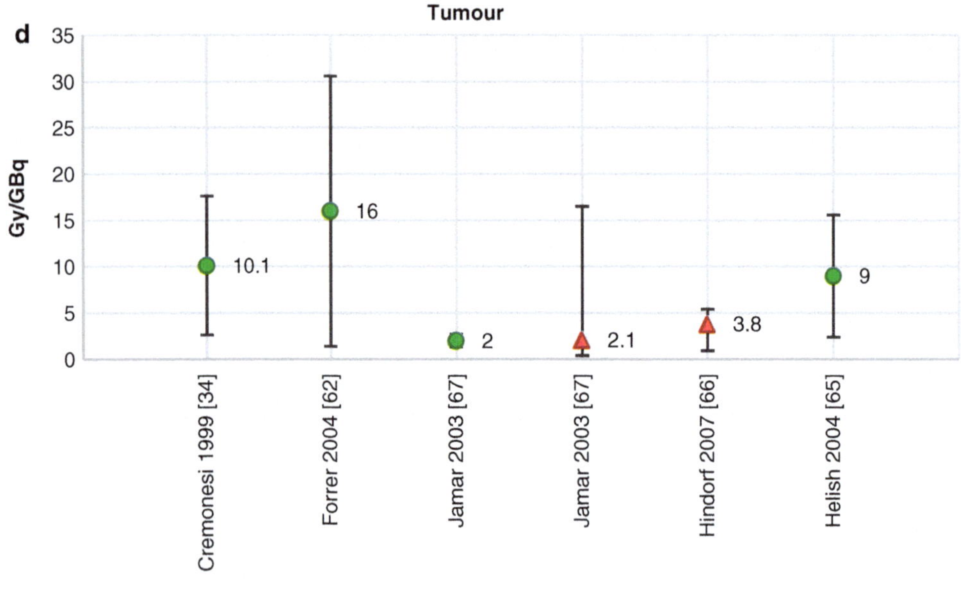

Fig. 23.1 (continued)

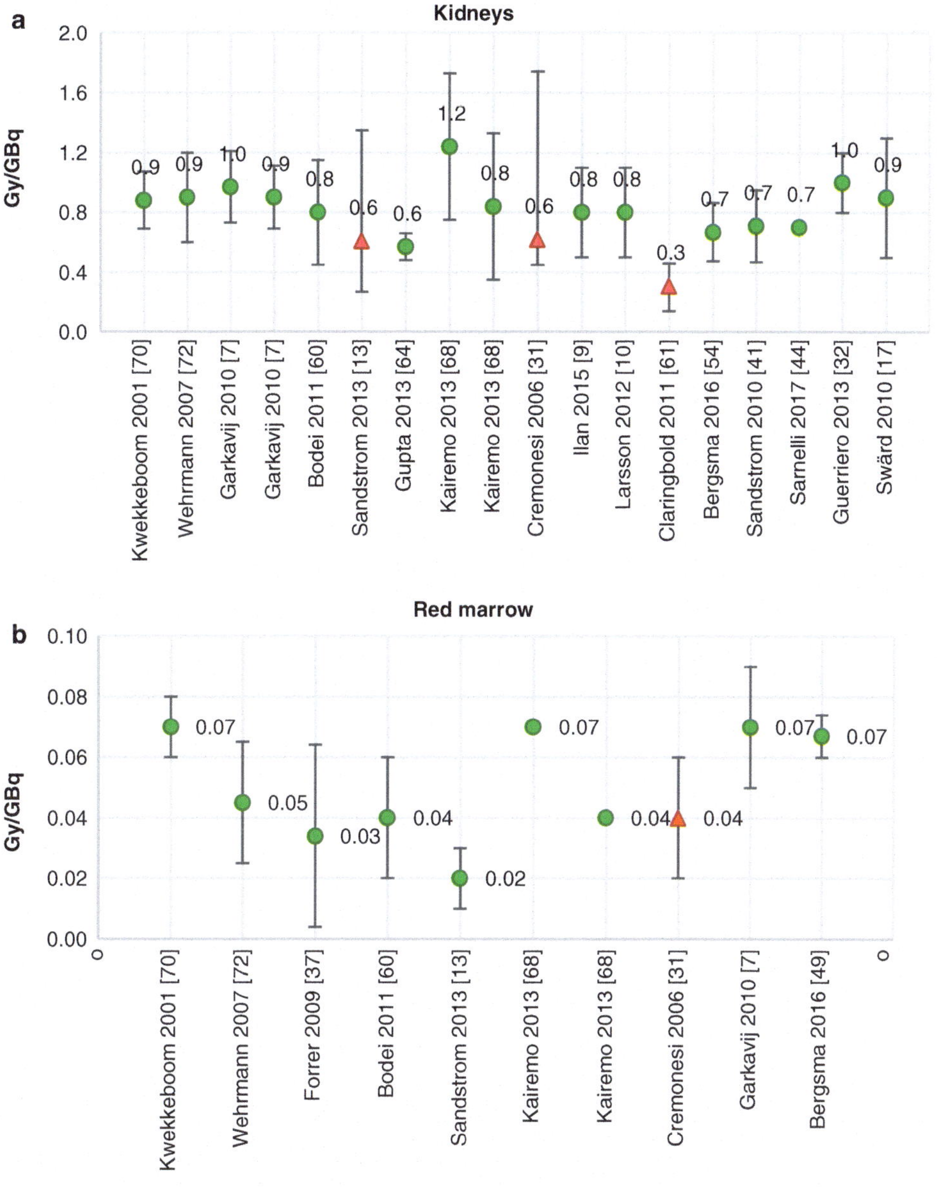

Fig. 23.2 Absorbed doses per unit activity (Gy/GBq) of ^{177}Lu-DOTATATE in kidneys (**a**), red marrow (**b**), other source organs—liver, spleen, urinary bladder and total body—(**c**), and tumour (**d**). Circles and corresponding error bars represent mean values and standard deviations; triangles and corresponding error bars represent median values and ranges of variability. In all cases, kidney absorbed doses include renal protection

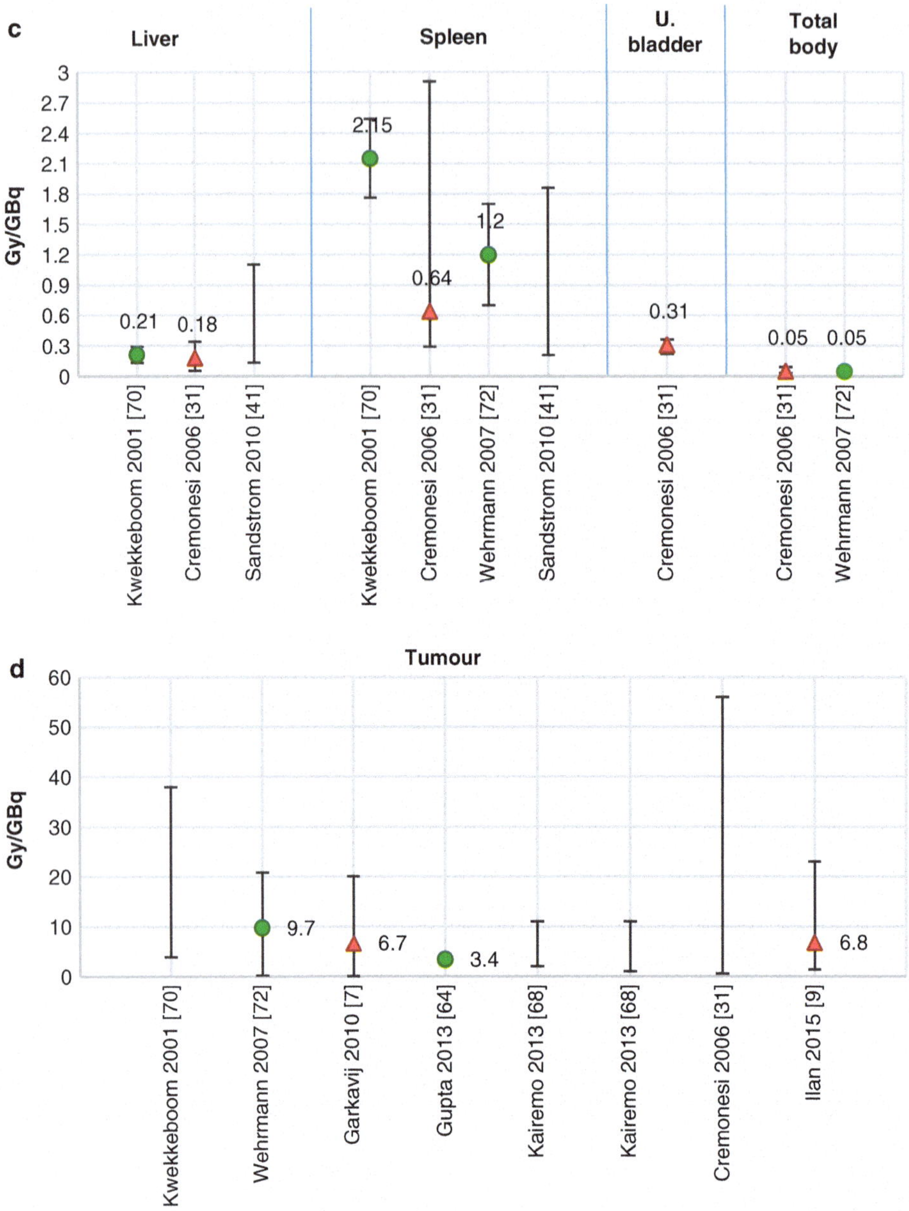

Fig. 23.2 (continued)

highly in tumours, testifying the need of personalised dosimetry.

Further to note is that the absorbed doses per unit activity of ^{177}Lu-DOTATATE are much lower (two- to fourfold) than for ^{90}Y-DOTATOC [28].

23.4.2 Comparison of Dosimetry Methods

Several authors have compared different methods for dosimetry, with the aim to identify the most accurate dosimetry and to establish the possible inaccuracy related to more convenient/simplified procedures.

Garkavij et al. and Sandström et al. compared planar and SPECT images of ^{177}Lu-PRRT, considering planar images corrected for scatter, background, attenuation, and response of the system, and SPECT images corrected for attenuation, scatter, and response of the system. In particular, for the kidneys, the dose differences observed indicated about a 20% overestimate when using elaborating planar vs. SPECT images [7, 41]. Moreover, differences of ~10–15% were derived when comparing planar images using two different background corrections [7, 41], of ~10% when comparing the hybrid (SPECT combined to planar images) with 3D SPECT methods [7] and ~10% when comparing 3D methods using different ways to draw the volumes of interest [41].

Larsson et al. focused on different planar dosimetric methods for the kidneys and studied the influence of the number of time points in ^{177}Lu-DOTATATE. The authors found a large interindividual variation—further enlarged in case of the lack of late acquisition on day 7—showing that personalised treatment planning with correction for individual organ sizes is warranted [10].

A further investigation about the most adequate timing for imaging and interpolation of the time-activity curve was carried out by Guerriero et al. [32] in both ^{177}Lu- and ^{90}Y-peptides. The authors also analysed the performance of a simplified dosimetry by means of only one to two scans and the influence of renal risk factors. They found that data should be collected at least up to ~100 h and ~70 h for ^{177}Lu- and ^{90}Y-PRRT, respectively, in order to avoid dose uncertainties even of ~40%, and that risk factors cause a significant 20% increase in dose.

Sandstrom et al. provided an interesting study focused on the method dependence, observer variability and kidney volumes of 3D dosimetry for ^{177}Lu-PRRT [14]. The methods based on a small volume of interest (VOI), on anatomical VOIs on CT and on thresholds on functional images rendered comparable results (within 5%), with small interobserver differences expressly for the small VOI method, which resulted to be preferable for calculating absorbed doses in solid organs.

23.4.3 Multiple Cycle Therapy and Variation of Dosimetry

Currently, PRRT trials of both ^{90}Y- and ^{177}Lu-radiopeptides are organised in multiple therapy cycles. This solution follows the first clinical experience on PRRT showing that single shot treatments could cause serious renal impairment, while cycles have demonstrated to lower toxicity incidence and/or severity for a same cumulative activity, especially in ^{90}Y-PRRT [42–44]. Such rationale, which has been confirmed by practice, relies on the different radiosensitivity of most tumours vs. the kidney tissue. As a consequence, cycles should allow to administer higher cumulative activities for a fixed renal risk, with the intent to improve the therapeutic outcome, based on the hypothesis that the irradiation of the renal parenchyma and of the tumours remains the same at each cycle. However, various authors have remarked the concern of possible changes in the biokinetics during the different cycles of therapy, which can occur to a negligible or relevant extent. Some studies have expressively compared the doses recorded at any cycle to the same patients. In particular, the study by Garkavij et al. on ^{177}Lu-DOTATATE showed that the first two of the four planned therapy cycles make the major contribution to the tumour absorbed dose, possibly due to a saturation of the peptide receptors, while the different cycles contribute on average equally, within 10%, to the absorbed dose to the kidneys [7]. These findings have been established also by other investigations [9]. Thus, the use of cycles increases the tolerability but at the cost of a lower cumulative irradiation of the tumour for a same absorbed dose to the kidneys. This means that an equilibrium has to be found between number of cycles (tolerability) and tumour irradiation (efficacy), as too many cycles might give no real therapeutic advantage and be less bearable from a practical point of view.

In any case, cycles are especially effective in ^{90}Y-PRRT, where occurrence of renal impairment has been confirmed [42–44].

23.4.4 Correlations with Renal Dose

The finding of dose-effect correlation between kidney absorbed doses and events of nephropathy is attributed to the group of Barone et al. who analysed the renal dosimetry of patients undergoing ^{90}Y-DOTATOC and included patient-specific mass adjustment [5]. This correlation had the typical sigmoidal trend of the normal tissue complication probability (NTCP) curve derived for external beam radiotherapy, but with a shift leading to higher cumulative doses tolerated in PRRT as compared to radiotherapy [18, 45]. Subsequent steps that improved the correlation analysis were the enrichment of the number of patients and the introduction of the biological effective dose (BED) concept [6, 46], according to the following formula:

$$\begin{aligned} BED &= \sum_i BED_i \\ &= \sum_i Di + b/a\, T_{1/2\,rep} / \left(T_{1/2\,rep} + T_{1/2\,eff}\right) Di^2 \end{aligned}$$

where D_i is the absorbed dose at the cycle i, α/β is the parameter relating the intrinsic radiosensitivity (α) and the potential sparing capacity (β) for a specified tissue and effect (in this case, the kidney), $T_{1/2rep}$ is the repair half-time of sublethal damage for the tissue and $T_{1/2eff}$ is the effective half-time of the radiopharmaceutical in that tissues. Considering the BED-effect correlation, the experimental curves from external beam radiotherapy and from ^{90}Y-PRRT for kidneys almost overlapped. A threshold BED of 33 Gy for kidney radiation damage and a BED of 44 Gy as the value associated to 50% of probability of damage were found [18].

This radiobiological model, in which the BED is not linear with absorbed dose, has the implication that the higher the number of cycles the lower the total BED for a same cumulative dose, thus the lower the nephrotoxicity induced [28]. This perfectly interpreted the clinical results of patients receiving therapy in multiple cycles without renal impairment as compared to the patients injected with high ^{90}Y-DOTATOC activity in one to two shots (e.g. 3.7 GBq/m^2 in two cycles) who developed high-grade toxicity [43, 47, 48]. Additionally, clinical experience provided evidence of safety up to a cumulative BED ~40 Gy to kidneys, and that risk factors lowered the tolerability to a BED threshold of ~28 Gy and encumbered the recovery of renal parameters [28, 42].

As regards ^{177}Lu-PRRT, the results available to date indicate a sporadic incidence of toxicity [36, 42, 49], thus impeding yet the construction of NTCP curves. In the majority of cases, ^{177}Lu-DOTATATE protocols conceived four cycles of 7.4 GBq each, which rarely reach the cumulative BED of 40 Gy that indicates risk in ^{90}Y-PRRT (see also Fig. 23.2a; the mean ± SD absorbed dose to the kidneys is 0.8 ± 0.1, leading to ~23 Gy with 29.6 GBq). Therefore, the kidney irradiation at such schedule could be still within the safe side, leaving room for further optimisation, as shown by Sandstrom et al. [13]. On the other hand, it is also possible that the NTCP curve for ^{90}Y-PRRT does not apply to ^{177}Lu-PRRT due to the different physical characteristics of the radionuclides, in particular the particle range, and the peptide localization, occurring preferably in the proximal tubuli (radioresistant cells), versus the glomeruli (radiosensitive cells). The short-range ^{177}Lu β-particles might irradiate more selectively the tubuli, while the long-range ^{90}Y β-particles may increase the irradiation of the glomeruli. Moreover, the inhomogeneous activity distribution could play an important role of sparing effect, as explained in the next paragraph [44, 50].

23.4.5 Kidney Dose Inhomogeneity

Kidney dosimetry is generally assessed by means of mean absorbed dose at organ level assuming uniform activity distribution. However, as interesting possible improvement, a sub-organ kidney dosimetry has been proposed, e.g. by the multiregion MIRD or OLINDA models, which allow to ascribe specific time-integrated activity coefficients to the kidney substructures [29, 51, 52]. Although some authors wished for the analysis of SPECT images [46], the determination of the activity proportion between renal cortex and medulla remains a tangible problem, being the SPECT resolution unable to provide a reliable activity distribution within the cortex, which is only few mm thick.

More detailed information about intra-renal distribution has been derived from the analysis of renal autoradiograms obtained from operated patients, previously administered with ^{111}In-octreotide [50]. In particular, the dose-volume histograms (DVH) based on the activity distribution were derived for ^{90}Y- and ^{177}Lu-peptides. For a same mean absorbed dose, the main difference was the much higher uniformity of the dose distribution for ^{90}Y as compared with ^{177}Lu, for which absorbed doses had a striped pattern in the cortex. Sarnelli et al. rescaled these DVH to the mean absorbed doses of clinical data and proposed a radiobiological model based on the equivalent uniform dose (EUD) to include the fraction of damaged cells in the calculation of the NTCP and to predict the possible kidney damage. The results showed that, due to the higher dose heterogeneity in case of ^{177}Lu, for a same mean absorbed dose with ^{90}Y and ^{177}Lu, the derived EUD, and hence NTCP, is lower for ^{177}Lu as compared to ^{90}Y. This model provides explanation of the higher kidney tolerability observed in the clinical experience even at mean absorbed doses attributable to thresholds for toxicity with ^{90}Y-DOTATOC [44].

23.4.6 Correlations with Tumour Response

Strong tumour dose-effect correlations are particularly difficult to be ascertained, as too many parameters concur to the response, such as histology, dimension, vascularization, radiosensitivity and activity distribution in the tumour. Said this, a first relationship between absorbed dose in NETs and tumour reduction has been observed by Pauwels et al. in 13 patients treated with ^{90}Y-DOTATOC, with a correlation coefficient of 0.5 [53]. Responding tumours could be identified as those receiving much higher doses compared to non-responding (~230 vs. ~40 Gy). More recently, Ilan et al. reported the results of a study in 30 patients affected by pancreatic NET and treated with ^{177}Lu-therapy. The authors applied accurate 3D dosimetry methods including correction for the partial volume effect. Excellent correlations between absorbed doses and tumour volume reduction were observed, with correlation coefficients of 0.6 and as high as 0.9 for tumour diameters larger than 2.2 cm and 4 cm, respectively [9].

If large series of data with specific radiobiological parameters and tumour characteristics are being collected, the outcome prediction will be certainly improved in the next future and enlarged to different tumours.

23.4.7 ^{90}Y or ^{177}Lu?

The choice of the most suitable radiopharmaceutical for PRRT cannot be generalised. It should be based instead on the individual characteristics that balance the cost-benefits effect, namely the possible renal toxicity and the tumour response.

In regard to toxicity, the previous paragraph "correlations with renal dose" has already anticipated that ^{177}Lu-peptides appear to be less nephrotoxic than ^{90}Y-peptides, at least in the protocols generally applied, in which the threshold limits for dose and BED are not generally reached [19, 36, 42, 54]. Despite that long-term data analysis of ^{90}Y- and ^{177}Lu-PRRT trials has been published, the intrinsic potential toxicity of the two radiopeptides is still to be elucidated. An ultimate comparison between ^{90}Y- and ^{177}Lu-radiopeptides would require randomised trials conceived to release the same cumulative BED—or at least the same cumulative absorbed dose—to the kidneys.

In regard to efficacy, the choice between ^{90}Y and ^{177}Lu should be based on the tumour extension, tumour localisation, uptake of normal tissues and targeting compound affinity. In principle, the physical characteristics of ^{177}Lu, with lower tissue penetration, make it more suitable for small tumours and micro-metastases, while the crossfire effect of ^{90}Y might be advantageous for the irradiation of larger and/or irregular lesions [28]. This rationale is laying the basis for clinical protocols proposing cocktails or tandem treatments of ^{177}Lu- and ^{90}Y-radiopeptides [55, 56]. To establish the proportion of ^{90}Y and ^{177}Lu activity, it should be taken into consideration that the absorbed dose per unit injected activity of ^{90}Y in kidneys and tumours is typically threefold or fourfold that of ^{177}Lu.

23.5 Future Perspectives

As future perspectives, simplified methods for dosimetry are to be considered, which are presently under study and will possibly provide new strategies for a reduced demand of data collection. For instance, trends of kinetics observed in extended groups of patients could be considered of reference, while quantification could require maybe one single acquisition. Of course, such possibility should be validated carefully, and the loss in accuracy established based on large series of data. Recently, an analytical method accepting the approximation of mono-exponential trends of the time-activity curves has been presented for ^{177}Lu-PRRT dosimetry with the request of just one image acquisition at 4 days p.i. (MRT dosimetry workshop, [57]). Although this method might need endorsement of ample data or might be restricted to certain groups of patients, it offers an interesting example of promising future standpoints, able to streamline the work of dosimetrists and clinicians and, not less importantly, the compliance of patients.

A further new issue that deserves citation in regard to tumour response is the monitoring of tumour gene activity levels by the measurement of circulating NET tumour transcripts (NETest), based on several marker genes. The results of preliminary studies confirmed that this test is able to assess the disease status and treatment efficacy with statistically significant higher accuracy and earlier time points as compared with other biomarkers (such as cromogranine A) and morphological/functional imaging [58, 59]. This offers precious information to be combined to dosimetry for tailored PRRT and attests the crucial role of interdisciplinarity, including dosimetry and genetic profile, allowing identifying responding patients or patient who will be more subject to side effects.

References

1. Bodei L, Cremonesi M, Kidd M, et al. Peptide receptor radionuclide therapy for advanced neuroendocrine tumors. Thorac Surg Clin. 2014;24(3):333–49.
2. Strosberg J, El-Haddad G, Wolin E, et al. Phase 3 trial of 177lu-dotatate for midgut neuroendocrine tumors. N Engl J Med. 2017;376(2):125–35.
3. van Essen M, Krenning EP, Kam BL, et al. Peptide-receptor radionuclide therapy for endocrine tumors. Nat Rev Endocrinol. 2009;5:382–93.
4. Baechler S, Hobbs RF, Prideaux AR, et al. Extension of the biological effective dose to the MIRD schema and possible implications in radionuclide therapy dosimetry. Med Phys. 2008;35:1123–34.
5. Barone R, Borson-Chazot F, Valkema R, et al. Patient-specific dosimetry in predicting renal toxicity with (90)Y-DOTATOC: relevance of kidney volume and dose rate in finding a dose-effect relationship. J Nucl Med. 2005;46(Suppl 1):99S–106S.
6. Dale R. Use of the linear-quadratic radiobiological model for quantifying kidney response in targeted radiotherapy. Cancer Biother Radiopharm. 2004;19:363–70.
7. Garkavij M, Nickel M, Sjogreen-Gleisner K, et al. 177Lu-[DOTA0,Tyr3] octreotate therapy in patients with disseminated neuroendocrine tumors: analysis of dosimetry with impact on future therapeutic strategy. Cancer. 2010;116:1084–92.
8. Gustafsson J, Brolin G, Cox M, et al. Uncertainty propagation for SPECT/CT-based renal dosimetry in (177)Lu peptide receptor radionuclide therapy. Phys Med Biol. 2015;60(21):8329–46.
9. Ilan E, Sandström M, Wassberg C, et al. Dose response of pancreatic neuroendocrine tumors treated with peptide receptor radionuclide therapy using 177Lu-DOTATATE. J Nucl Med. 2015;56(2):177–82.
10. Larsson M, Bernhardt P, Svensson JB, et al. Estimation of absorbed dose to the kidneys in patients after treatment with 177Lu-octreotate: comparison between methods based on planar scintigraphy. EJNMMI Res. 2012;2:49.
11. Lassmann M, Chiesa C, Flux G, et al. EANM dosimetry committee guidance document: good practice of clinical dosimetry reporting. Eur J Nucl Med Mol Imaging. 2011;38(1):192–200.
12. Ljungberg M, Celler A, Konijnenberg MW, et al. MIRD pamphlet no. 26: joint EANM/MIRD guidelines

for quantitative 177Lu SPECT applied for dosimetry of radiopharmaceutical therapy. J Nucl Med. 2016;57(1):151–62.
13. Sandstrom M, Garske-Roman U, Granberg D, et al. Individualized dosimetry of kidney and bone marrow in patients undergoing 177Lu-DOTA-octreotate treatment. J Nucl Med. 2013;54:33–41.
14. Sandström M, Ilan E, Karlberg A, et al. Method dependence, observer variability and kidney volumes in radiation dosimetry of (177)Lu-DOTATATE therapy in patients with neuroendocrine tumours. EJNMMI Phys. 2015;2(1):24.
15. Strigari L, Benassi M, Chiesa C, et al. Dosimetry in nuclear medicine therapy: radiobiology application and results. Q J Nucl Med Mol Imaging. 2011;55(2):205–21.
16. Strigari L, Konijnenberg M, Chiesa C, et al. The evidence base for the use of internal dosimetry in the clinical practice of molecular radiotherapy. Eur J Nucl Med Mol Imaging. 2014;41(10):1976–88.
17. Swärd C, Bernhardt P, Ahlman H, et al. [177Lu-DOTA 0-Tyr 3]-octreotate treatment in patients with disseminated gastroenteropancreatic neuroendocrine tumors: the value of measuring absorbed dose to the kidney. World J Surg. 2010;34(6):1368–72.
18. Wessels BW, Konijnenberg MW, Dale RG, et al. MIRD pamphlet no. 20: the effect of model assumptions on kidney dosimetry and response--implications for radionuclide therapy. J Nucl Med. 2008;49:1884–99.
19. Kwekkeboom DJ, de Herder WW, Kam BL, et al. Treatment with the radiolabeled somatostatin analog [177 Lu-DOTA 0,Tyr3]octreotate: toxicity, efficacy, and survival. J Clin Oncol. 2008;26:2124–30.
20. Eberlein U, Cremonesi M, Lassmann M. Individualized dosimetry for theranostics: necessary, nice to have, counterproductive? J Nucl Med. 2017;58 (Suppl 2):97S–103S.
21. Van Binnebeek S, Baete K, Vanbilloen B, et al. Individualized dosimetry-based activity reduction of 90Y-DOTATOC prevents severe and rapid kidney function deterioration from peptide receptor radionuclide therapy. Eur J Nucl Med Mol Imaging. 2014;41:1141–57.
22. Fabbri C, Sarti G, Cremonesi M, et al. Quantitative analysis of 90Y bremsstrahlung SPECT-CT images for application to 3D patient-specific dosimetry. Cancer Biother Radiopharm. 2009;24:145–54.
23. Minarik D, Sjögreen Gleisner K, Ljungberg M. Evaluation of quantitative (90)Y SPECT based on experimental phantom studies. Phys Med Biol. 2008;53:5689–703.
24. Minarik D, Ljungberg M, Segars P, Gleisner KS. Evaluation of quantitative planar 90Y bremsstrahlung whole-body imaging. Phys Med Biol. 2009;54:5873–83.
25. Fabbri C, Bartolomei M, Mattone V, et al. (90) Y-PET/CT imaging quantification for dosimetry in peptide receptor radionuclide therapy: analysis and corrections of the impairing factors. Cancer Biother Radiopharm. 2015;30(5):200–10.
26. Martí-Climent JM, Prieto E, Elosúa C, et al. PET optimization for improved assessment and accurate quantification of 90Y-microsphere biodistribution after radioembolization. Med Phys. 2014;41(9):092503.
27. Willowson KP, Tapner M, QUEST Investigator Team, et al. A multicentre comparison of quantitative (90) Y PET/CT for dosimetric purposes after radioembolization with resin microspheres: the QUEST phantom study. Eur J Nucl Med Mol Imaging. 2015;42(8):1202–22.
28. Cremonesi M, Botta F, Di Dia A, et al. Dosimetry for treatment with radiolabelled somatostatin analogues. A review. Q J Nucl Med Mol Imaging. 2010;54:3 7–51.
29. Stabin MG, Sparks RB, Crowe E. OLINDA/EXM: the second-generation personal computer software for internal dose assessment in nuclear medicine. J Nucl Med. 2005;46(6):1023–7.
30. Bolch WE, Eckerman KF, Sgouros G, et al. MIRD pamphlet no. 21: a generalized schema for radiopharmaceutical dosimetry--standardization of nomenclature. J Nucl Med. 2009;50(3):477–84.
31. Cremonesi M, Ferrari M, Bodei L, et al. Dosimetry in patients undergoing 177Lu-DOTATATE therapy with indications for 90Y- DOTATATE. Eur J Nucl Med Mol Imaging. 2006;33:S102.
32. Guerriero F, Ferrari ME, Botta F, et al. Kidney dosimetry in 177Lu and 90Y peptide receptor radionuclide therapy: influence of image timing, time-activity integration method, and risk factors. Biomed Res Int. 2013;2013:935351.
33. Siegel JA, Thomas SR, Stubbs JB, et al. MIRD pamphlet no. 16: techniques for quantitative radiopharmaceutical biodistribution data acquisition and analysis for use in human radiation dose estimates. J Nucl Med. 1999;40:37S–61S.
34. Cremonesi M, Ferrari M, Zoboli S, et al. Biokinetics and dosimetry in patients administered with (111) in-DOTA-Tyr(3)-octreotide: implications for internal radiotherapy with (90)Y-DOTATOC. Eur J Nucl Med. 1999;26:877–86.
35. Ljungberg M, Gleisner KS. Hybrid imaging for patient-specific dosimetry in radionuclide therapy. Diagnostics. 2015;5(3):296–317.
36. Bodei L, Kidd M, Modlin IM, et al. Gene transcript analysis blood values correlate with ^{68}Ga-DOTA-somatostatin analog (SSA) PET/CT imaging in neuroendocrine tumors and can define disease status. Eur J Nucl Med Mol Imaging. 2015;42(9):1341–52.
37. Forrer F, Krenning EP, Kooij PP, et al. Bone marrow dosimetry in peptide receptor radionuclide therapy with [177Lu-DOTA(0),Tyr(3)]octreotate. Eur J Nucl Med Mol Imaging. 2009;36:1138–46.
38. Valkema R, Pauwels S, Kvols LK, et al. Survival and response after peptide receptor radionuclide therapy with [90Y-DOTA0,Tyr3]octreotide in patients with advanced gastroenteropancreatic neuroendocrine tumors. Semin Nucl Med. 2006;36:147–56.
39. Bodei L, Mueller-Brand J, Baum RP, et al. The joint IAEA, EANM, and SNMMI practical guidance on

peptide receptor radionuclide therapy (PRRNT) in neuroendocrine tumours. Eur J Nucl Med Mol Imaging. 2013;40:800–16.
40. Rolleman EJ, Melis M, Valkema R, et al. Kidney protection during peptide receptor radionuclide therapy with somatostatin analogues. Eur J Nucl Med Mol Imaging. 2010;37(5):1018–31.
41. Sandström M, Garske U, Granberg D, et al. Individualized dosimetry in patients undergoing therapy with (177)Lu-DOTA-D-Phe (1)-Tyr (3)-octreotate. Eur J Nucl Med Mol Imaging. 2010;37:212–25.
42. Bodei L, Cremonesi M, Ferrari M, et al. Long-term evaluation of renal toxicity after peptide receptor radionuclide therapy with 90Y-DOTATOC and 177Lu-DOTATATE: the role of associated risk factors. Eur J Nucl Med Mol Imaging. 2008;35:1847–56.
43. Cybulla M, Weiner SM, Otte A. End-stage renal disease after treatment with 90Y-DOTATOC. Eur J Nucl Med. 2001;28(10):1552–4.
44. Sarnelli A, Guerriero F, Botta F, et al. Therapeutic schemes in177Lu and 90Y-PRRT: radiobiological considerations. Q J Nucl Med Mol Imaging. 2017;61(2):216–31.
45. Emami B, Lyman J, Brown A, et al. Tolerance of normal tissue to therapeutic irradiation. Int J Radiat Oncol Biol Phys. 1991;21:109–22.
46. Baechler S, Hobbs RF, Boubaker A, et al. Three-dimensional radiobiological dosimetry of kidneys for treatment planning in peptide receptor radionuclide therapy. Med Phys. 2012;39(10):6118–28.
47. Imhof A, Brunner P, Marincek N, et al. Response, survival, and long-term toxicity after therapy with the radiolabeled somatostatin analogue [90Y-DOTA]-TOC in metastasized neuroendocrine cancers. J Clin Oncol. 2011;29:2416–23.
48. Otte A, Weiner SM, Cybulla M. Is radiation nephropathy caused by yttrium-90? Lancet. 2002;359(9310):979.
49. Bergsma H, Konijnenberg MW, Kam BL, et al. Subacute haematotoxicity after PRRT with (177) Lu-DOTA-octreotate: prognostic factors, incidence and course. Eur J Nucl Med Mol Imaging. 2016;43(3):453–63.
50. Konijnenberg M, Melis M, Valkema R, et al. Radiation dose distribution in human kidneys by octreotides in peptide receptor radionuclide therapy. J Nucl Med. 2007;48:134–42.
51. Bouchet LG, Bolch WE, Blanco HP, et al. MIRD pamphlet no 19: absorbed fractions and radionuclide S values for six age-dependent multiregion models of the kidney. J Nucl Med. 2003;44(7):1113–47.
52. Green A, Flynn A, Pedley RB, et al. Nonuniform absorbed dose distribution in the kidney: the influence of organ architecture. Cancer Biother Radiopharm. 2004;19:371–7.
53. Pauwels S, Barone R, Walrand S, et al. Practical dosimetry of peptide receptor radionuclide therapy with (90)Y-labeled somatostatin analogs. J Nucl Med. 2005;46:92S–8S.
54. Bergsma H, Konijnenberg MW, van der Zwan WA, et al. Nephrotoxicity after PRRT with (177) Lu-DOTA-octreotate. Eur J Nucl Med Mol Imaging. 2016;43(10):1802–11.
55. Kunikowska J, Królicki L, Hubalewska-Dydejczyk A, et al. Clinical results of radionuclide therapy of neuroendocrine tumours with 90Y-DOTATATE and tandem 90Y/177Lu-DOTATATE: which is a better therapy option? Eur J Nucl Med Mol Imaging. 2011;38(10):1788–97.
56. Seregni E, Maccauro M, Chiesa C, et al. Treatment with tandem [90Y]DOTA-TATE and [177Lu]DOTA-TATE of neuroendocrine tumours refractory to conventional therapy. Eur J Nucl Med Mol Imaging. 2014;41(2):223–30.
57. Hänscheid H, Lapa C, Buck AK, et al. Dose mapping after endoradiotherapy with 177Lu-DOTATATE/-TOC by one single measurement after four days. J Nucl Med. 2017. https://doi.org/10.2967/jnumed.117.193706.
58. Bodei L, Kidd M, Paganelli G, et al. Long-term tolerability of PRRT in 807 patients with neuroendocrine tumours: the value and limitations of clinical factors. Eur J Nucl Med Mol Imaging. 2015b;42(1):5–19.
59. Bodei L, Kidd M, Modlin IM, et al. Measurement of circulating transcripts and gene cluster analysis predicts and defines therapeutic efficacy of peptide receptor radionuclide therapy (PRRT) in neuroendocrine tumors. Eur J Nucl Med Mol Imaging. 2016;43(5):839–51.
60. Bodei L, Cremonesi M, Grana CM, et al. Peptide receptor radionuclide therapy with (177) Lu-DOTATATE: the IEO phase I-II study. Eur J Nucl Med Mol Imaging. 2011;38(12):2125–35.
61. Claringbold PG, Brayshaw PA, Price RA, et al. Phase II study of radiopeptide 177Lu-octreotate and capecitabine therapy of progressive disseminated neuroendocrine tumours. Eur J Nucl Med Mol Imaging. 2011;38(2):302–11.
62. Forrer F, Uusijarvi H, Waldherr C, et al. A comparison of (111)In-DOTATOC and (111)In-DOTATATE: biodistribution and dosimetry in the same patients with metastatic neuroendocrine tumours. Eur J Nucl Med Mol Imaging. 2004;31:1257–62.
63. Forster GJ, Engelbach MJ, Brockmann JJ, et al. Preliminary data on biodistribution and dosimetry for therapy planning of somatostatin receptor positive tumours: comparison of 86Y-DOTATOC and 111In-DTPA-octreotide. Eur J Nucl Med. 2001;28:1743–50.
64. Gupta SK, Singla S, Thakral P, et al. Dosimetric analyses of kidneys, liver, spleen, pituitary gland, and neuroendocrine tumors of patients treated with 177Lu-DOTATATE. Clin Nucl Med. 2013;38:188–94.
65. Helisch A, Forster GJ, Reber H, et al. Pre-therapeutic dosimetry and biodistribution of 86Y-DOTA-Phe1-Tyr3-octreotide versus 111In-pentetreotide in patients

with advanced neuroendocrine tumours. Eur J Nucl Med Mol Imaging. 2004;31:1386–92.
66. Hindorf C, Chittenden S, Causer L, et al. Dosimetry for (90)Y-DOTATOC therapies in patients with neuroendocrine tumors. Cancer Biother Radiopharm. 2007;22:130–5.
67. Jamar F, Barone R, Mathieu I, et al. (86Y-DOTA0)-D-Phe1-Tyr3-octreotide (SMT487)--a phase 1 clinical study: pharmacokinetics, biodistribution and renal protective effect of different regimens of amino acid co-infusion. Eur J Nucl Med Mol Imaging. 2003;30:510–8.
68. Kairemo K, Kangasmaki A. 4D SPECT/CT acquisition for 3D dose calculation and dose planning in (177)Lu-peptide receptor radionuclide therapy: applications for clinical routine. Recent Results Cancer Res. 2013;194:537–50.
69. Kwekkeboom DJ, Kooij PP, Bakker WH, et al. Comparison of 111In-DOTA-Tyr3-octreotide and 111In-DTPA-octreotide in the same patients: biodistribution, kinetics, organ and tumor uptake. J Nucl Med. 1999;40:762–7.
70. Kwekkeboom DJ, Bakker WH, Kooij PP, et al. [177Lu-DOTAOTyr3]octreotate: comparison with [111In-DTPAo]octreotide in patients. Eur J Nucl Med. 2001;28(9):1319–25.
71. Rodrigues M, Traub-Weidinger T, Li S, et al. Comparison of 111In-DOTA-DPhe1-Tyr3-octreotide and 111In-DOTA-lanreotide scintigraphy and dosimetry in patients with neuroendocrine tumours. Eur J Nucl Med Mol Imaging. 2006;33:532–40.
72. Wehrmann C, Senftleben S, Zachert C, et al. Results of individual patient dosimetry in peptide receptor radionuclide therapy with 177Lu DOTA-TATE and 177Lu DOTA-NOC. Cancer Biother Radiopharm. 2007;22:406–16.

Guidelines on Radioisotope Treatment of Neuroendocrine Tumors

24

Federico Caobelli and Laura Evangelista

24.1 Introduction

The present chapter has the aim to provide the current position of radioimmunotherapy (RIT) for the treatment of neuroendocrine tumors (NETs), in the main national and international clinical guidelines. Table 24.1 reported a summary of clinical indications.

24.2 Comments and Suggestions

In the latest years, in patients affected by neuroendocrine tumors, RIT has gained worldwide interest, given the possibility of a targeted therapy in unresectable and/or metastatic disease, similar to what for years yielded in the management of thyroid carcinomas by means of 131-iodine. Despite this great interest, there is still lack of prospective, randomized clinical studies in the literature, resulting in generally poor level of evidence. As a consequence, the current guidelines only provide general indications based either on specialist board consensus or on retrospective, nonrandomized clinical studies.

While NANETS guidelines do not either mention RIT as a practical alternative in patients with neuroendocrine tumors, the BCCA guidelines recognize a role for RIT in patients with progressive and/or symptomatic metastatic NETs, provided that tumors are receptor positive (as proven by a 111-In pentetreotide or 123-I MIBG scan) and have a Ki-67 $\leq$ 20%. However, no precise indications are given, and patients may just be referred to RIT after a multidisciplinary specialist consensus. Most surprisingly, the assessment of receptor positivity is based on the demonstration of tumor uptake on classical planar, whole body scintigraphy based on the use of either 111-In Pentetreotide or 123-I MIBG scan. As this assessment has been effectively performed in the latest years taking advantages of the increased sensitivity and improved spatial resolution of 68-Ga DOTATOC positron emission tomography (PET)/computed tomography (CT), an update of these latter guidelines would be highly warranted.

Firstly in 2012, the ESMO guidelines found an initial, defined role for RIT, by providing an important, although still investigational role (level of evidence: IV), for selective internal irradiation therapy (SIRT was recommended in patients with liver metastases, while PRRT was suggested for patients with both functioning and nonfunctioning NETs with positive somatostatin receptor scintigraphy; see Table 24.1). According to this European guidelines, the primary tumor

F. Caobelli (✉)
Clinic of Radiology & Nuclear Medicine, Basel University Hospital, University of Basel, Basel, Switzerland
e-mail: Federico.caobelli@usb.ch

L. Evangelista
Nuclear Medicine and Molecular Imaging Unit, Veneto Institute of Oncology IOV – IRCCS, Padua, Italy

E. Bombardieri et al. (eds.), *Clinical Applications of Nuclear Medicine Targeted Therapy*,
https://doi.org/10.1007/978-3-319-63067-0_24

Table 24.1 A schematic information about the available guidelines on radioisotope treatment of NETs

	Name of guidelines	Year of pub.	Useful link	Clinical indications	Level/ grade of evidence[a]
1	ESMO [1]	2012	https://academic.oup.com/annonc/article-lookup/doi/10.1093/annonc/mds295	• SIRT with 90Y- microspheres can be indicated in selected patients with liver metastases from NETs • PRRT may be indicated in non-pancreatic NETs: – Grade 1 or 2 – Non-resectable, with metastases – Ki-67 <30%	IV
2	NANETS [2]	2013	https://www.nanets.net/2013-nanets-guidelines	No role for peptide receptor radionuclide therapy. Of note, the use of molecular imaging in the diagnosis and the follow-up are limited to 111In-pentetreotide scan	NA
3	BCCA	2013	http://www.bccancer.bc.ca/health-professionals/professional-resources/cancer-management-guidelines/gastrointestinal/neuroendocrine-tumors	Patients with progressive and/or symptomatic metastatic NETs whose tumors are receptor positive and have a Ki-67 ≤20% may be candidates for radionuclide therapy	IV
4	IAEA/EANM/SNMMI [3]	2013	http://www-pub.iaea.org/books/iaeabooks/8789/Practical-Guidance-on-Peptide-Receptor-Radionuclide-Therapy-PRRNT-for-Neuroendocrine-Tumours	Procedural guidelines • PRRT is indicated: – In tumors expressing SSTR-2 – NETs grade 1 or 2 – In metastatic or inoperable NETs – In selected cases, pheochromocytoma, paraganglioma, neuroblastoma, medullary thyroid carcinoma • PRRT is contraindicated in patients with: – Severe tumors expressing SSTR-2 – NETs grade 1 or 2 – In metastatic or inoperable NETs – In selected cases, pheochromocytoma, paraganglioma, neuroblastoma, medullary thyroid carcinoma – Reduced renal function – Severely compromised bone marrow • Patients with impaired renal function should preliminarily undergo a pretreatment with amino acids to prevent renal failure	IIB
5	NCCN	2015	https://www.nccn.org/professionals/physician_gls/f_guidelines.asp	• PRRT is indicated in patients with: – Well-differentiated non-pancreatic NETs (grade 1 or 2) – Metastatic carcinoid tumors refractory to octreotide • PRRT is not proven to be useful in pancreatic NETs	IIB

Table 24.1 (continued)

	Name of guidelines	Year of pub.	Useful link	Clinical indications	Level/ grade of evidence[a]
6	SCONET	2015		• 131I-MIBG is indicated as: – Adjuvant therapy after primary surgery – In metastatic disease (pheo-chromocytoma, paraganglioma, neuroblastoma) – Primary therapy in patients unfit for surgery, occasionally • PRRT is indicated: – To treat patients with soma-tostatin receptor-positive NETs (demonstrated by 111In-octreotide) and acceptable renal function	NA
7.	Canadian National Expert Group [4]	2015	NA	• PRRT is considered the standard systemic approach in patients with octreotide-avid disease • PRRT can be used in patients with MIBG/octreotide avid disease; • Adequate renal, hepatic, and bone marrow function • Good to excellent performance status • Moderate bulk disease • Progressive disease despite consid-eration or attempted use of other potentially less toxic therapies	NA
8	ENETS Consensus Guidelines Update for Gastroduodenal Neuroendocrine Neoplasms [5]	2016	www.enets.org/enets_guidelines.html	No data about RIT are available	NA
9	ENETS Consensus Guidelines Update for Neuroendocrine Neoplasm of the Jejunum and Ileum [6]	2016	www.enets.org/enets_guidelines.html	No data about RIT are available	NA
10	ENETS Consensus Guidelines Update for Management of Patients with Digestive Neuroendocrine Tumors: An Update [7]	2016	www.enets.org/enets_guidelines.html	No data about RIT are available	NA

[a]Level of evidence: *NA* = not available; *IA* evidence from meta-analysis of randomized controlled trials; *IB* evidence from at least one randomized controlled trial; *IIA* evidence from at least one controlled study without randomization; *IIB* evidence from at least one other type of quasi-experimental study; *III* evidence from nonexperimental descriptive studies, such as comparative studies, correlation studies, and case-control studies; *IV* evidence from expert committee reports or opinions or clinical experience of respected authorities or both

ESMO European Society of Medical Oncology, *NANETS* North American Neuroendocrine Tumor Society, *BCCA* BC Cancer Agency, *NCCN* National Comprehensive Cancer Network, *IAEA* International Atomic Energy Agency, *EANM* European Association of Nuclear Medicine and Molecular Imaging, *SNMMI* Society of Nuclear Medicine and Molecular Imaging, *ENETS* European Neuroendocrine Tumor Society, *SCONET* Scottish Neuroendocrine Tumour Group, *SIRT* selective Internal Radiotherapy, *PRRT* peptide receptor radionuclide therapy, *Ki67* proliferation index, *SSTR* somatostatin receptor, *MIBG* metaiodiobenzylguanidine, *RIT* radioimmunotherapy

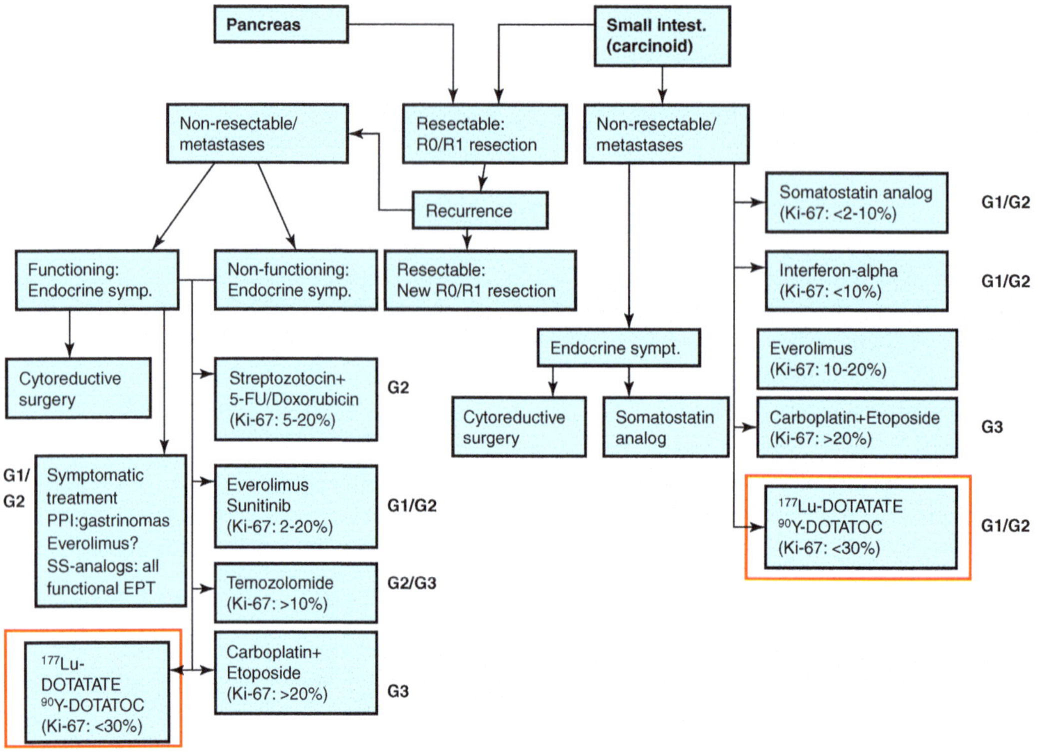

Fig. 24.1 Algorithm considering all possible therapeutic options in patients with neuroendocrine tumors, provided in ESMO Guidelines (2012)

site should not represent a discriminant, although the authors report higher response rates in pancreatic than small intestinal NETs, with the highest objective response rate in metastatic rectal NETs. For the first time, an algorithm has been provided (Fig. 24.1).

These indications partially differ from those in NCCN guidelines (2015). While confirming a possible important role for SIRT in patients with liver metastases, PRRT is not recommended in patients with pancreatic NETs. Capitalizing on more evidences from the literature, showing in most papers a bias in selection (i.e., randomized studies of radiolabeled somatostatin analogs have not yet been completed in patients with advanced pancreatic NETs), the authors reported only an investigational role for PRRT in patients with metastatic pancreatic NETs. Conversely, PRRT can be recommended in patients with non-pancreatic NETs. This recommendation was drawn considering a prospective and randomized study by Dobson and coworkers [8] featuring more than 200 patients with advanced midgut NETs, undergoing either 177Lutetium (177Lu)-DOTATATE or high-dose octreotide. In this trial, the PRRT was associated with a significant improvement in progression-free survival (PFS, not reached vs. 8.4 months; $p < 0.0001$) and with a significant higher rate of tumor response (18 vs. 3% in control group, $p < 0.001$). These observations have been confirmed in a recent randomized trial by Strosberg et al. [9], wherein, among patients with advanced midgut NETs, the treatment with 177Lu-DOTATATE resulted in significantly longer PFS and a significantly higher response rate than high-dose octreotide (PFS: 65.2% for PRRT vs. 10.8% for octreotide at 20 months, $p < 0.001$). Furthermore, a preliminary evidence of an overall survival benefit was demonstrated in an interim analysis (14 deaths in the PRRT group vs. 26 in the octreotide group). As long as new evidences are reported in the literature, a parallel update of the guidelines will be highly anticipated.

Nuclear medicine physicians can refer to current joint procedural guidelines formulated by IAEA, SNMMI, and EANM and published in 2013 [3]. These guidelines provide information about chemical and physical characteristics of the radiopharmaceuticals, about their kinetic and mechanism of action, also dealing with the procedural issues concerning personnel and facility, patient preparation and instruction, radiopharmaceutical labelling and administration, possible side effects of the treatment, and dosimetric features. Also in these procedures, there is a lack of clear and defined indications for PRRT. Nevertheless, the authors suggest that a PRRT can be considered in patients with NETs expressing SSTR-2 of grade 1 or 2, in patients with metastatic or inoperable NETs, and in selected cases of pheochromocytoma, paraganglioma, neuroblastoma, and medullary thyroid carcinoma. Although these indications are not based on randomized, prospective clinical trials but rather on a consensus among a multidisciplinary specialist panel, still they recognize for the first time a broader field of application for PRRT, not limited to classical defined NETs but also suitable for other types of cancer expressing somatostatin-like receptors. This latter aspect is of great importance, as it underlines the strategic importance of specific receptors to predict the feasibility and efficacy of a targeted therapy.

From the careful analysis of the abovementioned guidelines, several important aspects need to be considered:

1. There is a lack of evidence in literature about the impact of PRRT in NETs, particularly in pancreatic and non-pancreatic disease. To date, only advanced midgut NETs have been reported to benefit from a targeted PRRT in large, randomized clinical trials. More high-quality papers are highly warranted to expand on the clinical feasibility and efficacy of PRRT.
2. PRRT is to date not specifically recommended in well-defined clinical situations. Rather, it is suggested in patients for whom no other traditional clinical approaches demonstrate a clinical benefit, especially in patients with symptomatic metastatic NETs, expressing SSTR-2, accepted renal function, and with a ki67 < 30%. While this approach can be considered acceptable until new evidence is available, this introduces a possible bias for the evaluation of treatment efficacy, being applied in patients with advanced disease. The "compassionate use" of PRRT might mask a possible incremental benefit even in the earlier stages of the disease.
3. Surprisingly, the majority of the current guidelines do not consider the possible beneficial role of PET/CT using 68-Ga labelled somatostatin analogs for the in vivo assessment of the receptor status.
4. In all the analyzed guidelines, new updates are warranted on the basis of the recent results from the NETTER-1 trial [9].

References

1. Öberg K, Knigge U, Kwekkeboom D, Perren A, ESMO Guidelines Working Group. Neuroendocrine gastro-entero-pancreatic tumors: ESMO clinical practice guidelines for diagnosis, treatment and follow-up. Ann Oncol. 2012;23(Suppl 7):vii124–30.
2. Kunz PL, Reidy-Lagunes D, Anthony LB, Bertino EM, Brendtro K, Chan JA, North American Neuroendocrine Tumor Society, et al. Consensus guidelines for the management and treatment of neuroendocrine tumors. Pancreas. 2013;42:557–77.
3. Bodei L, Mueller-Brand J, Baum RP, Pavel ME, Hörsch D, O'Dorisio MS, et al. The joint IAEA, EANM, and SNMMI practical guidance on peptide receptor radionuclide therapy (PRRNT) in neuroendocrine tumours. Eur J Nucl Med Mol Imaging. 2013;40:800–16.
4. Singh S, Dev C, Kenneche H, Kocha W, Maroun J, Metrakos P, et al. Consensus recommendations for the diagnosis and management of pancreatic neuroendocrine tumors: guidelines from a Canadian National Expert Group. Ann Surg Oncol. 2015;22: 2685–99.
5. Delle Fave G, O'Toole D, Sundin A, Taal B, Ferolla P, Ramage JK, et al. ENETS consensus guidelines update for gastroduodenal neuroendocrine neoplasms. Neuroendocrinology. 2016;103:119–24.
6. Niederle B, Pape U-F, Costa F, Gross D, Kelestimur F, Knigge U, et al. ENETS consensus guidelines update for neuroendocrine neoplasms of the jejunum and ileum. Neuroendocrinology. 2016;103:125–38.

7. O'Toole D, Kianmanesh R, Caplin M. ENETS consensus guidelines update for management of patients with digestive neuroendocrine tumors: an update. Neuroendocrinology. 2016;103:117–8.
8. Dobson R, Vinjamuri S, Hsuan J, Banks M, Terlizzo M, Wieshmann H, et al. Treatment of orbital metastases from a primary midgut neuroendocrine tumor with peptide-receptor radiolabeled therapy using 177 lutetium-DOTATATE. J Clin Oncol. 2013;31: e272–5.
9. Strosberg J, El-Haddad G, Wolin E, Hendifar A, Yao J, Chasen B, et al. NETTER-1 trial investigators. Phase 3 trial of 177lu-dotatate for midgut neuroendocrine tumors. N Engl J Med. 2017;376:125–35.

Part IV

Prostate Cancer

25 Bone Metastases in Prostate Cancer

Maria Bonomi, Eleonora Cerchiaro, Elisa Villa, Lucia Rebecca Setti, Letizia Gianoncelli, Emanuele Micheli, and Giovanni Luca Ceresoli

Abstract

Bone metastases occur in more than 80% of men with metastatic prostate cancer. Affecting the structural integrity of the bone, they can lead to skeletal complications and pain, with a negative impact on patient quality of life and survival. The last decade has witnessed tremendous advances in the treatment of metastatic PCa. New therapeutic options that prolong overall survival are now available. The optimization of bone metastasis management (and prevention of skeletal morbidities) is therefore of paramount importance to improve clinical outcome. Some issues are still debated, such as the most effective radiologic or nuclear medicine technique to diagnose and monitor bone disease, the ideal surrogate circulating marker to assess response or progression to treatment, patient selection, as well as the optimal sequencing or combination of available therapeutic options. Several healthcare professionals play a role in the treatment of metastatic PCa. The presence of a multidisciplinary team for the discussion of treatment strategies for each patient should be the standard of care.

M. Bonomi (✉) • E. Cerchiaro • L. Gianoncelli
G.L. Ceresoli
Department of Medical Oncology, Cliniche Humanitas Gavazzeni, Bergamo, Italy
e-mail: maria.bonomi@gavazzeni.it

E. Villa
Department of Radiation Oncology, Cliniche Humanitas Gavazzeni, Bergamo, Italy

L.R. Setti
Department of Nuclear Medicine, Cliniche Humanitas Gavazzeni, Bergamo, Italy

E. Micheli
Department of Urology, Cliniche Humanitas Gavazzeni, Bergamo, Italy

25.1 Introduction

Prostate cancer (PCa) is the second most common malignancy in men and the fifth leading cause of death from cancer in men. In 2012 it accounted for an estimated 1.1 million of new diagnosis and 307,000 deaths worldwide, respectively (http://globocan.iarc.fr/Pages/fact_sheets_cancer.aspx).

At diagnosis, approximately 80% of patients present with localized disease and 4% with distant metastases, with 5-year relative survival rate of 100% and 28%, respectively [1].

E. Bombardieri et al. (eds.), *Clinical Applications of Nuclear Medicine Targeted Therapy*, https://doi.org/10.1007/978-3-319-63067-0_25

Androgen-dependent tumor growth is controlled by surgical or medical castration. Androgen deprivation therapy (ADT) is the cornerstone of the treatment of patients with advanced or metastatic hormone-sensitive PCa. This approach includes luteinizing hormone-releasing hormone (LHRH) antagonists or agonists and antiandrogens [2] (https://www.nccn.org/professionals/physician_gls/pdf/prostate.pdf). However, after initial response to ADT, in many men the disease will progress despite castration levels of testosterone to a castration-resistant status (CRPC) [3]. Up to 30% of patients can respond to additional hormonal manipulations, but responses are usually short lasting [4]. PCa was considered resistant to chemotherapy until the mid-1990s, when mitoxantrone with prednisone was shown to have a role in the palliative treatment of metastatic CRPC (mCRPC). Men with mCRPC experienced an improvement in pain and quality of life (QoL) if treated with mitoxantrone plus steroids compared with prednisone alone, although no survival benefit was detected [5, 6]. In 2004 docetaxel became the standard of care in mCRPC after two landmark randomized controlled trials (RCTs) demonstrated an improvement in overall survival (OS) vs mitoxantrone [7, 8].

The last few years have witnessed a revolution in the treatment of mCRPC, due to a better understanding of CRPC biology and the demonstration that after the progression to the castrate status (defined on serum testosterone levels), PCa cells remain dependent on androgens and on the androgen receptor (AR) signaling pathway [9].

Currently five agents besides docetaxel are approved for the treatment of mCRPC, based on improvement in OS in phase III RCTs. These include a cytotoxic agent (cabazitaxel [10]), two hormone-based therapies (abiraterone [11, 12] and enzalutamide [13, 14]), and a bone-targeting radiopharmaceutical (Ra 223 dichloride [15]). Sipuleucel-T, a therapeutic cancer vaccine, is currently approved only in the USA [16]. Zoledronate [17] and denosumab [18] are two osteoclast-inhibiting agents used in supportive care to prevent bone metastasis (BM)-related complications.

25.2 Bone Metastasis in Prostate Cancer

PCa has a propensity to metastasize to bone. In an autoptic study on 1589 men older than 40 years with PCa, hematogenous metastases were present in 35%, the most frequent site being bone (90%) [19]. According to a recent review of clinical records from over 50 US cancer centers, the incidence of BMs in patients affected by stage IV PCa was 44.5, 60.4, and 71.1% at 1, 3, and 5 years from diagnosis, respectively [20]. The most common sites of metastases are the spine, pelvis, and ribs, while the skull and long bones are less common [21, 22].

BMs often lead to pain and skeletal complications, generally referred as skeletal-related events (SREs). SREs include pathologic fractures, need for radiotherapy or surgery to bone, spinal cord compression, and hypercalcemia, although the latter may be of paraneoplastic origin [23]. In a large study of 721 patients with newly diagnosed skeletal metastases from PCa, 72 (10%) had SREs coincident with the diagnosis of BMs. Among the remaining 649 patients, 301 (46.4%) experienced SREs during follow-up [24].

BMs and SREs are associated with decreased QoL, limitations of self-sufficiency, and loss of social functioning [23, 25]. BMs and related morbidities also pose a significant economic burden with increased hospital admissions and healthcare cost [26, 27].

Finally the extent of bone involvement in mCRPC [28] and the incidence of SREs [29] correlate negatively with survival. In a Danish population-based study in men with PCa, 1-year survival rates were 87% for men with PCa and no BMs, 47% for men with BMs, and 40% in those with BMs and SREs. Five-year overall survival (OS) rates were 56%, 3%, and less than 1%, respectively [30]. In a SEER database review in PCa patients, the HR for risk of death was 6.6 for men with BMs but no SRE and 10.2 for men with BMs plus SRE, compared with men without BMs, respectively [31].

With the advent of new treatment options that prolong OS in mCRPC, the improvement of BM management and prevention of SREs and other complications is of paramount importance to improve clinical outcome and reduce the financial burden of the disease. Several healthcare professionals play a role in the management of metastatic PCa patients, including, not exhaustively, urologists, radiation oncologists, medical oncologists, nuclear medicine physicians, radiologists, orthopedic surgeons, and experts in palliative and supportive care. Patient selection, optimal treatment sequencing, and the possibility to combine different treatment modalities are still debated. In this setting a multidisciplinary approach, in which members may discuss the treatment strategies in different phases of the disease, should be the standard of care [32].

25.3 Pathophysiology of Bone Metastases

The structural integrity of normal bone is maintained by a continuous and dynamic process of bone remodeling: osteoclasts induce bone reabsorption, while osteoblasts are responsible for bone apposition [33].

The receptor activator of nuclear factor κ-B (RANK)-RANK ligand (RANKL)-osteoprotegerin (OPG) axis is the main regulator of the interactions between osteoblasts and osteoclasts. RANK is a transmembrane receptor expressed on the surface of osteoclast precursor cells. RANKL is produced by osteocytes, osteoblasts, and bone marrow stromal cells. Interaction of RANK and RANKL regulates differentiation, activity, and survival of osteoclasts. OPG is a soluble decoy receptor of RANKL produced by osteoblast and stromal cells. OPG binds to RANKL and blocks the interaction between RANK and RANKL, thereby limiting excessive osteoclast-mediated bone reabsorption [34].

Bone homeostasis is disrupted when PCa cells interact with normal bone cells and bone microenvironment [35]. As described by Paget's "seed and soil" theory in 1889, bone microenvironment, due to the abundance of cytokines and growth factors, is an ideal "soil" for PCa cells (i.e., the "seeds") to proliferate. Commonly the metastatic process is divided into four stages: (1) homing, (2) dormancy, (3) colonization, and (4) expansion [36].

The first step of the metastatic process is the homing of tumor cells to the bone matrix. Tumor cells that metastasize to bone exploit the same physiological mechanisms used by hematopoietic stem cells homing to bone. A well-known interaction involves the stromal-derived factor 1 (SDF-1) and the CXCR4 receptor, present on the surface of hematopoietic cells but also of PCa cells [36, 37]. Once tumor cells migrate in the extracellular bone matrix, they may remain quiescent or colonize [33, 36]. During the dormancy state, by engaging a reversible cell cycle arrest, tumor cell may become resistant to traditional chemotherapy agents that target rapidly dividing cells [37]. In the phase of colonization, tumor cells secrete paracrine factors that interfere both with osteoblasts and with osteoclasts. In the early phase of the metastatic process, osteolysis is predominant: tumor cells produce osteoclast-activating factors such as transforming growth factor-β (TGF-β), parathyroid-related peptide (PTHrp), and IL-6 that promote the stromal and osteoblastic production of RANKL. Activation of osteoclasts by the RANKL-RANK pathway induces osteolysis which in turn causes release from bone matrix of cytokines and growth factors that stimulate proliferation of cancer cells (the "vicious cycle") [35, 38]. Later on bone apposition becomes predominant due to the release by bone matrix and neoplastic cells of osteoblast-stimulating factors such as fibroblast growth factor (FGF), bone morphogenetic proteins (BMP), and endothelin 1 (ET1) [35, 38].

The excessive osteoblastic activity observed in PCa bone metastases leads to calcium entrapment in skeletal tissue ("bone hunger syndrome") and to a secondary hyperparathyroidism in response to calcium deficiency. This, in turn, causes a generalized osteoclast activation, not limited to metastatic sites [39]. Thus notwithstanding the mainly osteoblastic nature of bone metastases from PCa, bone reabsorption is also increased, favoring the occurrence of skeletal complications. Finally, treatment-related osteoporosis (e.g., caused by long-term ADT) should be mentioned as another cause of bone reabsorption, bone mass loss, and increased risk of SREs [40].

25.4 Diagnosis, Evaluation, and Monitoring of BMs

Diagnosis, evaluation, and monitoring of BMs are not always straightforward. Clinical, biochemical, and diagnostic tools are available for detecting bone lesions and evaluating their changes during therapy in metastatic PCa patients.

25.4.1 Clinical Evaluation

Pain is a very frequent symptom in PCa patients with BMs. Unidimensional rating tools such as visual analogue scales (VAS), categorical verbal or numerical rating scales (VRS or NRS), or multidimensional rating tools such as the brief pain inventory (BPI) have been validated and used in clinical trials [41]. Analgesic use can be recorded and coded using tools such as the WHO scale (0 no analgesics, 1 nonopioid analgesics, 2 opioid analgesics for mild-moderate pain, 3 opioids for moderate-severe pain). Quality of life (QoL) questionnaires generally include evaluation of pain [41]. The European Organisation for Research and Treatment of Cancer (EORTC) [42] and the Functional Assessment of Cancer Therapy (FACT) scale [43] QoL questionnaires have both been validated and have a PCa-specific module [44]. The incidence of symptomatic skeletal events (SSEs) is frequently used to measure bone involvement in clinical trials. In contrast to SRE, defined above, SSEs include only symptomatic events (i.e., symptomatic pathologic fracture or spinal cord compression, irradiation to bone, surgery to bone).

25.4.2 Circulating Tumor Markers

25.4.2.1 PSA

PSA has an absolute specificity for prostate tissue and is expressed by the majority of PCa. Being "organ specific," PSA is of limited utility in the diagnostic phase as possible increases may be due to other causes affecting the prostate gland than cancer [45]. In newly diagnosed patients, the main clinical practice guidelines recommend the use of PSA (in association with the Gleason score and clinical stage) to define risk groups [2, 46] (https://www.nccn.org/professionals/physician_gls/pdf/prostate.pdf). A value of PSA >10 or >20 ng/mL is per se a predictor of intermediate or high risk, respectively, and a bone scan should be always performed if PSA > 20 ng/ml (or T2 and >10 ng/ml) (https://www.nccn.org/professionals/physician_gls/pdf/prostate.pdf). After radical treatment for PCa (i.e., surgery or radiotherapy), PSA becomes "cancer specific" and is a very reliable marker as even small increases may indicate a relapse [45]. As the disease progresses, PCa becomes more heterogenous and may dedifferentiate leading to an extreme variability in PSA expression both between patients and within the same patient. This may limit the utility of PSA as a marker of disease in the advanced setting [45]. Recommendations from the Prostate Cancer Clinical Trials Working Group 2 (PCWG2) advise against using PSA measurements as the sole criterion for clinical decisions especially in the first 12 weeks of treatment during which a transient increase may occur in patients subsequently experiencing a PSA response or stabilization [47]. PSA progression, during or after therapy, is defined as a 25% or greater increase and an absolute increase in 2 ng/mL or more from the nadir, confirmed by a second value obtained 3 or more weeks late [48].

Notwithstanding possible limitations, PSA is currently used in everyday clinical practice to monitor the disease in metastatic patients. However, further investigations are needed to establish PSA-based surrogate criteria of response or progression to systemic therapies for mCRPC.

25.4.2.2 Bone Turnover Markers

The processes of osteolysis and osteogenesis are associated with the release of distinct biochemical markers that can be measured in blood or urine. For example, serum levels of carboxy [C]-terminal cross-linked telopeptides of type I collagen (CTX) and urinary concentrations of the amino terminal cross-linked telopeptides (NTX) are associated with osteolysis, whereas bone-specific alkaline phosphatase (b-ALP) and procollagen type I N-terminal peptides (PINP) are associated with osteogenesis. Some markers may be associated with both (e.g., osteocalcin) [49]. Therefore, on a theoretical point of view, markers of bone turnover (MBT) could be used to monitor ongoing osteolytic and osteoblastic activity in BMs. However MBT reflects rates of bone reabsorption and formation in the body as a whole, not being able to provide information on a specific lesion (i.e., BMs). Moreover they are bone specific and not cancer specific, reflecting alterations in skeletal metabolism caused by various neoplastic or nonneoplastic factors such as age, vitamin D deficiency, secondary hyperparathyroidism, or ADT, whose separate contribution cannot be distinguished [23, 50].

Nevertheless, the utility of MBT in monitoring metastatic bone disease, detecting patients at higher risk of progression (and skeletal-related complications), or identifying patients more likely to benefit from osteoclast-inhibiting agents has been widely studied [49, 50]. A retrospective analysis of data from phase III trials comparing zoledronate to placebo in mCRPC showed that elevated b-ALP levels were significantly associated with a shorter time to the first SRE [51] and shorter OS [52]. Similarly high NTX level correlated with higher risk of SREs, progression, and death [53]. Normalization of NTX during treatment with bisphosphonates (BPs) was related to a reduced risk of death, 50% improvement in SRE-free survival, and a trend toward an increased bone lesion progression-free survival compared to patients without normalization of NTX [54]. Recently, rapidly increasing bone ALP values were found to be an independent predictor of poor OS in CRPC [55]. Despite growing evidences of a potential application of MBT for diagnosis, prognosis, and monitoring therapy in cancer patients, the routine use of these markers cannot yet be recommended.

25.4.3 Conventional Radiology

Plain radiography can be used to evaluate symptomatic regions in the skeleton. However it will not detect lesions <1 cm or with loss of <50% of mineral content [23, 56] (https://www.nccn.org/professionals/physician_gls/pdf/prostate.pdf). Computed tomography (CT) is more sensitive and can detect smaller areas of trabecular destruction/invasion of the cortical bone [56]. However, assessing therapeutic response with CT scan can be difficult as bone structure rarely normalizes even in case of effective therapy. According to RECIST 1.1 criteria, bone lesions are nonmeasurable lesions, unless soft tissue component is associated [57]. Magnetic resonance imaging (MRI) detects the presence of tumor tissue in the bone marrow, before the osteoclastic/osteoblastic response takes effect, therefore allowing early detection of BMs and with effective monitoring of the disease and response to therapy [56, 58]. However, MRI requires advanced diagnostic techniques (available only in centers of excellence), longer duration of examination, and higher costs.

25.4.4 Nuclear Medicine

Conventional 99mTc-diphosphonate whole-body bone scintigraphy (BS) is widely used to image BMs because it is sensitive, relatively inexpensive, and available even in small centers [59]. It detects osteoblastic or mixed lesions, but is less sensitive on osteolytic ones. The major limitation of 99mTc-diphosphonate bone scintigraphy is its relatively low specificity and false-positive results in traumatic, degenerative, and infectious changes. The calculated range of sensitivity and specificity is 70–95% and 60–75%, respectively [60]. PET/CT techniques both with bone-targeting radiotracers (such as 18F-fluoride) [61, 62] and prostate cancer-targeting radiotracers (18F/11C-choline) [63] have shown a higher diagnostic accuracy in detecting BMs than conventional bone scan [60]. In the majority of the guidelines, bone scan is strongly recommended, despite the low sensitivity and specificity (https://www.nccn.org/professionals/physician_gls/pdf/prostate.pdf). On the contrary, the role of 18F-fluoride and choline PET/CT is still indeterminate, particularly in the staging phase. The relatively high cost of PET/CT techniques is the major limitation for a wide clinical application. Cost-effectiveness analyses should be carried out in order to evaluate the impact of these techniques on a wider perspective, taking into consideration also the possible improvements on patient management (early and correct diagnosis to avoid useless or ineffective treatments). Available guidelines do not provide well-defined criteria to assess response to therapy with nuclear medicine tools. According to PCWG2 [48], when the bone scan is the sole indicator, progression is defined when at least two or more new lesions are seen compared with a prior scan. If the scan findings are suggestive of a flare reaction, or apparent new lesion(s) may represent trauma, MRI or CT scan can be used as a confirmation. PCWG2 criteria were developed specifically for clinical trials and maybe not easy to apply in real-life context.

25.5 Bone-Targeting Agents for Metastatic Prostate Cancer

25.5.1 Zoledronic Acid

Zoledronic acid (ZA) is a third-generation bisphosphonate (BP) and is the first agent approved for the treatment of BMs from mCRPC. BPs have a chemical structure similar to normal bone matrix pyrophosphate, bind to hydroxyapatite crystal, and inhibit osteoclast bone reabsorption [64].

In a landmark phase III trial, patients with BMs from mCRPC were randomized to ZA (4 mg every 3 weeks) vs placebo. Initially the trial included also an 8 mg cohort, which was later reduced to 4 mg after evidence of excessive renal toxicity emerged. At the 24-month follow-up, ZA resulted in a lower incidence of SRE (38% vs 49%; p 0.028), prolonged time to first SRE (488 vs 321 days; $p < 0.009$), and reduced by 36% the percentage of patients that, having experienced a SRE on study, developed a subsequent SRE. ZA also improved pain control (according to patient-reported BPI) and was associated with decreased urinary levels of bone reabsorption markers (NTX, pyridinoline, and deoxypyridinoline) and serum levels of bone-specific ALP. No differences in objective response rate (ORR), time to radiological progression, or PSA changes within 30 days of progression were detected [17, 65]. On the basis of these results, ZA was approved for the treatment of patients with BMs from CRPC.

ZA has also been tested in hormone-sensitive PCa with BMs. In the CALBG90202 phase III placebo-controlled trial, early initiation of ZA was not associated with increased time to first SRE (median, 31.9 ms vs 29.8 ms; $p=0.39$). OS and PFS were similar. In an exploratory subgroup analysis, ZA was associated with longer time to first on-study SRE in men who experienced a SRE before study entry (median, 31.9 ms vs 17.9 ms) [66]. Similarly in the STAMPEDE trial (discussed in "Chemotherapy" section), a randomized controlled multiarm multistage trial recruiting men with high-risk, locally advanced, metastatic or recurrent PCa, the addition of ZA to ADT did not prolong time to first SRE [67].

In the adjuvant setting, ZA, administered every 3 months for 4 years, was not effective in preventing the incidence of BMs vs observation in patients with high-risk localized PCa (PSA > 20 ng/ml, Gleason score 8–10, or positive lymph nodes) [68].

Although the potential efficacy of ZA in the adjuvant or hormone-sensitive setting cannot be excluded in different populations or with different schedules than those used in the abovementioned trials, mCRPC is the only setting in which ZA has a proven efficacy.

25.5.2 Denosumab

Denosumab is a fully human monoclonal antibody against RANKL. It inhibits osteoclast-mediated bone destruction and increases bone mass [69].

Denosumab (120 mg subcutaneous every 4 weeks) was compared to ZA (4 mg endovenous every 4 weeks) in a phase III RCT. Time to first on-study SRE (primary endpoint) favored denosumab (median, 20.7 ms vs 17.1 ms p 0.00002). Denosumab also reduced bone turnover markers more than ZA and prolonged time to first and subsequent on-study SREs. No significant differences were detected for OS and PFS [18]. In a prespecified subgroup analysis, the incidence of SSEs (defined as radiation to bone, symptomatic pathologic fracture, surgery to bone, or symptomatic spinal cord compression) was analyzed as well. Denosumab reduced both the risk of developing first SSE (HR 0.78; 95% CI, 0.66–0.93; p 0.005) and first and subsequent SSEs (HR 0.78; 95% CI, 0.65–0.92; p 0.004) [70]. On the basis of these results, denosumab was approved to reduce SRE in metastatic PCa at a dose of 120 mg every 4 weeks. Although approval does not specify that the disease must be castration-resistant, no data are available in hormone-sensitive patients.

Denosumab was also assessed in high-risk nonmetastatic CRPC patients (defined as PSA > 8 ng/ml, PSA doubling time < 10 months or both). In a phase III RCT by Smith et al., 1432 patients were randomized to denosumab (120 mg sc every 4 weeks) or placebo. BM-free survival was 4.2 months longer with denosumab (median, 29.5 ms vs 25.2 ms, p 0.028). The incidence of symptomatic BMs was 9.6% in the denosumab group vs 13% in the placebo group (p 0.01). Biochemical markers of bone turnover decreased significantly with denosumab treatment compared with placebo. Osteonecrosis of the jaw occurred in 33 (5%) men receiving denosumab and in no patient in the placebo arm. Grade 3 or 4 hypocalcemia was reported in nine (1%) patients on denosumab vs two on placebo. No differences in OS and PFS were detected [71]. Despite a slight increase in BM-free survival, denosumab was not approved by FDA or EMA for this indication. Although not strictly related to the BM setting, it is worth mentioning that denosumab at a dose of 60 mg every 6 month has been approved to increase bone mass in nonmetastatic PCa patients receiving ADT at high risk for fracture. In the HALT 138 study, denosumab increased bone mineral density (BMD) of the lumbar spine by 5.6%, compared with a loss of 1.0% in the placebo group ($P < 0.001$). Denosumab was also associated with significant increases in BMD at the total hip, femoral neck, and distal third of the radius at all time points. Rates of adverse events were similar between the two groups [72].

Long-term treatment with BPs or denosumab can lead to peculiar side effects that can be prevented with appropriate patients' selection, monitoring, and proactive treatment.

ZA and denosumab are both associated with hypocalcemia. In the phase III RCT comparing these two agents, hypocalcemia was more frequent in the denosumab arm (any grade 13% vs 6%, $p < 0.0001$, grade 3–4 5% vs 1%) [18]. Supplementation with at least 500 mg calcium and 400 IU vitamin D daily is required in all patients treated with either denosumab or ZA (http://www.ema.europa.eu/docs/en_GB/document_library/EPAR_-_Product_Information/human/000336/WC500051730.pdf; http://www.ema.europa.eu/docs/en_GB/document_library/EPAR_-_Product_Information/human/002173/WC500110381.pdf).

Osteonecrosis of the jaw (ONJ) is defined as the presence of exposed bone in the maxillofacial region lasting for more than 8 weeks despite appropriate management in patients treated with BPs that have not received radiation to the bone [73]. In a pooled analysis of three RCTs comparing denosumab vs ZA in various solid tumors, the incidence of ONJ was 1.8% with denosumab vs 1.3% with ZA (p 0.13) [74]. Dental extractions and poor oral hygiene are well-known risk factors. A baseline dental evaluation is recommended. If invasive procedures are required, these agents should be withheld till complete healing [73].

ZA is potentially nephrotoxic: the risk of renal failure is directly related to the drug infusion time and dosage [75]. According to drug label, ZA dose should be reduced in case of impaired renal failure (30–60 ml/min) and is contraindicated in case of severe renal dysfunction (http://www.ema.europa.eu/docs/en_GB/document_library/EPAR_-_Product_Information/human/000336/WC500051730.pdf). No dose reduction is required for denosumab in case of mild renal function (http://www.ema.europa.eu/docs/en_GB/document_library/EPAR_-_Product_Information/human/002173/WC500110381.pdf).

Table 25.1 Summary of efficacy data from randomized trials on bone targeting agents approved for prostate cancer

Agent	Population	Treatment arms (no. of patients)	Primary endpoint	Results of primary outcome	Other outcomes
Zoledronic Acid (Saad 2002; Saad 2004)	mCRPC	Zoledronic acid 4 mg (214) vs. placebo (208) q 4 weeks	Proportion of patients with SRE	38% vs. 49% ($p = 0.028$)	Time to SRE 488 vs. 321 days (p 0.009) Significant reduction of urinary bone reabsorption markers w zoledronic acid (p 0.001)
Denosumab (Fizazi 2011)	mCRPC	Denosumab 120 mg (950) vs. zoledronic acid 4 mg (951) q 4 weeks	Time to first on study SRE	20.7 ms vs. 17.1 ms ($p = 0.0002$)	uNTX decrease week 13 −40.3% vs. −28.4% ($p < 0.0001$) ALP decrease week 13 −7.9% vs. −4.8% ($p < 0.0001$)
Denosumab (Smith 2009)	Nonmetastatic castration sensitive PCa	Denosumab 60 mg vs. placebo q 6 ms	BMD lumbar spine	+5.6% vs. −1.0% ($p < 0.001$)	Significant BMD increase at hip, femoral neck, and distal radius w denosumab ($p < 0.001$) Vertebral fracture at 36 ms 1.5% vs. 3.9% (p 0.006) Reduction of BMT at 36 ms w denosumab ($p < 0.001$)
Denosumab (Smith 2012)	Nonmetastatic CRPC	Denosumab 120 mg (716) vs. placebo (716) every 4 weeks	BMFS	29.5 ms vs. 25.2 ms (p 0.028)	Symptomatic bone metastasis 10% vs. 13% ($p = 0.03$) Reduction of BMT w denosumab ($p < 0.001$)
Ra223 (Parker 2013; Sartor 2014)	mCRPC	223Ra (614) vs. Placebo (307)	OS	14.9 ms vs. 11.3 ms (p 0.001)	Median time to SRE 9.8 ms vs. 5.6 ms ($p < 0.001$) Significant reduction and normalization of ALP levels with Ra223 ($p < 0.001$)

ALP alkaline phosphatase, *BMD* bone mineral density, *BMT* bone turnover markers, *BMFS* bone metastasis free survival, *mCRPC* metastatic castration resistant prostate cancer, *ONJ* osteonecrosis of the jaw, *OS* overall survival, *SRE* skeletal related adverse events, *uNTX* urinary amino terminal cross-linked telopeptides

25.5.3 Ra-223

In the pivotal phase III ALSYMPCA trial that leads to approval of Ra-223 in mCRPC, 921 patients with symptomatic mCRPC and 2 or more BMs (and no visceral involvement) were randomized to Ra-223 (six injections of 50 kBq/kg every 4 weeks) or placebo. Ra-223 significantly improved OS vs placebo (median, 14.9 ms vs 11.3 ms; HR 0.70; 95% CI 0.58–0.83; p 0.001). The benefit was evident in both docetaxel-naive and docetaxel-pretreated patients [15]. Ra-223 significantly prolonged time to first SSE (median, 15.6 ms vs 9.8 ms; HR, 0.66; 95% CI, 0.52–0.83; $P < 0.001$) [15]. SSEs occurred in 33% of patients in the Ra-223 group and 38% in the placebo group. Ra-223 reduced the risks of external radiotherapy for bone pain (HR 0.67; 95% CI, 0.53–0.85) and spinal cord compression (HR 0.52; 95% CI, 0.29–0.93), while there was no significant benefit in time to symptomatic pathological bone fracture and tumor-related orthopedic surgical intervention [76]. A summary of efficacy data from randomized trials on bone-targeting agents approved for PCa is reported in Table 25.1.

25.6 Chemotherapy

25.6.1 Docetaxel

Docetaxel is a semisynthetic taxane, approved for the treatment of mCRPC after the results of two landmark RCTs in 2004 demonstrated an OS improvement versus mitoxantrone.

In the TAX 327 trial, 1006 men with mCRPC (90% with BMs) received 10 mg of prednisone daily and were randomized to mitoxantrone 12 mg/m^2 every 3 weeks, or docetaxel 75 mg/m^2 every 3 weeks (3 W) or docetaxel 30 mg/m^2 weekly (W). At the final analysis, median OS was 19.2 months for the 3 W group vs 16.3 months in the mitoxantrone arm (p 0.004). Patients given W docetaxel had a median OS of 17.8 months (p 0.09 vs mitoxantrone) [77]. Three W docetaxel led to an improved QoL (according to FACT-P questionnaire) and to a reduction of pain (assessed with present pain inventory PPI), while the effect on pain control was not significant for W docetaxel. Adverse events were more common with 3W docetaxel. In fact, G3-G4 neutropenia was observed in 32%, 2%, and 22% of patients with 3W, W docetaxel, and mitoxantrone; febrile neutropenia occurred in 3, 0, and 2%, respectively [7]. The OS benefit with 3W docetaxel was confirmed in all patient subgroups, irrespectively of age, tumor burden, site of metastasis, bone involvement, and presence of disease-related symptoms [77].

In the SWOG 9916 phase III RCT, the association of estramustine and docetaxel led to an OS benefit vs mitoxantrone (17.5 ms vs 15.6 ms, p 0.02). PFS was also significantly superior (6.3 ms vs 3.2 ms, $p < 0.001$), as was PSA response. Radiologic response rate and pain relief were similar. Febrile neutropenia, nausea and vomiting, and cardiovascular events were more common in the docetaxel arm. Although HR for death and median OS in the docetaxel arm were similar to those reported in the TAX 327 study, the SWOG 9916 trial failed to meet its primary endpoint (33% improvement in median OS) [8].

Based on these results, there is a general consensus that weekly docetaxel schedule should not be adopted, with the possible exception of patients with poor performance status or at high risk of hematological toxicity (e.g., febrile neutropenia). The addition of estramustine seems to increase toxicity with no added benefit. Although enrolling a high percentage of patients with BMs (90%), none of these two RCTs included an analysis on SREs.

The impact of early docetaxel in association with ADT has been evaluated in three RCTs [67, 78, 79]. In the GETUG-AFU 15, median OS was not improved in hormone-sensitive mCRPC (80% with BMs) by the addition of docetaxel both in the overall and in the BMs population [78]. In the CHAARTED trial, the combination of docetaxel plus ADT leads to a 13.6-month increase in OS in overall population (median, 57.6 ms vs 44 ms; HR 0.61, 95% CI, 0.47–0.80; $p < 0.001$). A subgroup analysis showed a survival improvement with docetaxel in high-volume patients defined as the presence of visceral metastases or ≥4 bone lesions with ≥1 beyond the vertebral bodies and pelvis (49.2 ms vs 32.2 ms; HR, 0.60; 95% CI, 0.45–0.81; p 0.001), but not in low-volume disease [79]. No specific analysis on incidence and timing of SREs was reported in GETUG-AFU 15 and CHAARTED trials.

The STAMPEDE trial is an ongoing adaptive multiarm, multistage randomized controlled trial recruiting men with high-risk, locally advanced, metastatic or recurrent PCa. In three of the trial arms, patients were randomized to ADT plus zoledronic acid or ADT plus docetaxel or ADT plus docetaxel and zoledronic acid; all these arms were compared to the standard arm of ADT alone. Patients treated with ADT had a median OS of 71 months (5-year OS 55%). A statistically significant improvement in OS was detected in the ADT plus docetaxel arm, with a median OS of 81 months and a 5-year OS of 63% (HR 0.78, 95% CI 0.66–0.93; $p = 0.006$), and in the ADT plus docetaxel plus zoledronic acid group, with median OS of 76 months and a 5-year OS of 60% (HR 0.82, 95% CI 0.69–0.97; $p = 0.022$). No OS improvement was reported in patients treated with ADT plus zoledronic acid (HR 0.94, $p = 0.45$). A preplanned subset analysis in metastatic patients only showed similar results. Time to first SRE was improved in the docetaxel + ADT arm (HR 0.60; 95% CI 0.48–0.74, p 0.127×10^{-5}) and in docetaxel + zoledronic acid + ADT arm (HR 0.55, 95% CI 0.44–0.69 p 0.277×10^{-7}) but not in the zoledronic acid + ADT group. The mean time to SRE was 61.4 months in ADT only, 68 months in docetaxel + ADT, and 68.3 months in docetaxel + zoledronic acid + ADT arm [67].

According to the available evidences, the use of early docetaxel combined with ADT should be considered in selected hormone-naive metastatic PCa patients (i.e., high volume according to CHAARTED definition) presenting with distant metastases at or soon after diagnosis, fit to receive chemotherapy.

25.6.2 Cabazitaxel

In more recent years, cabazitaxel, a new-generation taxane, has been approved for mCRPC patients progressing during or after docetaxel treatment. In the TROPIC trial, 755 patients were randomized to mitoxantrone versus cabazitaxel, both in combination with low-dose prednisone. Cabazitaxel led to an improved OS (median 15.1 ms vs 12.7 ms, HR 0.70, 95% CI 0.59–0.83; $p < 0.0001$) and trial-specific PFS (defined as PSA, tumor or pain progression, or death). Cabazitaxel also improved PSA and tumor response, while pain response rate was not different in the two arms. The most common clinically significant grade ≥ 3 AEs with cabazitaxel were neutropenia and diarrhea [10]. A subsequent long-term analysis confirmed the superiority of cabazitaxel in terms of OS, but did not detect any clinical benefit in pain palliation (evaluated by PPI and analgesic score) [80].

With the aim to improve the toxicity profile, a 20 mg/m^2 dose of cabazitaxel was compared to the 25 mg/m^2 one in a noninferiority RCT, showing similar OS benefit with a more favorable toxicity profile [81]. In the FIRSTANA study, cabazitaxel (either 20 or 25/m^2) failed to prove superiority versus docetaxel in the first-line setting in mCRPC [82]. No data are available on the impact of cabazitaxel on prevention or delay of SREs.

25.7 Hormonal and Targeted Therapy

25.7.1 Abiraterone

Abiraterone acetate is a potent irreversible and selective inhibitor of the 17 alpha-hydroxylase C17.20-lyase (CYP17A1) that blocks androgen synthesis in adrenal glands, testicles, and prostate cancer [83]. Abiraterone is administered orally (1000 mg per day) and requires a concomitant low dose of prednisone (5 mg twice a day) to prevent side effects from the excess of mineralocorticoids associated with CYP17A1 blockade. Currently it is approved for the treatment of mCRPC (both chemonaive and progressing after chemotherapy).

In the COU-AA-301 phase III double-blind placebo-controlled RCT, 1195 patients (90% with BMs), who had relapsed after docetaxel-based treatment, were randomized to abiraterone vs placebo [12]. Abiraterone significantly improved OS (median 15.8 ms vs 11.2 ms, HR 0.74, 95% CI 0.64–0.86; $p < 0.001$) [84]. All the secondary endpoints (PSA response, radiologic PFS, and time to progression) favored the experimental arm. Mineralocorticoid-related adverse events such as fluid retention, hypokalemia, and hypertension were more common with abiraterone [12]. Abiraterone prolonged time to first SRE (median 25.0 ms vs 20.3 ms p 0.0001). Rates of patients with SRE were lower at 6, 12, and 18 months in the abiraterone group as was the overall rate of SRE adjusted for duration of treatment. In patients with significant pain at baseline, abiraterone provided a superior (45% vs 28%, p 0.0005) and faster palliation (median time to palliation 5.6 vs 13.7 ms, p 0.0018) of pain intensity [85].

Based on these positive results, the COU-AA-302 phase III double-blind placebo-controlled RCT was conceived to evaluate abiraterone in chemonaive mCRPC (1088 patients, 80% with BMs). In the overall population, radiographic PFS was statistically superior in the experimental arm (median, 16.5 ms vs 8.3 ms, HR 0.53, 95% CI 0.45–0.62; $p < 0.001$) [86]; OS, coprimary endpoint, also favored abiraterone (median 34.7 ms vs 30.3 ms, HR 0.81, 95% CI 0.70–0.93; p 0.0033) [11]. In patients with BMs only, median PFS was 20.7 vs 11.1 ms (HR 0.54, 95% IC 0.42–0.70) [87], while median OS was 38.9 vs 34.1 ms (HR 0.78, 95% IC 0.62–0.97) [11]. The presence of BMs only at baseline was a positive prognostic factor for an OS benefit with abiraterone in a multivariate analysis (with baseline PSA, LDH, ALP, hemoglobin, age, and ECOG performance status). Abiraterone improved median time to progression of mean pain intensity (26.7 ms vs 18.4 ms HR 0.82, 95% CI 0.67–1.00; p 0.049) and median time to progression of pain interference with daily activities (10.3 ms vs 7.4 ms; HR 0.79, 95% CI 0.67–0.93; p 0.005). Median time to progression of worst pain was also longer, but the difference was not significant [88]. The incidence of SREs was not reported.

A post hoc analysis evaluated the safety and efficacy of concomitant use of abiraterone and bone-targeting agents (mainly ZA). The addition of such agents was associated with longer OS (p 0.012), longer time to deterioration of PS, and longer time to opiate use for cancer pain. However, these results should be considered with caution considering the retrospective nature of the analysis and the small sample size [89].

25.7.2 Enzalutamide

Enzalutamide is a new-generation antiandrogen, with no agonistic activity and a greater affinity for the androgen receptor (AR) than first-generation antiandrogens like bicalutamide. By blocking the AR, it prevents its nuclear translocation, DNA binding, and recruitment of co-activators [90]. Similarly to abiraterone, enzalutamide is currently approved for the treatment of both chemonaive and chemotherapy-pretreated mCRPC patients.

In the AFFIRM trial, 1199 mCRPC patients progressing on or after docetaxel treatment (about 90% with BMs) were randomized to enzalutamide or placebo. Median OS was significantly improved with enzalutamide (18.4 ms vs 13.6 ms, HR 0.63 95% CI 0.53–0.75; $p < 0.001$) as were time to radiological and PSA progression. Among secondary endpoints, enzalutamide significantly delayed time to first SRE (16.7 ms vs 13.3 ms, $p < 0.001$) [13]. The risk of developing a SRE was lower with enzalutamide irrespective of BP and corticosteroid use [91]. Fatigue, diarrhea, and hot flashes were common in the enzalutamide group. Seizures were reported in five patients (0.6%) receiving enzalutamide [13].

In chemotherapy-naive mCRPC patients, enzalutamide showed a 68% reduction in the risk of PFS vs placebo ($p < 0.0001$) and a 23% reduction in the risk of death (HR 0.71, p 0.0002) [14]. Median rPFS was 20 vs 5.4 months, while median OS was 35.3 vs 31.3 months [92]. Among secondary endpoints, treatment with enzalutamide resulted in a reduction of SREs (32% vs 37% $p < 0.001$), while median time to first SRE was 31.1 vs 31.3 months. Median time to pain progression (according to the BPI-SF) was 5.7 ms with enzalutamide vs 5.6 ms with placebo ($p < 0.001$). At week 13, progression of pain was less common with enzalutamide (29 vs 42%, p 0.0001) [93]. In a prespecified subgroup analysis, enzalutamide improved rPFS vs placebo in patients with visceral and nonvisceral disease and low- or high-volume bone disease (< 4 vs 4 > BMs). Among patients with bone disease, the rPFS benefit was similar regardless of the burden of disease and the presence of visceral metastasis. Among patients with high-volume bone disease and no visceral metastasis, the OS benefit was similar to that of patients with low-volume bone disease, while in patients with visceral metastases, no OS benefit was detected [94]. A summary of primary and skeletal- and pain-related outcomes in selected phase III RCTs is reported in Table 25.2.

Table 25.2 Primary, bone and pain related endpoints in main phase III RCTs in metastatic prostate cancer

Agent	Population	Treatment arms (no. of patients)	Primary endpoint	Bone related endpoints	Pain related endpoints[a]
Docetaxel (Tannock 2004; Berthold 2008)	mCRPC	Mitoxantrone (337) vs. Docetaxel q21 (335) Docetaxel q7 (334)	OS: 16.3 ms mitoxantrone, 19.2 ms docetaxel q21 (p 0.004)[a], 17.8 ms docetaxel q7 (p 0.09)[a]	Not reported	Pain reduction: 22% mitoxantrone, 35% docetaxel q 21 (p 0.001)[a], 31% docetaxel q7 (p 0.018)[a]
Cabazitaxel (DeBono 2010)	mCRPC docetaxel pretreated	Cabazitaxel (378) vs. Mitoxantrone (377)	OS: 15.1 ms vs. 12.7 ms (HR 0.70 95% CI 0.59–0.83; $p < 0.0001$)	Not reported	Similar pain response rate and pain progression rate
Docetaxel (James 2016)	mHSPC	SOC (1184) vs. SOC + ZA (593) SOC + docetaxel (592) SOC + docetaxel + ZA (593)	OS: SOC 71 ms, SOC + ZA NR (p 0.45)[c], SOC + docetaxel 81 ms (p 0.006)[c], SOC + docetaxel + ZA 76 ms (p 0.022)[c]	Mean time to SRE: ADT 61.4 ms, docetaxel + ADT 68 ms (p 0.177 × 10−4), docetaxel + ZA + ADT 68.3 ms (p 0.24 × 10−5)	Not reported
Abiraterone (DeBono 2011; Fizazi 2012; Logothetis 2012)	mCRPC docetaxel pretreated	Abiraterone + PDN (797) vs. Placebo + PDN (398)	OS 15.8 ms vs. 11.2 ms (HR 0.74 95% CI 0.64–0.86; $p < 0.0001$)	Median time to SRE 25 ms vs. 20.3 ms (HR 0.61, p 0.0001) SRE rate per 100 pts/ys of exposure 24% vs. 46.1%	Pain intensity palliation: 45% vs. 28% (p 0.0005); Time to pain intensity palliation 5.6 ms vs. 13.7 ms (p 0.00018) Duration of palliation of pain intensity 4.2 ms vs. 2.1 ms (p 0.0056) Similar results with pain interference palliation Longer time to pain palliation and intensity progression
Abiraterone (Ryan 2013; Basch 2013; Ryan 2015)	mCRPC docetaxel naive	Abiraterone + PDN (546) vs. Placebo + PDN (542)	PFS 16.5 ms vs. 8.2 ms (HR 0.52 95% CI 0.45–0.61; $p < 0.001$) OS 34.7 ms vs. 30.3 ms (HR 0.81, 95% CI 0.70–0.93; p 0.0033)	Not reported	Median time to opiate use 33.4 ms vs. 23.4 ms ($p < 0.0001$) Median time to progression of mean pain intensity 26.7 ms vs. 18.4 ms (p 0.0490) Median time to progression of pain interference w daily activities 10.3 ms vs. 7.4 ms (p 0.005)

Table 25.2 (continued)

Agent	Population	Treatment arms (no. of patients)	Primary endpoint	Bone related endpoints	Pain related endpoints[a]
Enzalutamide (Scher 2012; Fizazi 2014)	mCRPC docetaxel pretreated	Enzalutamide (800) vs. Placebo (399)	OS 18.4 ms vs. 13.6 ms (HR 0.63 95% CI 0.53–0.75; $p < 0.001$)	Median time to SRE 16.7 ms vs. 13.7 ms (HR 0.69; $p < 0.001$)	Pain progression at week 13 28% vs. 39% (p 0.0018) Pain reduction at week 13 vs. baseline 45% vs. 7% (p 0.0079) Longer time to pain progression, significant reduction of pain severity and pain interference for enzalutamide
Enzalutamide (Beer 2014; Loriot 2015; Beer 2017)	mCRPC docetaxel naive	Enzalutamide (872) vs. Placebo (845)	rPFS 20 ms vs. 5.4 ms (HR 0.32 95% CI 0.28–0.37; $p < 0.0001$) OS 35.3 ms vs. 31.3 ms (HR 0.77 95% CI 0.67–0.88; p 0.0002)	Median time to SRE 31.1 ms vs. 31.3 ms (HR 0.72, $p < 0.001$) Pts with SRE 32% vs. 37% ($p < 0.001$)	Median time to progression of pain at its worst 5.7 vs. 5.6 ms (p 0.0001) Progression of pain at its worst at week 13 29% vs. 42% ($p < 0.0001$); at week 25 32% vs. 38% (p 0.068)

ADT androgen deprivation therapy, *mCRPC* metastatic castration resistant prostate cancer, *mHSPC* metastatic hormone-sensitive prostate cancer, *OS* overall survival, *PDN* prednisone, *PFS* progression free survival, *SOC* standard of care (i.e., androgen deprivation therapy), *SRE* skeletal related events, *ZA* zoledronic acid

[a]Exact definitions of pain related end point are reported in material and methods section of each trial

[b]Vs. mitoxantrone

[c]Vs. SOC

25.8 Cabozantinib

Cabozantinib is an oral multi-targeted tyrosine kinase inhibitor of multiple receptors including MET and VEGFR2. In a phase II randomized placebo-controlled discontinuation trial, mCRPC patients with stable disease after 12 weeks of treatment with cabozantinib were randomized to placebo vs cabozantinib. A marked increase in PFS was observed in the experimental arm (median PFS 23.9 vs 5.9 weeks; p 0.001). Response rate was 5%. Partial response on bone scan was seen in 68% of patients (12% complete response). Opioid use and pain improvement were recorded in 56% and 67% of patients, respectively. Bone scan improvement correlated with soft tissue response, pain response, and reduction in bone turnover markers. Besides a direct antitumor activity, inhibition of osteoblast uptake of radiotracer and reduced permeability caused by antiangiogenic effects are possible mechanisms of the observed bone scan response [95]. Unfortunately, cabozantinib failed to confirm its efficacy in two phase III RCTs. In COMET 1 (cabozantinib vs prednisone in mCRPC with BMs pretreated with docetaxel and either abiraterone or enzalutamide), cabozantinib did not improve OS vs placebo despite improving bone scan response at 12 weeks (42% vs 3%, $p < 0.001$) and PFS (5.6 months vs 2.8 months p 0.48). Time to first SSE (HR 0.62; 95% CI, 0.48–0.81 p 0.001) and rates of SSEs during the study also favored cabozantinib (cabozantinib, 14%; prednisone, 21%) [96]. In COMET 2 (same population as in COMET 1 but vs mitoxantrone in symptomatic patients requiring opioid use), cabozantinib did not improve pain control over mitoxantrone (primary endpoint) [97] .

25.9 Radiotherapy

Radiotherapy (RT) has an important role in the management of BMs, particularly for the "uncomplicated" ones, defined as the presence of painful lesions not associated with impending or existing pathologic fracture or existing spinal cord or cauda equina compression [98]. The primary goals of RT are palliation of pain, prevention of SREs, reduction of neurological symptoms due to spinal compression, and consequently improvement of QoL. The definition of the optimal dose and fractionation schedule is of paramount importance. Many factors should be considered such as patient performance status, life expectancy, need for long-term palliation, and expected toxicities. Several studies and meta-analyses were conducted to evaluate the efficacy of single- or multiple-fraction RT. Chow et al. [99] reviewed 25 randomized trials including 5263 patients. Complete and overall response rates for pain relief were similar in patients receiving either single- or multiple-fraction schedules, although retreatment rate was higher in single-fraction group. No differences in acute toxicities were reported. According to recently updated ASTRO guidelines [100], similar pain relief can be achieved following a single 8 Gy fraction, 20 Gy in 5, 24 Gy in 6, and 30 Gy in 10 fractions in patients with previously not irradiated symptomatic BMs, although retreatment rates are higher. Authors suggest, with high-quality evidence and strong recommendation, that a single-fraction RT should be considered in patients with limited life expectancy, in which a shorter treatment may be easier to complete [100].

Spinal cord is a challenging site of metastatic bone disease. Spinal metastases can be complicated by instability and compression of neural structures [101]. RT is generally the treatment of choice in patients with metastatic spinal cord compression (MSCC). Two RCT phase III trials were conducted to define the most effective radiation schedule in patients with MSCC and short life expectancy. Maranzano et al. [102] randomized 267 patients to short-course RT (8 Gy × 2 days) or to a split-course regimen (5 Gy × 3 days and 3 Gy × 5 days). No significant difference in response rate and OS was found, with similar toxicity. Authors concluded that a short-course regimen could be the more convenient choice for patients with MSCC and short life expectancy. The second trial compared two different short-course schedules (8 Gy single fraction versus 8 Gy × 2 fractions) in 303 patients. No differences in response rate were observed;

both regimens were well tolerated [103]. In patients with MSCC and long life expectancy, long-course RT (3 Gy × 10 or 2.5 Gy × 15 or 2 Gy × 20) provided a significant better local control versus short-course (8 Gy × 1 or 5 Gy × 4) (81% vs 61%, $p = 0.0005$). RT schedule had no significant impact on functional outcomes or OS. Acute toxicity was moderate [104]. Authors concluded that patients with a relatively favorable prognosis might have higher risk for local relapse and therefore may benefit from long-course RT. In another, more recent trial randomizing 203 patients with MSCC and poor and intermediate expected survival, a short-course RT with 4 Gy × 5 was not significantly inferior to 3 Gy × 10 fractions [105]. In selected patients with MSCC or impending spinal instability, surgical decompression and stabilization should be considered as the treatment of choice [101]. According to ASTRO guidelines, surgery does not obviate the need for postoperative RT in patients with MSCC [100], and prolonged schedules (30 Gy in ten fractions) are the preferred treatment in this setting.

The introduction of new treatments that prolong OS in metastatic PCa has increased the number of patients who may undergo retreatment with RT. Retreatment rates are about 20% and 8% in patients receiving single-fraction palliative and multifractionated RT, respectively [99]. In planning retreatment many factor should be considered: previous dose and schedule of RT, interval between first RT and recurrent symptoms, previous toxicity, dose constraints to organ at risk, and life expectancy. Retreatment can be considered in different settings: absence or only partial pain relief after previous RT or pain relapse after either partial or complete response to first-time RT [106]. In a recent review on available studies on RT retreatment, evaluating 645 patients, CR, PR, and ORR to retreatment were 20%, 50%, and 68%, respectively, comparable to the response rates for the first irradiation [107]. Toxicity and adverse events were underreported; however, no grades 3 and 4 were recorded, and the rates of pathologic fracture and spinal cord compression were comparable in initial RT treatments and in reirradiation. No consensus has been reached so far on the optimal timing and dose fractionation of retreatment. According to ASTRO guidelines [108], reirradiation for recurrent pain, both in spine and in peripheral lesions, should be considered at least 1 month after the initial treatment, emphasizing the adherence to normal tissue constraints. 8 Gy in a single fraction seems to be non-inferior in terms of both pain relief and decrease in SRE and less toxic than 20 Gy in multiple fractions [109].

Technological improvements and the introduction of image-guided RT (IGRT) have definitely improved the accuracy of treatment delivery, allowing the development of stereotactic techniques. Stereotactic body radiation therapy (SBRT) is a highly conformal external beam radiation technique able to deliver high radiation doses to small volumes and is an important chance for the treatment of oligometastatic patients and in retreatment setting, in particular for spinal metastases, in order to reduce toxicity to the spinal cord. Oligometastatic PCa patients have a better prognosis compared with those with a more extended disease. In a subgroup analysis of oligometastatic patients of the TROG 03.04 RADAR trial [110], patients with up to three BMs at the time of the first diagnosis of metastatic disease experienced a longer time to prostate cancer-specific mortality than patients with four or more BMs. Singh et al. [111] in a retrospective analysis on 369 patients found a significantly better survival in patients with less than five lesions. Several studies have shown that higher radiation doses produce high local control rates without severe toxicities, possibly delaying the start of androgen deprivation therapy [112–115]. Ost et al. [118] in a multi-institutional study found that a lower radiation dose predicted for a higher recurrence rate, with a 3-year local progression-free survival of 79% for patients treated with a biologically effective dose (BED) < 100 Gy versus 99% for patients treated with BED >100 Gy, without grade 3 toxicity. Further evaluation of SBRT in a prospective clinical trial will clarify the role in this setting.

25.10 Surgery

BMs and SREs are mainly managed with medical treatment and RT. However, surgery may play a role in selected cases [116]. Several factors should be considered in patient selection, either patient-related (performance status, life expectancy), disease-related (osseous and extraosseous tumor burden), or BM-related (single vs multiple, site, size, and osteolytic or osteoblastic predominance) [117]. Two main settings can be identified: (a) "curative," for single metastasis, onset after several years, in an otherwise healthy patient, and (b) "palliative," in case of impending or already-occurred fracture, MSCC, or painful lesions in a multi-metastatic patient. Techniques can be divided into resection techniques, which require wide R0 margin, and stabilization techniques of biomechanical value [116].

Decompression and stabilization are the most common procedures for vertebral metastases in patients with intermediate-good prognosis [118]. En bloc vertebrectomy of single dorsal or lumbar metastasis can be considered in very selected patients with excellent prognosis. Percutaneous vertebroplasty can stabilize the vertebral body in a minimally invasive way and relieve associated pain [116, 118].

For long bone fractures, resection and prosthetic reconstructions or intramedullary stabilization can be considered, according to the presence of pain, location, size, and osteoblastic or osteolytic nature of the metastasis [116]. For example, an osteolytic lesion of the neck of the femur, occupying more than two thirds of the entire bone fragment, could be a good candidate for resection and prosthetic reconstruction, while lesions located from the trochanteric area until the distal diaphysis in a pluri-metastatic patient may benefit more from an intramedullary stabilization.

Finally, percutaneous modalities like radiofrequency ablation, cryoablation, and high-intensity focused ultrasound and microwave can relieve pain and improve bone strength avoiding the risk of morbidity associated with open surgery [117].

Conclusions

BMs are very common in PCa. Their management should be optimized in order to prevent SREs and associated morbidities and improve patient QoL accordingly. Radiological diagnosis and monitoring of BMs in everyday clinical practice remain challenging, as well as the use of circulating biomarkers. Several healthcare professionals are involved in the management of metastatic PCa, and different treatment options can be offered. Patient selection, treatment sequencing, and association of different agents and modalities should be ideally discussed in a multidisciplinary team.

References

1. Zustovich F, Pastorelli D. Therapeutic management of bone metastasis in prostate cancer: an update. Expert Rev Anticancer Ther. 2016;16:1–13.
2. Parker C, Gillessen S, Heidenreich A, Horwich A, Esmo GC. Cancer of the prostate: ESMO clinical practice guidelines for diagnosis, treatment and follow-up. Ann Oncol. 2015;26(Suppl 5):v69–77.
3. Scher HI, Buchanan G, Gerald W, Butler LM, Tilley WD. Targeting the androgen receptor: improving outcomes for castration-resistant prostate cancer. Endocr Relat Cancer. 2004;11(3):459–76.
4. Newling DW. Re: secondary hormonal therapy for advanced prostate cancer. Eur Urol. 2006;49(5):925–6.
5. Tannock IF, Osoba D, Stockler MR, Ernst DS, Neville AJ, Moore MJ, et al. Chemotherapy with mitoxantrone plus prednisone or prednisone alone for symptomatic hormone-resistant prostate cancer: a Canadian randomized trial with palliative end points. J Clin Oncol. 1996;14(6):1756–64.
6. Kantoff PW, Halabi S, Conaway M, Picus J, Kirshner J, Hars V, et al. Hydrocortisone with or without mitoxantrone in men with hormone-refractory prostate cancer: results of the cancer and leukemia group B 9182 study. J Clin Oncol. 1999;17(8):2506–13.
7. Tannock IF, de Wit R, Berry WR, Horti J, Pluzanska A, Chi KN, et al. Docetaxel plus prednisone or mitoxantrone plus prednisone for advanced prostate cancer. N Engl J Med. 2004;351(15):1502–12.
8. Petrylak DP, Tangen CM, Hussain MH, Lara PN Jr, Jones JA, Taplin ME, et al. Docetaxel and estramustine compared with mitoxantrone and prednisone for advanced refractory prostate cancer. N Engl J Med. 2004;351(15):1513–20.
9. Mostaghel EA, Page ST, Lin DW, Fazli L, Coleman IM, True LD, et al. Intraprostatic androgens

and androgen-regulated gene expression persist after testosterone suppression: therapeutic implications for castration-resistant prostate cancer. Cancer Res. 2007;67(10):5033–41.
10. de Bono JS, Oudard S, Ozguroglu M, Hansen S, Machiels JP, Kocak I, et al. Prednisone plus cabazitaxel or mitoxantrone for metastatic castration-resistant prostate cancer progressing after docetaxel treatment: a randomised open-label trial. Lancet. 2010;376(9747):1147–54.
11. Ryan CJ, Smith MR, Fizazi K, Saad F, Mulders PF, Sternberg CN, et al. Abiraterone acetate plus prednisone versus placebo plus prednisone in chemotherapy-naive men with metastatic castration-resistant prostate cancer (COU-AA-302): final overall survival analysis of a randomised, double-blind, placebo-controlled phase 3 study. Lancet Oncol. 2015;16(2):152–60.
12. de Bono JS, Logothetis CJ, Molina A, Fizazi K, North S, Chu L, et al. Abiraterone and increased survival in metastatic prostate cancer. N Engl J Med. 2011;364(21):1995–2005.
13. Scher HI, Fizazi K, Saad F, Taplin ME, Sternberg CN, Miller K, et al. Increased survival with enzalutamide in prostate cancer after chemotherapy. N Engl J Med. 2012;367(13):1187–97.
14. Beer TM, Armstrong AJ, Rathkopf DE, Loriot Y, Sternberg CN, Higano CS, et al. Enzalutamide in metastatic prostate cancer before chemotherapy. Lancet Oncol. 2014;371(5):424–33.
15. Parker C, Nilsson S, Heinrich D, Helle SI, O'Sullivan JM, Fossa SD, et al. Alpha emitter radium-223 and survival in metastatic prostate cancer. N Engl J Med. 2013;369(3):213–23.
16. Kantoff PW, Higano CS, Shore ND, Berger ER, Small EJ, Penson DF, et al. Sipuleucel-T immunotherapy for castration-resistant prostate cancer. N Engl J Med. 2010;363(5):411–22.
17. Saad F, Gleason DM, Murray R, Tchekmedyian S, Venner P, Lacombe L, et al. A randomized, placebo-controlled trial of zoledronic acid in patients with hormone-refractory metastatic prostate carcinoma. J Natl Cancer Inst. 2002;94(19):1458–68.
18. Fizazi K, Carducci M, Smith M, Damiao R, Brown J, Karsh L, et al. Denosumab versus zoledronic acid for treatment of bone metastases in men with castration-resistant prostate cancer: a randomised, double-blind study. Lancet. 2011;377(9768):813–22.
19. Bubendorf L, Schopfer A, Wagner U, Sauter G, Moch H, Willi N, et al. Metastatic patterns of prostate cancer: an autopsy study of 1,589 patients. Hum Pathol. 2000;31(5):578–83.
20. RKW H, Wade SW, Reich A, Pirolli MA, Liede A, Lyman GH. Incidence of bone metastases in U.S. patients with solid tumors. J Clin Oncol. 2016;34:e13099.
21. Wang C, Shen Y, Zhu S. Distribution features of skeletal metastases: a comparative study between pulmonary and prostate cancers. PLoS One. 2015;10(11):e0143437.
22. Kakhki VR, Anvari K, Sadeghi R, Mahmoudian AS, Torabian-Kakhki M. Pattern and distribution of bone metastases in common malignant tumors. Nucl Med Rev Cent East Eur. 2013;16(2):66–9.
23. Coleman R, Body JJ, Aapro M, Hadji P, Herrstedt J, Esmo GWG. Bone health in cancer patients: ESMO clinical practice guidelines. Lancet Oncol. 2014;25(Suppl 3):iii124–37.
24. Oster G, Lamerato L, Glass AG, Richert-Boe KE, Lopez A, Chung K, et al. Natural history of skeletal-related events in patients with breast, lung, or prostate cancer and metastases to bone: a 15-year study in two large US health systems. Support Care Cancer. 2013;21(12):3279–86.
25. Weinfurt KP, Li Y, Castel LD, Saad F, Timbie JW, Glendenning GA, et al. The significance of skeletal-related events for the health-related quality of life of patients with metastatic prostate cancer. Ann Oncol. 2005;16(4):579–84.
26. Hagiwara M, Delea TE, Saville MW, Chung K. Healthcare utilization and costs associated with skeletal-related events in prostate cancer patients with bone metastases. Prostate Cancer Prostatic Dis. 2013;16(1):23–7.
27. Pockett RD, Castellano D, McEwan P, Oglesby A, Barber BL, Chung K. The hospital burden of disease associated with bone metastases and skeletal-related events in patients with breast cancer, lung cancer, or prostate cancer in Spain. Eur J Cancer Care. 2010;19(6):755–60.
28. Sabbatini P, Larson SM, Kremer A, Zhang ZF, Sun M, Yeung H, et al. Prognostic significance of extent of disease in bone in patients with androgen-independent prostate cancer. J Clin Oncol. 1999;17(3):948–57.
29. Saad F, Lipton A, Cook R, Chen YM, Smith M, Coleman R. Pathologic fractures correlate with reduced survival in patients with malignant bone disease. Cancer. 2007;110(8):1860–7.
30. Norgaard M, Jensen AO, Jacobsen JB, Cetin K, Fryzek JP, Sorensen HT. Skeletal related events, bone metastasis and survival of prostate cancer: a population based cohort study in Denmark (1999 to 2007). J Urol. 2010;184(1):162–7.
31. Sathiakumar N, Delzell E, Morrisey MA, Falkson C, Yong M, Chia V, et al. Mortality following bone metastasis and skeletal-related events among men with prostate cancer: a population-based analysis of US Medicare beneficiaries, 1999–2006. Prostate Cancer Prostatic Dis. 2011;14(2):177–83.
32. Valdagni R, Van Poppel H, Aitchison M, Albers P, Berthold D, Bossi A, et al. Prostate cancer unit initiative in Europe: a position paper by the European school of oncology. Crit Rev Oncol Hematol. 2015;95(2):133–43.
33. Weilbaecher KN, Guise TA, McCauley LK. Cancer to bone: a fatal attraction. Nat Rev Cancer. 2011;11(6):411–25.
34. Boyle WJ, Simonet WS, Lacey DL. Osteoclast differentiation and activation. Nature. 2003;423(6937):337–42.

35. Msaouel P, Pissimissis N, Halapas A, Koutsilieris M. Mechanisms of bone metastasis in prostate cancer: clinical implications. Best Pract Res Clin Endocrinol Metab. 2008;22(2):341–55.
36. Autio KA, Morris MJ. Targeting bone physiology for the treatment of metastatic prostate cancer. Clin Adv Hematol Oncol. 2013;11(3):134–43.
37. Pedersen EA, Shiozawa Y, Pienta KJ, Taichman RS. The prostate cancer bone marrow niche: more than just 'fertile soil'. Asian J Androl. 2012;14(3):423–7.
38. Vignani F, Bertaglia V, Buttigliero C, Tucci M, Scagliotti GV, Di Maio M. Skeletal metastases and impact of anticancer and bone-targeted agents in patients with castration-resistant prostate cancer. Cancer Treat Rev. 2016;44:61–73.
39. Berruti A, Dogliotti D, Tucci M, Scarpa RM, Angeli A. Hyperparathyroidism due to the so-called bone hunger syndrome in prostate cancer patients. J Clin Endocrinol Metab. 2002;87(4):1907–12.
40. Smith MR. Treatment-related osteoporosis in men with prostate cancer. Clin Cancer Res. 2006;12(20 Pt 2):6315s–9s.
41. Caraceni A, Cherny N, Fainsinger R, Kaasa S, Poulain P, Radbruch L, et al. Pain measurement tools and methods in clinical research in palliative care: recommendations of an expert working Group of the European Association of palliative care. J Pain Symptom Manag. 2002;23(3):239–55.
42. Aaronson NK, Ahmedzai S, Bergman B, Bullinger M, Cull A, Duez NJ, et al. The European Organization for Research and Treatment of cancer QLQ-C30: a quality-of-life instrument for use in international clinical trials in oncology. J Natl Cancer Inst. 1993;85(5):365–76.
43. Cella DF, Tulsky DS, Gray G, Sarafian B, Linn E, Bonomi A, et al. The functional assessment of cancer therapy scale: development and validation of the general measure. J Clin Oncol. 1993;11(3):570–9.
44. Chu D, Popovic M, Chow E, Cella D, Beaumont JL, Lam H, et al. Development, characteristics and validity of the EORTC QLQ-PR25 and the FACT-P for assessment of quality of life in prostate cancer patients. J Comp Eff Res. 2014;3(5):523–31.
45. Payne H, Cornford P. Prostate-specific antigen: an evolving role in diagnosis, monitoring, and treatment evaluation in prostate cancer. Urol Oncol. 2011;29(6):593–601.
46. Mottet N, Bellmunt J, Bolla M, Briers E, Cumberbatch MG, De Santis M, et al. EAU-ESTRO-SIOG guidelines on prostate cancer. Part 1: screening, diagnosis, and local treatment with curative intent. Eur Urol. 2017;71(4):618–29.
47. Thuret R, Massard C, Gross-Goupil M, Escudier B, Di PM, Bossi A, et al. The postchemotherapy PSA surge syndrome. Ann Oncol. 2008;19(7):1308–11.
48. Scher HI, Halabi S, Tannock I, Morris M, Sternberg CN, Carducci MA, et al. Design and end points of clinical trials for patients with progressive prostate cancer and castrate levels of testosterone: recommendations of the prostate cancer clinical trials working group. J Clin Oncol. 2008;26(7):1148–59.
49. Coleman R, Costa L, Saad F, Cook R, Hadji P, Terpos E, et al. Consensus on the utility of bone markers in the malignant bone disease setting. Crit Rev Oncol Hematol. 2011;80(3):411–32.
50. Bertoldo F. Markers of bone turnover in bone metastasis from prostate cancer. In: Bone metastases from prostate cancer. Cham: Springer; 2017. p. 13–23.
51. Smith MR, Cook RJ, Coleman R, Brown J, Lipton A, Major P, et al. Predictors of skeletal complications in men with hormone-refractory metastatic prostate cancer. Urology. 2007;70(2):315–9.
52. Cook RJ, Coleman R, Brown J, Lipton A, Major P, Hei YJ, et al. Markers of bone metabolism and survival in men with hormone-refractory metastatic prostate cancer. Clin Cancer Res. 2006;12(11 Pt 1):3361–7.
53. Coleman RE, Major P, Lipton A, Brown JE, Lee KA, Smith M, et al. Predictive value of bone resorption and formation markers in cancer patients with bone metastases receiving the bisphosphonate zoledronic acid. J Clin Oncol. 2005;23(22):4925–35.
54. Lipton A, Cook R, Saad F, Major P, Garnero P, Terpos E, et al. Normalization of bone markers is associated with improved survival in patients with bone metastases from solid tumors and elevated bone resorption receiving zoledronic acid. Cancer. 2008;113(1): 193–201.
55. Metwalli AR, Rosner IL, Cullen J, Chen Y, Brand T, Brassell SA, et al. Elevated alkaline phosphatase velocity strongly predicts overall survival and the risk of bone metastases in castrate-resistant prostate cancer. Urol Oncol. 2014;32(6):761–8.
56. Heindel W, Gubitz R, Vieth V, Weckesser M, Schober O, Schafers M. The diagnostic imaging of bone metastases. Dtsch Arztebl Int. 2014;111(44):741–7.
57. Eisenhauer EA, Therasse P, Bogaerts J, Schwartz LH, Sargent D, Ford R, et al. New response evaluation criteria in solid tumours: revised RECIST guideline (version 1.1). Eur J Cancer. 2009;45(2):228–47.
58. Hwang S, Panicek DM. Magnetic resonance imaging of bone marrow in oncology, part 2. Skelet Radiol. 2007;36(11):1017–27.
59. Love C, Din AS, Tomas MB, Kalapparambath TP, Palestro CJ. Radionuclide bone imaging: an illustrative review. Radiographics. 2003;23(2):341–58.
60. Bombardieri E, Setti L, Kirienko M, Antunovic L, Guglielmo P, Ciocia G. Which metabolic imaging, besides bone scan with 99mTc-phosphonates, for detecting and evaluating bone metastases in prostatic cancer patients? An open discussion. Q J Nucl Med Mol Imaging. 2015;59(4):381–99.
61. Hillner BE, Siegel BA, Hanna L, Duan F, Quinn B, Shields AF. 18F-fluoride PET used for treatment monitoring of systemic cancer therapy: results from the National Oncologic PET registry. J Nucl Med. 2015;56(2):222–8.
62. Langester WR, Rezaee A, Beheshiti M. Nuclear medicine modalities to image bone metastases with bone-targeting agents: conventional scintigraphy and positron-emission tomography. In: Bone metastases from prostate cancer. Cham: Springer International; 2017. p. 61–74.

63. Incerti EM, Mapelli P, Picchio M. Detection of bone metastases and 7 evaluation of therapy response in prostate cancer patients by radiolabelled choline PET/C. In: Bone metastases from prostate cancer. Cham: Springer International; 2017. p. 75–85.
64. Roelofs AJ, Thompson K, Gordon S, Rogers MJ. Molecular mechanisms of action of bisphosphonates: current status. Clin Cancer Res. 2006;12(20 Pt 2):6222s–30s.
65. Saad F, Gleason DM, Murray R, Tchekmedyian S, Venner P, Lacombe L, et al. Long-term efficacy of zoledronic acid for the prevention of skeletal complications in patients with metastatic hormone-refractory prostate cancer. J Natl Cancer Inst. 2004;96(11):879–82.
66. Smith MR, Halabi S, Ryan CJ, Hussain A, Vogelzang N, Stadler W, et al. Randomized controlled trial of early zoledronic acid in men with castration-sensitive prostate cancer and bone metastases: results of CALGB 90202 (alliance). J Clin Oncol. 2014;32(11):1143–50.
67. James ND, Sydes MR, Clarke NW, Mason MD, Dearnaley DP, Spears MR, et al. Addition of docetaxel, zoledronic acid, or both to first-line long-term hormone therapy in prostate cancer (STAMPEDE): survival results from an adaptive, multiarm, multistage, platform randomised controlled trial. Lancet. 2016;387(10024):1163–77.
68. Wirth M, Tammela T, Cicalese V, Gomez Veiga F, Delaere K, Miller K, et al. Prevention of bone metastases in patients with high-risk nonmetastatic prostate cancer treated with zoledronic acid: efficacy and safety results of the Zometa European study (ZEUS). Eur Urol. 2015;67(3):482–91.
69. Lipton A, Goessl C. Clinical development of anti-RANKL therapies for treatment and prevention of bone metastasis. Bone. 2011;48(1):96–9.
70. Smith MR, Coleman RE, Klotz L, Pittman K, Milecki P, Ng S, et al. Denosumab for the prevention of skeletal complications in metastatic castration-resistant prostate cancer: comparison of skeletal-related events and symptomatic skeletal events. Ann Oncol. 2015;26(2):368–74.
71. Smith MR, Saad F, Coleman R, Shore N, Fizazi K, Tombal B, et al. Denosumab and bone-metastasis-free survival in men with castration-resistant prostate cancer: results of a phase 3, randomised, placebo-controlled trial. Lancet. 2012;379(9810):39–46.
72. Smith MR, Egerdie B, Hernandez Toriz N, Feldman R, Tammela TL, Saad F, et al. Denosumab in men receiving androgen-deprivation therapy for prostate cancer. N Engl J Med. 2009;361(8):745–55.
73. Ruggiero SL, Dodson TB, Assael LA, Landesberg R, Marx RE, Mehrotra B. American Association of Oral and Maxillofacial Surgeons position paper on bisphosphonate-related osteonecrosis of the jaws--2009 update. J Oral Maxillofac Surg. 2009;67(5 Suppl):2–12.
74. Saad F, Brown JE, Van PC, Ibrahim T, Stemmer SM, Stopeck AT, et al. Incidence, risk factors, and outcomes of osteonecrosis of the jaw: integrated analysis from three blinded active-controlled phase III trials in cancer patients with bone metastases. Ann Oncol. 2012;23(5):1341–7.
75. Tanvetyanon T, Stiff PJ. Management of the adverse effects associated with intravenous bisphosphonates. Ann Oncol. 2006;17(6):897–907.
76. Sartor O, Coleman R, Nilsson S, Heinrich D, Helle SI, O'Sullivan JM, et al. Effect of radium-223 dichloride on symptomatic skeletal events in patients with castration-resistant prostate cancer and bone metastases: results from a phase 3, double-blind, randomised trial. Lancet Oncol. 2014;15(7):738–46.
77. Berthold DR, Pond GR, Soban F, de WR, Eisenberger M, Tannock IF. Docetaxel plus prednisone or mitoxantrone plus prednisone for advanced prostate cancer: updated survival in the TAX 327 study. J Clin Oncol. 2008;26(2):242–5.
78. Gravis G, Fizazi K, Joly F, Oudard S, Priou F, Esterni B, et al. Androgen-deprivation therapy alone or with docetaxel in non-castrate metastatic prostate cancer (GETUG-AFU 15): a randomised, open-label, phase 3 trial. Lancet Oncol. 2013;14(2):149–58.
79. Sweeney CJ, Chen YH, Carducci M, Liu G, Jarrard DF, Eisenberger M, et al. Chemohormonal therapy in metastatic hormone-sensitive prostate cancer. N Engl J Med. 2015;373(8):737–46.
80. Bahl A, Oudard S, Tombal B, Ozguroglu M, Hansen S, Kocak I, et al. Impact of cabazitaxel on 2-year survival and palliation of tumour-related pain in men with metastatic castration-resistant prostate cancer treated in the TROPIC trial. Ann Oncol. 2013;24(9):2402–8.
81. De Bono J, Hardy-Bessard A, Kim C, et al. Phase III non-inferiority study of cabazitaxel 20 mg/m2 versus 25 mg/m2 in patients with metastatic castration-resistant prostate cancer previously treated with docetaxel. J Clin Oncol. 2016;34:5008.
82. Sartor O, Oudard S, Sengelov L, et al. Cabazitaxel versus docetaxel in chemotherapy-naïve patients with metastatic castration-resistant prostate cancer: a three-arm phase III study (FIRSTANA). J Clin Oncol. 2016;34:5006.
83. Logothetis CJ, Efstathiou E, Manuguid F, Kirkpatrick P. Abiraterone acetate. Nat Rev Drug Discov. 2011;10(8):573–4.
84. Fizazi K, Scher HI, Molina A, Logothetis CJ, Chi KN, Jones RJ, et al. Abiraterone acetate for treatment of metastatic castration-resistant prostate cancer: final overall survival analysis of the COU-AA-301 randomised, double-blind, placebo-controlled phase 3 study. Lancet Oncol. 2012;13(10):983–92.
85. Logothetis CJ, Basch E, Molina A, Fizazi K, North SA, Chi KN, et al. Effect of abiraterone acetate and prednisone compared with placebo and prednisone on pain control and skeletal-related events in patients with metastatic castration-resistant prostate cancer:

exploratory analysis of data from the COU-AA-301 randomised trial. Lancet Oncol. 2012;13(12): 1210–7.
86. Ryan CJ, Smith MR, de Bono JS, Molina A, Logothetis CJ, de Souza P, et al. Abiraterone in metastatic prostate cancer without previous chemotherapy. N Engl J Med. 2013;368(2):138–48.
87. Rathkopf DE, Smith MR, De Bono JS, Logothetis CJ, Shore ND, De Souza P, et al. Updated interim efficacy analysis and long-term safety of abiraterone acetate in metastatic castration-resistant prostate cancer patients without prior chemotherapy (COU-AA-302). Eur Urol. 2014;66(5):815–25.
88. Basch E, Autio K, Ryan CJ, Mulders P, Shore N, Kheoh T, et al. Abiraterone acetate plus prednisone versus prednisone alone in chemotherapy-naive men with metastatic castration-resistant prostate cancer: patient-reported outcome results of a randomised phase 3 trial. Lancet Oncol. 2013;14(12):1193–9.
89. Saad F, Shore N, Van PH, Rathkopf DE, Smith MR, de Bono JS, et al. Impact of bone-targeted therapies in chemotherapy-naive metastatic castration-resistant prostate cancer patients treated with abiraterone acetate: post hoc analysis of study COU-AA-302. Eur Urol. 2015;68(4):570–7.
90. Tran C, Ouk S, Clegg NJ, Chen Y, Watson PA, Arora V, et al. Development of a second-generation antiandrogen for treatment of advanced prostate cancer. Science. 2009;324(5928):787–90.
91. Fizazi K, Scher HI, Miller K, Basch E, Sternberg CN, Cella D, et al. Effect of enzalutamide on time to first skeletal-related event, pain, and quality of life in men with castration-resistant prostate cancer: results from the randomised, phase 3 AFFIRM trial. BJU Int. 2014;15(10):1147–56.
92. Beer TM, Armstrong AJ, Rathkopf D, Loriot Y, Sternberg CN, Higano CS, et al. Enzalutamide in men with chemotherapy-naive metastatic castration-resistant prostate cancer: extended analysis of the phase 3 PREVAIL study. Eur Urol. 2017;71(2):151–4.
93. Loriot Y, Miller K, Sternberg CN, Fizazi K, De Bono JS, Chowdhury S, et al. Effect of enzalutamide on health-related quality of life, pain, and skeletal-related events in asymptomatic and minimally symptomatic, chemotherapy-naive patients with metastatic castration-resistant prostate cancer (PREVAIL): results from a randomised, phase 3 trial. Lancet Oncol. 2015;16(5):509–21.
94. Evans CP, Higano CS, Keane T, Andriole G, Saad F, Iversen P, et al. The PREVAIL study: primary outcomes by site and extent of baseline disease for enzalutamide-treated men with chemotherapy-naive metastatic castration-resistant prostate cancer. Eur Urol. 2016;70(4):675–83.
95. Smith MR, Sweeney CJ, Corn PG, Rathkopf DE, Smith DC, Hussain M, et al. Cabozantinib in chemotherapy-pretreated metastatic castration-resistant prostate cancer: results of a phase II nonrandomized expansion study. J Clin Oncol. 2014;32(30):3391–9.
96. Smith M, Bono JD, Sternberg C, Moulec SL, Oudard S, Giorgi UD, et al. Phase III study of cabozantinib in previously treated metastatic castration-resistant prostate cancer: COMET-1. J Clin Oncol. 2016;34(25):3005–13.
97. Basch EM, Scholz M, De Bono JS, Vogelzang NJ, et al. Final analysis of COMET-2: Cabozantinib (Cabo) versus mitoxantrone/prednisone (MP) in metastatic castration-resistant prostate cancer (mCRPC) patients (pts) with moderate to severe pain who were previously treated with docetaxel (D) and abiraterone (a) and/or enzalutamide (E). J Clin Oncol. 2015;33:141.
98. Cheon PM, Wong E, Thavarajah N, Dennis K, Lutz S, Zeng L, et al. A definition of "uncomplicated bone metastases" based on previous bone metastases radiation trials comparing single-fraction and multi-fraction radiation therapy. J Bone Oncol. 2015;4(1):13–7.
99. Chow E, Zeng L, Salvo N, Dennis K, Tsao M, Lutz S. Update on the systematic review of palliative radiotherapy trials for bone metastases. Clin Oncol (R Coll Radiol). 2012;24(2):112–24.
100. Lutz S, Balboni T, Jones J, Lo S, Petit J, Rich SE, et al. Palliative radiation therapy for bone metastases: update of an ASTRO evidence-based guideline. Pract Radiat Oncol. 2017;7(1):4–12.
101. Delank KS, Wendtner C, Eich HT, Eysel P. The treatment of spinal metastases. Dtsch Arztebl Int. 2011;108(5):71–9. quiz 80
102. Maranzano E, Bellavita R, Rossi R, De AV, Frattegiani A, Bagnoli R, et al. Short-course versus split-course radiotherapy in metastatic spinal cord compression: results of a phase III, randomized, multicenter trial. J Clin Oncol. 2005;23(15): 3358–65.
103. Maranzano E, Trippa F, Casale M, Costantini S, Lupattelli M, Bellavita R, et al. 8Gy single-dose radiotherapy is effective in metastatic spinal cord compression: results of a phase III randomized multicentre Italian trial. Radiother Oncol. 2009;93(2):174–9.
104. Rades D, Lange M, Veninga T, Stalpers LJ, Bajrovic A, Adamietz IA, et al. Final results of a prospective study comparing the local control of short-course and long-course radiotherapy for metastatic spinal cord compression. Int J Radiat Oncol Biol Phys. 2011;79(2):524–30.
105. Rades D, Segedin B, Conde-Moreno AJ, Garcia R, Perpar A, Metz M, et al. Radiotherapy with 4 Gy x 5 versus 3 Gy x 10 for metastatic epidural spinal cord compression: final results of the SCORE-2 trial (ARO 2009/01). J Clin Oncol. 2016;34(6):597–602.
106. Chow E, JS W, Hoskin P, Coia LR, Bentzen SM, Blitzer PH. International consensus on palliative radiotherapy endpoints for future clinical trials in bone metastases. Radiother Oncol. 2002;64(3): 275–80.
107. Wong E, Hoskin P, Bedard G, Poon M, Zeng L, Lam H, et al. Re-irradiation for painful bone

metastases - a systematic review. Radiother Oncol. 2014;110(1):61–70.
108. Lutz S, Berk L, Chang E, Chow E, Hahn C, Hoskin P, et al. Palliative radiotherapy for bone metastases: an ASTRO evidence-based guideline. Int J Radiat Oncol Biol Phys. 2011;79(4):965–76.
109. Chow E, van dLYM, Roos D, Hartsell WF, Hoskin P, Wu JS, et al. Single versus multiple fractions of repeat radiation for painful bone metastases: a randomised, controlled, non-inferiority trial. Lancet Oncol. 2014;15(2):164–71.
110. Sridharan S, Steigler A, Spry NA, Joseph D, Lamb DS, Matthews JH, et al. Oligometastatic bone disease in prostate cancer patients treated on the TROG 03.04 RADAR trial. Radiother Oncol. 2016;121(1):98–102.
111. Singh D, Yi WS, Brasacchio RA, Muhs AG, Smudzin T, Williams JP, et al. Is there a favorable subset of patients with prostate cancer who develop oligometastases? Int J Radiat Oncol Biol Phys. 2004;58(1):3–10.
112. Ahmed KA, Barney BM, Davis BJ, Park SS, Kwon ED, Olivier KR. Stereotactic body radiation therapy in the treatment of oligometastatic prostate cancer. Front Oncol. 2012;2:215.
113. Ost P, Jereczek-Fossa BA, NV A, Zilli T, Muacevic A, Olivier K, et al. Progression-free survival following stereotactic body radiotherapy for oligometastatic prostate cancer treatment-naive recurrence: a multi-institutional analysis. Eur Urol. 2016;69(1):9–12.
114. Decaestecker K, De MG, Lambert B, Delrue L, Fonteyne V, Claeys T, et al. Repeated stereotactic body radiotherapy for oligometastatic prostate cancer recurrence. Radiat Oncol. 2014;9:135.
115. Berkovic P, De MG, Delrue L, Lambert B, Fonteyne V, Lumen N, et al. Salvage stereotactic body radiotherapy for patients with limited prostate cancer metastases: deferring androgen deprivation therapy. Clin Genitourin. 2013;11(1):27–32.
116. Luzzati A, Scotto G, Perrucchini G, Zoccali C. Surgery: treatment of oligometastatic disease. In: Bone metastases from prostate cancer. Cham: Springer; 2017. p. 147–61.
117. Agarwal MG, Nayak P. Management of skeletal metastases: an orthopaedic surgeon's guide. Indian J Orthop. 2015;49(1):83–100.
118. Shibata H, Kato S, Sekine I, Abe K, Araki N, Iguchi H, et al. Diagnosis and treatment of bone metastasis: comprehensive guideline of the Japanese Society of Medical Oncology, Japanese Orthopedic association, Japanese Urological Association, and Japanese Society for Radiation Oncology. ESMO Open. 2016;1(2):e000037.

26 Radiopharmaceuticals for Bone Metastases

Benedetta Pagano and Sergio Baldari

Abstract

Bone-seeking radiopharmaceuticals play a significant role in the treatment of metastatic pain as an alternative, or in addition, to classic palliative treatment.

Until a few years ago, radionuclides for the management of prostate cancer consisted of several beta-emitting agents, such as strontium (^{89}Sr), phosphorus (^{32}P) and samarium (^{153}Sm) as well as rhenium (^{186}Re and ^{188}Re), which only exhibit a palliative effect in patients with extensive skeletal disease.

Radium (^{223}Ra) dichloride represents a new generation of radiopharmaceuticals, being the first targeted alpha-emitting agent approved, which improves overall survival, postpones skeletal-related events (SREs) and controls bone pain.

Conjugates of bisphosphonates (BP) with macrocyclic chelators open new possibilities in bone-targeted radionuclide imaging and therapy, when labelled with positron and beta-emitting radiometals. [^{68}Ga/^{177}Lu]DOTA^{ZOL} appears to be the best leading compound showing fast blood clearance, low uptake in soft tissue and high accumulation in the skeleton.

Prostate-specific membrane antigen (PSMA) is an attractive target for diagnosis and therapy of prostate cancer. ^{177}Lu-PSMA-617 is a new treatment option, which is not solely directed to bone metastases, but also demonstrates "antitumour" activity with limited and well-tolerated side effects.

26.1 Introduction

Bone pain due to skeletal metastases is one of the complications experienced by the majority of patients suffering from prostate cancer. These patients receive palliative care to improve quality of life. Bone-seeking radiopharmaceuticals play

B. Pagano (✉) • S. Baldari
Nuclear Medicine Unit, AOU Policlinico "G. Martino", Messina, Italy
e-mail: btt.pagano@gmail.com

E. Bombardieri et al. (eds.), *Clinical Applications of Nuclear Medicine Targeted Therapy*,
https://doi.org/10.1007/978-3-319-63067-0_26

a significant role in the treatment of metastatic pain as an alternative, or in addition, to classic palliative treatment.

The choice of the radiopharmaceutical is based on the physical properties of the radionuclide, in relation to the extent of metastatic disease and bone marrow reserve and on availability in individual countries. Ionizing radiation can be selectively delivered to areas of increased osteoblastic activity, allowing the targeting of multiple metastases simultaneously, including both symptomatic and asymptomatic lesions. The goal of such irradiation is to kill tumour cells in the bone while sparing normal bone marrow, the site of haematopoiesis.

Until a few years ago, radionuclides for the management of prostate cancer consisted of several beta-emitting agents, such as strontium (^{89}Sr), phosphorus (^{32}P) and samarium (^{153}Sm) as well as rhenium (^{186}Re and ^{188}Re), which only exhibit a palliative effect in patients with extensive skeletal disease. Radium (^{223}Ra) dichloride represents a new generation of radiopharmaceuticals and a fundamental advance for nuclear medicine application, being the first targeted alpha-emitting agent approved, which improves overall survival, postpones skeletal-related events (SREs) and controls bone pain.

The insertion of radium in the armamentarium for the therapy of bone metastases has created enthusiasm regarding the contribution of nuclear medicine for improved management of prostate cancer patients. The great effort of chemists, pharmacists, biologists, physicists and physicians is the key to progress in bone therapy benefitting from an increased understanding of both physiological and pathological molecular processes. Among the more recent and developing applications, the theranostic approach covers a major role, where therapy is closely supported by imaging.

Conjugates of bisphosphonates (BP) with macrocyclic chelators represent an excellent example, opening new possibilities in bone-targeted radionuclide imaging and therapy, when labelled with positron and beta-emitting radiometals. Lutetium (^{177}Lu) complexes of macrocyclic BPs might become options for therapy of skeletal metastases in the near future (such as 1,4,7,10-tetraazacyclododecane-1,4,7,10 tetracetic acid (DOTA)-based zoledronate), showing fast blood clearance, low uptake in soft tissue and a high accumulation in the skeleton.

Furthermore, thanks to recent developments in radiopharmaceutical chemistry, prostate-specific membrane antigen (PSMA) targeting has arisen as a key strategy for the development of several selective molecular agents. PSMA is highly and specifically expressed on the surface of prostate tumour cells and represents a promising theranostic target for radioligand imaging and therapy beyond metastatic bone disease. ^{177}Lu-PSMA-617 is a new treatment option for metastatic castrate-resistant prostate cancer (mCRPC), which is not solely directed to bone metastases, but also demonstrates "antitumour" activity with limited and well-tolerated side effects.

26.2 Evolving Role of Targeted Radionuclide Therapy in Bone Metastases

Radionuclide therapy is indicated for the treatment of bone pain due to skeletal metastases associated with an osteoblastic response on bone scintigraphy; it is also indicated for the treatment of painful skeletal metastases, inadequately treated by analgesics, intolerant to analgesics and hormone resistant (metastatic castrate-resistant prostate cancer, mCRPC) [1].

The treatment of patients with bone metastases has dramatically changed over the last few years, due to new therapeutic approaches addressed to obtaining pain control, reducing skeletal morbidity and, most importantly, increasing survival rate. A possible therapy can be based on the use of radiopharmaceuticals systemically administered to slow or reverse bone metastatic progression. Bone-homing radiopharmaceuticals are taken up in areas of high bone turnover, including areas with high osteoblastic activity [2].

Although a large number of such radiotracers have been developed and have undergone preliminary biological investigations, only few radiopharmaceuticals have been administered in human patients and find regular use in clinics.

The reasons rely probably on the competition with application of "classic" medical approaches and the lack of general consensus on the use of radioactive compounds. Furthermore, most radiopharmaceuticals show only partial benefits over the disease while requiring specific handling procedures, thus restricting application to nuclear medicine departments. Last but not least, regulatory and clinical development aspects should be considered for introductions into clinical practice, together with economic interests from the major pharmaceutical companies [3].

Radiopharmaceuticals for the treatment of bone metastases are particular with respect to standard therapies regarding mechanism of action. Treatment success depends on matching the pathophysiologic characteristics of the target tissue to a specific radiopharmaceutical. Once the chemical structure of a potential new radiotracer has been identified for a specific biological target, the next step is to synthesize the desired compound by coupling an emitting nuclide suitable for therapy.

For calcium mimetic and phosphate agents, it is the radionuclide itself which delivers the therapeutic emission on bone lesion, which shows elevated uptake because of altered matrix turnover.

This is the case of the first use of systemic radionuclide therapy, with the advent of strontium (^{89}Sr) in the 1940s, which was quickly followed by the discovery of phosphorus (^{32}P) as a potential radiotherapeutic agent for metastatic bone cancers. However, the use of ^{32}P-phosphate became increasingly unpopular due to its high bone marrow toxicity, whereas ^{89}Sr was approved in Europe in 1992 for treatment of painful bone metastases [4–6].

In a poor therapeutic context, several agents have been designed and developed during the last two decades, such as rhenium phosphonate complexes (^{186}Re and ^{188}Re) that show similar indications but also shorter half-lives. However, despite the fact that a considerable number of radiolabelled molecules have been introduced into clinical trials, only a few have reached clinical approval in nuclear medicine. The late 1990s saw the authorization of samarium (^{153}Sm) in an attempt to utilize several advantages over the radioisotopes mentioned above, culminating in the evolution of novel α-emitting radium (^{223}Ra) as the radiopharmaceutical of great potential. $^{223}RaCl_2$ is the first radiopharmaceutical drug to demonstrate a prolongation of overall survival of patients with prostate cancer [7, 8].

26.2.1 The Ideal Radiopharmaceutical for Bone Pain Palliation

The success of a radiopharmaceutical being used for bone pain palliation depends on several factors, such as feasibility of production or sourcing of the radioisotope, nuclear decay characteristics, molecular structure and feasibility of formulation of the radiopharmaceutical, pharmacokinetic behaviour in vivo, logistics of distribution and cost-effectiveness [9].

When designing therapeutic radiotracers, the following key factors are taken into account: choice of the target indicative or representative of the pathology, identification of the lead compound/structure with specificity for the target, selection of the radionuclide and labelling strategy to synthesize the desired chemical structure. In addition, to allow the radioactivity to distribute into bone lesions, radiotracers should ideally exhibit rapid and quantitative absorption to bone matrix, high affinity and selectivity for the target, in vivo stability and absence of radioactive metabolites and favourable pharmacokinetic and pharmacodynamic properties in relation to radionuclide half-life [10].

The half-life of the radionuclide in a radiotracer should correlate with the kinetic of the process to investigate. In other words, the radiotracer, after injection, should reach the bone matrix and interact quantitatively with the target, in a time frame that must be consistent with the radionuclide half-life to avoid an unnecessary radiation burden on patients [11, 12].

However, most radiotracers are significantly metabolized in vivo. The nature and degree of the metabolism (biological half-life) of a radiolabelled compound depend on its molecular structure, and this can have a significant influence on radioactive distribution and, eventually, on the reliability of the therapeutic effects [13].

Typically, radiopharmaceuticals must meet several specifications in order to fulfil clinical requirements, including high specific activity, high radiochemical and radionuclide purity and high radiochemical yield. No-carrier-added (NCA) radionuclides are ideal to obtain high specific activity radiotracer. This will ensure that radioactive carrier molecules are delivered to the tumour, thus improving the delivery of radiation absorbed dose per unit of injected activity [14].

Specific activity is an important parameter to assess during radiotracer development, and it is defined as the amount of radioactivity per unit mass of a radiolabelled compound. This mass includes the mass of the radioactive product and the mass of its nonradioactive counterpart. Every radioactive molecule is characterized by a specific activity; however, its evaluation may not be critical for all application with radiotracers. On the other hand, specific activity becomes crucial when the radioactive and nonradioactive molecules contained in the radiotracer batch may produce undesired pharmacodynamics-toxicological effects as well as target occupancy [15].

Trabecular bone is considered a large capacity site and does not require a radionuclide with very high specific activity. For this reason, the need of a radionuclide with high specific activity for treatment of bone metastases is less pressing than other targeted therapies. Under this premise, medium-low specific activity radionuclide can generally be used for palliative treatment of bone metastases [16].

Several factors, regarding pharmaceutical requirements for human use, are also imposed by drug regulatory authorities. Current radiopharmaceutical development shares much with standard drug discovery and development practices, and although therapeutic radiopharmaceuticals are generally administered only a few times in a patient's lifetime and adverse reactions are extremely rare, the safety profile of a new radiotracer has to be demonstrated and validated. This assessment includes the evaluation of pharmacological and toxicological activity of the therapeutic preparation (including any component other than the labelled tracer) and the estimation of the absorbed radiation activity to prove a favourable risk-to-benefit ratio [12].

Ideally, the emission characteristics of a therapeutic radionuclide should match the lesion size/volume to be treated to focus energy within the tumour rather than in the tissue surrounding the lesion.

Although beta-emitting radiopharmaceuticals used for the treatment of painful bone metastases differ in physical and biochemical characteristics, several studies reported differences in onset and duration of response, but did not report significant differences in response rate or bone marrow toxicity. The onset of response is rapid after treatment with short-lived isotopes (^{153}Sm-EDTMP, ^{186}Re-HEDP and ^{188}Re-HEDP) and prolonged for a few weeks after treatment with long-lived isotopes (^{89}Sr, ^{32}P). The duration of response is longer for long-lived radioisotopes than for short-lived isotopes. Therefore, patients with progressive disease and pain, for whom rapid relief is required, are best treated with short-lived isotopes with acceptable toxicity and easy repeatability, while patients with better prognosis and better clinical condition may be treated with long-lived isotope [16].

26.2.2 Classification and Mechanism of Action of Bone-Seeking Radiopharmaceuticals

Therapeutic bone-seeking agents can be divided into two principal chemical classes:

- Calcium mimetics and phosphate
- Phosphonate chelating agent or non-calcium analogues (bone seekers with different mechanism of uptake into the bone)

The mechanism of uptake varies depending on the chemical behaviour of the radiopharmaceutical. The first class behaves like Ca^{2+} analogues ($^{223}RaCl_2$ and $^{89}SrCl_2$) or phosphate anion ($Na^{32}PO_4$). These species target the bone because of their periodic similarity to natural constituents. They do not need a non-radioactive substance as a carrier to reach the target, and accumulate at high concentrations at sites of active bone remodelling, where osteoblastic activity is increased.

On the other hand, non-calcium analogues show no natural affinity for bone and thus need to be complexed with a chelator (organic phosphates and diphosphonate) to which the radioisotopes are chemically attached, in order to be chemisorbed in bone hydroxyapatite crystals $Ca_5(PO_4)_3(OH)$ by forming hydroxide bridges. The carriers are hydroxyethylidene diphosphonate (HEDP) or etidronate for ^{186}Re and ^{188}Re and ethylenediamine tetramethylene phosphonate (EDTMP) or lexidronam for ^{153}Sm [17–20].

A further evolution to this second approach is represented by the use of novel bisphosphonates chelated at 1,4,7,10-tetraazacyclododecane-1,4,7,10 tetracetic acid (DOTA), which is opening new possibilities in the theranostic field, as they can be used as both imaging and therapy agents depending on the radionuclide employed when labelled. Following positron emission tomography (PET) examinations utilizing ^{68}Ga-labelled analogues, radioligand therapy with lutetium (^{177}Lu)-labelled macrocyclic bisphosphonates may have great potential in the treatment of painful skeletal metastases [21, 22].

Other than the fact that the mechanism of most radiopharmaceuticals is based on the well-known matrix turnover, the exact therapeutic effect of bone-seeking radiopharmaceuticals is not fully understood. A possible explanation is that radiation-induced tumour necrosis decreases the number of cells involved in inflammatory and immunological reactions, consequently reducing chemical mediators such as growth factors and cytokines that increase pain perception [23–25]. Therefore, in many patients, the use of opiates and other analgesics is considerably reduced.

26.2.3 The Choice of a Radionuclide with Appropriate Emission Properties

The first radiopharmaceuticals were formulated containing beta-emitting radionuclides, while during the last decade, alpha emitters have become important for the design of new agents for therapy. The differences between alpha and beta particles are energy, tissue range, linear energy transfer (LET) and number of DNA hits needed for cell killing. In general, for therapeutic purposes, alpha particles are preferred to beta particles. They are characterized by higher energy, higher LET and a short range in tissues, resulting in a dense deposition of energy very close to the origin of decay [3, 26–28].

However, the relative radiosensitivity of tumour cells can depend on several factors, including the local environment (e.g. state of oxygenation) and the quality of the radiation to which they are exposed. This fact is particularly relevant considering that bone is a hypoxic tissue. It would appear that, at the same dose, high LET radiation is more destructive, as energy is transferred to a small region of the cell. Therefore, it impacts on the DNA damage which, being concentrated, is more difficult to repair than diffused DNA damage.

Radiobiology demonstrates that cytotoxicity due to the effect of alpha particles is more effective than beta particles, leading to cell death in fewer interactions. The short range of tissue penetration of alpha particles has another important consequence: lower irradiation of neighbouring areas. In the case of bone metastases treatment, this implies lower myelotoxicity [11, 29].

26.2.4 Development of New Molecular Targets with Application Both in Imaging and Therapy

For a long time, radiopharmaceuticals for prostate cancer therapy were limited to bone lesions because of the specificity to the matrix. The latest application has been developed in order to overcome this limitation providing widespread therapeutic action similar to those of the classic pharmaceuticals.

The development of new therapeutic agents for prostate cancer follows a modern approach based on two main steps: first, the identification of the biological process indicative of the pathology and second, the identification of the molecular target best representing the process. This target will virtually represent the chemist's workbench for the design of the proper chemical structures.

Prostate-specific membrane antigen (PSMA) is an attractive target for diagnosis and therapy of prostate cancer since expression levels are directly correlated to metastatic and hormone-refractory cancers. PSMA is a transmembrane protein, also known as glutamate carboxypeptidase (GCPII), which is anchored in the cell membrane of prostate epithelial cells and overexpressed at all tumour stages on the surface of prostate tumour cells in comparison to benign prostatic tissue. Radiolabelling of small molecular weight PSMA inhibitors with ^{177}Lu has been obtained (such as ^{177}Lu-PSMA-617), and results of several clinical studies have been published [30, 31].

26.3 Radiopharmaceuticals for Bone Metastases

26.3.1 Calcium Mimetics and Phosphate

26.3.1.1 Strontium [^{89}Sr] Dichloride

Strontium (^{89}Sr) dichloride ($^{89}SrCl_2$, commercial name Metastron®) is used for providing palliative care to patients suffering from bone pain due to skeletal metastasis. It was the first radiopharmaceutical to be approved in the European Union in 1992 (GE Healthcare, United Kingdom) and is indicated for men with hormone-relapsed prostate cancer and painful bone metastases, especially in those who are unlikely to receive myelosuppressive chemotherapy (Clinical guideline [CG175] January 2014) [32, 33].

^{89}Sr has a long physical half-life of 50.7 days and decays to stable yttrium (^{89}Y) by emitting beta particles with maximum energy *E*(max) = 1.492 MeV, mean energy *E*(mean) = 0.58 MeV and only 0.01% gamma emission, with energy of 909 keV. The therapeutic effects derive from beta particles, which have maximum tissue penetration range of approximately 7 mm [10, 34–37].

Physical characteristics of bone-seeking radionuclides are shown in Table 26.1.

The standard recommended activity is 1.48 MBq/Kg for all patients, where administration of larger activities of this radiopharmaceutical results in higher myelosuppression. Toxicity is generally limited to a temporary reduction in leucocyte and platelet counts [3, 19].

Strontium is one of the alkaline earth metals and a member of family IIA in the periodic table, as is calcium. It acts as a calcium mimic and accumulates at sites of high osteoblastic activity through incorporation into mineralizing collagen during new bone formation. The sites of osteoblastic bone metastases show higher accumulation and longer retention compared to areas of normal bone in the same patient. Symptomatic improvement usually occurs within 6 weeks after i.v. injection, with a mean duration of relief of 3–6 months in approximately 50–60% of patients [8, 38, 39]. Retreatment for responders

Table 26.1 Physical characteristics of bone-seeking radionuclides

Radionuclides		Half-life (days)	Particle emission E(max) (MeV)	Energy gamma (γ) particles (MeV)	Maximum tissue penetration (mm)
Beta emitter	Strontium-89	50.7	β 1.492 (99.99%)	0.910 (0.01%)	7
	Phosphorus-32	14.3	β 1.710 (100%)	–	8.5
	Samarium-153	1.95	β 0.807 (21%)	0.103 (28%)	4
	Rhenium-186	3.8	β 1.077 (72%)	0.137 (9%)	5
	Rhenium-188	0.7	β 2.118 (72%)	0.155 (15%)	10
	Lutetium-177	6.73	β 0.497 (78.7%)	0.208 (11%)	1.7
	Yttrium-90	2.67	β 2.284 (100%)	–	11
Alpha emitter	Radium-223	11.4	7.39 (95.3%)	0.82 (1.1%)	<0.1

Table 26.2 Summary of the key clinical outcomes of different radiopharmaceuticals

Radiopharmaceutical	Pain response to therapy (%)	Duration of therapeutic response (months)	Recommended therapeutic activity	Main elimination route
$^{89}SrCl_2$	60–80	3–6	1.48 MBq/kg	Urinary
$^{223}RaCl_2$	50–60	2–3	0.055 MBq/kg	Intestinal
$Na^{32}PO_4$	50–70	2–4	370–444 MBq	Urinary
^{153}Sm-EDTMP	62–84	3–4	37 MBq/kg	Urinary
^{186}Re-HEDP	77–90	2–4	1295 MBq	Urinary
^{188}Re-HEDP	64–77	3–6	2960–3300 MBq	Urinary

is possible at intervals of not less than 3 months. The success of ^{89}Sr in providing this benefit probably relates to the long effective half-life of this radiopharmaceutical in the bone. After intravenous injection, $^{89}SrCl_2$ is excreted by both the genitourinary (80%) and gastrointestinal (20%) systems. Urinary excretion is greater in the first 2 days following injection, and approximately 30–35% of the radiopharmaceutical remains in the bone after 90 days [20, 36].

Table 26.2 shows summary of the key clinical outcomes of different radiopharmaceuticals.

^{89}Sr is usually produced via ^{88}Sr(n, γ)^{89}Sr reaction, but the need for highly enriched target material to avoid formation of concomitant radionuclidic impurities makes this radioisotope quite expensive.

It can also be produced using the ^{89}Y(n, p)^{89}Sr route. This nuclear reaction suffers from very low cross-section, thus making the agent expensive and thereby unaffordable for the majority of patients. In fact, the production of ^{89}Sr with reasonable yield and specific activity suitable for therapeutic applications is difficult in reactors [14, 18].

Although $^{89}SrCl_2$ has been proven to be efficacious in retarding, as well as controlling bone pain, haematological toxicity becomes a relevant impediment to the widespread use of this radiopharmaceutical. Several observations suggest higher and often delayed myelotoxicity for ^{89}Sr. However, as widely confirmed in literature data, the percentage of early haematological complications is accounting for approximately 25% of cases. The degree of bone marrow suppression appears associated with the proportion of ^{89}Sr accumulated and retained in the bone. The risk of such complications increases proportionally to not only every administered dose of radioisotope but also is a result of prior or concurrent treatment with other anticancer modalities such as radiotherapy, chemotherapy, hormonotherapy or symptomatic pain treatment, etc. Unfortunately, each of these combinations is related to an increase in probability of side effects [38].

26.3.1.2 Radium [^{223}Ra] Dichloride

Radium (^{223}Ra) dichloride ($^{223}RaCl_2$, Alpharadin) represents a new generation of bone-targeting agents to significantly improve patient overall survival while reducing pain and symptomatic skeletal events (SSEs).

On 13 November 2013, the European Union approved the use of $^{223}RaCl_2$ (with the brand name Xofigo®, Bayer Pharma AG, Germany) for the treatment of patients with mCRPC, symptomatic bone metastases and unknown visceral metastatic disease, on the basis of the results of the ALpharadin in SYMPtomatic Prostate CAncer (ALSYMPCA) trial [40–42].

^{223}Ra is widely used, as its decay chain and half-life ($T_{1/2}$ = 11.4 days) have good characteristics for biomedical application. The alpha particle range is less than 100 µm (less than 10 cell diameters) which minimizes damage to the surrounding normal tissue [10, 43] (Table 26.1).

^{223}Ra decays via a chain of short-lived daughter radionuclides to stable lead (^{207}Pb), producing four alpha particles for each atom with high energy deposition (each composed of two protons and two neutrons) and two beta particles with a total decay energy of 28 MeV: 95.3% of the energy is due to alpha emissions (energy range of 5.0–7.5 MeV). The fraction emitted as beta particles is 3.6% and only 1.1% of the energy emitted is gamma rays. The first three

Table 26.3 Decay of radium-223 dichloride ($^{223}RaCl_2$)

Nuclide	Alpha energy	Beta energy	$T_{1/2}$
Ra-223	5.64 MeV	–	11.4 day
Rn-219	6.75 MeV	–	4.0 s
Po-215	7.39 MeV	–	1.8 ms
Pb-211	–	0.45 MeV	36.1 min
Bi-211	6.55 MeV	–	2.17 min
Tl-207	–	0.49 MeV	4.8 min
Pb-207 stable			

alpha emissions occur within 5 s: in this period, significant translocation between organs does not happen. However, it is likely to occur during the last alpha decay (^{211}Pb decay to ^{211}Bi with a $t_{1/2}$ of 36 min) [12, 44–46].

Table 26.3 shows decay of radium-223 dichloride.

^{223}Ra is administered intravenously in its cationic form ($^{223}Ra^{++}$) bound to dichloride ($2Cl^-$) forming the radiopharmaceutical $^{223}RaCl_2$, soluble in water. The use of $^{223}RaCl_2$ is simple and easy, it does not require lengthy preparation and handling (ready-to-use), and it can be administered in a hospital outpatient setting. $^{223}RaCl_2$ is a sterile solution, which is supplied in single-dose vials. The recommended dosing schedule is one intravenous injection every 4 weeks for 6 months (for a total of six injections), with an activity per injection of 55 kBq/kg body weight. The volume of the administered agent to achieve the required dose must be calculated using a combination of patient body weight (kg), radioactive concentration of the product (1100 kBq/mL) at reference date (given on the vial) and decay correction factor to correct for physical decay of ^{223}Ra [47, 48].

^{223}Ra is a therapeutic alpha particle-emitting pharmaceutical that acts as a calcium mimetic by forming complexes with the bone mineral hydroxyapatite in areas of high bone turnover, thereby directly targeting the areas of bone metastases. Alpha particles induce a highly localized biological effect, producing non-repairable double-stranded DNA breaks and subsequent cell killing, while limiting damage to the surrounding normal tissue; undesired off-target effects in the bone environment, especially on bone marrow cells, are minimized. It appears that alpha particles are more cytotoxic than beta particles, especially under hypoxic conditions, and because of their higher biological efficacy, the required activity is lower than that of beta particles. The high linear energy transfer of alpha emitters is 80 keV/μm [43, 49–51].

Repeated administration of $^{223}RaCl_2$ results in pain responses of 50–60%. In general, ^{223}Ra is well tolerated, and myelosuppression is one of the most significant adverse events [52, 53]. The total skeletal uptake of ^{223}Ra in patients with osteoblastic bone lesions is estimated to range between 40 and 60% of the administered dose, and ^{223}Ra uptake in bone increased up to 24 h without significant redistribution of daughter nuclides from bone (2% at 6 h and <1% at 3 days) [28, 54].

^{223}Ra is an isotope that decays and is not metabolized. After intravenous injection, it is rapidly cleared from the blood (10 min). It is taken up primarily into the bone or is excreted by the intestine (without significant uptake in nontarget organs such as the heart, liver and spleen); less than 1% of the activity can be found in the blood at 24 h. Approximately 63–76% of injected radioactivity is eliminated from the body within 7 days. The principal route of excretion is through the gastrointestinal tract (about 51% at 24 h), while urinary excretion is negligible (approximately 5%) [55–58] (Table 26.2).

^{223}Ra is produced relatively inexpensively, readily and in large amounts from the decay of actinium-227 (^{227}Ac) (half-life 21.7 years) using a long-term ^{227}Ac-based generator system (^{227}Ac is produced by neutron irradiation of the available ^{227}Ra). The comparatively longer half-life of ^{223}Ra provides sufficient time for the preparation of the agent, its distribution to distant places and administration to patients [2].

The use of $^{223}RaCl_2$ in different clinical conditions needs to be thoroughly evaluated to maximize the advantages of each available treatment in a multidisciplinary, individualized approach to the patient. In other words, a deeper insight into the mechanism of action on the tumour microenvironment may provide the rationale for an association of $^{223}RaCl_2$ with other drugs and their sequential use in clinical practice [49, 59–62].

26.3.1.3 Sodium Phosphate [^{32}P]

Phosphorus (^{32}P) was introduced for treatment of metastatic bone pain in 1942 and was the most widely used radiotracer until the 1980s.

^{32}P is a beta emitter radiopharmaceutical with physical half-life of 14.3 days, E(max) = 1.71 MeV, E(mean) = 0.696 MeV and the maximum tissue penetration range of approximately 8.5 mm [10, 34] (Table 26.1).

^{32}P is absorbed in the particles of hydroxyapatite, one of the major constituents of bone matrix, and causes cell death when it decays to stable sulphur (^{32}S). The radiopharmaceutical is usually administered either through an intravenous pathway (such as sodium orthophosphate, $Na^{32}PO_4$) or by oral route. The monograph "sodium phosphate (^{32}P) injection" is reported in both the European and US Pharmacopeia [63, 64].

The administered therapeutic activity generally varies between 185 and 370 MBq when injected intravenously and between 370 and 444 MBq when delivered through oral route. Following administration, 85% of the activity is incorporated into the bone matrix with pain palliation in 50–70% of patients and a mean response duration of 2–4 months, but it is also associated with a 20–30% incidence of significant bone marrow toxicity [35, 36] (Table 26.2).

This radionuclide can be prepared by neutron activation of natural phosphorus $^{31}P(n,\gamma)^{32}P$ (100% abundance) or sulphur $^{32}S(n,p)^{32}P$ (95.02%). The nuclear reactor using (n,p) reaction employing ^{32}S as the target material yields ^{32}P in no-carrier-added form; however, several hundred grams of sulphur target are required in order to produce GBq quantities of ^{32}P. Furthermore, specific activity can be considerably reduced by the introduction of ^{31}P impurities during the radiochemical processing. Due to the low production cross-section and the large irradiation volumes required, the cost of ^{32}P is considerably high.

^{32}P can also be produced by direct neutron capture using elemental phosphorous as the target, which is a simpler and more cost-effective method. This production involves comparatively simple radiochemical processing, thereby reducing the processing time and radiation exposure. However, ^{32}P produced via this route is of very low specific activity and hence not suitable for many applications [36, 65].

The long half-life of ^{32}P displays favourable nuclear properties for the supply of this radiopharmaceutical to nuclear medicines far from its production site without much loss of activity due to radioactive decay. However, unfortunately, despite its efficacious nature, as well as economic availability, the use of the agent steadily declined due to the high tissue penetration range of the emitted radioactive particles, which causes severe bone marrow toxicity including myelosuppression and pancytopenia [37].

26.3.2 Phosphonate Chelating Agents or Non-calcium Analogues

26.3.2.1 Samarium [^{153}Sm] Lexidronam Pentasodium

Samarium (^{153}Sm) is a member of the lanthanide series labelled EDTMP (ethylene diamine tetramethylene phosphonic acid, lexidronam), commonly known by the trade name Quadramet®. It is a beta-emitting radiopharmaceutical that was approved by the European Union in 1998 (CIS Bio International, France) for alleviating bone pain in cancer patients suffering from skeletal metastases [66].

^{153}Sm emits beta particles with a half-life of 1.95 days, E(max) = 0.807 MeV and E(mean) = 0.23 MeV; the maximum tissue penetration range of the beta particles is approximately 4 mm [16, 34]. It is also a gamma emitter of 103 keV (28%) that allows correlation with conventional technetium-99 m (^{99m}Tc) bone scans (Table 26.1). Notably, the gamma emission from this agent enables localization of bone metastases through imaging, making this bone-seeking radioisotope useful for both diagnostic and therapeutic purposes [8, 35].

^{153}Sm-EDTMP is administered intravenously as pentasodium salt with molecular mass of 696 g mol^{-1}. EDTMP is a polydentate ligand that chelates $^{153}SmCl_2$ (1:1) by forming four O-^{153}Sm bonds and two N-^{153}Sm bonds. It is bone-seeking as EDTMP contains four phosphonate moieties

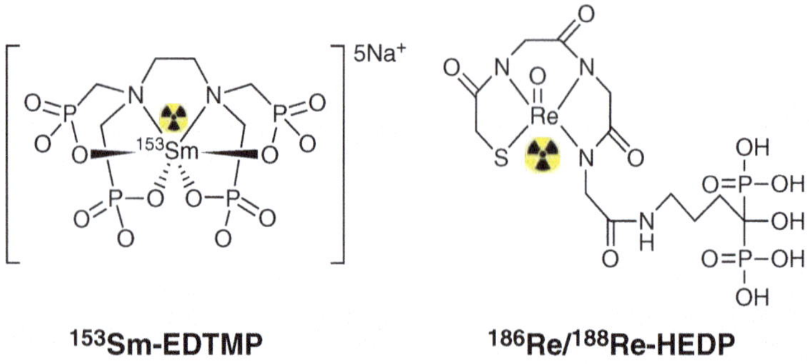

Fig. 26.1 Chemical structures of non-calcium analogues

and is structurally similar to bisphosphonates. Figure 26.1 shows chemical structures of non-calcium analogues.

The ability of bisphosphonates to target bone is due to their great affinity for inorganic hydroxyapatite in sites of accelerated bone turnover. It is proven that as ^{153}Sm-EDTMP readily chelates calcium cations, the compound accumulates in the metastatic sites where metabolism, and thus calcium levels, is high. The cytotoxic irradiation delivered by the beta decay of ^{153}Sm kills malignant cells in the bone and thus can relieve pain [18].

However, the chelating properties of EDTMP produce a reduction in blood calcium levels, and this led to the development of a ^{153}Sm-Ca/Na-EDTMP complex which, due to the presence of added calcium in the formulation, prevents the decrease in plasma calcium levels and is now considered safer. The addition of calcium to the formulation reduces the potential toxicity without changing the biodistribution [67].

^{153}Sm-EDTMP given at 37 MBq/kg leads to pain reduction in 62–84% of evaluated patients for as long as 2–4 months. The radiation dose to the red marrow from activity in the blood is assumed negligible [3, 36–39].

The relatively shorter half-life of ^{153}Sm (compared to ^{89}Sr and ^{186}Re) enables faster radiation delivery and rapid clearance from the body after intravenous injection, making it a suitable radionuclide for bone-targeted treatment. Approximately half of the injected dose is excreted into the urine after 6–7 h. The remaining dose (<45%) is deposited in bone with little accumulation in soft tissue, such as the liver. Metastatic lesions can accumulate about five times more ^{153}Sm-EDTMP than healthy bone tissue. Less than 1% of the injected dose remains in the blood 5 h post injection [39, 66, 68] (Table 26.2).

^{153}Sm can be produced from neutron capture of natural or isotopically enriched ^{153}Sm (as Sm_2O_3) in a nuclear reactor. Due to the large thermal neutron capture cross-section of ^{152}Sm(n,γ)^{153}Sm reaction, ^{153}Sm can be produced in large quantities and with high specific activity. The reaction is high yielding (>99%) and creates only trace amounts of by-products europium-152 (^{152}Eu) and europium-154 (^{154}Eu). Because Sm^{+3} metal has some distribution to the liver, lung and spleen, it is important that ^{153}Sm-EDTMP preparations be of high quality, with little or no unchelated Sm^{+3} to avoid liver uptake and potential hepatotoxicity [2, 69].

The simple postirradiation radiochemical processing and easy formulation of the radiopharmaceutical, either by using a freeze-dried kit or in situ at the hospital radiopharmacy, make this agent attractive for large-scale commercial utilization. However, one of the major drawbacks associated with the agent comes from the comparatively shorter half-life of ^{153}Sm which causes significant loss of activity due to radioactive decay. This in turn necessitates production and handling of a much higher quantity of radioactivity to deliver the desired dose to the end user [9].

26.3.2.2 Rhenium [^{186}Re/^{188}Re] etidronate

Rhenium-186 (^{186}Re) and rhenium-188 (^{188}Re) are two isotopes linked to hydroxyethylidene diphosphonate (HEDP, the generic name of this chelator is etidronate) and are bone-seeking radiopharmaceuticals used for radiometabolic treatment of painful bone metastases (Fig. 26.1).

These radiopharmaceuticals show no natural affinity to the bone and need to be complexed with a chelator (organic phosphates) to be chemisorbed into calcium atoms in bone hydroxyapatite crystals by forming hydroxide bridges in a hydrolysis reaction.

Interestingly, the chemical properties of rhenium are similar to technetium as both these elements exist in group VIIB of the periodic table and label the carrier molecule with either ^{186}Re and ^{188}Re for target radiotherapy or the most used imaging radionuclide, technetium-99 m (^{99m}Tc) [70].

However, though technetium and rhenium possess a chemical analogy with each other, it is known that rhenium complexes are more difficult to prepare than technetium analogues. Rhenium complexes have a higher tendency to reoxidize back to perrhenate than the analogous technetium complexes. This reoxidation, and consequently, the presence of high radiochemical impurities in the final product, is one of the major hindrances in the development of rhenium radiopharmaceuticals [28].

Rhenium [^{186}Re]etidronate

In the late 1980s, ^{186}Re-HEDP was identified as a potential agent for palliative treatment of bone metastases. ^{186}Re is a beta emitter with E(max) = 1.077 MeV, E(mean) = 0.349 MeV and 137 keV (9%) gamma emission. Its short half-life ($T_{1/2}$ = 3.8 days) and the maximum tissue penetration range of approximately 5 mm make it a potentially useful isotope in patients with poor bone marrow reserve (Table 26.1). The availability of suitable energy gamma photons helps in dosimetric and pharmacokinetic evaluation of the agent, without adding any significant additional radiation dose burden to the patient [10, 34].

The agent is administered intravenously with high dose ranging from 1.48 to 3.33 GBq (in the published European Association of Nuclear Medicine guidelines, the recommended dose of ^{186}Re-HEDP is 1295 GBq) and has exhibited a response rate of 77–90% [18, 71].

The mean duration of pain relief is 2–4 months. It binds to plasma proteins in a time-dependent interaction and reaches peak skeletal uptake 3 h after intravenous administration. Following administration of ^{186}Re-HEDP, around 70% of the radioactivity is excreted in the urine over 72 h. This radiopharmaceutical is retained longer in the reactive bone around the lesion than in normal bone. ^{186}Re-HEDP has been reported to be characterized by less clinically significant haematological toxicity than ^{153}Sm-EDTMP and by more suitable physical characteristics for imaging than ^{89}Sr [8, 72] (Table 26.2).

^{186}Re can be produced either in a nuclear reactor or in a particle accelerator (cyclotron). The former method utilizes neutron capture of enriched ^{185}Re, ^{185}Re(n,γ)^{186}Re. In the latter method, ^{186}Re is obtained mainly via proton bombardment of natural tungsten (^{186}W) as a target [19, 73].

Rhenium [^{188}Re]etidronate

^{188}Re-HEDP is currently considered a very attractive candidate for a wide variety of therapeutic applications. ^{188}Re emits beta particles with E(max) = 2.118 MeV, E(mean) = 0.78 and 15% of gamma rays with energy of 155 keV which are adequate for therapy and imaging, respectively. Its physical half-life is 17 h (0.7 days), and the maximum tissue penetration range of the beta particles is approximately 10 mm [16, 34] (Table 26.1).

The higher beta energy of this isotope offers the potential for lethal insults to tumour cells in the region of decay, and emission of gamma photons is an added benefit that permits evaluation of biodistribution, pharmacokinetics and dosimetry [20].

As previously reported, it is necessary to add a carrier when preparing ^{188}Re-HEDP to allow accumulation in bone. ^{188}Re-HEDP is administered with a dose of 2.96–3.33 GBq through the intravenous route. Multiple administrations of the agent in patients, up to a maximum of eight times, have been performed with an interval of 8 weeks between two successive administrations, and this is reported to enhance pain palliation of patients with a response rate of 64–77% and a mean duration of 3–6 months. However, the high energy of beta particles of ^{188}Re emission is reported to cause considerable bone marrow suppression [9, 35] (Table 26.2).

The production method of choice for ^{188}Re is by the decay of the longer-lived tungsten-188

(^{188}W) parent ($T_{1/2}$ = 69.4 days), which is produced in a nuclear reactor by irradiation of tungsten oxide. The decay chain from a 100% pure target ^{186}W according to neutron flux and irradiation time shows the origin of some of the radioactive contaminants present in the generator [70].

Preparation of ^{188}Re from a $^{188}W/^{188}Re$ generator is interesting, as it provides a long-term source for NCA ^{188}Re in nuclear medicine departments. ^{188}Re is eluted with a saline solution in the form of sodium perrhenate ($Na^{188}ReO_4$), and the chromatographic generator with alumina is suitable for high specific activity ^{188}W. The 24-h postgenerator ^{188}Re elution ingrowth of 62% and high elution yields (75–85%) result in daily yields of about 50%, with consistently low ^{188}W parent breakthrough ($<10^{-6}$). Simple postelution concentration methods have been developed to provide very high radioactive concentration solutions of ^{188}Re for radiolabelling. The radionuclidic and chemical properties of rhenium, and the possibility of obtaining ^{188}Re in-house and on demand, make this generator system ideal for many applications [74].

The availability of the $^{188}W/^{188}Re$ generator is especially important for providing a reliable source of this versatile therapeutic radioisotope to remote sites, especially in developing regions, which involve long distances and expensive distribution costs. The development of new chemical strategies allows to obtain ^{188}Re radiopharmaceutical in very high yields and in physiological conditions and gives a novel attractive prospective to the development of new radiopharmaceuticals for therapy [75, 76].

On the other hand, the limited availability of reactors in the world for the production of ^{188}W, coupled with the long irradiation period required to produce the isotope in sufficient quantity, makes the $^{188}W/^{188}Re$ generator expensive, and this may consequently restrict the affordable availability of this useful radionuclide [14].

26.4 The Role of Bisphosphonates

Several bisphosphonates (BP) (formerly referred to as diphosphonates) are used for bone pain. A phosphonate is formed by a non-ionic bond between a carbon and a phosphorus atom. They inhibit osteoclast-induced resorption by binding to bone mineral through the phosphate moiety, interfere with osteoclast activation and also induce osteoclast apoptosis. Meanwhile, these bisphosphonates have been shown also to stimulate osteoblast differentiation and hence new bone formation.

Clinically bisphosphonates reduce the risk of developing skeletal complications of metastatic disease including hypercalcemia and pathologic fracture. They delay the progression of existing bone metastases and reduce the development of new lesions. Bisphosphonates appear to have a beneficial effect on bone pain [16, 40]. Taking into account the pharmaceutical class of bisphosphonates, it is thought to bind them to a chelator and label with radionuclides.

^{177}Lu-EDTMP was one of the most common administered bone-targeting agents for palliative care. Although the results of using this complex in clinical studies indicated significant pain relief in metastatic patients, EDTMP complexes have shown low in vivo stability and thus dissociate which result in liver accumulation and high toxicity. As a consequence, new compounds with improved characteristics have been developed [77].

26.4.1 DOTA-Based Bisphosphonate for Bone Targeting

DOTA-bisphosphonates can be used as imaging and therapy agents, when labelled with positron and beta-emitting radiometals. Their theranostic potential has been explored using ^{177}Lu for the treatment of widespread, progressive and painful skeletal metastases refractory to conventional treatment [32].

DOTA is an excellent lanthanide-chelating moiety, which has the specific advantages of binding trivalent (III) metal and allowing nearly quantitative radiolabelling yields of lanthanides under mild conditions with the formation of a stable Lu complex [12].

New DOTA-based molecules have been successfully prepared, such as (4-{[bis-(phosphonomethyl)) carbamoyl]methyl}-7,10-bis(carboxy methyl)-1,4,7,10-tetraazacyclododec-1-yl)acetic acid (BPAMD) [77].

BPAMD is a simple DOTA-α-H-bisphosphonate conjugate whose complexes have been proven to effectively seek bone tissue. In contrast to open-chain chelating agents such as HEDP and EDTMP, macrocyclic tetraaza ligands can complex the positron-emitting PET radionuclide ^{68}Ga(III), as well as the therapeutic low-energy beta emitter ^{177}Lu(III). ^{177}Lu-BPAMD is now becoming more widely used, both in experimental preclinical work and in patients for treatment of bone metastases, and a kit for eventual regular production in hospitals has been developed [78].

^{177}Lu is chosen for its physical properties, emitting a short-range (0.2–0.3 mm) beta particle *E*(max) = 0.49 MeV) with maximum tissue penetration range less than 2 mm, as well as gamma radiation, which allows the scintigraphic evaluation of biodistribution and dosimetry. Its half-life is 6.71 days, and it decays to stable hafnium (^{177}Hf). The relatively low radiation energy results in less penetration into the marrow, hence less bone marrow toxicity, while a relatively short half-life offers a faster rate of dose delivery for therapeutic purposes [79, 80].

^{177}Lu is produced by simple ^{176}Lu(n,γ)^{177}Lu reaction with high specific activity and excellent radionuclidic purity even using medium-high flux research reactors. On the other hand, ^{177}Lu can be produced with high specific activity via the indirect method by neutron irradiation of ^{176}Yb. Since 2016, it is available commercially as $^{177}LuCl_3$ with marketing authorization [25, 34, 81].

However, ^{177}Lu-BPAMD efficiency may be further improved as more than half of the injected dose is rapidly eliminated from the body. To evaluate the possibility to delay body clearance in bone-targeting radiotherapy, a new class of "DOTA-BP retard" tracers was synthesized and evaluated in vitro and in vivo. The new ligand 1,4,7,10-tetraazacyclododececane, 1-(glutaric acid)-4,7,10-triacetic acid (DOTAGA) is bound to an albumin-binding moiety and has a significant blood concentration and high affinity for hydroxyapatite [21, 82].

Recently, based on the established pharmaceuticals pamidronate (3-aminopropyl-1-hydroxy-1,1-bis[phosphonic acid]) and zoledronate ([1-hydroxy-2-(1H-imidazol-1-yl)-ethylidene] bisphosphonic acid), two new DOTA-α-OH-bisphosphonates (DOTA^{PAM} and DOTA^{ZOL}) have been successfully synthesized and show significantly improved accumulation in the skeleton [83].

Chemical structures of DOTA-based bisphosphonates are shown in Fig. 26.2.

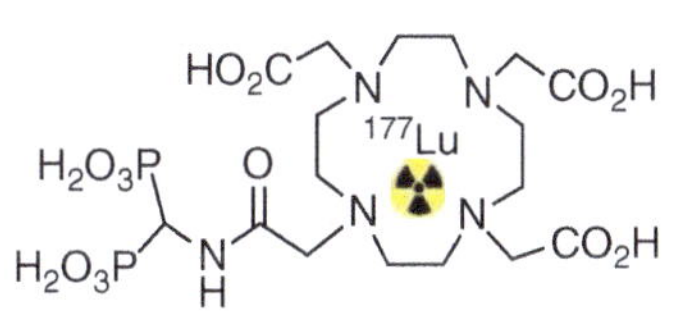

^{177}Lu-BPAMD

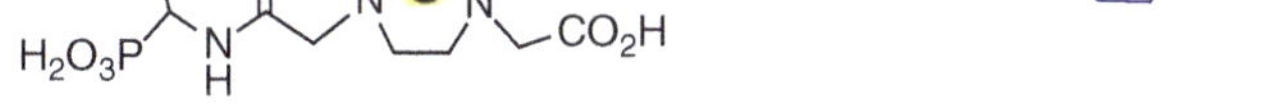

^{177}Lu-DOTAGA-albumin

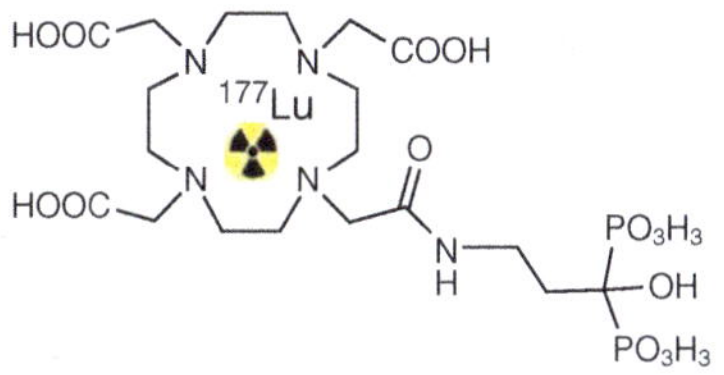

^{177}Lu-DOTA^{PAM}

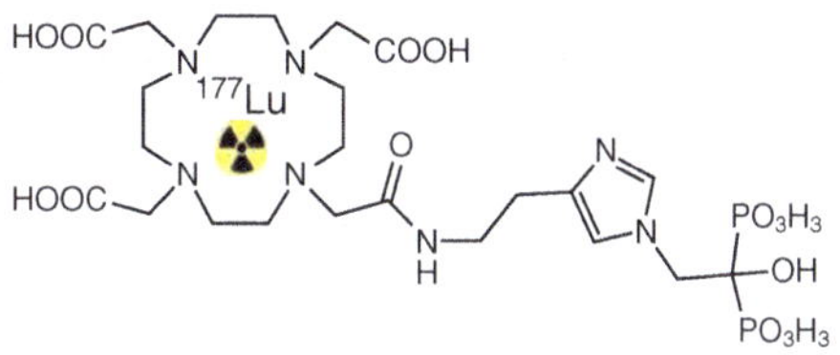

^{177}Lu-DOTA^{ZOL}

Fig. 26.2 Chemical structures of DOTA-based bisphosphonates

In particular, zoledronic acid containing an imidazole ring belongs to the class of bisphosphonates and acts primarily on bone mineral. It is an inhibitor of osteoclastic bone resorption, which alters the bone marrow microenvironment, making it less conducive to tumour cell growth, anti-angiogenic activity and anti-pain activity. In addition, zoledronic acid also possesses several antitumour properties that contribute to its overall efficacy in the treatment of metastatic bone disease [84].

Therefore, the compound $DOTA^{ZOL}$ seems quite suitable for the use of the theranostic pair $^{68}Ga/^{177}Lu$ to both detect and treat bone diseases. The overall change of the Me(III)-DOTA-moiety results in two different complexes, the six-dentate ^{68}Ga complex and the seven-dentate ^{177}Lu complex, and contributes to the pharmacology of the whole molecule. In particular, [$^{68}Ga/^{177}Lu$] $DOTA^{ZOL}$ appears to be the best leading compound showing fast blood clearance, low uptake in soft tissue and high accumulation in the skeleton [22]. This class of bisphosphonate enables an increased tumour to healthy bone ratio, which might end up in an improved therapeutic success [16, 40].

26.5 Beyond Bone Seekers: New Radiopharmaceuticals for Prostate Cancer

Because of high incidence, and the morbidity and mortality associated with prostate-derived cancer, the development of new technologies continues to be an important goal for the accurate detection and treatment of localized prostate cancer, lymphatic involvement and metastases.

Targeted therapy using bone-seeking agents such as $^{89}SrCl_2$, ^{153}Sm-EDTMP or ^{188}Re-HEDP has been in use for over 30 years for palliative treatment of advanced prostate cancer patients. However, this class of tracers is not taken up by the primary or soft tissue lesions. The discovery and cloning of PSMA have opened the possibility of using it as the target for radiopharmaceuticals [85].

26.5.1 PSMA-Targeted Radionuclide Therapy of Prostate Cancer

PSMA (glycoprotein II or *N*-acetyl-L-aspartyl-L-glutamate peptidase) is expressed in high levels on prostate-derived cells and is an important target for visualization and treatment of prostate cancer: the ideal target is highly expressed on tumour cell surfaces and only lightly expressed (or not expressed) on normal tissues. Therefore, important clinical factors include the highest tumour radiation dose with concomitant low radiation dose to nontarget tissues, primarily including the kidneys, lachrymal gland and salivary glands [86].

Two distinct approaches have been used for targeting PSMA: the first approach takes advantage of the macromolecular protein structure of PSMA to provide specific monoclonal antibodies as targeting vectors, and the second approach takes advantage of the enzyme activity of PSMA and uses radiolabelled enzyme inhibitors or binding agents as target-seeking agents. However, the first approach is slowly becoming overshadowed by the second approach which utilizes radiolabelled small molecules targeting the enzyme activity of PSMA [87].

Among the different types of inhibitor molecules developed as part of drug discovery, the dipeptide Lys-urea-Glu appears to be the most successful to be used as the pharmacophore in radiopharmaceutical development. Therefore, the availability of these types of small molecular weight inhibitors exhibiting high uptake in prostate cancer has opened the possibility of radiolabelling them with therapeutic radionuclides. One essential requirement is that the radionuclide must be available either as no carrier added (NCA) or with high specific activity [2, 88].

Since 2013, commercial availability of PSMA-617 has helped in the use of [^{177}Lu]PSMA-617 in multiple centres in different parts of the world. PSMA-617 consists of Glu-urea motif and chelator DOTA, separated by a lipophilic linker region. DOTA chelator can be labelled with radionuclides, for example, ^{68}Ga and ^{177}Lu, and used for both imaging and therapy. In order to prevent relevant kidney toxicity, the treatment regimen. The ^{177}Lu-PSMA-617 treatment regimen is limited to four to six cycles of approximately 5.9 GBq (range 3–8 GBq), generally at a minimum 6-week intervals, in order to prevent relevant kidney toxicity. Dose calculations for individual patients have been determined from a combination of disease burden, patient weight and renal function which is based on initial dosimetric studies. Several publications reported PSA response rates of 70–80% in patients receiving up to three cycles of ^{177}Lu-PSMA-617 [89–93].

Currently, a DOTA version (DOTAGA-(I-y)fk(Sub-KuE) of the same PSMA-617 has been synthesized and has shown promising properties when labelled with ^{177}Lu, such as accumulation in prostate cancer lesions and low kidney retention. Clinical trials have demonstrated the beneficial effect of DOTAGA-for-DOTA substitution and of using a D-amino acid peptide linker on PSMA affinity and metabolic stability and thus uptake and clearance kinetics, respectively. Furthermore, the substitution of one of the D-phenylalanine residues in the peptidic linker by 3-iodo-D-tyrosine has improved the interaction of the tracer molecule with a remote binding site. The use of this compound is proposed for both imaging and therapeutic applications and thus designated PSMA I&T acronym (i.e. PSMA for Imaging & Therapy).

Chemical structures of small-molecule PSMA inhibitors are shown in Fig. 26.3.

It allows fast and high-yield labelling with ^{68}Ga(III) and ^{177}Lu(III), high PSMA affinity and enhanced internalization into PSMA-expressing cells. With the possibility of ^{177}Lu-based therapy, PSMA I&T opens new perspectives for theranostic approaches in the management of prostate cancer [94].

Thus far, ^{177}Lu is emerging as the isotope for therapy of prostate cancer, as its radiochemistry is well understood, and ^{177}Lu, having high specific activity, both NCA and carrier added (CA), is available from several sources [95].

In the future, ^{90}Y ($T_{1/2}$ = 2.7 days), the high-energy beta emitter (2.284 MeV), may also

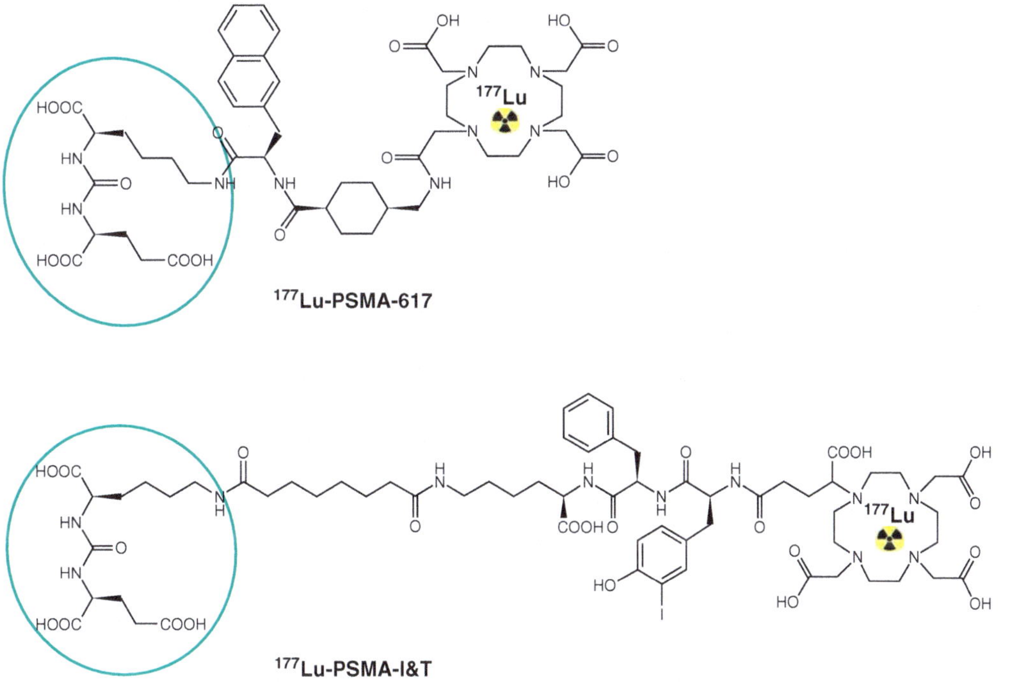

Fig. 26.3 Chemical structures of small-molecule PSMA inhibitors

emerge as an alternative to ^{177}Lu since many of the prostate metastases are bulk tumours and the beta particles emitted by ^{90}Y have a range up to 11 mm in tissue. ^{90}Y obtained from $^{90}Sr/^{90}Y$ generator is NCA and might be efficacious for therapy [31, 34].

Furthermore, interest is also emerging for the evaluation of PSMA targeting with ligands labelled with alpha-particle emitting radioisotopes, such as actinium (^{225}Ac) and bismuth (^{213}Bi). These studies are in progress and will be reported in the near future. However, the highly localized ionization of alpha particles would suggest that such PSMA-targeted agents will be more effective to treat micrometastases and will not have any "crossfire" radiation exposure, as seen with beta particle emitters such as ^{177}Lu or ^{90}Y for larger mass irradiation.

In conclusion, it can be foreseen that radiolabelled enzyme inhibitors and binding agents targeting PSMA are poised to have a significant role in the theranostic management of prostate cancer patients [29, 96–98].

26.5.1.1 Concluding Remarks and Prospects

Over the years, efforts have been undertaken to identify radionuclides with improved physical properties for use in palliative care of metastatic bone pain, as well as to develop better bone-seeking agents to be radiolabelled with promising radionuclides.

The management of refractory metastatic prostate cancer has recently seen impressive advances thanks to the development of novel radiopharmaceuticals both for diagnosis and therapy. It may be considered the new strategy for the treatment of painful bone metastases with high therapeutic efficacy and low complications and side effects. NCA radionuclides are ideal to obtain high specific activity radiopharmaceuticals, and this will ensure that radioactive carrier molecules are delivered to the tumour. Furthermore, targeted alpha particles have some theoretical advantages, given their small radius of damage and high linear energy transfer. Towards that end, $^{223}RaCl_2$ is a step in the right direction, but there is much more to be done, given that ^{223}Ra only targets osteoblastic bone lesions.

However, if nuclear medicine therapy is to sustain the expected growth rate, it is essential to ensure steady production and reliable supply of therapeutic radionuclides at affordable costs. To ensure wider distribution, the radionuclide should have a relatively longer half-life or be available from a radionuclide generator system having a parent with a relatively longer half-life.

Therefore, several aspects need to be considered when choosing the radiopharmaceutical to use for target tumour radiotherapy. This should go beyond the inevitable analysis of costs and logistics, and should include an analysis of the radionuclide's physical properties, as well as the size of the lesions to be treated and the patient's clinical condition and life expectancy, in order to optimize therapeutic efficacy.

In the future, personalized therapies are expected to guide the treatment for patients (especially targeted treatments) and to significantly improve healthcare delivery and reduce costs.

In particular, the increased awareness for the quality and safety of radiopharmaceuticals and the need for confirmation that the therapeutic agent has to provide clinically useful data contributed to making widespread use of new agents very challenging. In this scenario, academic investigators play a major role in the design and synthesis of therapeutic agents whose development must be in line with the emerging needs of the public health system, but which must also be economically sustainable for companies.

PSMA is a promising target for directing new therapies. Radioactive PSMA ligand, which is directly internalized into tumour cells, will be effective in delivering high doses for systemic radiotherapy. Thus, PSMA targeting is complementary to currently approved drugs and can be effective when targeting the androgen receptor axis fails.

Key Points

- Bone-seeking radiopharmaceuticals play a significant role in the treatment of metastatic pain as an alternative, or in addition, to classic palliative treatment. Ionizing radiation can be selectively delivered to areas of increased osteoblastic activity, allowing the targeting of multiple metastases. The goal of such irradiation is to kill tumour cells in the bone while sparing normal bone marrow, the site of haematopoiesis.

- Until a few years ago, radionuclides for the management of prostate cancer consisted of several beta-emitting agents, such as strontium (^{89}Sr), phosphorus (^{32}P) and samarium (^{153}Sm) as well as rhenium (^{186}Re and ^{188}Re), which only exhibit a palliative effect in patients with extensive skeletal disease.
- Radium (^{223}Ra) dichloride represents a new generation of radiopharmaceuticals and a great advance for nuclear medicine application, being the first targeted alpha-emitting agent approved, which improves overall survival, postpones skeletal-related events (SREs) and controls bone pain.
- Conjugates of bisphosphonates (BP) with macrocyclic chelators open new possibilities in bone-targeted radionuclide imaging and therapy, when labelled with positron and beta-emitting radiometals. [^{68}Ga/^{177}Lu]DOTA^{ZOL} appears to be the best leading compound showing fast blood clearance, low uptake in soft tissue and high accumulation in the skeleton.
- Prostate-specific membrane antigen (PSMA) is an attractive target for diagnosis and therapy of prostate cancer since expression levels are directly correlated to metastatic and hormone-refractory cancers. ^{177}Lu-PSMA-617 is a new treatment option, which is not solely directed to bone metastases but also demonstrates "antitumour" activity with limited and well-tolerated side effects.

References

1. Liepe K, Shinto A. From palliative therapy to prolongation of survival: $^{223}RaCl_2$ in the treatment of bone metastases. Ther Adv Med Oncol. 2016;8(4):294–304.
2. Maffioli L, Florimonte L, Costa DC, et al. New radiopharmaceutical agents for the treatment of castration-resistant prostate cancer. Q J Nucl Med Mol Imaging. 2015;59:420–38.
3. Guerra Liberal FDC, Tavares AAS, Tavares JMRS. Palliative treatment of metastatic bone pain with radiopharmaceuticals: a perspective beyond Strontium-89 and Samarium-153. Appl Rad Isotope. 2016;110:87–99.
4. Bienz M, Saad F. Management of bone metastases in prostate cancer: a review. Curr Opin Support Palliat Care. 2015;9:261–7.
5. Blacksburg SR, Witten MR, Haas JA. Integrating bone targeting radiopharmaceuticals into the management of patients with castrate-resistant prostate cancer with symptomatic bone metastases. Curr Treat Options in Oncol. 2015;16:11.
6. Liepe K, Runge R, Kotzerke J. The benefit of bone-seeking radiopharmaceuticals in the treatment of metastatic bone pain. J Cancer Res Clin Oncol. 2005;131:60–6.
7. Bellmunt J. Tackling the bone with alpha emitters in metastatic castration-resistant prostate cancer patients. Eur Urol. 2013;63:198–200.
8. Goyal J, Antonarakis ES. Bone-targeting radiopharmaceuticals for the treatment of prostate cancer with bone metastases. Cancer Lett. 2012;323:135–46.
9. Das T, Banerjee S. Radiopharmaceuticals for metastatic bone pain palliation: available options in the clinical domain and their comparisons. Clin Exp Metastasis. 2016;34(1):1–10.
10. Srivastava SC, Mausner LF. Therapeutic radionuclides: production, physical characteristics, and applications. In: Baum RP, editor. Therapeutic nuclear medicine. Heidelberg: Springer; 2013.
11. Lewis B, Sartor O. Radiation-based approaches for therapy and palliation of advanced prostate cancer. Curr Opin Urol. 2012;22:183–9.
12. Knapp FF, Dash A. Radiopharmaceuticals for therapy. India: Springer; 2016.
13. Sartor O, Hoskin P, Bruland ØS. Targeted radionuclide therapy of skeletal metastases. Cancer Treat Rev. 2013;39:18–26.
14. Das T, Pillai MRA. Options to meet the future global demand of radionuclides for radionuclide therapy. Nucl Med Biol. 2013;40:23–32.
15. Riondato M, Eckelman WC. In: Ciarmiello A, Mansi L, editors. Radiopharmaceuticals. PET-CT and PET-MRI in neurology. SWOT analysis applied to hybrid imaging, vol. 4. Part I ed. Switzerland: Springer; 2016. p. 31–58.
16. Silberstein EB. Teletherapy and radiopharmaceutical therapy of painful bone metastases. Semin Nucl Med. 2005;35:152–8.
17. van Dodewaard-de JM, Oprea-Lager DE, Hooft L, et al. Radiopharmaceuticals for palliation of bone pain in patients with castration- resistant prostate cancer metastatic to bone: a systematic review. Eur Urol. 2016;70:416–26.
18. Rubini G, Nicoletti A, Rubini D, Niccoli A. Radiometabolic treatment of bone-metastasizing cancer:

from ^{186}Renium to ^{223}Radium. Cancer Biother Radiopharm. 2013;29(1):1–11.
19. Finlay IG, Mason MD, Shelley M. Radioisotopes for the palliation of metastatic bone cancer: a systematic review. Lancet Oncol. 2005;6(6):392–400.
20. Lewington VJ. Bone-seeking radionuclides for therapy. J Nucl Med. 2005;46:38S–47S.
21. Bergmann R, Meckel M, Kubíček V, et al. ^{177}Lu-labelled macrocyclic bisphosphonates for targeting bone metastasis in cancer treatment. EJNMMI Res. 2016;6:5.
22. Meckel M, Bergmann R, Miederer M, Roesch F. Bone targeting compounds for radiotherapy and imaging: *me(III)-DOTA conjugates of bisphosphonic acid, pamidronic acid and zoledronic acid. EJNMMI Radiopharmacy Chem. 2016;1:14.
23. Rachner TD, Jakob F, Hofbauer LC. Cancer-targeted therapies and radiopharmaceuticals. Bonekey Reports. 2015;4:707.
24. Hofbauer LC, Rachner TD, Coleman RE, Jakob F. Endocrine aspects of bone metastases. Lancet Diabetes Endocrinol. 2014;2(6):500–12.
25. Mantyh PW. Bone cancer pain: from mechanism to therapy. Curr Opin Support Palliat Care. 2014;8(2):83–90.
26. Abi-Ghanem AS, McGrath MA, Jacene HA. Radionuclide therapy for osseous metastases in prostate. Cancer Semin Nucl Med. 2015;45:66–80.
27. Baidoo KE, Yong K, Brechbiel M. Molecular pathways: targeted alpha-particle radiation therapy. Clin Cancer Res. 2013;19(3):530–7.
28. Florimonte L, Dellavedova L, Maffioli LS. Radium-223 dichloride in clinical practice: a review. Eur J Nucl Med Mol Imaging. 2016;43(10): 1896–909.
29. Sartor O. Radiopharmaceuticals: a path forward. Eur Urol. 2016;70:427–8.
30. Emmett L, Kathy Willowson K, et al. Lutetium-177 PSMA radionuclide therapy for men with prostate cancer: a review of the current literature and discussion of practical aspects of therapy. J Med Radiat Sci. 2017;64(1):52–60.
31. Afshar-Oromieh A, Hetzheim H, Kratochwil C, et al. The theranostic PSMA ligand PSMA-617 in the diagnosis of prostate cancer by PET/CT: biodistribution in humans, radiation dosimetry, and first evaluation of tumor lesions. J Nucl Med. 2015;56:1697–705.
32. Clinical guideline [CG175]. 2014. http://www.nice.org.uk/guidance/cg175
33. Italian Medicines Agency, European Public Assessment Report (EPAR) Strontium [^{89}Sr] dichloride (last updated 10 June 2016. http://www.aifa.gov.it/en.
34. Delacroix D, Guerre JP, Leblanc P, Hickman C. Radionuclide and radiation protection data handbook. Radiat Prot Dosim. 2002;98:1.
35. Lam MGEH, de Klerk JMH, van Rijk PP, Zonnenberg BA. Bone seeking radiopharmaceuticals for palliation of pain in cancer patients with osseous metastases. Anti Cancer Agents Med Chem. 2007;7: 381–97.
36. Ogawa K, Washiyama K. Bone target radiotracers for palliative therapy of bone metastases. Curr Med Chem. 2012;19:3290–300.
37. Pandit-Taskar N, Batraki M, Divgi CR. Radiopharmaceutical therapy for palliation of bone pain from osseous metastases. J Nucl Med. 2004;45:1358–65.
38. Paes FM, Ernani V, Hosein P, Serafi ni AN. Radiopharmaceuticals: when and how to use them to treat metastatic bone pain. J Support Oncol. 2011;9:197–205.
39. Morris MJ, Scher HI. Clinical approaches to osseous metastases in prostate cancer. Oncologist. 2003;8(2):161–73.
40. Gravalos C, Rodriguez C, Sabino A, et al. SEOM clinical guideline for bone metastases from solid tumours (2016). Clin Transl Oncol. 2016;18:1243–53.
41. Nilsson S. Radionuclide therapies in prostate cancer: integrating radium-223 in the treatment of patients with metastatic castration-resistant prostate. Cancer Curr Oncol Rep. 2016;18:14.
42. Tucci M, Scagliotti GV, Vignani F. Metastatic castration-resistant prostate cancer: time for innovation. Future Oncol. 2015;11(1):91–106.
43. Harrison MR, Wong TZ, Armstrong AJ, George DJ. Radium-223 chloride: a potential new treatment for castration-resistant prostate cancer patients with metastatic bone disease. Cancer Manag Res. 2013;5:1–14.
44. El-Amm J, Aragon-Ching JB. Radium-223 for the treatment of castration-resistant prostate cancer. Oncol Targets Therap. 2015;8:1103–9.
45. Pandit-Taskar N, Larson SM, Carrasquillo JA. Bone-seeking radiopharmaceuticals for treatment of osseous metastases, part 1: a therapy with ^{223}Ra-dichloride. J Nucl Med. 2014;55:268–74.
46. Jadvar H, Quinn DI. Targeted alpha-particle therapy of bone metastases in prostate cancer. Clin Nucl Med. 2013;38:966–71.
47. European Medicines Agency (EMA) European Public Assessment Report (EPAR) radium [^{223}Ra] dichloride (last updated 2016). http://www.ema.europa.eu/ema/.
48. Lien LME, Tvedt B, Heinrich D. Treatment of castration-resistant prostate cancer and bone metastases with radium-223 dichloride. Int J Urol Nurs. 2015;9:3–13.
49. Buroni FE, Persico MG, Pasi F, et al. Review radium-223: insight and perspectives in bone-metastatic castration-resistant prostate cancer. Anticancer Res. 2016;36:5719–30.
50. Parker C, Nilsson S, Heinrich D, et al. Alpha emitter radium-223 and survival in metastatic prostate cancer. N Engl J Med. 2013;369:213–23.
51. Ryan CJ, Saylor PJ, Everly JJ, Sartor O. Bone-targeting radiopharmaceuticals for the treatment of bone-metastatic castration-resistant prostate cancer: exploring the implications of new data. Oncologist. 2014;19(10):1012–8.
52. Nilsson S. Radium-223 dichloride for the treatment of bone metastatic castration-resistant prostate cancer: an evaluation of its safety. Expert Opin Drug Saf. 2015;14(7):1127–36.

53. Sartor O, Coleman R, Nilsson S, et al. Effect of radium-223 dichloride on symptomatic skeletal events in patients with castration-resistant prostate cancer and bone metastases: results from a phase 3, double-blind, randomised trial. Lancet Oncol. 2014;15:738–46.
54. Shore ND. Radium-223 dichloride for metastatic castration-resistant prostate cancer: the urologist's perspective. Urology. 2015;85(4):717–24.
55. Cheetham PJ, Petrylak DP. Alpha particles as radiopharmaceuticals in the treatment of bone metastases: mechanism of action of radium-223 chloride (Alpharadin) and radiation. Oncology (Williston Park). 2012;26(4):330–41.
56. Coleman R. Treatment of metastatic bone disease and the emerging role of radium-223. Semin Nucl Med. 2016;46:99–104.
57. Shirley M, McCormack PL. Radium-223 dichloride: a review of its use in patients with castration resistant prostate cancer with symptomatic bone metastases. Drugs. 2014;74:579–86.
58. Wieder HA, Lassmann M, Allen-Auerbach MS, et al. Clinical use of bone-targeting radiopharmaceuticals with focus on alpha-emitters. World J Radiol. 2014;6(7):480–5.
59. Bombardieri E, Evangelista L, Ceresoli GL, Boccardo F. Nuclear medicine and the revolution in the modern management of castration-resistant prostate cancer patients: from ^{223}Ra-dichloride to new horizons for therapeutic response assessment. Eur J Nucl Med Mol Imaging. 2016;43:5–7.
60. El-Amm J, Freeman A, Patel N, Aragon-Ching JB. Bone-targeted therapies in metastatic castration-resistant prostate cancer: evolving paradigms. Prostate Cancer. 2013;2013:210686.
61. Iagaru AH, Mittra E, Colletti PM, Jadvar H. Bone-targeted imaging and radionuclide therapy in prostate cancer. J Nucl Med. 2016;57:19S–24S.
62. Baldari S, Boni G, Bortolus R, et al. Management of metastatic castration-resistant prostate cancer: a focus on radium-223 opinions and suggestions from an expert multidisciplinary panel. Crit Rev. Oncol Hematol. 2017;113:43–51.
63. European Pharmacopoeia 5.0 "Sodium phosphate (^{32}P) injection" (Ph Eur monograph 0284) (01/2005).
64. USP monographs: Sodium phosphate P 32 solution. 2005. USP29-NF2:1727.
65. Vimalnath KV, Shetty P, Chakraborty S, et al. Practicality of production of 32P by direct neutron activation for its utilization in bone pain palliation as $Na_3[^{32}P]PO_4$. Cancer Biother Radiopharm. 2013;28:423–8.
66. Sartor O, Reid RH, Hoskin PJ, et al. Samarium-153-lexidronam complex for treatment of painful bone metastases in hormone refractory prostate cancer. Urology. 2004;63:940–5.
67. European Medicines Agency (EMA) European Public Assessment Report (EPAR) Samarium [^{153}Sm] lexidronam (last updated 2015). http://www.ema.europa.eu/ema.
68. Paes FM, Serafini AN. Systemic metabolic radiopharmaceutical therapy in the treatment of metastatic bone pain. Semin Nucl Med. 2010;40:89–104.
69. Anderson P. Samarium for osteoblastic bone metastases and osteosarcoma. Expert Opin Pharmacother. 2006;7:1475–86.
70. Pillai MRA, Dash A, Knapp FF Jr. Rhenium-188: availability from the ^{188}W/^{188}Re generator and status of current applications. Curr Radiopharm. 2012;5:228–43.
71. Bodei L, Lam M, Chiesa C, et al. EANM procedure guideline for treatment of refractory metastatic bone pain. Eur J Nucl Med Mol Imaging EANM. 2008;35(10):1934–40.
72. Minutoli F, Herberg A, Spadaro P. [^{186}Re]-HEDP in the palliation of painful bone metastases from cancers other than prostate and breast. Q J Nucl Med Mol Imaging. 2006;50:355–62.
73. Knapp FF Jr, Beets AL, Pinkert J, et al. Rhenium radioisotopes for therapeutic radiopharmaceutical development. Inter seminar on therapeutic applications of radiopharmaceuticals (IAEA-SR-209), Hyderabad, India. 1999.
74. Boschi A, Uccelli L, Pasquali M, et al. 188 W/188Re generator system and its therapeutic applications. J Chemom. 2014;2014:529406.
75. Argyrou M, Valassi A, Andreou M, Lyra M. Rhenium-188 production in hospitals, by W-188/re-188 generator, for easy use in radionuclide therapy. Int J Mol Imaging. 2013;2013:290750.
76. Liepe K, Kropp J, RungeR KJ. Therapeutic efficiency of rhenium-188-HEDP in human prostate cancer skeletal metastases. Br J Cancer. 2003;89:625–9.
77. Yousefnia H, Zolghadri S, Sadeghi HR. Preparation and biological assessment of 177Lu-BPAMD as a high potential agent for bone pain palliation therapy: comparison with 177Lu-EDTMP. J Radioanal Nucl Chem. 2015;307:1243–51.
78. Meckel M. Macrocyclic bisphosphonates for PET-diagnosis and endoradiotherapy of bone metastases [Dissertation]; 2014.
79. Banerjee S, Pillai MRA, Knapp FF Jr. Lutetium-177 therapeutic radiopharmaceuticals-linking chemistry, radiochemistry and practical applications. Chem Rev. 2015;115:2934–74.
80. Dash A, Pillai MRA, Knapp FF. Production of ^{177}Lu for targeted radionuclide therapy: available options. Nucl Med Mol Imaging. 2015;49:85–107.
81. European Medicines Agency (EMA) European Public Assessment Report (EPAR) Lutetium (^{177}Lu) chloride (last updated 2017). http://www.ema.europa.eu/ema.
82. Meckel M, Kubíček V, Hermann P, et al. A DOTA based bisphosphonate with an albumin binding moiety for delayed body clearance for bone targeting. Nucl Med Biol. 2016;43:670–8.
83. Rasheed R, Lodhi NA, Khalid M, et al. Radiosynthesis, and in-vivo skeletal localization of ^{177}Lu-zoledronic acid as novel bone seeking therapeutic radiopharmaceutical. J Anesth Clin Res. 2015;6:516.

84. European Medicines Agency (EMA) European Public Assessment Report (EPAR) Zoledronic acid (last updated 2016). http://www.ema.europa.eu/ema.
85. Kiess AP, Banerjee SR, Mease RC, et al. Prostate-specific membrane antigen as a target for cancer imaging and therapy. Q J Nucl Med Mol Imaging. 2015;59:241–68.
86. Baum RP, Kulkarni HR, Schuchardt C, et al. ^{177}Lu-labeled prostate-specific membrane antigen radioligand therapy of metastatic castration-resistant prostate cancer: safety and efficacy. J Nucl Med. 2016;57:1006–13.
87. Pillai MRA, Nanabala R, Joy A, et al. Radiolabeled enzyme inhibitors and binding agents targeting PSMA: effective theranostic tools for imaging and therapy of prostate cancer. Nucl Med Biol. 2016;43:692–720.
88. Wüstemann T, Bauder-Wüst U, Schäfer M, et al. Design of internalizing PSMA-specific Glu-ureido-based radiotherapeuticals. Theranostics. 2016; 6(8):1085–95.
89. Nanabala R, Sasikumar A, Joy A, Pillai MRA. Preparation of [^{177}Lu]PSMA-617 using carrier added (CA) 177Lu for radionuclide therapy of prostate cancer. J Nucl Med Radiat Ther. 2016;7:306.
90. Tagawa ST, Milowsky MI, Morris M, et al. Phase II study of lutetium-177-labeled anti-prostate-specific membrane antigen monoclonal antibody J591 for metastatic castration-resistant prostate. Cancer Clin Cancer Res. 2013;19(18):5182–91.
91. Rahbar K, Ahmadzadehfar H, Kratochwil C. German multicenter study investigating ^{177}Lu-PSMA-617 radiology and therapy in advanced prostate cancer patients. J Nucl Med. 2017;58:85–90.
92. Rahbar K, Bode A, Weckesser M, et al. Radioligand therapy with ^{177}Lu-PSMA-617 as a novel therapeutic option in patients with metastatic castration resistant prostate. Cancer Clin Nucl Med. 2016;41:522–8.
93. Kratochwil C, Giesel FL, Stefanova M. PSMA-targeted radionuclide therapy of metastatic castration-resistant prostate cancer with ^{177}Lu-labeled PSMA-617. J Nucl Med. 2016;57:1170–6.
94. Afshar-Oromieh A, Babich JW, Kratochwil C. The rise of PSMA ligands for diagnosis and therapy of prostate cancer. Nucl Med. 2016;57:79S–89S.
95. Heck MM, Retz M, D'Alessandria C, et al. Systemic radioligand therapy with ^{177}Lu-PSMA-I&T in patients with metastatic castration-resistant prostate cancer. J Urol. 2016;196(2):382–91.
96. Weineisen M, Schottelius M, Simecek J, et al. ^{68}Ga- and ^{177}Lu-labeled PSMA I&T: optimization of a PSMA-targeted theranostic concept and first proof-of-concept human studies. J Nucl Med. 2015;56: 1169–76.
97. Chatalic KLS, Heskamp S, Konijnenberg M, et al. Towards personalized treatment of prostate cancer: PSMA I&T, a promising prostate-specific membrane antigen-targeted theranostic agent. Theranostics. 2016;6(6):849–61.
98. Barrio M, Fendler WP, Czernin J, Herrmann K. Prostate specific membrane antigen (PSMA) ligands for diagnosis and therapy of prostate cancer. Expert Rev. Mol Diagn. 2016;16(11):1177–88.

27 Targeted Therapy with Radium-223 of Bone Metastases

Sergio Baldari, Alessandro Sindoni, Laura Evangelista, and Emilio Bombardieri

Abstract

^{223}Ra is a targeted alpha therapy approved for treatment of metastatic prostate cancer with symptomatic bone metastases and without known visceral metastases. It documented an overall survival benefit, increased time to symptomatic skeletal event, improved quality of life and good safety profile in the pivotal trial ALSYMPCA.

The patient suitable for treatment must present at least two sites of osseous localization at bone scan, with no visceral involvement and lymph nodal disease within 3 cm diameter (short axis).

First data from clinical practice and from expanded access program confirmed safety and efficacy and highlighted that early use is related to completion of six cycles and better clinical outcome.

During treatment, it is important to evaluate pain response, clinical outcome, complete blood count and ALP at each cycle, while PSA must be assessed only every three cycles. Imaging modalities should be repeated at baseline (to select the right patient) and after at least 8 weeks from last administration (to assess the disease response); only in case of clinical suspicion of relapse, the same modalities could be repeated during treatment to exclude a disease progression.

S. Baldari (✉) • A. Sindoni
Department of Biomedical and Dental Sciences, and of Morphological and Functional Images, University of Messina, Messina, Italy
e-mail: sbaldari@unime.it

L. Evangelista
Veneto Institute of Oncology IOV – IRCCS, Padua, Italy

E. Bombardieri
Department of Nuclear Medicine, Humanitas Gavazzeni Hospital, Bergamo, Italy

27.1 Physical and Biological Properties of ^{223}Ra

^{223}Ra is a targeted alpha therapy that documented a survival benefit in metastatic castration-resistant prostate cancer [1]; it is an alpha-emitting radionuclide, with a calcium mimetic behaviour, which belongs to the alkali earth metals in the periodic table. Emitted energy distribution is α-energy (average) = 5.78 MeV (accounts for

E. Bombardieri et al. (eds.), *Clinical Applications of Nuclear Medicine Targeted Therapy*,
https://doi.org/10.1007/978-3-319-63067-0_27

93.5% of emitted energy), <4% as beta particles and <2% as γ radiation. Combined energy for the complete decay of ^{223}Ra and daughters is equal to 28 MeV; some γ (0.9 MeV total) is also emitted.

Tissue range for ^{223}Ra is inferior to 100 μm (α) with respect to several mm for β-particles, and it is characterized by a higher linear transfer energy ranging 100–200 keV/μm with respect to that of β-particles, which is inferior to 1 keV/μm: this high energy deposition of α-particles in a very small tissue range is able to cause irreversible double-strand DNA breaks [2, 3]. Other than DNA damage, the high energy determines the production of highly toxic radicals and chemicals for cells. Since energy of α-particles is released in a very short range in tissue, the targeted cells receive higher absorbed radiation doses than adjacent healthy cells, which permit to spare near-critical structure and, in particular, bone marrow [4].

In vitro experiments have demonstrated that the lethal effect is not cell type specific and is also delivered on multidrug resistant cells; moreover, it produces G2 arrest and causes a dose-dependent inhibition of differentiation of the osteoclasts [5–7]. In mice model bearing intratibial LNCaP or LuCaP 58 tumours and administered with ^{223}Ra, the inhibition of tumour-induced osteoblastic bone growth and protection of normal bone architecture leading to reduced bone volume were documented. ^{223}Ra resulted in lower PSA values and reduced total tissue and tumour areas.

A decreased number of osteoblasts and osteoclasts and reduced level of the bone formation marker PINP were observed. ^{223}Ra therapy exhibits a dual targeting mode of action that induces tumour cell death and suppresses tumour-induced pathological bone formation, both essential players in the destructive vicious cycle of osteoblastic bone metastasis in prostate cancer [8].

27.2 Castration-Resistant Prostate Cancer

Prostate cancer is the most common solid malignant tumour in men and represents the second cause of cancer-related deaths in this sex [9]. Men with localized prostate cancer are treated with surgery or radiation therapy. However, at follow-up, biochemical recurrence (increase in PSA levels) can occur, and, in this setting, localization of disease is important for patients' management, which may include active surveillance, systemic therapy, localized salvage therapy or both systemic and localized treatments. The term "castration resistant" is used when a measurable progression of disease occurs in the setting of castrate levels of testosterone, manifesting itself with PSA increase or imaging abnormalities at computed tomography, magnetic resonance imaging or nuclear medicine techniques. Up to 20% of patients with metastatic prostate cancer develop CRPC within 5 years; prevalence CRPC has been estimated to be 17.8% among patients with prostate cancer [10]. In the majority of patients affected by CRPC, bone is the site of metastatic involvement. Bone metastases are cause of decreased quality of life, pain and disability with increased treatment cost and, finally, also death. The major concerns in these patients are skeletal-related events (SREs), manifesting with spinal cord compression and pathological fractures. Available treatments for metastatic CRPC (mCRPC) include chemotherapy with docetaxel or cabazitaxel, androgen synthesis inhibitors abiraterone acetate, androgen receptor blocker enzalutamide and immunotherapy with sipuleucel-T [11]. Although these drugs have provided interesting results, additional studies are needed to define potential combinations and optimal sequencing. Since bone is a frequent site of metastatic involvement, significant efforts in developing approaches for bone metastases have been made and are ongoing with the aim to reduce pain and limit complications and SREs. Bisphosphonates, zoledronic acid [12] and mostly antibodies to RANKL (denosumab) have demonstrated to delay SREs [13], but they have not shown significant impact in patients' survival.

Palliative therapy using [^{186}Re]hydroxyethylidene diphosphonate (HEDP) was extensively performed in patients with bone metastases from prostate and breast cancers [14].

^{89}Sr-chloride showed significant results when used with the aim of palliating pain from bone metastases, in particular metastatic prostate or breast cancer, resulting in pain relief in 60–92% of patients [15–21]. Since ^{153}Sm alone has no affinity for bone, the isotope is chelated to ethylene diamine tetramethylene phosphonate (EDTMP) for targeting bone.

The absorbed dose and relative biological effectiveness (EBR) of ^{223}Ra to lesions per unit administered activity was much higher than that of other bone-seeking radiopharmaceuticals, but considering a standard administration of 21 MBq (six injections of 50 kBq/kg to a 70-kg patient), the mean cumulative value of absorbed dose and relative biological effectiveness was about 19 Gy and was therefore in the range of those of other radiopharmaceuticals [20].

In the wave of novel therapies for mCRPC which has characterized the last years, a renewed attention towards the potential role of targeted α-therapy has been established in the set of patients affected by bone metastases from mCRPC.

27.3 ^{223}Ra in Symptomatic Prostate Cancer Clinical Trial

In phase I and II studies involving patients with bone metastases [22, 23], safety and tolerability of ^{223}Ra had been previously evaluated. The first phase I trial enrolled breast and prostate cancer patients with skeletal metastases (15 prostate and 10 breast cancer ones) for receiving a single IV injection of ^{223}Ra: five patients were included at each of the dosages, 46, 93, 163, 213 or 250 kBq/kg, and followed for 8 weeks [22]. A phase II trial enrolled patients with hormone-refractory prostate cancer and bone pain needing external-beam radiotherapy, who were randomized to four administrations of ^{223}Ra (50 kBq/kg, 33 patients) or placebo (31 patients), given every 4 weeks [23].

In 2013, Parker et al. [24] assessed efficacy and safety of ^{223}Ra compared to placebo, in addition to the best standard of care, in men with CRPC and bone metastases. In this phase III study, they randomly assigned 921 patients who had received, were not eligible to receive, or declined docetaxel, in a 2:1 ratio, to receive six injections of ^{223}Ra (50 kBq/kg b.w. intravenously) or matching placebo. Time interval between each injection was 4 weeks. The primary end point was overall survival; the main secondary efficacy end points were the time to the first symptomatic skeletal, time to PSA and ALP progression, PSA and ALP responses, safety and quality of life. At the interim analysis, which involved 809 patients and was performed when 314 deaths had occurred, ^{223}Ra significantly improved overall survival with respect to placebo (median, 14.0 months vs. 11.2 months; $P = 0.002$). The updated analysis, performed when 528 deaths had occurred and involving 921 patients, confirmed the ^{223}Ra survival benefit (median, 14.9 months vs. 11.3 months; $P < 0.001$). Also considering all main secondary efficacy end points, a benefit of radium-233 with respect to placebo was found. ^{223}Ra significantly prolonged the time to the first symptomatic skeletal event (median, 15.6 months vs. 9.8 months; $P < 0.001$), the time to an increase in the total alkaline phosphatase level ($P < 0.001$) and the time to an increase in the PSA level ($P < 0.001$). More patients in the ^{223}Ra group than in the placebo group experienced a decrease in the total alkaline phosphatase and PSA levels. About safety, ^{223}Ra was associated with low myelosuppression rates and few adverse events.

^{223}Ra demonstrated to prolong median OS with respect to placebo, regardless of previous docetaxel use. However, patients previously treated with docetaxel had a higher incidence of grades 3–4 thrombocytopenia with ^{223}Ra with respect to placebo, whereas the incidences of grades 3–4 anaemia were associated with bone involvement at baseline in both arms of treatment. In ^{223}Ra and placebo patients who received subsequent chemotherapy (142 patients for ^{223}Ra and 64 placebo), evaluation of haemoglobin, neutrophils and thrombocytes showed similar findings up to 18 months following the start of chemotherapy, and only a low percentage of cases in both groups showed grades 3–4 haematological toxicities: from this evaluation, chemotherapy after ^{223}Ra, regardless of prior docetaxel treatment, is well tolerated in patients with CRPC and symptomatic bone metastases [25].

Recently, Alva et al. [26] identified potential clinical variables associated with outcomes after ^{223}Ra therapy in 145 patients. 74/145 (or 51%) received six cycles of treatment. In their study, survival was highly associated with receiving all six doses, and the receipt of six doses was also associated with ECOG PS of 0–1, lower baseline PSA and pain level, no prior abiraterone/enzalutamide, <5 bone scan index value and normal alkaline phosphatase. In 72 patients with baseline pain evaluation, pain declined in 51% after one dose and increased in 7%. PSA declined ≥50% in 16% of cases, whereas alkaline phosphatase declined ≥25% in 48% and ≥50% in 23% of patients. Bone scan index declined in 17/25 (or 68%) who had bone scan available at treatment follow-up. Grade ≥ 3 neutropenia, anaemia and thrombocytopenia occurred in 4% (n = 114), 4% (n = 125) and 5% (n = 123), respectively. They concluded that patients earlier in their disease course with <5 bone scan index, low pain score and good ECOG performance status are optimal candidates for ^{223}Ra.

27.4 ^{223}Ra Dichloride: Indication and Patient Management

^{223}Ra is indicated for the treatment of adults with castration-resistant prostate cancer, symptomatic bone metastases and no known visceral metastases.

Before considering a patient for this treatment modality, it is mandatory to check eligibility and verify osseous metastases on a recent bone scan. Patients must present at least two sites of bone metastases demonstrated at bone scintigraphy[a] with ^{99m}Tc-diphosphonate performed before to start therapy with ^{223}Ra. As an alternative, ^{18}F-NaF PET/CT can be used because it has demonstrated a higher diagnostic performance than bone scintigraphy. To exclude visceral metastases, a computed tomography (CT) imaging and/or positron emission tomography (PET)/CT after administration of ^{18}F/^{11}C-choline or ^{68}Ga-prostate-specific membrane antigen (PSMA) in selected cases must be performed. These imaging modalities consent to verify also the presence of nodal disease (the presence of malignant lymph nodes greater than 3 cm short axis represents exclusion criteria for treatment) (Table 27.1). Diagnostic examinations have to be done within 3 months before starting treatment.

Pain must be assessed through specific questionnaires and scales; according to ALSYMPCA inclusion criteria and approved label, patient must present a WHO pain ≥1 (=assumption of nonsteroidal anti-inflammatory or antalgic EBRT in the previous 12 weeks; in the ALSYMPCA trial, 44% of enrolled pts presented a WHO pain = 1). According to Brief Pain Inventory-Short Form (BPI-SF) question 3, the referred pain in the last 24 h must be ≥2 (the score 2–3 corresponds to a mildly symptomatic disease, while the score from 4 to 10 is from moderate to severe pain) (Tables 27.1 and 27.4).

Haematological evaluation must be performed at baseline and prior to every radiopharmaceutical administration. Before the first administration, the absolute neutrophil count should be ≥1.5 × 10^9/l, the platelet count ≥100 × 10^9/l and haemoglobin ≥10.0 g/dl. Before subsequent administrations, the absolute neutrophil count should be ≥1.0 × 10^9/l and the platelet count ≥50 × 10^9/l. In patients with persistent impairment in these values within 6 weeks after the last administration of ^{223}Ra despite receiving standard of care, treatment with ^{223}Ra should only be continued after a benefit/risk balance [27].

In the presence of compromised bone marrow functionality related to prior cytotoxic therapies (chemotherapy and/or radiotherapy) or prostate cancer patients with advanced diffuse bone infiltration, treatment should be performed with caution because these patients have a higher risk of haematological toxicity. In "superscan" condition, patients can be treated with ^{223}Ra after careful evaluation. Other comorbidities have to be evaluated, such as inflammatory bowel disease (a condition that can be worsened because of faecal ^{223}Ra excretion) and spinal cord compression and fractures (which have to be stabilized before starting treatment). Osteonecrosis of the jaw, often related to previous treatment with zoledronic acid or denosumab, is not an absolute contraindication to ^{223}Ra administration, but it represents a condition to be carefully evaluated.

There aren't any known interactions with other drugs nor contraindication in patients with renal or hepatic impairment. No dosage adjustment is required in older patients, and no differences in

Table 27.1 Characteristics of patients suitable for ^{223}Ra treatment

Characteristics	Definition
Bone-dominant castrate-resistant prostate cancer (CRPC)	At least two sites of bone metastases were demonstrated at bone scintigraphy[a] with ^{99m}Tc-diphosphonate performed before to start therapy with ^{223}Ra
Presence of symptomatic bone metastasis	Identified by: – The assumption of specific pharmacologic agents, such as FANS or opioids (WHO scale ≥1;) and/or – BPI-SF ≥2 (the score 2–3 corresponds to a mild pain, the score ≥4 is an intense pain)
Adequate medullary function	Before the administration of ^{223}Ra, please check: – Absolute neutrophil count (ANC) (should be ≥1.5 × 10⁹/l) – Platelet count (should be ≥100 × 10⁹/l) – Haemoglobin (should be ≥10.0 g/dl) Before the administration of ^{223}Ra (after the first cycle), please check: – ANC (should be ≥1.0 × 10⁹/l) – Platelet count (should be ≥50 × 10⁹/l) (If the above-mentioned values remain abnormal until 6 weeks from the last administration, Ra223 should be continued after a benefit/risk balance
No visceral metastases[b] (an absolute contraindication to the treatment)	Liver, lung and central nervous system (CNS)
Presence of lymph node metastases[b]	Only lymph node metastases with a diameter <3 cm are allowed

[a]Bone scintigraphy is useful because the uptake of ^{99m}Tc-phosphonate is similar to that of ^{223}Ra, therefore similar to calcium. As an alternative, ^{18}F-NaF PET/CT can be used because it has demonstrated a higher diagnostic performance than bone scintigraphy

[b]To exclude the presence of visceral metastases or to assess the presence of lymph node dissemination, it is recommended to perform a thorax-abdominal computed tomography (CT) with contrast enhancement or a PET/CT with radiolabelled choline. The examination should be performed at least 3 months before to start ^{223}Ra treatment. PET/CT does not exclude the execution of bone scintigraphy, before to start ^{223}Ra treatment

terms of efficacy in patients <65 years vs. >65 years resulted in the ALSYMPCA trial.

^{223}Ra is contraindicated in patients who experience life-threatening complications despite supportive care approaches. In fact, therapeutic decision-making should consider all the aspects of the patient's overall clinical state, such as age, performance status, comorbidities, other available therapeutic options in the disease setting and patient's choice. Attention must be taken considering disease aggressiveness in accordance with extent of metastases, presence of visceral metastases, presence of pain, time from diagnosis, PSA kinetic and ADT response duration. The most appropriate patients may be those with lower burden of bone disease and good bone marrow reserve [28] since ^{223}Ra administration is limited only by haemoglobin levels <10 mg/dl. In chemo-naïve patients, physician should consider the presence of pain: in symptomatic patients, the use of abiraterone acetate and enzalutamide is not indicated [28], and in this set of patients, excluding those with visceral metastases and/or with relevant nodal involvement (nodes ≥3 cm), mCRPC patients may receive docetaxel or ^{223}Ra [28]. Ideal candidates for ^{223}Ra treatment are patients with mildly symptomatic bone metastasis, limited burden of disease and a long PSA doubling time (e.g. ≥6 months), or with comorbidities contraindicating the use of chemotherapy, or in patients refusing chemotherapy [28]: interestingly, as mentioned above, ^{223}Ra allows subsequent docetaxel therapy [29]. In patients already treated with docetaxel, physician should consider its toxicities: for example, patients experiencing relevant toxicities may be not good candidates for cabazitaxel, while the toxicity profiles of the new hormonal agents or ^{223}Ra could favour their use in the setting of symptomatic patients without visceral metastases and relevant nodal involvement (nodes ≥3 cm) [28]. By contrast, in patients with aggressive disease after docetaxel failure, cabazitaxel could be proposed. If abiraterone or enzalutamide was administered as first-line therapy for mCRPC, valid therapeutic options include docetaxel and ^{223}Ra if indicated [28]. Additionally, if the choice is between ^{223}Ra and a new generation hormonal agent, the presence of relevant comorbidities should be evaluated, since the use of enzalutamide may be limited by either clinical history of seizure or concomitant administration of drugs that act on CYP3A4, CYP2C9 and CYP2C19 [28], and the presence of severe cardiovascular disease or uncontrolled diabetes suggests caution in the use of abiraterone: in this setting, ^{223}Ra is an alternative valid approach [28]. Moreover, consideration about sequencing of the available active agents in mCRPC is needed: medical literature suggests a relationship between the development of resistance to new hormonal agents and the upregulation of androgen receptors; ^{223}Ra efficacy is not related to androgen receptor pathways and to the known pathways involved in drugs' resistance [28].

Before starting treatment, a complete bone disease staging must be performed as described above. Pain evaluation, dosage of alkaline phosphatase and complete blood count should be repeated at baseline and each cycle; PSA should be tested at baseline and, during treatment, only if clinically indicated (Table 27.2).

Imaging must be repeated at the end of six cycles, after at least 8 weeks from last administration, to avoid the phenomenon of bone flare at scan. Visceral status of disease with CT scan or choline PET is generally repeated at the same time (+8 weeks from last cycle), but if clinically suggested, it could be performed also after third cycle, in case of clinical suspicion of disease progression. It is mandatory to use the same imaging modalities applied at baseline (Table 27.2).

A signed consent form should be obtained after showing the features of the treatment to the patient or patient's caregiver and answering all their questions. ^{223}Ra should be handled following both radiation safety and pharmaceutical quality requirements. Aseptic precautions should be taken. Dose calibrator measurement may be required. The volume to be administered is calculated on the basis of patient's body weight (kg), dosage level (55 kBq/kg body weight according to National Institute of Standards and Technology [30]), activity at reference date (6.6 MBq or 1100 kBq/ml) and decay correction factor to correct for physical decay of ^{223}Ra. Double gloves should be worn. Floor, chair and table have to be protected from eventual contamination. Saline flushes and an IV pole with 500 ml saline and primed tubing should be available. The saline flow has to be connected through a

Table 27.2 Preparation of patients for the treatment with ^{223}Ra

Biochemical analysis	Imaging evaluation	Medical condition
Baseline serum ALP Baseline serum PSA	Bone scintigraphy	In older patients, the dosage should not be rearranged (no differences in terms of efficacy in patients aged <65 years vs. aged >65 years, in the ALSYMPCA trial)
Serum testosterone (in order to confirm the presence of *castration-resistant disease*)	CT scan or radiolabelled choline PET/CT scan[a]	In patients with liver dysfunction, the dosage should not be rearranged, because ^{223}Ra is not metabolized by the liver and it is not eliminated by the bile
		In patients with renal failure, the dosage should not be rearranged because the urinary excretion is minimal (<5%)
		In patients with inflammatory bowel disease (Crohn disease or ulcerative colitis), the risk/benefit ratio should be considered, because ^{223}Ra has an intestinal elimination (>75%)
		In patients with a "superscan," ^{223}Ra is not contraindicated, but a careful evaluation of the performance status and medullary reserve is required
		In patients with a potential medullary compression or bone fracture, the stabilization is recommended before to start the treatment with ^{223}Ra
		There are no limitations regarding previous treatments, like chemotherapy or others. In accordance with phase II trial (ALSYMPCA), both patients before and after chemotherapy are eligible for the therapy with ^{223}Ra

ALP alkaline phosphatase, *PSA* prostate-specific antigen
[a]*See* Table 27.1

three-way stopcock and should be stopped, and then ^{223}Ra should be administered up to 1 min by the physician. Also central venous catheter could be used for administration. A therapeutic activity of 55 kBq per kg body weight is recommended. Then saline flushes are connected and pushed. Then all the tubing and the radioisotope syringe are placed in an appropriate container and left in a red biohazard bag for measuring eventual residual. Technologist's and physician's hands and feet have also to be preserved from potential contamination. Before patient demission, general status evaluation with heart rate and blood pressure has to be performed. A report indicating cycle's number administered activity and basic information on clinical indication and laboratory data. The patient is scheduled for the next cycles 28 days later. The most frequently observed adverse reactions (≥10%) in patients receiving ^{223}Ra were diarrhoea, nausea, vomiting and thrombocytopenia. Rare serious adverse reactions were thrombocytopenia and neutropenia. It is mandatory to evaluate complete blood count and other markers such as serum alkaline phosphatase (ALP), serum PSA, lactate dehydrogenase and bone-specific alkaline phosphatase. Restaging is recommended after the completion of six cycles of ^{223}Ra, but the revaluation can be performed earlier if suspicious clinical symptoms occur.

The patient should avoid prolonged contact with children and pregnant women during the first week after each administration. It is recommended that he follows behavioural norms to avoid contamination (by using gloves if it is necessary to clean urine, stool or vomit and when touching or washing dirty clothes). Toilet should be flushed twice after each use. Possible incontinence must be checked by physicians, to give complete information to patients and their caregivers. Underwear used during the first week after each ^{223}Ra administration and any clothing soiled with urine, stool or blood should be washed separately).

If a patient dies within 7 days from last administration, cremation must be postponed or burial used instead [31].

Diagnostic imaging workup in CRPC includes nuclear medicine (bone scintigraphy, PET/CT) and radiological techniques (CT, magnetic resonance imaging). Nuclear medicine techniques may be used to assess response in bone metastases treated with ^{223}Ra, either with bone scintigraphy or with PET/CT imaging. Among last techniques, changes in large metastatic deposits after ^{223}Ra therapy have been reported, with a dramatic drop of radiopharmaceutical lesions' accumulation either of ^{18}F-choline [11] or ^{68}Ga-PSMA [32, 33] in responders together with a reduction of PSA and ALP. This phenomenon cannot be simply explained by tumour cell irradiation but also by an effect on the microenvironment including vessels and stroma, which induces tumour regression in both osteolytic and osteoblastic tumours [7], opening the way for the use of ^{223}Ra also for other malignancies.

How to calculate 223Ra dose

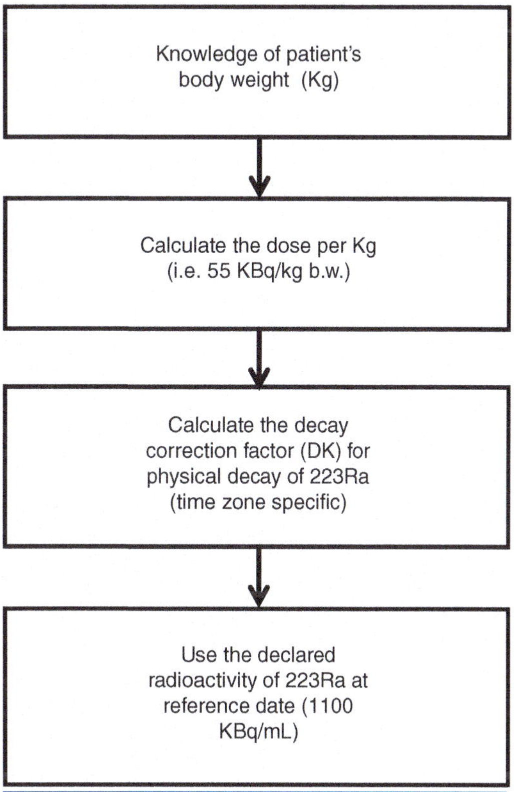

Example:

- A 79 years-old patient (b.w. 70 Kg)
- 223Ra dose will be admistered after 1 day from the date of calibration.
- The volume that we have to inject will be:

70 (b.w. of patient)
55 kBq/b.w.
DK=0.94
(70x55)/(0.94x1100)= 3850/1034=**3.72mL of volume**

27.5 Response Evaluation

Response evaluation after ^{223}Ra therapy can be followed by several biomarkers and bone scintigraphy (Table 27.3). ALP is a biomarker of osteoblastic activity and its serum levels are often incremented in mCRPC patients. High serum ALP levels are related to an increased risk of SREs and mortality. It can be used for evaluating treatment response, disease progression and survival in mCRPC patients [34–39]. Major reduction of ALP levels with respect to PSA ones reflects the differences between the two biomarkers: in fact, if ALP levels are linked to bone metabolism and are therefore influenced by a bone-targeted treatment as ^{223}Ra, serum PSA is an expression of overall disease evolution and is less influenced by a targeted therapy.

Considering disease markers for response evaluation, such as serum PSA and bone metabolism indices (bone and total ALP) together with bone scan, it has been found that ALP represents the most accurate marker for evaluating response to treatment, whereas in some patients serum PSA levels can increase at the end of the treatment. Bone scan is accurate and has a high sensibility in detection of bone metastases. Additionally, it can show new findings, since some lesions can be characterized by metabolic response, whereas new lesions can appear after the end of ^{223}Ra therapy. In this setting, combination with other medical approaches can be useful. It should be considered that flare response can occur, since some patients can experience an increase in disease biomarkers (PSA and ALP) together with a worsening of pain after the starting of the treatment, but followed by an improvement at bone scintigraphy and a subsequent reduction of disease biomarkers and pain:

Table 27.3 Evaluation of response to ^{223}Ra treatment

Test	Time
ALP	Baseline After 3 months At the end of therapy
Complete blood count (CBC)	Every 1 month before ^{223}Ra administration[a]
PSA	Baseline During treatment, if requested by nuclear medicine physician, only for monitoring the presence of visceral involvement[b]
CT or radiolabelled choline PET/CT	Only in case of visceral progression
Bone scintigraphy	Baseline After 2–3 months from the end of treatment
Pain score test	*See* Table 27.4

ALP alkaline phosphatase, *PSA* prostate specific antigen

[a]CBC is suggested at each cycle for assessing the eligible of patients (*see* Table 27.2)

[b]PSA can falsely increase during ^{223}Ra therapy (flare phenomena), but it represents a marker of a potential visceral progression

Table 27.4 Pain scales for the assessment of life quality

Method	Grade	Meaning
ECOG	0	Fully active, able to carry on all pre-disease performance without restriction
	1	Restricted in physically strenuous activity but ambulatory and able to carry out work of a light or sedentary nature, e.g. light house work, office work
	2	Ambulatory and capable of all self-care but unable to carry out any work activities; up and about more than 50% of waking hours
	3	Capable of only limited self-care; confined to bed or chain more than 50% of waking hours
	4	Completely disabled; cannot carry on any self-care; totally confined to bed or chair
	5	Dead
WHO	0	No pain at rest on movement
	1	No pain at rest, mild on movement (mild analgesic action, i.e. paracetamol)
	2	Mild pain at rest, moderate on movement (weak opiate/NSAID and consider paracetamol)
	3	Continuous pain at rest, severe on movement (morphine or other strong agent; and consider weak opiate/NSAID/paracetamol)
EQ-5D	1	Mobility
	2	Self-care
	3	Usual activities
	4	Pain/discomfort
	5	Anxiety/depression

flare phenomenon can occur up to 12 weeks after the starting of ^{223}Ra therapy. On this way, progression of disease should be considered at least in cases with ≥2 bone lesions after flare occurrence and should be confirmed by a bone scan performed 6 weeks later [40]. An interesting aspect of bone scan is represented by the calculation of the bone scan index, which allows to assess more precisely the extent of metastatic disease [41].

On the other hand, patients who underwent multiple prior chemotherapy schemes, ECOG ≥2 and lower haemoglobin levels have more advanced disease and are less likely to reach the recommended six administrations; oppositely, the completion of treatment is associated with higher efficacy (Fig. 27.1) and longer overall survival [42].

Even if CT is the classical imaging technique used to detect cancer and to assess disease status through "Response Evaluation Criteria In Solid Tumors" (RECIST criteria), it cannot be used to assess response to therapy in bone metastases: in fact, even if it permits to evaluate osseous architecture, bone structure rarely normalizes even with completely effective therapy [43]. Additionally, the occurrence of worsening bone sclerosis on CT is occasionally and erroneously classified as disease progression, without considering CT flare response [43]. The superiority of MRI for detection of bone metastases with respect to CT has been demonstrated. Diffusion-weighted imaging (DWI) sequences are able to detect changes in water diffusion: if normal fatty marrow is replaced with highly dense cellularity, normal water movements among cell membranes

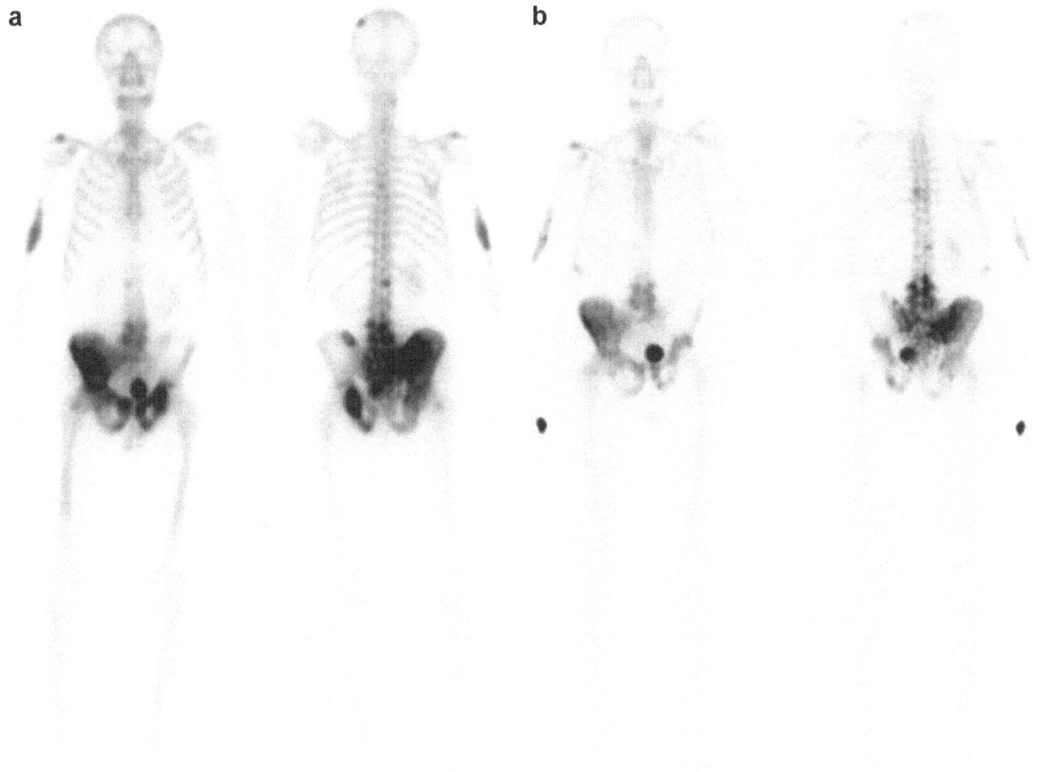

Fig. 27.1 Pretreatment (**a**) and post-treatment (**b**) bone scintigraphy of a 73-year-old patient affected by castration-resistant prostate cancer (Gleason 9) with bone metastases who underwent six administrations of $^{223}RaCl_3$ at the therapeutic activity of 55 kBq/kg b.w

are limited. Moreover, changes in water mobility occur in response to treatment. However, benign conditions may show high signal intensity on DWI images, and, on the contrary, false-negative findings may occur, mainly in sclerotic or calcified metastases. On this way, MRI is a reliable tool for confirming stable disease or corroborating progressive disease if new lesions appear or if a sclerotic lesion has a new peripheral halo [43].

New nuclear imaging techniques are now available to better assess patients' condition and treatment response. First of all, ^{18}F-fluoride may be considered, since it is a bone-seeking radiopharmaceutical which is used for PET/CT imaging: in particular, it has shown higher sensibility, higher specificity and higher accuracy than bone scintigraphy [44]. The spreading of nuclear medicine centres using new tracers, such as ^{18}F-choline/^{11}C-choline and ^{68}Ga-PSMA, offers additional opportunities to better evaluate disease status of patients.

Choline PET/CT has demonstrated agreement with PSA changes in patients with progressive disease but has some limitations in identifying patients with partial or complete response to therapy: in fact, the uptake normalization is not always related to the disappearance of the cancer lesion, since it could represent the effect of a stable or nonmetabolic lesion [43]. In contrast, the appearance of new areas of uptake does not always correlate with certain progression, but they can be an expression of the well-known flare phenomenon [43]. So, choline PET/CT should be repeated within 3 months if a flare phenomenon is suspected. Advantages of ^{68}Ga-PSMA PET/CT are the sensitive detection of lesions, even at low PSA levels (i.e. PSA <1 ng/ml), small lymph node metastases and central bone and liver metastases due to tumour/non-tumour ratio [43].

Finally, the main markers to be used for monitoring the response to treatment are:

- Pain reduction: its evaluation is mandatory, in association with quality of life evaluation.
- Serum PSA: it should not be used as specific marker for treatment response, since it reflects the general evolution of the disease.
- Serum ALP: it should be considered the most important marker.
- Bone scintigraphy: its usefulness is indisputable, not only to evaluate the patient at the end of the treatment but also in an "ad interim" intent in cases which elicit strong clinical suspicion of bone disease progression.

During treatment, diagnostic imaging should not be performed systematically but in the set of a multidisciplinary evaluation which considers also clinical and laboratory data. However, a clear worsening clinical condition justifies evaluation by means of imaging modalities.

On the basis of clinical evidence, the following lines have to be followed:

- Continue treatment and stop it only in cases with major side effects or clinical deterioration.
- Consider all available clinical sign and symptoms.
- Keep an eye on overall patients' conditions.

Conclusions

^{223}Ra is a calcium mimetic targeted alpha therapy and permits delivery of high radiation energy at sites of active bone turnover due to metastatic spreading. Literature experiences have demonstrated increased overall survival and decreased time to skeletal-related events with ^{223}Ra-dichloride, with additional benefits involving also other disease biomarkers. The integration of ^{223}Ra into the management of mCRPC may improve OS also by the additional and sequential chemotherapy. This leads to consider what is the best sequence of drugs or if a combined therapy could be used. The nonoverlapping mechanism of action and the safety of ^{223}Ra may allow new combination strategies in an era of releasing of novel innovative drugs, moving from symptomatic and more diffuse bone disease to an earlier phase characterized by asymptomatic/limited bone disease or in the set of patients with visceral disease and bone involved. Finally, further studies are needed in the metastatic bone setting from other solid malignancies besides prostate cancer. These questions require a more accurate evaluation of ^{223}Ra's action and a dosimetric approach beyond activity/weight criteria: interestingly, lesions with ^{99m}Tc-MDP contrast ratio higher than 10, not overlapping the gastrointestinal tract, are generally visible on ^{223}Ra images acquired at 24 h after the administration, and possibly eligible for dosimetric studies [45].

Key Points

- ^{223}Ra delays time to symptomatic skeletal-related events and prolongs overall survival in men affected by metastatic castration-resistant prostate cancer (mCRPC) and more than two painful bone metastases.
- $^{223}RaCl_2$ is the only radiopharmaceutical that has demonstrated to give a benefit in overall survival, regardless of previous docetaxel use.
- Patients earlier in their disease course with <5 bone scan index, low pain score and good ECOG performance status are optimal candidates for ^{223}Ra.
- Men who underwent multiple prior chemotherapy schemes, ECOG ≥2 and lower haemoglobin levels have more advanced disease and are less likely to reach the recommended six administrations; on the other hand, the completion of treatment is associated with higher efficacy and longer overall survival.
- Prostate-specific antigen trend should not be used to determine response or duration of treatment, whereas ALP represents the most accurate marker for evaluating response to treatment.

References

1. Picciotto M, Franchina T, Russo A, Ricciardi GRR, Provazza G, Sava S, Baldari S, Caffo O, Adamo V. Emerging role of Radium-223 in the growing therapeutic armamentarium of metastatic castration-resistant prostate cancer. Expert Opin Pharmacother. 2017;18:899–908.
2. Kassis AI. Therapeutic radionuclides: biophysical and radiobiologic principles. Semin Nucl Med. 2008;38:358–66.
3. Harrison MR, Wong TZ, Armstrong AJ, George DJ. Radium-223 chloride: a potential new treatment for castration-resistant prostate cancer patients with metastatic bone disease. Cancer Manag Res. 2013;5:1–14.
4. Logothetis CJ, Gallick GE, Maity SN, et al. Molecular classification of prostate cancer progression: foundation for marker-driven treatment of prostate cancer. Cancer Discov. 2013;3:849–61.
5. Henriksen G, Breistøl K, Bruland ØS, Fodstad Ø, Larsen RH. Significant antitumor effect from bone-seeking, alpha-particle emitting (223)Ra demonstrated in an experimental skeletal metastases model. Cancer Res. 2002;62:3120–5.
6. Suominen MI, Rissanen JP, Käkönen R, Fagerlund KM, Alhoniemi E, Mumberg D, Ziegelbauer K, Halleen JM, Käkönen SM, Scholz A. Survival benefit with radium-223 dichloride in a mouse model of breast cancer bone metastasis. J Natl Cancer Inst. 2013;105:908–16.
7. Abou DS, Ulmert D, Doucet M, Hobbs RF, Riddle RC, Thorek DL. Whole-body and microenvironmental localization of Radium-223 in naïve and mouse models of prostate cancer metastasis. J Natl Cancer Inst 2016; 108: pii: djv380.
8. Suominen MI, Fagerlund KM, Rissanen JP, Konkol YM, Morko JP, Peng ZQ, Alhoniemi EJ, Laine SK, Corey E, Mumberg D, Ziegelbauer K, Käkönen SM, Halleen JM, Vessella RL, Scholz A. Radium-223 inhibits osseous prostate cancer growth by dual targeting of cancer cells and bone microenvironment in mouse models. Clin Cancer Res. 2017;23(15):4335–46.
9. Siegel RL, Miller KD, Jemal A. Cancer statistics, 2015. CA Cancer J Clin. 2015;65:5–29.
10. Alemayehu B, Buysman E, Parry D, Becker L, Nathan F. Economic burden and healthcare utilization associated with castration-resistant prostate cancer in a commercial and medicare advantage US patient population. J Med Econ. 2010;13:351–61.
11. Ritch CR, Cookson MS. Advances in the management of castration resistant prostate cancer. BMJ. 2016;355:i4405.
12. Saad F, Gleason DM, Murray R, Tchekmedyian S, Venner P, Lacombe L, Chin JL, Vinholes JJ, Goas JA, Chen B. Zoledronic acid prostate cancer study group: a randomized, placebo-controlled trial of zoledronic acid in patients with hormone-refractory metastatic prostate carcinoma. J Natl Cancer Inst. 2002;94:1458–68.
13. Fizazi K, Beuzeboc P, Lumbroso J, Haddad V, Massard C, Gross-Goupil M, Di Palma M, Escudier B, Theodore C, Loriot Y, Tournay E, Bouzy J, Laplanche A. Phase II trial of consolidation docetaxel and samarium-153 in patients with bone metastases from castration-resistant prostate cancer. J Clin Oncol. 2009;27:2429–35.
14. Minutoli F, Herberg A, Spadaro P, Restifo Pecorella G, Baldari S, Aricò D, Altavilla G, Baldari S. [186Re] HEDP in the palliation of painful bone metastases from cancers other than prostate and breast. Q J Nucl Med Mol Imaging. 2006;50:355–62.
15. Fuster D, Herranz D, Vidal-Sicart S, et al. Usefulness of strontium-89 for bone pain palliation in metastatic breast cancer patients. Nucl Med Commun. 2000;21:623–6.

16. Kraeber-Bodéré F, Campion L, Rousseau C, et al. Treatment of bone metastases of prostate cancer with strontium-89 chloride: efficacy in relation to the degree of bone involvement. Eur J Nucl Med. 2000;27:1487–93.
17. Ashayeri E, Omogbehin A, Sridhar R, et al. Strontium 89 in the treatment of pain due to diffuse osseous metastases: a university hospital experience. J Natl Med Assoc. 2002;94:706–11.
18. Gunawardana DH, Lichtenstein M, Better N, et al. Results of strontium-89 therapy in patients with prostate cancer resistant to chemotherapy. Clin Nucl Med. 2004;29:81–5.
19. Liepe K, Kotzerke J. A comparative study of 188Re-HEDP, 186Re-HEDP, 153Sm-EDTMP and 89Sr in the treatment of painful skeletal metastases. Nucl Med Commun. 2007;28:623–30.
20. Pacilio M, Ventroni G, De Vincentis G, Cassano B, Pellegrini R, Di Castro E, Frantellizzi V, Follacchio GA, Garkavaya T, Lorenzon L, Ialongo P, Pani R, Mango L. Dosimetry of bone metastases in targeted radionuclide therapy with alpha-emitting (223)Ra-dichloride. Eur J Nucl Med Mol Imaging. 2016;43:21–33.
21. Correa-González L, Arteaga de Murphy C, Pichardo-Romero P, Pedraza-López M, Moreno-García C, Correa-Hernández L. (153)Sm-EDTMP for pain relief of bone metastases from prostate and breast cancer and other malignancies. Arch Med Res. 2014;45:301–8.
22. Nilsson S, Larsen RH, Fosså SD, Balteskard L, Borch KW, Westlin JE, Salberg G, Bruland OS. First clinical experience with alpha-emitting radium-223 in the treatment of skeletal metastases. Clin Cancer Res. 2005;11:4451–9.
23. Nilsson S, Franzén L, Parker C, Tyrrell C, Blom R, Tennvall J, Lennernäs B, Petersson U, Johannessen DC, Sokal M, Pigott K, Yachnin J, Garkavij M, Strang P, Harmenberg J, Bolstad B, Bruland OS. Bone-targeted radium-223 in symptomatic, hormone-refractory prostate cancer: a randomised, multicentre, placebo-controlled phase II study. Lancet Oncol. 2007;8:587–94.
24. Parker C, Nilsson S, Heinrich D, Helle SI, O'Sullivan JM, Fosså SD, Chodacki A, Wiechno P, Logue J, Seke M, Widmark A, Johannessen DC, Hoskin P, Bottomley D, James ND, Solberg A, Syndikus I, Kliment J, Wedel S, Boehmer S, Dall'Oglio M, Franzén L, Coleman R, Vogelzang NJ, O'Bryan-Tear CG, Staudacher K, Garcia-Vargas J, Shan M, Bruland ØS, Sartor O, ALSYMPCA Investigators. Alpha emitter radium-223 and survival in metastatic prostate cancer. N Engl J Med. 2013;369:213–23.
25. Sartor O, Hoskin P, Coleman RE, et al. Chemotherapy following radium-223 dichloride treatment in ALSYMPCA. Prostate. 2016;76:905–16.
26. Alva A, Nordquist L, Daignault S, George S, Ramos J, Albany C, Isharwal S, McDonald M, Campbell G, Danchaivijitr P, Yentz S, Anand A, Yu EY. Clinical correlates of benefit from Radium-223 therapy in metastatic castration resistant prostate cancer. Prostate. 2017;77:479–88.
27. ema.europa.eu. Summary of product characteristics. http://www.ema.europa.eu/docs/en_GB/document_library/EPAR__Product_Information/human/002653/WC500156172.pdf. Accessed Mar 2017.
28. Baldari S, Boni G, Bortolus R, CAffo O, Conti G, De Vincentis G, Monari F, Procopio G, Santini D, Seregni E, Valdagni R. Management of metastatic castration-resistant prostate cancer: a focus on radium-223. Crit Rev Oncol Hematol. 2017;113:43–51.
29. Sartor AO, Heinrich D, Mariados N. Radium-223 (Ra-223) re-treatment (Re-tx): first experience from an international, multicenter, prospective study in patients (Pts) with castration-resistant prostate cancer and bone metastases (mCRPC). J Clin Oncol. 2016;34(Suppl 2S):197. Dent Abstr
30. Zimmerman BE, Bergeron DE, Cessna JT, Fitzgerald R, Pibida L. Revision of the NIST standard for (223)Ra: new measurements and review of 2008 data. J Res Natl Inst Stand Technol. 2015;120:37–57.
31. Prior JO, Gillessen S, Wirth M, Dale W, Aapro M, Oyen WJG. Radiopharmaceuticals in the elderly cancer patient: practical considerations, with a focus on prostate cancer therapy: a position paper from the International Society of Geriatric Oncology Task Force. Eur J Cancer. 2017;77:127–39.
32. Miyazaki KS, Kuang Y, Kwee SA. Changes in skeletal tumor activity on (18)F-choline PET/CT in patients receiving (223)radium radionuclide therapy for metastatic prostate cancer. Nucl Med Mol Imaging. 2015;49:160–4.
33. Ahmadzadehfar H, Schlenkhoff CD, Rogenhofer S, Yordanova A, Essler M. 68Ga-PSMA-11 PET represents the tumoricidal effect of 223Ra in a patient with castrate-resistant metastatic prostate cancer. Clin Nucl Med. 2016;41:695–6.
34. Seibel MJ. Biochemical markers of bone turnover: part I: biochemistry and variability. Clin Biochem Rev. 2005;26:97–122.
35. Jung K, Lein M, Stephan C, Von Hösslin K, Semjonow A, Sinha P, Loening SA, Schnorr D. Comparison of 10 serum bone turnover markers in prostate carcinoma patients with bone metastatic spread: diagnostic and prognostic implications. Int J Cancer. 2004;111:783–91.
36. Berruti A, Tucci M, Mosca A, Tarabuzzi R, Gorzegno G, Terrone C, Vana F, Lamanna G, Tampellini M, Porpiglia F, Angeli A, Scarpa RM, Dogliotti L. Predictive factors for skeletal complications in hormone-refractory prostate cancer patients with metastatic bone disease. Br J Cancer. 2005;93:633–8.
37. Smith MR, Cook RJ, Coleman R, Brown J, Lipton A, Major P, Hei YJ, Saad F. Predictors of skeletal complications in men with hormone-refractory metastatic prostate cancer. Urology. 2007;70:315–9.
38. Cook RJ, Coleman R, Brown J, Lipton A, Major P, Hei YJ, Saad F, Smith MR. Markers of bone metabolism and survival in men with hormone-refractory metastatic prostate cancer. Clin Cancer Res. 2006;12(11 Pt 1):3361–7.

39. Som A, Tu SM, Liu J, Wang X, Qiao W, Logothetis C, Corn PG. Response in bone turnover markers during therapy predicts overall survival in patients with metastatic prostate cancer: analysis of three clinical trials. Br J Cancer. 2012;107:1547–53.
40. Fox JJ, Morris MJ, Larson SM, Schöder H, Scher HI. Developing imaging strategies for castration resistant prostate cancer. Acta Oncol. 2011;50(Suppl 1):39–48.
41. Dennis ER, Jia X, Mezheritskiy IS, Stephenson RD, Schoder H, Fox JJ, Heller G, Scher HI, Larson SM, Morris MJ. Bone scan index: a quantitative treatment response biomarker for castration-resistant metastatic prostate cancer. J Clin Oncol. 2012;30: 519–24.
42. Sartor O, Coleman RE, Nilsson S, et al. 3-year follow-up of chemotherapy following radium-223 dichloride (Ra-223) in castration-resistant prostate cancer (CRPC) patients (Pts) with symptomatic bone metastases (Mets) from ALSYMPCA. Presented at: European Cancer Congress 2015. Vienna, Austria: Poster session. Abstract 2510.
43. Evangelista L, Bertoldo F, Boccardo F, Conti G, Menchi I, Mungai F, Ricardi U, Bombardieri E. Diagnostic imaging to detect and evaluate response to therapy in bone metastases from prostate cancer: current modalities and new horizons. Eur J Nucl Med Mol Imaging. 2016;43:1546–62.
44. Withofs N, Grayet B, Tancredi T, Rorive A, Mella C, Giacomelli F, Mievis F, Aerts J, Waltregny D, Jerusalem G, Hustinx R. ^{18}F-fluoride PET/CT for assessing bone involvement in prostate and breast cancers. Nucl Med Commun. 2011;32:168–76.
45. Pacilio M, Cassano B, Chiesa C, Giancola S, Ferrari M, Pettinato C, Amato E, Fioroni F, Lorenzon L, Pellegrini R, Di Castro E, Pani R, Cremonesi M. The Italian multicentre dosimetric study for lesion dosimetry in (223)Ra therapy of bone metastases: calibration protocol of gamma cameras and patient eligibility criteria. Phys Med. 2016;32:1731–7.

Novel Approaches of Treatment with Radium-223 Targeted Therapy

28

Giovanni Luca Ceresoli, Letizia Gianoncelli, Maria Bonomi, Eleonora Cerchiaro, and Emilio Bombardieri

Abstract

The role of radium-223 (Ra-223) in metastatic castration-resistant prostate cancer (mCRPC) with bone metastases and no visceral disease is well established in clinical practice. Treatment with Ra-223 is well tolerated and significantly improves overall survival and time to first symptomatic skeletal event. Several questions, however, remain open. Patient selection is critical, and treatment assessment is challenging. There is no standard imaging, and PSA has limited usefulness in this setting.

Furthermore, the optimal schedule and dosing of Ra-223 remain to be defined by current trials. Combined treatments with AR-targeting agents such as abiraterone and enzalutamide will probably extend the use of Ra-223 to cases with concomitant bone and visceral disease. Due to ist peculiar mechanism of action and good toxicity profile, Ra-223 is being explored beyond mCRPC in several other neoplasms with predominant bone disease.

28.1 Current Practice of Ra-223

28.1.1 The ALSYMPCA Trial: Data and Post Hoc Analyses

Most patients with metastatic castration-resistant prostate cancer (mCRPC) have radiological evidence of bone metastases, often leading to symptomatic skeletal events (SSEs) such as pain and fractures and to decreased survival and quality of life (QoL) [1]. Radium-223 (Ra-223) has been approved worldwide for clinical use in patients with mCRPC and at least two symptomatic bone

G.L. Ceresoli (✉)
Department of Medical Oncology, Cliniche Humanitas Gavazzeni, Bergamo, Italy

Thoracic and GU Oncology Unit, Cliniche Humanitas Gavazzeni, Bergamo, Italy
e-mail: giovanni_luca.ceresoli@gavazzeni.it

L. Gianoncelli • M. Bonomi • E. Cerchiaro
Department of Medical Oncology, Cliniche Humanitas Gavazzeni, Bergamo, Italy

E. Bombardieri
Department of Nuclear Medicine, Cliniche Humanitas Gavazzeni, Bergamo, Italy

E. Bombardieri et al. (eds.), *Clinical Applications of Nuclear Medicine Targeted Therapy*,
https://doi.org/10.1007/978-3-319-63067-0_28

metastases and no visceral disease, in a time in which the therapeutic landscape for patients with mCRPC has rapidly changed due to the introduction of several other active drugs in this setting [2]. In the pivotal ALSYMPCA trial, a Phase III randomized, double-blind placebo-controlled study, 921 patients were randomized to receive Ra-223 at the dose of 50 kBq/kg versus placebo for 6 cycles repeated at 4-week intervals [3]. Eligibility criteria included the presence of at least two symptomatic bone metastases, the absence of visceral disease except for a lymph nodal disease <3 cm, and a confirmed status of mCRPC. Patients were eligible irrespective of prior docetaxel treatment and were stratified according to prior docetaxel, bisphosphonate use, and levels of alkaline phosphatase (ALP). Primary endpoint of the study was overall survival (OS), while secondary endpoints were time to first SSE, safety, and QoL.

Ra-223 was associated with a significantly longer OS as compared to the matched placebo; median OS was improved by 3.6 months, with a hazard ratio (HR) of 0.70 (95% CI 0.58–0.83, $p < 0.001$). Moreover, median time to first SSE was prolonged by 5.8 months, with an HR of 0.66 (95% CI 0.52–0.83, $p < 0.001$). The risks of external beam radiation therapy (EBRT) for bone pain (HR 0.67, 95% CI 0.53–0.85) and spinal cord compression (HR = 0.52, 95% CI 0.29–0.93) were reduced with Ra-233 compared with placebo. Conversely, Ra-223 treatment did not significantly reduce the risk of symptomatic pathological bone fracture or the need for tumor-related orthopedic surgical intervention [4]. Patients treated with Ra-223 had also a meaningful improvement in QoL, measured according to two validated instruments: the general EuroQoL 5D (EQ-5D) and the disease-specific Functional Assessment of Cancer Therapy-Prostate (FACT-P) scores [5]. Health-care resource use, including hospitalization events and days, was prospectively collected in ALSYMPCA. Significantly fewer Ra-223 versus placebo patients (37.0 vs 45.5%, $p = 0.016$) had at least one hospitalization event. There were significantly fewer hospitalization days per patient for Ra-223 (4.44 versus 6.68, respectively, $p = 0.004$). The reduction in hospitalization days with Ra-223 was observed both before first SSE and after SSE [6].

In the ALSYMPCA trial, eligible patients were required to have symptomatic disease; however, symptomatic was broadly defined, in that opioid use was not required and patients were defined as minimally symptomatic if they had regular use of any analgesic medication or if they had received EBRT in the 12 weeks before randomization. Additional analyses included time to first opioid use, time to first EBRT for bone pain, and safety of concomitant EBRT [7]. At baseline, 408 (44%) patients had no pain and no analgesic use or mild pain with non-opioid therapy (World Health Organization ladder pain score 0–1 [non-opioid subgroup]), and 513 (56%) had moderate pain with occasional opioids or severe pain with regular daily opioids (World Health Organization ladder pain score 2–3 [opioid subgroup]). Ra-223 significantly prolonged OS and significantly reduced the risk of SSEs versus placebo regardless of baseline opioid use. Time to first opioid use for bone pain was significantly delayed with Ra-223 versus placebo (HR = 0.62, 95% CI 0.46–0.85, $p = 0.002$). Adverse event incidence was similar between opioid subgroups. During the study, 30% of Ra-223 patients and 34% of placebo patients received EBRT for bone pain. Ra-223 significantly reduced the risk of needing EBRT for bone pain versus placebo (HR = 0.67, 95% CI 0.53–0.85, $p = 0.001$). No differences were observed in the safety profile (particularly as regards myelosuppression) between patients who did and did not receive concomitant EBRT for bone pain during the study [7].

Ra-223 showed a favorable toxicity profile, with a low incidence of grade 3–4 toxicities. The most frequent adverse events were minor gastrointestinal side effects and mild neutropenia and thrombocytopenia. A severe anemia was observed in 13% of patients and a thrombocytopenia in 6% of patients, but their rate was similar in the placebo arm [3]. A post hoc analysis of the toxicity pattern in the ALSYMPCA trial [8] showed that the risk of a severe thrombocytopenia was associated with prior use of docetaxel and with lower basal levels of platelets and hemoglobin and that an increased risk of grade 2–4 anemia was related to the presence of more than six bone metastases and to a higher PSA at treatment start. Neutropenia events were too few in placebo patients for a comparative analysis. There was no significant association between hematologic toxicities and number of Ra-223 injections received (4–6 versus 1–3).

Patients were enrolled in the ALSYMPCA trial independently of the prior use of docetaxel. Overall, 526 (57%) of 921 randomly assigned patients had received previous docetaxel treatment (352 in the Ra-223 and 174 in the placebo group), and 395 (43%) had not (262 in the Ra-223 and 133 in the placebo group). A prespecified subgroup analysis revealed that the OS benefit was maintained in both docetaxel-pretreated and docetaxel-naïve patients, with a similar hazard ratio [9]. Namely, in patients with previous docetaxel use, Ra-223 prolonged median OS from 11.3 to 14.4 months (HR 0.70, 95% CI 0.56–0.88; $p = 0.002$), while in patients without previous docetaxel use, mOS was 16.1 months with Ra-223 versus 11.5 months in the placebo group (HR 0.69, 0.52–0.92; $p = 0.01$). The benefit of Ra-223 compared with placebo was seen in both docetaxel subgroups for most main secondary efficacy endpoints; however, time to first SSE was reduced in patients with previous docetaxel use, but the difference was not significant in those with no previous docetaxel use. Patients pretreated with docetaxel had a higher incidence of grade 3–4 thrombocytopenia with Ra-223 than with placebo (9 versus 3%), whereas the incidence was similar between treatment groups among patients with no previous docetaxel use (3 versus 1%). On the contrary, the incidence of grade 3–4 anemia and neutropenia was similar between the Ra-223 and placebo groups within both docetaxel subgroups [9].

Current international guidelines recommend Ra-223 as an option in both pre-and post-docetaxel settings. Interestingly, no safety concern was identified in an exploratory analysis of prospectively collected data from ALSYMPCA trial in patients who received subsequent chemotherapy after Ra-223 or placebo [10]. Therefore, the use of chemotherapy following Ra-223 seems feasible and effective. These observations suggest the opportunity of an earlier use of Ra-223 itself, when tumor burden is limited, hemoglobin level is adequate, and patients are more likely to complete the planned treatment [11].

28.1.2 The Ra-223 Expanded Access Program

The expanded access program was a Phase IIIB trial conducted after the closure of ALSYMPCA and before regulatory approval [12]. Overall, 839 patients with mCRPC and at least 2 bone metastases were treated with Ra-223 at the dose of 50 kBq/kg delivered every 4 weeks for up to 6 cycles. As in the ALSYMPCA trial, limited lymph node metastases were allowed. Notably, also asymptomatic cases could participate in the study. Moreover, other concomitant anticancer treatments (such as denosumab, abiraterone, and enzalutamide) were admitted. Safety and OS were the primary endpoints of the study, which were evaluable in 696 patients. Median OS was 16 months. Ra-223 was generally well tolerated, with no new safety concerns as compared to the ALSYMPCA trial. In particular, grade 3–4 adverse events were observed in 37% of patients; grade 3 anemia occurred in 12%, grade 3–4 thrombocytopenia in 3%, and grade 3–4 neutropenia in 2% [12]. Several prognostic factors were highlighted in this large "real-life" series of patients treated with Ra-223. Patients with hemoglobin ≥ 10 g/dL and with normal serum total ALP had a significantly longer OS, as well as patients with good Eastern Cooperative Oncology Group (ECOG) performance status (PS) (0–1 versus 2) and patients with no or mild baseline pain (as opposed to moderate to severe pain) [12]. Importantly, in the early access program, patients were allowed to receive other oncological treatments concomitantly to Ra-223. In a post hoc exploratory analysis on this population, a longer OS was found in patients who received Ra-223 with concomitant denosumab and in those who received concomitant abiraterone, enzalutamide, or both, than in patients treated with Ra-223 alone. These findings are under evaluation in specifically designed prospective, randomized clinical trials.

28.1.3 Patient Selection and Response Assessment with Ra-223

28.1.3.1 Imaging

Imaging has a key role in the proper selection and monitoring of patients who are candidates to Ra-223. The goal of imaging in this setting is to evaluate skeletal disease and to rule out the onset of visceral disease at the same time [13]. In the ALSYMPCA trial, a bone scintigraphy with ^{99m}TC-diphosphonate and a contrast-enhanced CT scan were performed at screening for patient selection; however, no imaging modalities were scheduled during and after treatment. Indeed, there are no established criteria to evaluate bone disease; in fact, bone metastases are considered as non-target lesions by RECIST criteria [14]. The evaluation of bone metastases by CT scan is challenging [15]. Two main options are offered by molecular imaging: bone-targeting tracers (i.e., ^{99m}Tc-phosphonate and ^{18}F-fluoride) and cancer-targeting agents (^{11}C/^{18}F-choline, ^{68}Ga-PSMA) [16]. Some preliminary data seem to indicate more advantages of cancer-targeting over bone-targeting tracers. In fact, cancer-targeting radiopharmaceutical agents can assess cancer metabolism both at bone level and in the viscera and are less influenced by the flare phenomenon than bone-targeting radiotracers. On the other hand, interpretation of cancer-targeting PET/CT scans after Ra-223 is often challenging due to the occurrence of mixed responses, in which a few lesions disappear while other apparently progress [17].

28.1.3.2 Biomarkers

In an exploratory analysis of biomarker dynamics in the ALSYMPCA trial, increase of total ALP and lactate dehydrogenase (LDH) was associated with the risk of death, while prostate-specific antigen (PSA) changes were not [18]. PSA levels typically continue to rise during the early phase of treatment courses. A PSA flare phenomenon during treatment with Ra-223 has been described and can be misinterpreted as therapeutic failure [19, 20]. A decline in PSA is usually observed in responding patients only after at least 4 or 5 months of treatment. PSA test is therefore not recommended in response assessment during therapy with Ra-223; particularly, treatment with Ra-223 should not be discontinued on the occurrence of an asymptomatic PSA rise not supported by a radiological disease progression. On the contrary, in the ALSYMPCA trial, a decrease in total ALP levels was almost always observed in responding patients during treatment with Ra-223. Namely, a decline of ALP at week 12 was associated with an improvement in OS, with a difference in median OS of 7.4 months (17.8 versus 10.4 months) and an HR of 0.45 (95% CI 0.34–0.61, $p < 0.0001$) [18].

28.1.3.3 Patient Selection and Response Evaluation for Ra-223 in Clinical Practice

Based on the data of the ALSYMPCA trial and of the expanded access program, treatment with Ra-223 should be proposed to patients with mCRPC, ≥2 detectable symptomatic bone metastases, and no visceral disease. Lymph nodal disease up to 3 cm of diameter in short axis is allowed. Symptomatic patients include cases with regular assumption of analgesic medication (non-opioid or opioid) or pain-free after recent palliative EBRT for cancer-related bone pain.

Prior docetaxel is allowed, but patients should be treated as early as possible, avoiding very advanced cases with poor PS, severe pain, or "bulky" disease (appearing as a "superscan" at nuclear medicine imaging), who are at higher risk of treatment failure, early development of visceral disease, and hematologic toxicity. Risk factors for severe hematologic adverse events should be identified, and patients at higher risk should be monitored carefully [11].

Few established data are available to guide imaging evaluation of response to Ra-223. Patients should be screened at baseline at least with a thoracic and abdominal contrast-enhanced CT scan to rule out visceral disease and with a bone scintigraphy with ^{99m}Tc-phosphonate to identify bone metastases. ^{11}C/^{18}F-choline or ^{68}Ga-PSMA PET/CT can substitute or complement CT scan [16,

17]. An interim CT or PET/CT scan after 3 administrations of Ra-223 is advisable in patients at high risk of visceral progression (generally characterized by higher bone disease volume, higher Gleason score, and shorter PSA doubling time). After conclusion of treatment with Ra-223, patients should be evaluated with a new bone scintigraphy with ^{99m}Tc-phosphonate and with a CT or PET/CT scan, according to previous imaging. Baseline, interim, and final evaluations of ALP and LDH are recommended. Importantly, clinical benefit and pain control, as well as hematologic parameters to monitor toxicity, should be evaluated at each treatment cycle. As previously discussed, PSA test should not be used to measure response during therapy with Ra-223 [11].

28.2 Therapeutic Challenges and New Scenarios of Ra-223

28.2.1 Biology and Mechanism of Action of Ra-223

The potential of Ra-223 in the treatment of mCRPC has been exploited only partially, and its role in the therapeutic management of this disease is yet to be fully established [11, 21]. Much remains to be learned about the biology by which Ra-223 exerts its clinical effect. Understanding this biology will likely yield the identification of additional therapeutic opportunities.

It is well known that prostate cancer cells induce a unique osteogenic program, which underlies their high bone tropism [22]. Prostate cancer cells activate bone development pathways in osteoblasts, leading to their proliferation and differentiation. In turn, these activated osteoblasts produce soluble factors that promote prostate cancer growth, thus favoring bone metastases. Osteoblasts also activate osteoclasts via RANK/RANKL, generating the "vicious cycle" of prostate cancer bone metastases, as osteoclasts induce turnover of the bone microenvironment, further stimulating growth of prostate cancer cells and creating a "niche" for metastatic growth [22–24].

Treatment with Ra-223 improves OS and delays SSEs, and a decrease in bone metabolism markers such as ALP is observed in responding patients; however, it does not appreciatively impact PSA. It has been hypothesized therefore that Ra-223 might act by targeting of the bone microenvironment, as opposed to having a directly tumoricidal effect [25].

Recently, Suominen et al. have reported the results of a preclinical study with two different prostate cancer xenograft models, demonstrating marked tumor growth suppression and inhibition of tumor-induced bone alteration in Ra-223-treated animals [26]. The same authors had previously reported similar findings with Ra-223 treatment in a mouse model of osteolytic breast cancer bone metastasis, suggesting that Ra-223 might be effective regardless of the primary tumor origin and the type of tumor-induced pathological effects on the bone [27]. They conclude that Ra-223 therapy likely possesses a dual mode of action, which inhibits tumor growth and suppresses tumor-induced abnormal bone formation, both essential players in the destructive vicious cycle of osteoblastic bone metastasis in prostate cancer [26].

Ra-223 was recently shown to induce T-cell-mediated lysis in human prostate, breast, and lung carcinoma cells [28]. There is increasing interest into the interaction between radiation therapy and the host immune system [28–31]. Radiation promotes the release of danger signals and chemokines that can recruit inflammatory cells into the tumor microenvironment, including antigen-presenting cells that activate cytotoxic T-cell functions. On the other hand, radiation can attract immunosuppressive cells into the tumor microenvironment. Several questions regarding the interaction between radiation and immunotherapy remain unanswered. The effects of different types of radiation (photons, protons, alfa, beta), as well as the issues of optimal radiation dose, schedules, and field size, are under active investigations in several tumor models, and preliminary trials on cancer patients are ongoing [31]. Additional preclinical studies in immunocompetent animal models are required to evaluate the immunotherapeutic effects of Ra-223 in prostate cancer and the possible efficacy of Ra-223 in combination with immune checkpoint inhibitors.

Finally, alpha radiation induces cell death by causing both single- and double-stranded DNA breaks. Combining DNA-damaging treatments such as platinum-based chemotherapy or PARP (polyADP ribose polymerase) inhibitors with Ra-223 may also offer opportunities for achieving therapeutic synergy. It has also proposed that single-agent Ra-223, as reported for PARP inhibitors [32], may be more effective in patients whose tumors harbor defects in DNA repair genes [21].

In conclusion, all these modern insights on the mechanism of action of Ra-223 strongly support the role of combination regimens of Ra-223 with other compounds, including bone-targeting agents (zoledronic acid, denosumab), agents targeting the androgen receptor pathway (abiraterone, enzalutamide), chemotherapy (docetaxel), immune checkpoint inhibitors, and PARP inhibitors.

28.2.2 Long-Term Safety

Treatment with Ra-223 is so far considered safe also in a long-term period of observation. No reports of late toxicity or secondary cancers (such as acute myeloid leukemia, myelodysplastic syndromes, or new primary bone cancer) were reported in 571 patients treated with Ra-223 in the ALSYMPCA trial over a 3-year follow-up period [33]. The most common adverse events at an interim analysis at 1.5 years were hematologic; however, myelosuppression incidence was <3%, and there were no grade 3 or 4 non-hematologic adverse events except for one pathological fracture (<1%).

The REASSURE study aims to provide further information in the evaluation of long-term toxicities [34]. REASSURE is a global, multicenter, prospective, uncontrolled, observational cohort study documenting data from patients with mCRPC receiving Ra-223 in a routine clinical practice setting. A total of 1334 patients will be enrolled and followed up to 7 years. The primary endpoint of the REASSURE trial is long-term safety, including incidence of secondary primary malignancies and long-term bone marrow suppression. Secondary endpoints are OS and pain assessment, as determined by patient responses on the "Brief Pain Inventory short form" (BPI-SF) questionnaire [35].

REASSURE was set up as a regulatory requirement to FDA and EMA to evaluate the long-term safety of Ra-223. The proposed 7-year timeline is based on the finding from the "Spiess study" [36], which follows up the health of 899 patients treated from 1945 to 1955 in Germany with multiple injections of the short-lived alpha-particle emitter Ra-224. The patients suffered predominantly from ankylosing spondylitis and tuberculosis. The most striking consequence of that treatment was the occurrence of 56 malignant bone tumors. They appeared in a temporal wave that peaked between 7 and 8 years after exposure [36].

28.2.3 Dose and Duration of RA-223 Treatment

At the currently approved dosage of 50 kBq/kg for 6 monthly injections, Ra-223 is well tolerated, with minimal hematologic toxicity. However, the current regimen was established based on limited dose escalation studies, and a maximum tolerated dose (MTD) has not been established. Therefore, the optimal dose and schedule of Ra-223 remain to be determined.

A Phase II, international, multicenter randomized study conducted on 360 patients from approximately 110 centers worldwide has assessed different doses and regimens of Ra-223 [37]. Eligibility criteria mirrored those of the ALSYMPCA trial, including a confirmed diagnosis of mCRPC, with ECOG PS 0–2, two or more skeletal metastases, adequate bone marrow function, and absence of visceral metastases or lymph node lesions >3 cm in short axis. The standard dose of 50 kBq/kg for 6 cycles was compared with the same dose for 12 cycles and with 6 cycles of high-dose Ra-223 at 80 kBq/kg. The primary endpoint of the trial was SSE-free survival. Secondary endpoints were safety, radiological PFS, OS, and pain control. Exploratory endpoints included PSA and ALP levels and a quantitative bone scan analysis. A prolonged follow-up to 7 years from treatment was planned in order to monitor long-term safety. The study has closed its enrollment in September 2015 and the first results are awaited soon.

On the other hand, a recent international, single-arm, open-label multicenter Phase II study in mCRPC with ≥2 bone metastases has explored the benefit of re-treatment with Ra-223 in patients who had already received 6 cycles and progressing thereafter with no visceral disease [38]. Re-treatment consisted of 6 further cycles of Ra-223, administered at the standard dose of 50 kBq/kg at 4-week intervals. Eligibility criteria for re-treatment with Ra-223 included an ECOG PS 0–2 and an adequate hematologic function. No chemotherapy was allowed after the first Ra-223 treatment. The primary endpoint of the trial was safety. Overall, 44 patients were included. Twenty-nine (66%) completed all the 6 re-treatment injections. No new safety concerns were noted; only two patients had grade 3 hematologic adverse events. Median radiological PFS was 9.9 months; interestingly, only one patient in this group had bone progression, and most progressions were at soft tissue sites.

28.2.4 Combination of RA-223 with Other Anticancer Drugs

The unique mechanism of action of Ra-223 does not overlap with other available treatments, and the drug is suitable for both sequencing and combination studies. Combination therapy may improve outcomes without increasing toxicities.

28.2.4.1 Androgen Receptor (AR)-Targeting Agents

As already discussed in this chapter, in a post hoc exploratory analysis of the early access program, patients receiving Ra-223 in combination with abiraterone, enzalutamide, or both had a significantly longer OS as compared to patients treated with Ra-223 alone, with no significant increase of toxicity [12]. Both Ra-223 and AR-targeting therapies increase OS and prolong the time to first SSE in mCRPC [3, 39–48]. Moreover, Ra-223 and AR-targeting agents act by distinct mechanisms and have likely non-overlapping mechanisms of resistance and noncumulative adverse effects.

Two large Phase III trials are testing the combination of one AR-targeting agent plus Ra-223 versus the same agent alone. The ERA 223 study [49] is a double-blind, placebo-controlled study testing abiraterone combined with either Ra-223 or placebo in chemo-naïve mCRPC patients with ECOG PS 0–1 and asymptomatic or mildly symptomatic bone metastases. Patients were stratified according to geographical region, concomitant use of bisphosphonates or denosumab, and ALP baseline levels. The primary endpoint of the trial was SSE-free survival. Secondary endpoints included OS, radiographic PFS (rPFS), safety, time to opiate use for cancer pain, time to pain progression, and health-related QoL. The study accrual was closed in September 2016, after the enrollment of 806 pts, and results are awaited soon. The PEACE-III trial is an open-label, Phase III study testing enzalutamide alone versus the combination of enzalutamide with Ra-223 in a similar patient cohort [50]. The primary endpoint of the study is rPFS. This endpoint may be perceived as risky, as although enzalutamide impacts rPFS, the impact of Ra-223 on rPFS is unknown. Secondary endpoints include OS, prostate cancer-specific survival, and time to first SSE. The PEACE-III trial is sponsored by the EORTC (European Organization for Research and Treatment of Cancer); 560 patients will be accrued by the end of 2017.

28.2.4.2 Docetaxel

The combination of docetaxel with Ra-223 has a strong rationale, as both these compounds have an OS benefit, one agent targets the bone while the other the tumor itself, and radiation and chemotherapy may have mutually amplifying antitumor effects. Issues that can arise when combining these treatments include safety, optimal dosing, sequencing, duration, and patient selection.

A Phase I/II randomized trial of Ra-223 plus docetaxel in mCRPC patients with bone metastases has been recently reported [51]. This trial included a dose escalation study followed by a Phase II randomized expansion study. In the expansion study, the dose of docetaxel selected for the Ra-223 combination arm was lower (60 mg/m^2) than the docetaxel alone arm (75 mg/m^2) due to greater toxicities observed with the higher dose of docetaxel in the Phase I part of the trial. Overall, 53 patients with ≥2 bone metastases were randomized 2:1 to Ra-223 (at standard dose for 6 cycles) plus docetaxel (at 60 mg/m^2 every 3 weeks for 10 cycles) versus docetaxel at 75 mg/m^2 every 3 weeks for 10 cycles, with step-down option to 60 mg/m^2. Total ALP, PSA, and several bone resorption and formation markers were analyzed at week 19 (after 3 Ra-223 injections) and 3 weeks after the end of treatment. At these doses, hematologic adverse events were higher in the single-agent docetaxel arm. On the contrary, patients in the combination arm had a greater decline in total ALP and in bone formation markers. Due to the small patient number, data are very preliminary, and further analysis and correlation with clinical outcomes in a larger study are warranted [52].

28.2.4.3 Other Agents

Other combinations of Ra-223 are being explored in patients with mCRPC.

It has been demonstrated that mCRPC can carry genomic alterations that interfere with DNA repair [32, 53–56]. Some of these DNA repair defects, including BRCA2 loss and ATM aberrations, have been associated with sensitivity to platinum derivatives and PARP inhibitors. Particularly, treatment with the PARP inhibitor olaparib in patients whose prostate cancer was no longer responding to standard treatments and who had defects in DNA repair genes led to a high response rate [32]. Platinum-based chemotherapy is generally not used for the treatment of mCRPC, since several studies have failed to show a survival benefit in unselected patients [57]. Nevertheless, responses to single-agent chemotherapy with a platinum analogue such as satraplatin have been reported [58]. Alpha radiation induces cell death by both single- and double-stranded DNA breaks. Inhibitors of DNA damage repair pathways may synergize with Ra-223 in inducing tumor cell death. Clinical trials combining Ra-223 with PARP inhibitors are being planned. Namely, a Phase IB trial of Ra-223 and niraparib in patients with mCRPC is ongoing. There will be 3 dose levels of niraparib combined with standard doses of Ra-223 to be evaluated for safety [59].

Based on the upcoming evidence that radiation therapy is able to induce the activation of antitumor immune responses [30, 31], there is great interest in combining Ra-223 with immunotherapy. Importantly, Ra-223 has no potentially overlapping toxicities with most immunotherapies. One critical issue of clinical trial design is selecting appropriate endpoints, as initial changes in tumor burden may not reflect survival benefit during treatment with immunotherapy [60].

The combination of radiation and vaccination has been found to increase the induction of antitumor antibody responses compared with radiation alone [61]. Based on this rationale, an ongoing trial is examining the combination of sipuleucel-T with Ra-223 [62]. Another possible mechanism of radiation is the upregulation of the immune checkpoint PD-1/PD-L1 pathway [30]. Several trials combining PD-1/PD-L1 inhibitors and Ra-223 are being planned. A randomized Phase II study evaluating the addition of pembrolizumab to Ra-223 has been proposed [63]. Patients previously treated with enzalutamide or abiraterone will be randomized to the combination versus Ra-223 alone. Primary endpoint of the study is the identification of immune changes in the tumor microenvironment in the two treatment arms (by a bone biopsy at baseline and at 8 weeks). Secondary endpoints include OS, PFS, and safety. Another study was designed to assess the safety and tolerability of atezolizumab when given in combination with Ra-223 in mCRPC patients who have progressed after treatment with an AR inhibitor. An adaptive design is planned to first investigate the tolerability of concurrent administration, with both treatments to begin in the first cycle. However, if the combination is not tolerated, additional cohorts may be enrolled to evaluate the tolerability of Ra-223 (to begin in cycle 1) with delayed atezolizumab (to begin in cycle 2 or 3) [64].

28.2.5 Treatment with Ra-223 in Other Indications Beyond mCRPC

Due to its mechanism of action and the favorable toxicity profile, several studies are exploring the potential of Ra-223, mainly in combination with other agents, in other cancers with a dominant bone disease [65, 66].

28.2.5.1 Castration-Sensitive Prostate Cancer

As already discussed for mCRPC, an earlier use of Ra-223 in the clinical history of prostate cancer should probably exploit the full therapeutic potential of this agent, minimizing at the same time the risk of treatment failure and toxicity. The setting of metastatic castration-sensitive prostate cancer (mCSPC) with bone metastases is therefore particularly attractive, although until now substantially unexplored. A randomized Phase II study is ongoing comparing androgen deprivation therapy (ADT) versus ADT plus Ra-223 at standard doses. According to the study plan, 204 patients will be randomized in a 2:1 design and stratified according to ALP levels and to the extent of disease (<6 skeletal metastases with no visceral disease versus ≥6 skeletal metastases or presence of visceral localizations) [67]. The primary endpoint of the trial is rPFS, while secondary endpoints include OS, time to first SSE, safety, and QoL.

28.2.5.2 Breast Cancer

Ra-223 is being explored also beyond prostate cancer. A Phase II exploratory trial was reported in 23 heavily pretreated patients with metastatic breast cancer with progressing bone-dominant disease and no longer candidates for further endocrine therapy [68]. Patients received Ra-223 at the dose of 50 kBq/kg every 4 weeks for 4 cycles. Coprimary endpoints of the study were levels of urinary N-telopeptide of type 1 (uNTX-1) and serum bone ALP (bALP). Secondary endpoints were safety and metabolic response assessed by FDG PET/CT. Treatment was safe and well tolerated, with minimal hematologic toxicity. Ra-223 significantly reduced the bone markers from baseline to end of treatment. Median uNTX-1 change was −10.1 nmol bone collagen equivalents/mmol creatinine (−32.8%; $p = 0.0124$); median bALP change was −16.7 ng/mL (−42.0%; $p = 0.0045$). Twenty of 23 patients had FDG PET/CT, identifying 155 hypermetabolic osteoblastic bone lesions at baseline; 50 lesions showed metabolic decrease after 2 Ra-223 injections (for a 32.3% metabolic response rate at week 9), persisting after the treatment period (with 41.5% metabolic response rate at week 17). Based on this preliminary evidence, two Phase II, double-blind, placebo-controlled randomized studies have been launched in breast cancer patients with bone-predominant disease and candidates to hormonal therapy [69, 70]. In both trials patients are randomized to hormonal therapy versus hormonal therapy plus Ra-223, with SSE-free survival as the primary endpoint. The first study (NCT02258464) [69] will assess efficacy and safety of Ra-223 in 227 patients with HER2-negative, hormone receptor-positive breast cancer with at least 2 bone metastases, treated with hormonal treatment background therapy. Presence of visceral metastases is allowed. Patients must have received at least one line of hormonal therapy in the metastatic setting and must be eligible for further standard of care endocrine treatment. Furthermore, they must have experienced no more than 2 SREs prior to study entry and be on therapy with either bisphosphonate or denosumab. Finally, patients who have either received chemotherapy for metastatic disease or are considered to be appropriate candidates for chemotherapy as current treatment for metastatic breast cancer are excluded from the study. The second study (NCT02258451) [70] has very similar design and eligibility criteria; however, patients must have experienced recurrent or progressive disease following treatment with a non-steroidal aromatase inhibitor (letrozole or anastrozole) in an adjuvant or metastatic setting and will be treated with exemestane plus everolimus in combination with Ra-223, versus the same hormonal therapy plus a matching placebo. The target accrual will be 323 patients.

28.2.5.3 Other Cancers with Bone Involvement

Finally, there are also preliminary studies in other cancers with extensive bone involvement, such as osteosarcoma [71–75], multiple myeloma [76], urothelial tumors [77], and metastatic radioiodine-refractory thyroid cancer [78].

Osteosarcoma is a cancer characterized by formation of primitive bone matrix by the malignant cells per se; therefore, both skeletal and visceral metastases of osteosarcoma can be osteoblastic [71]. Bone scintigraphy by ^{99m}Tc-phosphonate is routinely done at diagnosis to evaluate primary tumor uptake and rule out distant metastases. Preclinical studies in mice with human osteosarcoma xenografts and in dogs with osteosarcoma have shown that Ra-223 may act as a low toxic, highly efficacy targeted agent for this tumor [72]. Based on this background, a Phase I dose escalation clinical trial of Ra-223 (at 50, 75, and 100 kBq/kg) has started for patients with progressive, locally recurrent, or metastatic osteosarcoma, with no standard curative options available and with at least one indicator lesion avid on ^{99m}Tc-phosphonate scan. Molecular imaging with ^{99m}Tc scan, FDG PET, or sodium fluoride-18 (NaF) PET was done at baseline and at restaging. Overall, 18 patients were enrolled. Treatment was well tolerated, with one case of G3 thrombocytopenia seen at 100 kBq/kg. A validated bone pain survey demonstrated a reduction in bone pain. The recommended dose for using Ra-223 in osteosarcoma was 100 kBq/kg monthly [73, 74]. A case showing early activity of Ra-223 and the first clinical evidence of an alpha particle with blood-brain barrier penetration has been published [75]. This patient received 3 infusions of Ra-223 at the dose of 75 kBq/kg at 4-week intervals. A clinical reduction in bone pain and no grade 3–4 toxicities were reported. Post-treatment imaging showed response to therapy at most sites, including a left cerebellar metastasis.

Multiple myeloma is an atypical disease to consider for Ra-223 treatment, given that it has mainly lytic bone involvement. However, bisphosphonates and denosumab, as well as bortezomib, may alter the bone matrix of the disease, potentially leading to a better target for Ra-223 [65]. This is the rationale of an ongoing Phase 1b/II trial [76], aiming to evaluate safety and efficacy of Ra-223 dichloride in combination with bortezomib and dexamethasone in early relapsed multiple myeloma.

Finally, the efficacy of Ra-223 is under evaluation in combination with immunotherapy with atezolizumab in a single-arm pilot trial in patients with urothelial carcinoma with bone metastases progressing after platinum-based chemotherapy [77] and as a single agent in a Phase II trial in radioactive iodine-refractory bone metastases from differentiated thyroid cancer [78].

Conclusions

In conclusion, the use of Ra-223 in mCRPC with bone metastases and no visceral disease is well established in clinical practice. In this setting Ra-223 prolongs OS and time to first SSE and improves QoL. At standard dose Ra-223 is safe and pretty well tolerated. Patient selection is critical, in order to avoid hematologic toxicity. Patients should be treated as early as possible, avoiding to leave treatment with Ra-223 for the last phase of the metastatic disease. Treatment assessment is challenging. There is no standard imaging, although molecular imaging, especially with tumor-targeting tracers, warrants further evaluation. Clinical benefit and ALP levels remain the main drivers of assessment and should always be considered. PSA has limited usefulness in this setting.

The potential of Ra-223 in the treatment of mCRPC has yet to be fully established. Several trials are ongoing to define the optimal schedule and dosing of Ra-223 in mCRPC. Combined treatments, especially with AR-targeting agents such as abiraterone and enzalutamide, are promising, and the results of Phase III trial are eagerly awaited.

Due to ist peculiar mechanism of action and good toxicity profile, Ra-223 is being explored beyond mCRPC in several other neoplasms with predominant bone disease, including mCSPC and metastatic breast cancer.

Key points

- Radium-223 (Ra-223) prolongs overall survival and reduces skeletal events in patients with metastatic castration-resistant prostate cancer (mCRPC) with bone metastases and no visceral disease.
- Patient selection and response assessment are challenging. There is no standard imaging, although molecular imaging is promising. PSA has limited usefulness in this setting.
- Several trials are ongoing to define the optimal schedule and dosing of Ra-223 in mCRPC.
- The combination of Ra-223 with other agents, such as AR-targeting agents, is promising.
- Ra-223 is being explored beyond mCRPC in several other neoplasms with predominant bone disease.

References

1. Saad F, Clarke N, Colombel M. Natural history and treatment of bone complications in prostate cancer. Eur Urol. 2006;49:429–40.
2. Attard G, Parker C, Eeles RA, et al. Prostate cancer. Lancet. 2016;387:70–82.
3. Parker C, Nilsson S, Heinrich D, et al. Alpha emitter radium-223 and survival in metastatic prostate cancer. N Engl J Med. 2013;369:213–23.
4. Sartor O, Coleman R, Nilsson S, et al. Effect of radium-223 dichloride on symptomatic skeletal events in patients with castration-resistant prostate cancer and bone metastases: results from a phase 3, double-blind, randomised trial. Lancet Oncol. 2014;15:738–46.
5. Nilsson S, Cislo P, Sartor O, et al. Patient-reported quality-of-life analysis of radium-223 dichloride from the phase III ALSYMPCA study. Ann Oncol. 2016;27:868–74.
6. Parker C, Zhan L, Cislo P, et al. Effect of radium-223 dichloride (Ra-223) on hospitalisation: an analysis from the phase 3 randomised Alpharadin in Symptomatic Prostate Cancer Patients (ALSYMPCA) trial. Eur J Cancer. 2017;71:1–6.
7. Parker C, Finkelstein SE, Michalski JM, et al. Efficacy and safety of radium-223 dichloride in symptomatic castration-resistant prostate cancer patients with or without baseline opioid use from the phase 3 ALSYMPCA trial. Eur Urol. 2016;70:875–83.
8. Vogelzang NJ, Coleman RE, Michalski JM, et al. Hematologic safety of radium-223 dichloride: baseline prognostic factors associated with myelosuppression in the ALSYMPCA trial. Clin Genitourin Cancer. 2017;15:42–52.
9. Hoskin P, Sartor O, O'Sullivan JM, et al. Efficacy and safety of radium-223 dichloride in patients with castration-resistant prostate cancer and symptomatic bone metastases, with or without previous docetaxel use: a prespecified subgroup analysis from the randomised, double-blind, phase 3 ALSYMPCA trial. Lancet Oncol. 2014;15:1397–406.
10. Sartor O, Hoskin P, Coleman RE, et al. Chemotherapy following radium-223 dichloride treatment in ALSYMPCA. Prostate. 2016;76:905–16.
11. Bombardieri E, Ceresoli GL, Setti L, et al. Role of radium-223 in the treatment of metastatic castration resistant prostate cancer (mCRPC): clinical practice and future perspectives. Clin Oncol. 2016;1:1173.
12. Saad F, Carles J, Gillessen S, et al. Radium-223 and concomitant therapies in patients with metastatic castration-resistant prostate cancer: an international, early access, open-label, single-arm phase 3b trial. Lancet Oncol. 2016;17:1306–16.
13. Etchebehere E, Brito AE, Rezaee A, et al. Therapy assessment of bone metastatic disease in the era of radium 223. Eur J Nucl Med Mol Imaging. 2017;44(Suppl 1):84–96. [Epub ahead of print]
14. Evangelista L, Bertoldo F, Boccardo F, et al. Diagnostic imaging to detect and evaluate response to therapy in bone metastases from prostate cancer: current modalities and new horizons. Eur J Nucl Med Mol Imaging. 2016;43:1546–62.
15. Messiou C, Cook G, Reid AH, et al. The CT flare response of metastatic bone disease in prostate cancer. Acta Radiol. 2011;52:557–61.
16. Gorin MA, Rowe SP, Denmeade SR. Clinical applications of molecular imaging in the management of prostate cancer. PET Clin. 2017;12:185–92.
17. Uprimny C, Kroiss A, Nilica B, et al. 68-Ga-PSMA ligand PET versus 18F-NaF PET: evaluation of response to Ra-223 therapy in a prostate cancer patient. Eur J Nucl Med Mol Imaging. 2015;42:362–3.
18. Sartor O, Coleman RE, Nilsson S, et al. An exploratory analysis of alkaline phosphatase, lactate dehydrogenase, and prostate-specific antigen dynamics in the phase 3 ALSYMPCA trial with radium-223. Ann Oncol. 2017;28:1090–7.
19. McNamara MA, George DJ. Pain, PSA flare, and bone scan response in a patient with metastatic castration-resistant prostate cancer treated with radium-223, a case report. BMC Cancer. 2015;15:371.
20. De Vincentis G, Follacchio GA, Frantellizzi V, et al. Prostate-specific antigen flare phenomenon during 223-Ra-dichloride treatment for bone metastatic castration-resistant prostate cancer: a case report. Clin Genitourin Cancer. 2016;14:e529–33.
21. Miyahira AK, Morris M, Soule HR, PCF Radium-223 Scientific Working Group. Meeting report from the Prostate Cancer Foundation scientific working group on radium-223. Prostate. 2017;77:245–54.
22. Bertoldo F. Biology and pathophysiology of bone metastasis in prostate cancer. In: Bertoldo, et al., editors. Bone metastases from prostate cancer. Switzerland: Springer; 2017.
23. Hensel J, Thalmann GN. Biology of bone metastases in prostate cancer. Urology. 2016;92:6–13.

24. Gartrell BA, Coleman R, Efstathiou E, et al. Metastatic prostate cancer and the bone: significance and therapeutic options. Eur Urol. 2015;68:850–8.
25. Wang N, Docherty FE, Brown HK, et al. Prostate cancer cells preferentially home to osteoblast-rich areas in the early stages of bone metastasis: evidence from in vivo models. J Bone Miner Res. 2014;29:2688–96.
26. Suominen MI, Fagerlund KM, Rissanen JP, et al. Radium-223 inhibits osseous prostate cancer growth by dual targeting of cancer cells and bone microenvironment in mouse models. Clin Cancer Res. 2017;23(15):4335–46. [Epub ahead of print]
27. Suominen MI, Rissanen JP, Käkönen R, et al. Survival benefit with radium-223 dichloride in a mouse model of breast cancer bone metastasis. J Natl Cancer Inst. 2013;105:908–16.
28. Malamas AS, Gameiro SR, Knudson KM, Hodge JW. Sublethal exposure to alpha radiation (223Ra dichloride) enhances various carcinomas' sensitivity to lysis by antigen-specific cytotoxic T lymphocytes through calreticulin-mediated immunogenic modulation. Oncotarget. 2016;7:86937–47.
29. Kroemer G, Galluzzi L, Kepp O, et al. Immunogenic cell death in cancer therapy. Annu Rev Immunol. 2013;31:51–72.
30. Weichselbaum RR, Liang H, Deng L, Fu YX. Radiotherapy and immunotherapy: a beneficial liaison? Nat Rev Clin Oncol. 2017;14:365–79.
31. Loi M, Desideri I, Greto D, et al. Radiotherapy in the age of cancer immunology: current concepts and future developments. Crit Rev Oncol Hematol. 2017;112:1–10.
32. Mateo J, Carreira S, Sandhu S, et al. DNA-repair defects and olaparib in metastatic prostate cancer. N Engl J Med. 2015;373:1697–708.
33. Parker C, Vogelzang NJ, Sartor O, et al. 3-year safety follow-up of radium-223 dichloride (Ra-223) in patients with castration-resistant prostate cancer (CRPC) and symptomatic bone metastases from ALSYMPCA. J Clin Oncol. 2015;33(suppl 7):195.
34. Observational study for the evaluation of long-term safety of radium-223 used for the treatment of metastatic castration resistant prostate cancer (REASSURE). NCT02141438. www.clinicaltrials.gov.
35. Cleeland CS, Gonin R, Hatfield AK, et al. Pain and its treatment in outpatients with metastatic cancer. N Engl J Med. 1994;330:592–6.
36. Nekolla EA, Kellerer AM, Kuse-Isingschulte M, et al. Malignancies in patients treated with high dose of radium-224. Radiat Res. 1999;152(suppl 6):S3–7.
37. A three arm randomized, open-label phase II study of radium-223 dichloride 50 kBq/kg (55 kBq/kg after implementation of NIST update) versus 80 kBq/kg (88 kBq/kg after implementation of NIST update), and versus 50 kBq/kg (55 kBq/kg after implementation of NIST update) in an extended dosing schedule in subjects with castration-resistant prostate cancer metastatic to the bone. NCT02023697. www.clinicaltrials.gov.
38. Sartor O, Heinrich D, Mariados N, et al. Radium-223 (Ra-223) re-treatment: first experience from an international, multicenter, prospective study in patients with castration-resistant prostate cancer and bone metastases (mCRPC). J Clin Oncol. 2016;34 (suppl 2S):197.
39. de Bono JS, Logothetis CJ, Molina A, et al. Abiraterone and increased survival in metastatic prostate cancer. N Engl J Med. 2011;364:1995–2005.
40. Fizazi K, Scher HI, Molina A, et al. Abiraterone acetate for treatment of metastatic castration-resistant prostate cancer: final overall survival analysis of the COU-AA-301 randomised, double-blind, placebo-controlled phase 3 study. Lancet Oncol. 2012;13:983–92.
41. Scher HI, Fizazi K, Saad F, et al. Increased survival with enzalutamide in prostate cancer after chemotherapy. N Engl J Med. 2012;367:1187–97.
42. Ryan CJ, Smith MR, de Bono JS, et al. Abiraterone in metastatic prostate cancer without previous chemotherapy. N Engl J Med. 2013;368:138–48.
43. Beer TM, Armstrong AJ, Rathkopf DE, et al. Enzalutamide in metastatic prostate cancer before chemotherapy. N Engl J Med. 2014;371:424–33.
44. Logothetis CJ, Basch E, Molina A, et al. Effect of abiraterone acetate and prednisone compared with placebo and prednisone on pain control and skeletal-related events in patients with metastatic castration-resistant prostate cancer: exploratory analysis of data from the COU-AA-301 randomised trial. Lancet Oncol. 2012;13:1210–7.
45. Loriot Y, Miller K, Sternberg CN, et al. Effect of enzalutamide on health-related quality of life, pain, and skeletal-related events in asymptomatic and minimally symptomatic, chemotherapy-naive patients with metastatic castration-resistant prostate cancer (PREVAIL): results from a randomised, phase 3 trial. Lancet Oncol. 2015;16:509–21.
46. Gartrell BA, Saad F. Managing bone metastases and reducing skeletal related events in prostate cancer. Nat Rev Clin Oncol. 2014;11:335–45.
47. Gartrell BA, Coleman R, Efstathiou E, et al. Metastatic prostate cancer and the bone: significance and therapeutic options. Eur Urol. 2015;68:850–8.
48. Vignani F, Bertaglia V, Buttigliero C, et al. Skeletal metastases and impact of anticancer and bone-targeted agents in patients with castration-resistant prostate cancer. Cancer Treat Rev. 2016;44:61–73.
49. A phase III randomized, double-blind, placebo-controlled trial of radium-223 dichloride in combination with abiraterone acetate and prednisone/prednisolone in the treatment of asymptomatic or mildly symptomatic chemotherapy-naïve subjects with bone predominant metastatic castration-resistant prostate cancer (ERA III). NCT02043678. www.clinicaltrials.gov.
50. A randomized multicenter Phase III trial comparing enzalutamide vs. a combination of Ra-223 and enzalutamide in asymptomatic or mildly symptomatic castration resistant prostate cancer patients metastatic to bone (PEACE III). NCT02194842. www.clinicaltrials.gov.

51. Morris MJ, Loriot Y, Sweeney C, et al. Updated results: a phase I/IIa randomized trial of radium-223 + docetaxel versus docetaxel in patients with castration-resistant prostate cancer and bone metastases. J Clin Oncol. 2016;34(suppl):5075.
52. A phase I/IIa study of safety and efficacy of Alpharadin® with docetaxel in patients with bone metastasis from castration-resistant prostate cancer. NCT01106352. www.clinicaltrials.gov.
53. Grasso CS, YM WU, Robinson DR, et al. The mutational landscape of lethal castrate resistant prostate cancer. Nature. 2012;487:239–43.
54. Beltran H, Yelensky R, Frampton GM, et al. Targeted next-generation sequencing of advanced prostate cancer identifies potential therapeutic targets and disease heterogeneity. Eur Urol. 2013;63:920–6.
55. Gundem G, Van Loo P, Kremeyer B, et al. The evolutionary history of lethal metastatic prostate cancer. Nature. 2015;520:353–7.
56. Evans JR, Zhao SG, Chang SL, et al. Patient-level DNA damage and repair pathway profiles and prognosis after prostatectomy for high-risk prostate cancer. JAMA Oncol. 2016;2:471–80.
57. Hager S, Ackermann CJ, Joerger M, et al. Anti-tumour activity of platinum compounds in advanced prostate cancer—a systematic literature review. Ann Oncol. 2016;27:975–84.
58. Sternberg CN, Petrylak DP, Sartor O, et al. Multinational, double-blind, phase III study of prednisone and either satraplatin or placebo in patients with castrate refractory prostate cancer progressing after prior chemotherapy: the SPARC trial. J Clin Oncol. 2009;27:5431–8.
59. Phase IB trial of radium-223 and niraparib in patients with castrate resistant prostate cancer (RAPARP). NCT03076203. www.clinicaltrials.gov.
60. Menis J, Litière S, Tryfonidis K, Golfinopoulos V. The European Organization for Research and Treatment of Cancer perspective on designing clinical trials with immune therapeutics. Ann Transl Med. 2016;4:267.
61. Nesslinger NJ, Ng A, Tsang KY, et al. A viral vaccine encoding prostate-specific antigen induces antigen spreading to a common set of self-proteins in prostate cancer patients. Clin Cancer Res. 2010;16:4046–56.
62. A phase 2 study of sipuleucel-T with or without radium-223 in men with asymptomatic or minimally symptomatic bone-metastatic castrate-resistant prostate cancer. NCT02463799. www.clinicaltrials.gov.
63. A randomized, Phase II study evaluating the addition of pembrolizumab (MK-3475) to Radium-223 in metastatic castration-resistant prostate cancer (mCRPC). NCT03093428. www.clinicaltrials.gov.
64. A phase Ib, open-label study of the safety and tolerability of atezolizumab in combination with Radium-223 dichloride in patients with castrate-resistant prostate cancer who have progressed following treatment with an androgen pathway inhibitor. NCT02814669. www.clinicaltrials.gov.
65. Humm JL, Sartor O, Parker C, et al. Radium-223 in the treatment of osteoblastic metastases: a critical clinical review. Int J Radiat Oncol Biol Phys. 2015;91:898–906.
66. Coleman R. Treatment of metastatic bone disease and the emerging role of radium-223. Semin Nucl Med. 2016;46:99–104.
67. Androgen deprivation therapy with or without radium-223 dichloride in patients with newly diagnosed metastatic prostate cancer with bone metastases: Hoosier Cancer Research Network GU13-170. NCT02582749. www.clinicaltrials.gov.
68. Coleman R, Aksnes AK, Naume B, et al. A phase IIa, nonrandomized study of radium-223 dichloride in advanced breast cancer patients with bone-dominant disease. Breast Cancer Res Treat. 2014;145:411–8.
69. A phase II randomized, double-blind, placebo-controlled trial of radium-223 dichloride versus placebo when administered to metastatic HER2 negative hormone receptor positive breast cancer subjects with bone metastases treated with hormonal treatment background therapy. NCT02258464. www.clinicaltrials.gov.
70. A phase II randomized, double-blind, placebo-controlled trial of radium-223 dichloride in combination with exemestane and everolimus versus placebo in combination with exemestane and everolimus when administered to metastatic HER2 negative hormone receptor positive breast cancer subjects with bone metastases. NCT02258451. www.clinicaltrials.gov.
71. Anderson PM, Subbiah V, Rohren E. Bone-seeking radiopharmaceuticals as targeted agents of osteosarcoma: Samarium-153-EDTMP and radium-223. Adv Exp Med Biol. 2014;804:291–304.
72. Bruland OS, Nilsson S, Fisher DR, Larsen RH. High-linear energy transfer irradiation targeted to skeletal metastases by the alpha-emitter 223Ra: adjuvant or alternative to conventional modalities? Clin Cancer Res. 2006;12:6250s–7s.
73. Phase I dose escalation of monthly intravenous Ra-223 dichloride in osteosarcoma. NCT 01833520. www.clinicaltrials.gov.
74. Subbiah V, Anderson PM, Kairemo K, et al. Alpha particle radium-223 dichloride (223RaCl2) in high risk osteosarcoma. J Clin Oncol. 2016;34(suppl):11029.
75. Subbiah V, Anderson P, Rohren E. Alpha Emitter radium 223 in high-risk osteosarcoma: first clinical evidence of response and blood-brain barrier penetration. JAMA Oncol. 2015;1:253–5.
76. A phase 1b/2 trial to evaluate the safety and efficacy of radium-223 dichloride (BAY88-8223) in combination with bortezomib and dexamethasone in early relapsed multiple myeloma. NCT02928029. www.clinicaltrials.gov.
77. Pilot trial of radium-223 and atezolizumab in patients with urothelial carcinoma with bone metastases who have had disease progression after platinum-based chemotherapy. NCT03208712. www.clinicaltrials.gov.
78. Single arm phase II trial evaluating the efficacy of radium-223 in radioactive iodine refractory bone metastases from differentiated thyroid cancer. NCT02390934. www.clinicaltrials.gov.

Check for updates

29 Dosimetry

Massimiliano Pacilio, Elisabetta Verdolino, Bartolomeo Cassano, and Giuseppe De Vincentis

Abstract

Improved overall survival and very low toxicity indicate that ^{223}Ra-dichloride therapy may provide a new standard of care for patients with castration-resistant prostate cancer metastatic to the bone. The high linear energy transfer (LET) of α-radiation results in greater biological effectiveness than β-radiation, giving rise to cytotoxicity that is independent of dose rate, cell cycle growth phase, and oxygen concentration. Due to the α-particle high LET and short range (of a few cell diameters in tissue), microdosimetry seems almost always necessary; however, the feasibility of macrodosimetry for organs and lesions has recently been demonstrated, providing new opportunities in the clinical routine not yet explored. With the low activity of the registered use, bone lesion macrodosimetry appeared more feasible than organ dosimetry and more effective for investigating possible relationships between absorbed dose and biological/clinical effect, as response is often observed in clinical practice, whereas toxicities are mild to moderate in intensity and easily manageable with symptomatic and supportive treatments. The first injection of the treatment can be used as if it were a pretreatment tracer activity, and just three scan acquisitions are required (with a duration of about 20–30 min each), as well as other conventional imaging (such as ^{99m}Tc-diphosphonate WB scan and CT study), with a limited burden for patients and staff. A lesion/soft tissue contrast ratio on ^{99m}Tc-MDP WB scan higher than 10 would imply detectability on ^{223}Ra spot scans. A specific preparation of the patient is not required, apart from the necessary informed consent.

M. Pacilio (✉)
Department of Medical Physics, Azienda Ospedaliera Universitaria Policlinico Umberto I, Rome, Italy
e-mail: M.Pacilio@policlinicoumberto1.it

E. Verdolino • B. Cassano
Postgraduate School of Medical Physics, "Sapienza" University of Rome, Rome, Italy

G. De Vincentis
Department of Radiological, Oncological and Anatomo Pathological Sciences, "Sapienza" University of Rome, Rome, Italy

E. Bombardieri et al. (eds.), *Clinical Applications of Nuclear Medicine Targeted Therapy*,
https://doi.org/10.1007/978-3-319-63067-0_29

The correlations of the absorbed dose to lesions with the biological/clinical effects are still under consideration; however, in the perspective of the availability of new fractionation regimens, the dosimetric approach would allow a dosimetry-based choice of the administration scheduling, opening the way to dosimetry-guided radiometabolic therapy of bone metastases with α-emitters.

29.1 Introduction

^{223}Ra is a short-lived (half-life 11.4 days) α-emitter, used to develop ^{223}Ra-dichloride, that targets metastatic bone disease, accumulating in areas of increased bone turnover. ^{223}Ra-dichloride has received marketing authorization as Xofigo© (Bayer HealthCare) from European Commission and approval by the US Food and Drug Administration for the treatment of patients affected by metastatic bone disease from castration-resistant (hormone-refractory) prostate cancer (CRPC/HRPC). ^{223}Ra decays through a cascade of short-lived α-emitting and β-emitting progeny, with a total emitted energy of about 28 MeV per starting atom through complete decay of the progeny to stable lead. On average, four alpha particles and two beta particles are emitted. The absorbed dose per unit cumulated activity imparted by ^{223}Ra and its daughters is higher than conventional beta emitters, and the high linear energy transfer (LET) of alpha radiation results in greater biological effectiveness than beta radiation, giving rise to cytotoxicity that is independent of dose rate, cell cycle growth phase, and oxygen concentration [1]. ^{223}Ra emits also photons useful for imaging: X-rays mainly at 81, 84, and around 95 keV (abundances of 15.0%, 24.7%, and about 10.8%, respectively) and gammas at 154, 269, 324, and 338 keV (abundances of 5.7%, 13.9%, 4.0%, and 2.8%, respectively). The low abundance of photonic emissions and the low amount of activity administered (registered use, 55 kBq/kg) produce an insufficient counting rate to acquire SPECT data in a time frame that is comfortable for the patient, but despite the low number of emitted photons, quantitative planar imaging with gamma camera is feasible [2–4], and dosimetric studies for organs and bone lesions have been recently published [5–7]. Activity quantification could be performed by planar imaging, basing on the approach reported by the MIRD Pamphlet No. 16 [8], i.e., using conjugated or single-view counting, performing background subtraction and corrections for attenuation and scatter, as also previously reported [5, 6]. Due to the low count statistics, the use of multiple energy windows for scatter correction is not advisable, but the pseudo-extrapolation number method could be used to correct simultaneously for attenuation and scatter in planar imaging [8]. The registered use of ^{223}Ra-dichloride (6 injections of 55 kBq/kg, administered every 4 weeks) does not foresee dosimetric studies. In principle, a dosimetric approach should be requested to perform treatment optimization and personalization. Currently, the possibility of activity escalation is also being studied, and a three-arm, randomized, open-label phase II study is ongoing (Bayer protocol 88-8223/16507), comparing clinical outcomes from 12 injections of 50 kBq/kg or 6 injections of 80 kBq/kg with the standard administration schedule. In this perspective, the dosimetric approach would allow a dosimetry-based choice of the fractionation regimen, opening the way to dosimetry-guided radiometabolic therapy of bone metastases with α-emitters.

29.2 Goal of Dosimetry in Treatment with ^{223}Ra-Dichloride Therapy

Microdosimetry provides a conceptual framework for a systematic analysis of the stochastic distribution of energy deposits in irradiated matter, based on a priori biodistribution information obtained from preclinical or, when the subcellular distribution is also relevant, cell-based studies. With the high LET and short range (of a few cell diameters in tissue) of alpha particles, the conventional dosimetry (or macrodosimetry) is apparently less important, whereas stochastic variations in the energy deposited in cell nuclei become more relevant because of the microscopic target size, low number of alpha particle traversals, and variation in LET along the alpha particle track [9]. In this scenario the MIRD committee [1] recommends cell-level and microdosimetry calculations. The rationale for using microdosimetry is traditionally based on a quantitative criterion (the Kellerer criterion) suggesting that microdosimetry should be applied when the relative deviation of the distribution of specific energy within a specified target exceeds 20% [1]. In the context of in vitro irradiation with alpha particles, microdosimetry seems almost always necessary, but in the clinical routine, its usefulness is more questionable. MIRD pamphlet 22 [1] indicates that microdosimetry would be adequate mainly for nontargeted tissues, in which mean absorbed doses are smaller. Possible alternative criteria for the microdosimetric approach could be the failure of macrodosimetry to describe the experimental observations or the evident possibility of obtaining further information in addition to the macrodosimetric analysis. The simultaneous use of these two phenomenological approaches could provide useful parameters to properly describe and predict biological outcomes [9]. However, it has only recently been demonstrated the feasibility of macrodosimetry in ^{223}Ra-dichloride therapy, and this provides new opportunities not yet explored.

The possibility of radiation-induced myelotoxicity was carefully investigated in past studies. Considering a relative biological effectiveness (RBE) of 5 for α-radiation, taking into consideration the radium daughter products, the RBE-weighted absorbed dose for deterministic biological effects (unit Gy as proposed by the ICRP in ICRP Publication 103) [10] is about 1.4 Gy for an injection of 3850 kBq (corresponding to 55 kBq/kg in a 70 kg patient) [11]. Since absorbed doses in the range 2–4 Gy are usually associated with severe myelosuppression in radioimmunotherapy, significant myelotoxicity could be foreseen for a standard treatment with ^{223}Ra-dichloride (six administrations). Nevertheless, hematological toxicity is unlikely; indeed no grade 4 toxicities and infrequent grade 3 toxicities (using National Cancer Institute Common Toxicity Criteria [12]) have been observed [13, 14]. Dose-limiting hematologic toxicity was not observed up to administration of 250 kBq/kg [15]. Microdosimetry could explain these results. In a recent study, the percentage of cells receiving a potentially toxic absorbed dose (2 or 4 Gy) as a function of the average absorbed dose over the marrow cavity was calculated, obtaining that (1) the cellular absorbed dose has a heterogeneous distribution strongly dependent on the position of the cell within the marrow cavity, and (2) increasing the average marrow cavity absorbed dose (by increasing the administered activity) results in only a small increase in potential marrow toxicity (i.e., the number of cells receiving more than 2 or 4 Gy) for a range of average marrow cavity absorbed doses from 1 to 20 Gy [16].

Chittenden et al. [5] evaluated absorbed dose to organs by in vivo imaging and biokinetic sampling during a Phase 1, open-label study, administrating 100 kBq/kg of body weight. In this study [5], twice the activity of the standard protocol was administered, and no specific uptake was observed in most organs (e.g., kidneys or liver). Therefore, organ dosimetry determined from activity retention measurements obtained by in vivo imaging seems less feasible with the registered administration schedule, except for the gut, whereas urine collection would allow the estimation of the cumulated activity in kidneys and bladder. Considering also that nonhematological toxicities (such as diarrhea, fatigue, nausea), although are more common than myelotoxicity, are also mild to moderate in intensity and easily manageable with symptomatic and supportive treatments [13–15, 17], at present, organ dosimetry seems less useful in the current clinical practice. Nevertheless, it deserves to be studied in the perspective of increasing activity per fraction and total injected activity.

Lesion macrodosimetry has proved more feasible with the registered administration protocol [6, 7]; moreover, local or global response is observed in most patients. The terms "local response" can mean reduction of lesion uptake, or lesion diameter, whereas "global response" can be referred to either clinical (e.g., alkaline phosphatase) or radiological indicators (e.g., number of detectable lesions or extension of the osseous disease), as well as time to symptomatic skeletal events or overall survival. Therefore, lesion macrodosimetry appears more effective for the purpose of investigating possible relationships between absorbed dose and observed biological/clinical effect in current clinical practice.

Lesion dosimetry would also have not negligible economic implications. In the perspective of performing activity escalation, it could increase the efficacy of the treatment helping a more adequate choice for the administration schedule. Currently, it could help to avoid useless treatment, especially once a possible correlation between absorbed dose and local response will be established.

29.3 The Practical Implementation of Dosimetry in Treatment with ^{223}Ra-Dichloride Therapy

The use of pretreatment administration of a tracer activity for dosimetric patient-specific studies is not included in the registered use of ^{223}Ra-dichloride. However, the first injection of the treatment can be used to perform patient-specific dosimetry as if it were a pretreatment tracer activity, so the total absorbed dose can then be estimated multiplying by 6 the absorbed dose measured after the first injection.

The dosimetric studies based on in vivo sampling published until now involved planar scintigraphic imaging (whole-body and spot views), whole-body counting with external probes, CT studies, blood urine, and fecal collection [5–7]. Lesion dosimetry can be performed using only CT studies and scintigraphic whole-body (WB) and spot views [6, 7]. This section will only deal with lesion dosimetry, whereas more details for organ dosimetry can be found in the literature [5].

^{223}Ra imaging for lesion dosimetry used mainly single- (82 keV) or double-peak acquisitions (both 82 and 154 keV, always 20% wide) [5–7]. The conjugated view method is recommended as it offers improvements over the single-view procedures, providing corrections for source thickness and attenuation, without the need to determine the source depth in the patient body [8]. In Fig. 29.1, an example of serial ^{223}Ra images after the first injection of ^{223}Ra-dichloride is reported [6].

Pretreatment ^{99m}Tc-diphosphonate WB scan and CT study are required for dosimetric studies. A good correlation between ^{99m}Tc-MDP and ^{223}Ra-dichloride uptake was previously reported (see Fig. 29.2) [6], so ^{99m}Tc-diphosphonate WB scan can be used for lesion contouring and to foresee lesion detectability on ^{223}Ra images.

Due to the low quality of ^{223}Ra images (partial volume effects and low count statistics), lesions observable on the pretreatment WB scan are sometimes not detectable on ^{223}Ra scintigrams. A preliminary study performed by univariate receiving operating characteristic (ROC) analysis showed that, using the lesion/soft tissue contrast ratio (CR) on ^{99m}Tc-MDP WB scan as score value and visible/non-visible lesions on ^{223}Ra spot scans (acquired at 24 h) as true positive/true negative group, the AUC was 0.972, and the optimal score value was 10, corresponding to a maximum accuracy of 92%. Figure 29.3 reports the AUC curve and the accuracy as a function of CR on ^{99m}Tc-MDP WB scan [2].

Obviously, a CR higher than 10 would be a necessary but not sufficient condition for the eligibility of a given lesion for the dosimetric study, because other factors could affect the possibility to perform dosimetry, such as biokinetics (which could affect visibility on subsequent serial images), count statistics of the acquisitions, sensitivity of the gamma camera for ^{223}Ra, lesion size, etc. Nevertheless, accounting for the variability of lesion effective half-times observed until now, and provided to standardize the ROI drawing on late serial images as indicated in the literature [6], with an acquisition time of 30 min

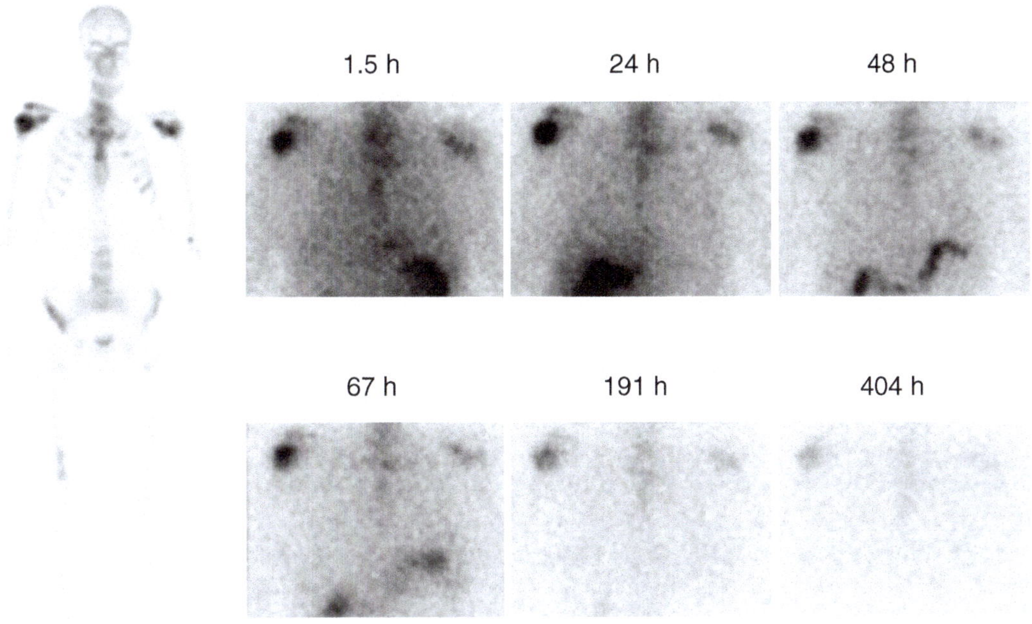

Fig. 29.1 ^{99m}Tc-MDP WB scan (on the left) and a series of anterior static images obtained at different times after administration of ^{223}Ra-dichloride. The static images were acquired at 1.5, 24, 48, 67, 191, and 404 h [6]

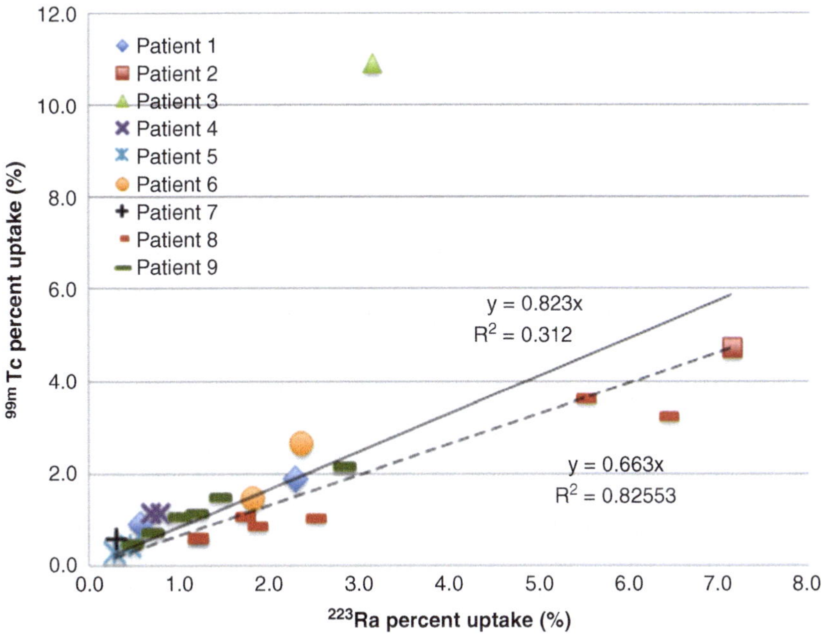

Fig. 29.2 Correlation between ^{99m}Tc and ^{223}Ra percent uptake. Two regression lines are shown, one relating to all the data (continuous line) and the other after removing the outlier (green triangle, dashed line) [6]

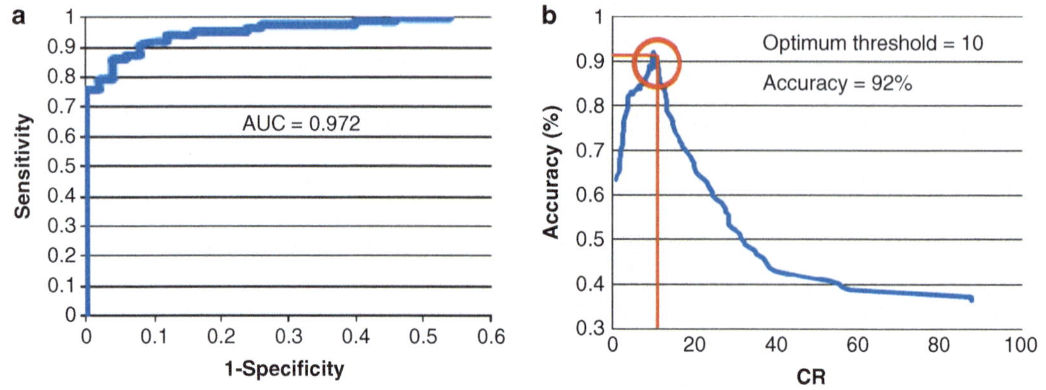

Fig. 29.3 Univariate ROC analysis: (**a**) ROC curve referred to the visibility of lesion on ^{223}Ra images acquired 24 h after the administration, using the contrast ratio (CR) lesion/soft tissue on the ^{99m}Tc-MDP WB scan as score value; (**b**) accuracy as function of the CR (adapted from [2])

and a gamma camera sensitivity for ^{223}Ra not lower than about 45 cps/MBq, a CR threshold of 10 should have a good predictive value in relation to the possibility to perform dosimetry [2]. The studies published until now used a gamma camera having the aforementioned sensitivity, and ^{223}Ra spot scans for temporal sampling [6, 7]. However, gamma cameras having twice the sensitivity [3] and lower scan speed are widespread, allowing also ^{223}Ra WB scans (preliminary studies not yet published).

Two-phase (uptake and washout) lesion biokinetics was observed in some cases, but the uptake effective half-life was short (at most, 2–3 h), and the percentage differences in the cumulated activity obtained with a biexponential curve (with respect to the monoexponential one) were small (mostly lower than 10%), so according to MIRD pamphlet no. 16 [8], the wash-in phase can be neglected in most cases, avoiding the early acquisitions without greatly affecting dosimetric accuracy [6]. The monoexponential fitting adequately described the washout phase; therefore, just three time points are needed. The optimal time sampling could be between 24 and 36 h, between 48 and 60 h, and between 7 and 15 days, considering that later than 15 days from the administration, most of lesions detected by ^{223}Ra spot scans are no longer visible [6, 7]. Figure 29.4 shows biokinetic data recently published [6].

Each lesion to be studied should be detectable on a CT scan, because contouring should be performed for a better estimation of the lesion volume. Lesion mass can be estimated as the product of the volume obtained from delineation on the CT image and the mean lesion density. The density of the bone tumors could be derived from the CT images in terms of Hounsfield units, but the range of variation previously reported was limited (1.34–1.59 g/cm^3) [18], so a mean density of 1.4 g/cm^3 (corresponding to the skeleton mean density) [19] can be assumed. The absorbed doses to the lesions can be easily evaluated as the product of the cumulated activity and the self-irradiation S-factor corresponding to the lesion mass [20].

To summarize, eligible lesions for dosimetry should be visible on ^{223}Ra images and CT studies. A specific preparation of the patient is not required, apart from the necessary informed consent after explaining the aims of the dosimetric approach and the need to undergo imaging for three times after the first administration (e.g., three static acquisitions on the chosen anatomic region, with a duration of about 20–30 min) [6].

29.4 Feasibility in the Routine

The main critical factor remains the methodology for lesion contouring. Accurate lesion contouring is of main importance, and even though ^{99m}TC WB scan helps, ROI positioning on ^{223}Ra images may be challenging, above all for late (more noisy) images. A procedure based on image

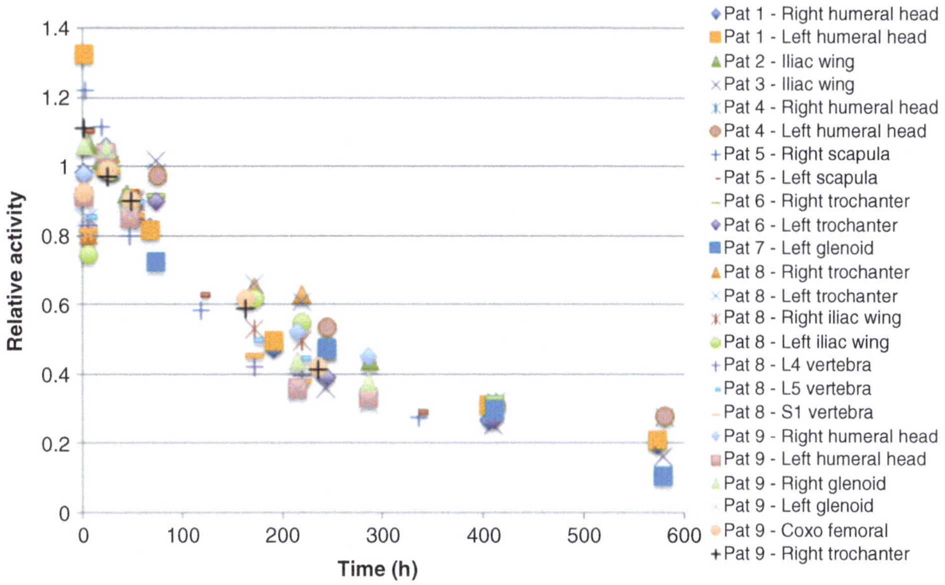

Fig. 29.4 Activities normalized to $t = 24$ h as a function of acquisition time for all the lesions studied in [6] (for each lesion, the 24-h normalization value was calculated from the corresponding biexponential biokinetic fit)

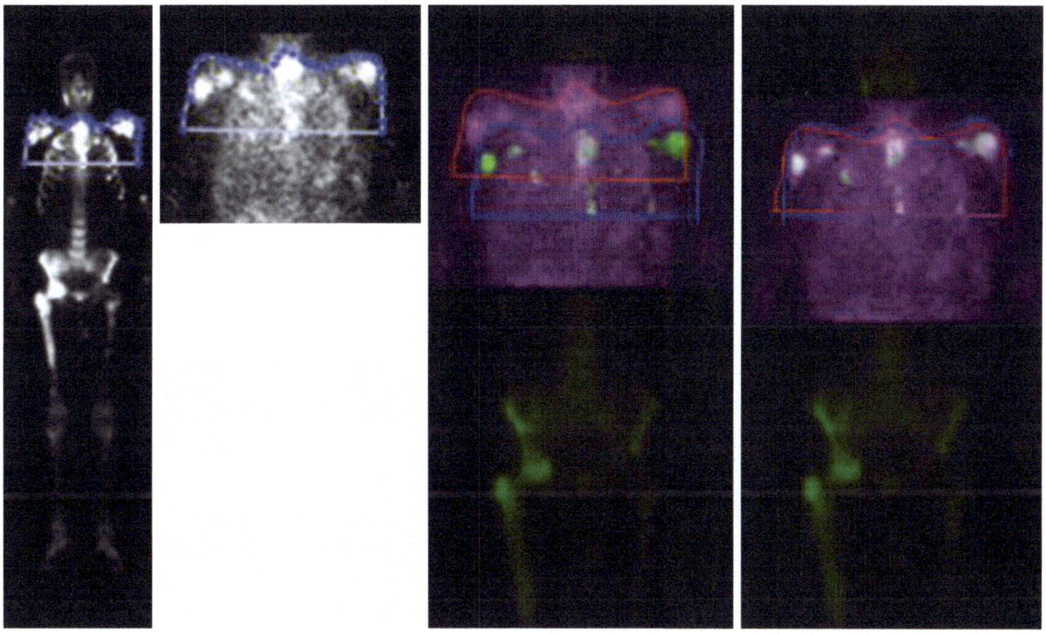

Fig. 29.5 Example of coregistration between a ^{99m}Tc-MDP WB image and a ^{223}Ra spot scan (acquired at 1.5 h after administration, anterior view), using an in-house developed MATLAB toolkit, delineating shoulders, and body contour [7]

coregistration between ^{223}Ra spot (or WB) and ^{99m}TC WB scan can surely increase the accuracy of ROI positioning. Figure 29.5 shows an example of a coregistration procedure between ^{99m}TC WB and ^{223}Ra spot scans, using an in-house developed MATLAB toolkit [6, 7]. However, the lack of tools for this specific purpose would be likely to create some difficulties.

An additional critical factor for dosimetry could be the need of gamma camera calibration: the wide variation obtained for calibration factors and transmission curve parameters among several gamma cameras highlights the need to perform individual calibration for each imaging system [2–4]. The calibration procedure would require at least measurements of calibration factors, transmission curves, and recovery coefficients to correct for partial volume effects, and this could take several hours, because the shortage of ^{223}Ra activity can lengthen the time of acquisition. Sometimes, sensitivity variations with the source-detector distance were also observed, so if single-view counting is used, distance sensitivity dependency should be assessed and taken into account, whereas for the conjugated method, the sensitivity dependence from the source-detector distance is relatively unimportant [3].

The possibility to perform dosimetry for more than one administration should be also considered, because appreciable variations among repeated inter-fraction absorbed dose assessments have been observed. As an example, Fig. 29.6 reports the four absorbed dose assessments (after the first, third, fifth, and sixth administration) for four lesions in a patient. The percent standard deviation of absorbed dose reached 21% [7]. However, a good enough estimation could also be obtained multiplying by 6 the mean value of absorbed dose derived from some (not necessarily all) administrations, distributed during the whole treatment.

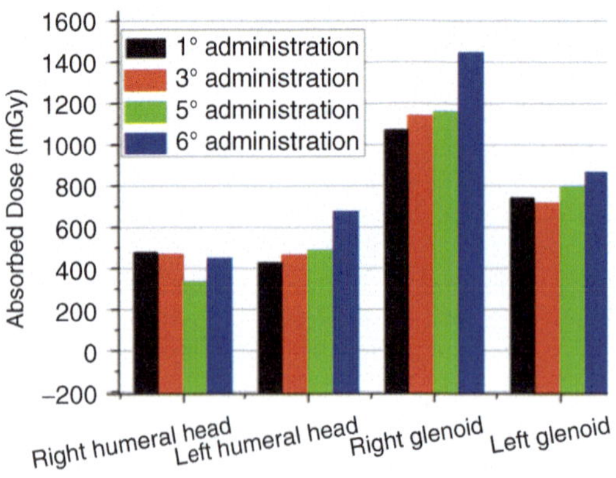

Fig. 29.6 Dosimetric assessments for right and left humeral head, right and left glenoid, performed after the first, third, fifth, and sixth injection of ^{223}Ra-dichloride for one treated patient [7]

Nevertheless, the routine dosimetric procedures would not require dedicated equipment (just gamma cameras and CT), would not be technically difficult (single- or double-peak acquisition of WB and spot scans), and would not be time-consuming (acquisition of just three spot scans with a duration of about 20–30 min each), requiring just an initial investment of time for developing an adequate contouring methodology and calibrating the gamma camera. The only additional item, which falls outside the standard clinical practice, is the need of a transmission image of the patient, required for correcting attenuation across the patient body, through the lesion ROI. It could be acquired by a transmission scan with a flood source, but the use of a CT scout scan is easier, its signal-to-noise ratio is high, the time required for acquisition is less than a minute, and the spatial resolution is exquisite [21].

29.5 Short Review

Main results in the literature for lesion dosimetry are reported in [6, 7]. The mean effective half-life ($T_{1/2eff}$) of ^{223}Ra was 8.2 days, with a range of 5.5–11.4 days (9 patients, 24 lesions), showing high interpatient variability. Values of absorbed dose to lesion were also reported; however, those studies aimed to demonstrate the feasibility of dosimetry, focusing mainly on procedures for lesion contouring and biokinetic sampling. The published values of absorbed dose were obtained using just the ^{223}Ra *S*-value, without taking into account the contributions for the daughters of the decay chain. However, the decay chain daughters greatly contribute to the lesion irradiation. The first daughter product (^{219}Rn) has a so short half-life (4 s) that nearly all ^{219}Rn activity produced in bone volume stays with the parent ^{223}Ra, similarly also for the next decay product, ^{215}Po, having a half-life less than 0.01 s. As regards the third decay product, it

Table 29.1 Mean values of effective half-lives in bone metastases, mean values of the ratio of the lesion of self-irradiation *S*-values between ^{223}Ra and a given radionuclide, administered activity per cycle, number of cycles usually performed as standard procedure, mean values of D_{RBE} per unit of administered activity, and cumulative D_{RBE} for a standard treatment are reported for the different therapeutical radiopharmaceuticals, together with the references for the information provided

Radiopharmaceutical	$T_{1/2eff}$ (days)	*S*-values ratio[a]	RBE	A_{adm}/cycle (MBq)	No. of cycles	D_{RBE}/A_{adm} (mGy/MBq)	D_{RBE} (Gy)
^{153}Sm-EDTMP	1.9[b]	94	1	2590[c]	1	4[d]	10.4
^{186}Re-HEDP	1.5[e]	85	1	1300[f]	1	33[g]	42.9
^{188}Re-HEDP	0.66[h]	38	1	3120[h]	1	3.8[h]	11.9
^{89}Sr-Cl_2	>25[i]	47	1	148[j]	1	230[k]	34.0
^{223}Ra-Cl_2	7.7[l]	1	5	3.85[c]	6	4675[l]	108

The cumulative D_{RBE} associated to a standard treatment with ^{223}Ra-dichloride has been calculated by multiplying the mean D_{RBE} per unit of administered activity (referred to the first injection) and the total activity injected to a 70 kg patient (23.1 MBq, obtained as six administrations of 55 kBq/kg)

[a]The mean value of the ratio between the ^{223}Ra self-irradiation *S*-value and that of a given radionuclide, in the range 1–6000 g, data from Stabin et al. [20]

[b]The physical half-time of ^{153}Sm

[c]The administered activity to a 70 kg patient

[d]A maximum value derived from data of van Rensburg et al. [24]

[e]Calculated with the mean biologic half-time for prostate lesions reported by Lewington [25]

[f]Usual administered activity reported by Lewington [25]

[g]Mean value derived from Maxon et al. [26, 27]

[h]Mean value reported by Liepe et al. [28]

[i]Resulting from the minimum biologic half-time for osteoblastic metastases reported by Lewington [25]

[j]The licensed activity reported by Lewington [25]

[k]The mean value reported by Blake et al. [18]

[l]Mean value from unpublished results

is possible that ^{211}Pb (with a half-life of 36 min) may localize to the liver, as stated in ICRP 67 [22]. The final radionuclides of the decay chain, ^{211}Bi, ^{211}Po, and ^{207}Tl, have half-lives of less than 5 min, so they could only marginally affect the biodistribution of radionuclides within the body [11]. For instance, the potential ^{211}Bi to localize in the liver was explored by Carrasquillo et al. [23] by imaging of the 351-keV emission, with inconclusive results. Hence it is generally assumed that the localization of all daughter products follows that of the ^{223}Ra [5]. Deriving the *S*-values from Olinda/EXM [20], the ratio between the total S-factor (including daughter contributes) and that from just ^{223}Ra is about 4.7 in a wide range of mass (1 g to 10 kg).

Currently, the results for lesion dosimetry are being updated. Estimations on 20 patients, 38 lesions, yielded the following preliminary results (unpublished results): mean $T_{1/2eff}$ was 7.7 days, with a range of 4.2–11.4 days; the mean absorbed dose for one administration was 3.6 Gy (without accounting for RBE), with a range of 0.8–9.7 Gy, whereas considering also a RBE of 5, the total RBE-weighted absorbed dose for deterministic biological effects (D_{RBE}, for a whole treatment) was 108 Gy, with a range of 24–291 Gy. Table 29.1 shows, for different therapeutic radiopharmaceuticals, mean effective half-lives in bone metastases, mean lesion self-irradiation S-value ratios between ^{223}Ra and the given radionuclide, administered activities per cycle, numbers of cycles usually performed as standard procedure, mean values of D_{RBE} per unit of administered activity, and total D_{RBE} for standard treatments, together with the references for the information provided (adapted from [6]).

Several examples of local response of bone metastases (in terms of reduction of lesion uptake or lesion diameter) are often observed in clinical practice [7]. However, possible correlation of the absorbed dose to lesions with the biological/clinical effects is still under consideration.

Conclusion

Except for an initial investment of time for developing an adequate contouring methodology and calibrating the gamma camera, lesion dosimetry in ^{223}Ra-dichloride therapy is feasible, does not require dedicated equipment (just gamma cameras and CT), and does not present technical difficulties (just single- or double-peak acquisition of WB and spot scans are needed). Three scan acquisitions are required (with a duration of about 20–30 min each), as well as other conventional diagnostic procedures such as ^{99m}Tc-diphosphonate WB scan and CT study, with a limited burden for patients and staff. A specific preparation of the patient is not required, apart from the necessary informed consent for the dosimetric approach, explaining the need to undergo imaging for three times after the first administration. The possibility to perform dosimetry for more than one administration of ^{223}Ra-dichloride could be also considered, due to possible inter-fraction variability for absorbed dose to lesions; however, dosimetric assessments should be performed at least after the first injection. The correlations of the absorbed dose to lesions with the biological/clinical effects are still under consideration; however, there are concrete possibilities to find them, due to the results of local response frequently observed in common clinical practice. In the perspective of the availability of new fractionation regimens, the dosimetric approach would allow a dosimetry-based choice of the administration scheduling, opening the way to dosimetry-guided radiometabolic therapy of bone metastases with α-emitters.

References

1. Sgouros G, Roeske JC, McDevitt MR, Palm S, Allen BJ, Fisher DR, et al. MIRD pamphlet no. 22 (abridged): radiobiology and dosimetry of α-particle emitters for targeted radionuclide therapy. J Nucl Med. 2010;51:311–28.
2. Pacilio M, Cassano B, Chiesa C, Giancola S, Ferrari M, Pettinato C, et al. The Italian multicentre dosimetric study for lesion dosimetry in ^{223}Ra therapy of bone metastases: calibration protocol of gamma cameras and patient eligibility criteria. Phys Med. 2016;32:1731–7.
3. Pacilio M, Cassano B, Pellegrini R, Di Castro E, Zorz A, De Vincentis G, et al. Gamma camera calibrations for the Italian multicentre study for lesion dosimetry in ^{223}Ra therapy of bone metastases. Phys Med. 2017. https://doi.org/10.1016/j.ejmp.2017.04.019.
4. Hindorf C, Chittenden S, Aksnes AK, Parker C, Flux GD. Quantitative imaging of ^{223}Ra-chloride (Alpharadin) for targeted alpha-emitting radionuclide therapy of bone metastases. Nucl Med Commun. 2012;33:726–32.
5. Chittenden S, Hindorf C, Parker CC, Lewington VJ, Pratt BE, Johnson B, et al. Phase 1, open-label study of the biodistribution, pharmacokinetics and dosimetry of Radium-223 dichloride (223Ra dichloride) in patients with hormone refractory prostate cancer and skeletal metastases. J Nucl Med. 2015;56:1304–9.
6. Pacilio M, Ventroni G, De Vincentis G, Cassano B, Pellegrini R, Di Castro E, et al. Dosimetry of bone metastases in targeted radionuclide therapy with alpha-emitting ^{223}Ra-dichloride. Eur J Nucl Med Mol Imaging. 2016;43:21–33.
7. Pacilio M, Ventroni G, Cassano B, Ialongo P, Lorenzon L, Di Castro E, et al. A case report of image-based dosimetry of bone metastases with Alpharadin (^{223}Radichloride) therapy: inter-fraction variability of absorbed dose and follow-up. Ann Nucl Med. 2016;30:163–8.
8. Siegel JA, Thomas SR, Stubbs JB, Stabin MG, Hays MT, Koral KF, et al. MIRD Pamphlet No. 16: techniques for quantitative radiopharmaceutical biodistribution data acquisition and analysis for use in human radiation dose estimates. J Nucl Med. 1999;40:37s–61s.
9. Chouin N, Bardies M. Alpha-particle microdosimetry. Curr Radiopharm. 2011;4:266–80.
10. ICRP. Publication 103: the 2007 recommendations of the International Commission on Radiological Protection. Ann ICRP. 2007;2007:37.
11. Lassmann M, Nosske D. Dosimetry of ^{223}Ra-chloride: dose to normal organs and tissues. Eur J Nucl Med Mol Imaging. 2013;40:207–12.
12. CTEP. Common terminology criteria for adverse events (CTCAE) v4.0. Bethesda, MD: Cancer Therapy Evaluation Program, National Cancer Institute; 2015. http://ctep.cancer.gov/protocolDevelopment/electronic_applications/ctc.htm. Accessed 20 Dec 2016.
13. Nilsson S, Larsen RH, Fossa SD, Balteskard L, Borch KW, Westlin JE, et al. First clinical experience with a-emitting radium-223 in the treatment of skeletal metastases. Clin Cancer Res. 2005;11:4451–9.
14. Nilsson S, Franzen L, Parker C, Tyrrell C, Blom R, Tennvall J, et al. Bone-targeted radium-223 in symptomatic, hormone-refractory prostate cancer: a randomised, multicentre, placebo-controlled phase II study. Lancet Oncol. 2007;8:587–94.
15. Bruland ØS, Nilsson S, Fisher DR, Larsen RH. High-linear energy transfer irradiation targeted to skeletal metastases by the alpha-emitter ^{223}Ra: adjuvant or

alternative to conventional modalities? Clin Cancer Res. 2006;12:6250s–7s.
16. Hobbs RF, Song H, Watchman CJ, Bolch WE, Aksnes AK, Ramdahl T, et al. A bone marrow toxicity model for Ra-223 α-emitter radiopharmaceutical therapy. Phys Med Biol. 2012;57:3207–22.
17. Parker CC, Pascoe S, Chodacki A, O'Sullivan JM, Germà JR, O'Bryan-Tear CG, et al. A randomized, double-blind, dose-finding, multicenter, phase 2 study of radium chloride (Ra 223) in patients with bone metastases and castration-resistant prostate cancer. Eur Urol. 2013;63:189–97.
18. Blake GM, Zivanovic MA, Blaquiere RM, Fine DR, McEwan AJ, Ackery DM. Strontium-89 therapy: measurement of absorbed dose to skeletal metastases. J Nucl Med. 1988;29:549–57.
19. Cristy M, Eckerman KF. Specific absorbed fractions of energy at various ages from internal photon sources. Technical Report ORNL/TM-8381/V1. Oak Ridge, TN: Oak Ridge National Laboratory; 1987.
20. Stabin MG, Sparks RB, Crowe E. OLINDA/EXM: the second-generation personal computer software for internal dose assessment in nuclear medicine. J Nucl Med. 2005;46:1023–7.
21. Minarik D, Sjogreen K, Ljungberg M. A new method to obtain transmission images for planar whole-body activity quantification. Cancer Biother Radiopharm. 2005;20:72–6.
22. International Commission on Radiological Protection (ICRP). Age-dependent doses to members of the public from intake of radionuclides: part 2 ingestion dose coefficients. ICRP publication 67. Oxford: ICRP; 1992.
23. Carrasquillo JA, O'Donoghue JA, Pandit-Taskar N, Humm JL, Rathkopf DE, Slovin SF, et al. Phase I pharmacokinetic and biodistribution study with escalating doses of Ra-dichloride in men with castration-resistant metastatic prostate cancer. Eur J Nucl Med Mol Imaging. 2013;40:1384–93.
24. van Rensburg AJ, Alberts AS, Louw WKA. Quantifying the radiation dosage to individual skeletal lesions treated with samarium-153-EDTMP. J Nucl Med. 1998;39:2110–5.
25. Lewington VJ. Bone-seeking radionuclides for therapy. J Nucl Med. 2005;46:38S–47S.
26. Maxon HR, Schroder LE, Thomas SR, Hertzberg VS, Deutsch EA, Scher HI, Samaratunga RC, Libson KF, Williams CC, Moulton JS. Re-186(Sn) HEDP for treatment of painful osseous metastases: initial clinical experience in 20 patients with hormone-resistant prostate cancer. Radiology. 1990;176:155–9.
27. Maxon HR, Schroder LE, Hertzberg VS, Thomas SR, Englaro EE, Samaratunga R, Smith H, Moulton JS, Williams CC, Ehrhardt GJ, et al. Rhenium-186(Sn) HEDP for treatment of painful osseous metastases: results of a double-blind crossover comparison with placebo. J Nucl Med. 1991;32:1877–81.
28. Liepe K, Hliscs R, Kropp J, Runge R, Knapp FF Jr, Franke WG. Dosimetry of ^{188}Re-hydroxyethylidene diphosphonate in human prostate cancer skeletal metastases. J Nucl Med. 2003;44:953–60.

30 Guidelines on Radioisotope Treatment of Bone Metastases in Prostate Cancer

Robert Murphy and Laura Evangelista

30.1 Introduction

Radium-223 (Ra-223), strontium-89 (Sr-89), and samarium-153 (Sm-153) are radiopharmaceuticals approved in the United States and elsewhere for the treatment of painful skeletal metastases in select populations (Tables 30.1 and 30.2). The primary aim of this chapter is to provide a cohesive educational review of practice recommendations for these agents using guidelines from professional societies, prescribing information, and published observations. Older agents, such as phosphorus-32 (P-32), and experimental agents or agents not approved in the United States, such as rhenium-186-HEDP, rhenium-188-HEDP, and Sn-117m-diethylenetriaminepentaacetic acid, are not discussed.

This review is for educational purposes only and does not substitute for the information provided in the package inserts for radium-223 [1], strontium-89 [2], and samarium-153 [3], does not substitute for published guidelines, nor should be considered an exhaustive examination of all of the published data on these agents. Furthermore, prescribing information can change, and it is critical for providers to continuously seek the most up-to-date information. Regulations established by the United States Nuclear Regulatory Commission for the medical use of byproduct material are not reviewed [4].

R. Murphy
Department of Radiology, Mayo Clinic, Rochester, MN, USA
e-mail: murphy.robert@mayo.edu

L. Evangelista (✉)
Veneto Institute of Oncology IOV – IRCCS, Padua, Italy
e-mail: laura.evangelista@iov.veneto.it

30.2 Ra-223 Mechanism of Action

Radium-223 (Ra-223) is a radioactive alkaline earth metal (in the same group as calcium) that decays to lead-207 with approximately 95% of energy released as four alpha particles [5]. When administered intravenously, it concentrates in the skeleton, particularly in areas of bone turnover [6–9]. The alpha particles deposit a large amount of energy over a very short range (2–10 cell diameters). This results in difficult to repair, double-stranded DNA breaks and local tumor cell death while mostly sparing nearby bone marrow [10]. Sr-89 and Sm-153 also target the skeleton, but their beta particles have a much longer maximal range (about 8 mm and 3 mm respectively) into adjacent, normal tissue [2, 3, 11]. Therefore, the biophysical profile of Ra-223 is the most ideal of the three agents for the treatment of prostate cancer metastases to the skeleton.

Several professional societies have recently published evidence-based guidelines for the use of radium-223 dichloride (commercial name, Xofigo)

E. Bombardieri et al. (eds.), *Clinical Applications of Nuclear Medicine Targeted Therapy*,
https://doi.org/10.1007/978-3-319-63067-0_30

Table 30.1 Radium-223 therapy guidelines and package insert links

Professional society guidelines	Links
American Urological Association (AUA)—2015	https://www.auanet.org/education/guidelines/castration-resistant-prostate-cancer.cfm
Canadian Urological Association (CUA)	http://pubmedcentralcanada.ca/pmcc/articles/PMC4455631/
Canadian Urological Oncology Group (CUOG)—2015	
Cancer Care Ontario (CCO)—2017	http://www.sciencedirect.com/science/article/pii/S093665551730033X
European Association of Urology (EAU)	http://www.sciencedirect.com/science/article/pii/S0302283816304699
European Society for Radiotherapy and Oncology (ESTRO)	
International Society of Geriatric Oncology (SIOG)—2017	
European Society for Medical Oncology (ESMO)—2015	https://academic.oup.com/annonc/article/26/suppl_5/v69/344382/Cancer-of-the-prostate-ESMO-Clinical-Practice
National Comprehensive Cancer Network (NCCN)—2017	https://www.nccn.org/professionals/physician_gls/pdf/prostate.pdf
Package inserts	
Radium-223 (Xofigo)—2016 update	https://www.accessdata.fda.gov/scripts/cder/daf/index.Cfm?event=overview.process&ApplNo=203971
Strontium-89 (Metastron)—2013	https://www.accessdata.fda.gov/scripts/cder/daf/index.cfm?event=overview.process&applno=020134
Samarium 153 (Quadramet)—2014	http://www.lantheus.com/products/overview/quadramet/
General summary	Ra-223 is appropriate for the treatment of castrate-resistant prostate cancer in patients with symptomatic skeletal metastases and no known visceral metastases, regardless of whether or not the patient has received prior docetaxel therapy. Patients with good performance status are more likely to complete therapy, and consideration should be given to the risks vs. benefits of therapy in regard to the patient's overall status and goals. Sequencing with other therapies remains a topic of investigation. Bone marrow function must be followed during therapy

Table 30.2 Commercial radiotracers for prostate cancer therapy

Isotope	Radium-223 [1]	Strontium-89 [2]	Samarium-153 [3]
Commercial name and manufacturer	Xofigo	Metastron	Quadramet
	Bayer HealthCare Pharmaceuticals	GE Healthcare	Lantheus Medical Imaging
Indication	Treatment of symptomatic skeletal metastases in men with castration-resistant prostate ca and no visceral metastases	Pain palliation of confirmed bone metastases	Pain palliation of skeletal metastases that are visible on radionuclide bone scans
Dose	55 kBq (1.49 μCi)/kg body weight every month for 6 months	148 MBq (4 mCi) or 1.5–22 MBq (40–60 μCi)/kg body weight	37 MBq (1.0 mCi)/kg

Table 30.2 (continued)

Isotope	Radium-223 [1]	Strontium-89 [2]	Samarium-153 [3]
Min required blood counts for therapy (from [36])			
Platelet × 10(9)/L	100 first dose; 50 subsequent does	At least 60 (preferably 100)	At least 60 (preferably 100)
ANC × 10(9)/L	1.5 first dose; 1.0 subsequent doses	Greater than 2.0	Greater than 2.0
WBC	No information	At least 2.4–3.0 (preferably 5.0)	At least 2.4–3.0 (preferably 5.0)
Hg (g/dL)	10 first dose; No info for subsequent doses	Greater than 10	Greater than 10
Therapeutic particle	Alpha (5–7.5 MeV), 4 emitted per Ra-223	Beta (0.583 MeV average) from [38]	Beta (0.233 MeV average)
Soft tissue range	Less than 100 μm	Approximately 8 mm maximum	Approximately 3 mm maximum
Physical $T_{1/2}$	11.4 days	50.5 days	1.93 days
Excretion	Majority fecal. About 5% in urine	Approximately 2/3 urinary and 1/3 fecal	Majority urine

ca cancer

as therapy in men with castrate-resistant prostate cancer metastatic to the skeleton (Table 30.1).

The recommendations are based primarily on data from the Alpharadin in Symptomatic Prostate Cancer Patients (ALSYMPCA), phase 3, randomized, double-blinded clinical trial [12]. This trial demonstrated increased median survival (14.9 vs. 11.3 months) and delayed median time to the first symptomatic skeletal event (15.6 vs. 9.8 months) in men with metastatic castrate-resistant prostate cancer (mCRPC) and good functional status who received Ra-223 therapy vs. men who received placebo.

30.3 Intended Patient Population for RA-223 Therapy

In light of data from the ALSYMPCA trial, approval by the US Food and Drug Administration (FDA) is limited to patients with symptomatic skeletal metastases from castrate-resistant prostate cancer and no known visceral metastases [1]. Ra-223 has no benefit in men with prostate cancer metastases that do not involve the skeleton. Men with skeletal metastases and visceral metastases, such as liver, brain, and peritoneum, are not ideal candidates for Ra-223 therapy. These patients usually have poor functional status and may not be able to complete a six-month course of Ra-223 therapy. Furthermore, Ra-223 only targets the skeleton, and concurrent therapy with docetaxel and other agents that affect visceral disease is considered investigational at this time. Men with skeletal metastases and extensive nodal disease (e.g., widespread or greater than 3 cm in short-axis diameter) are also currently considered not to be appropriate candidates for Ra-223 therapy. This may evolve in the future as more advanced therapy protocols are elucidated which combine Ra-223 with other drugs [13]. This topic is discussed further below.

The majority of professional societies specify that Ra-223 therapy is appropriate when castrate-resistant bone metastases become symptomatic. The AUA suggests that "symptomatic" can be interpreted as requiring opiates for pain management [14]. Other leaders in practice suggest a holistic approach in which the effects of pain on the quality of life are taken into account [15]. In the ALSYMPCA trial, symptomatic was defined as requiring the regular use of analgesic medication or external beam radiation therapy (ERBT) for bone pain within 12 weeks before randomization [12].

It has been noted that patients with high metastatic burden and who have undergone multiple other therapies have difficulty completing the full course of six Ra-223 injections [16]. In the ALSYMPCA trial, 87% of patients in the treatment arm had Eastern Cooperative Oncology Group (ECOG) performance scores of only 0 or 1 [12]. Accordingly, the AUA suggests that Ra-223 therapy should be reserved for individuals with good performance status except in situations where poor performance status is directly related to bone metastases [14]. EAU, ESTRO, and SIOG jointly indicate that performance status, extent of disease, and comorbidities should be considered [17].

30.4 Sequencing of RA-223 with Other Therapies

Depending on clinical parameters, abiraterone (to inhibit androgen synthesis), enzalutamide (to inhibit the androgen receptor signaling pathway), and chemotherapy (usually docetaxel) are the primary therapeutic choices for metastatic castrate-resistant prostate cancer that is not limited to the skeleton [18]. Sipuleucel-T is an additional option outside of the European Union.

All of the above professional societies indicate that Ra-223 can be considered before and after chemotherapy (particularly docetaxel) in men with castrate-resistant prostate cancer metastatic to bone. The National Institute for Health Care Excellence (NICE) in England states that docetaxel should be used in those patients who can tolerate it before Ra-223 is considered [19]. However, the Prostate Cancer Radiographic Assessments for Detection of Advanced Recurrence II (RADAR II) Working Group suggests chemotherapy should not be given as a first-line agent for metastatic castrate-resistant prostate cancer except in specific situations such as high-volume disease [20]. It has been noted that the incidences of grades 3 and 4 thrombocytopenia and neutropenia are higher in patients who receive Ra-223 and who have had prior therapy with docetaxel (8.9% thrombocytopenia; 3.2% neutropenia) compared to those who receive Ra-223 and who have not had prior therapy with docetaxel (2.8% thrombocytopenia; 0.8% neutropenia) [21]. There is growing recognition that early treatment with Ra-223 may be a preferred course of action [18].

Abiraterone and enzalutamide can be given before or after Ra-223. Co-administration of Ra-223 with abiraterone and enzalutamide is the subject of clinical trials (e.g., NCT02043678/ERA223, NCT02194842/mCRPC-PEACEIII, NCT 02034552, NCT02225704, NCT02097303) [22], although this is already done in some clinical practice settings since the mechanisms of action are different [15, 20]. Sequencing of Ra-223 therapy with sipuleucel-T, which has limited availability, is discussed further by Crawford et al. [20]. Concurrent administration of chemotherapy (e.g., docetaxel) and Ra-223 is not appropriate outside of a clinical trial (e.g., NCT01106352) [22] due to concern for potential harmful bone marrow suppression.

External beam radiation to select painful bone metastases is acceptable during Ra-223 therapy [20, 23]. The potential for unacceptable myelosuppression from concurrent use of hemibody radiation or other systemic therapeutic radionuclides (e.g., Sm-153 and Sr-89) with Ra-223 has not been studied [21]. Pathologic fractures and spinal cord compression should be treated by standard care (e.g., orthopedic fixation, external beam radiation therapy) before initiating or resuming Ra-223 therapy [21].

30.5 Other RA-223 Considerations

The full-dose regimen for Xofigo currently approved by the US Food and Drug Administration (FDA) is 55 kBq (1.49 μCi) per kg body weight administered every 4 weeks for a total of 6 injections [1]. The original package insert released in 2013 listed 50 kBq/kg body weight as the administered dose, but this was changed in 2016 to 55 kBq/kg body weight following reassessment of the National Institute of Standards and Technology (NIST) traceable reference material for Ra-223 [24]. Extension of therapy beyond these parameters is the subject of ongoing research (NCT02023697) [22]. Another consideration for future evaluation is whether or not dosing based on height rather than weight would be more appropriate since the skeleton is the target for Ra-223 [25].

The absolute neutrophil count (ANC) should be at least 1.5 × 10(9)/L, the platelet count should be at least 100 × 10(9)/L, and the hemoglobin level should be at least 10.0 g/dL before the first administration of drug (Table 30.2). The ANC should be at least 1.0 × 10(9) and the platelet count at least 50 × 10(9)/L before subsequent administrations. The NCCN guidelines comment that the minimal platelet criterion for subsequent therapy might be too low in practice [26]; no additional elaboration is made. The next round of therapy should be delayed if the ANC has not recovered to at least 1.0 × 10(9) and platelets to 50 × 10(9)/L during the typical 4-week interval between injections. If values have not recovered by 6–8 weeks since the last administration of Ra-223, then therapy should be terminated [1]. In ALSYMPCA, 1.3, 2.2, and 6.3% of patients treated with Ra-223 experienced grade 3–4 leukopenia, neutropenia, and thrombocytopenia vs. 0.3, 0.7, and 2.0% in the placebo arm [21].

Administered Ra-223 not taken up by the skeleton is predominantly eliminated in feces, and safety of use in patients with Crohn disease, ulcerative colitis, and severe constipation has not been evaluated [1]. A patient treated with Ra-223 and who has unmanageable fecal incontinence is a potential radiation safety issue for caregivers. In ALSYMPCA, 25.0, 35.5, and 18.5% of patients treated with Ra-223 experienced diarrhea, nausea, and vomiting vs. 15.0, 34.6, and 13.6% in the placebo arm [21]. The package insert advises that safety has not been assessed in patients with several renal impairment (creatinine clearance less than 30 mL/min), moderate hepatic dysfunction, or severe hepatic dysfunction [1]. Fortunately, the kidneys and liver are not major routes of elimination.

There are no specific contact restrictions for patients treated with Ra-223 since most decay energy (approximately 95%) is released as alpha particles with a range of only about 100 μm (2–10 cell diameters) in tissue. Minor amounts of beta radiation (3.6%) and high-energy photons (1.1%) are released [27]. Realistically, the only potential source of significant exposure to others is through inadvertent ingestion of bodily excretions, particularly feces. Thus, patient instructions focus on good bathroom hygiene, hand washing, and the use of gloves to clean up spills. It is advised that sexually active men should wear condoms for a week after therapy due to the potential for a small amount of radiotracer to be transferred in semen [27]. Males and female partners are advised to use contraception until 6 months have elapsed following therapy due to the potential effect of radiation on spermatogenesis [21].

Use of biochemical markers and imaging to monitor the efficacy of ongoing Ra-223 therapy remains a topic of investigation. It is common for PSA to continue to rise during treatment, and it is the general consensus that rising PSA during therapy does not warrant discontinuation before the full course of six injections is completed. Rapidly rising PSA may be an indicator of the development of visceral disease and should prompt a CT scan. If rising PSA is determined to be due to development of visceral/nodal metastases, Crawford et al. [20] suggest adding abiraterone or enzalutamide as concurrent therapy. Alkaline phosphatase is a promising biomarker that is being further elucidated [18, 20, 25, 28]. Bone scan response is still a topic of research (NCT02034552) [22]. Further investigation is needed to evaluate the utility of more advanced imaging methods, such as choline PET-CT, to monitor Ra-223 therapy response. Pain flares are common during treatment [16] and should not prompt early termination of therapy.

A case report in the literature [29] describes a patient who experienced an infiltration of Ra-223 into his hand during therapy and developed acantholytic squamous cell cancer at the same location 4 months later. As of this writing, the authors are otherwise unaware of any other secondary malignancies attributable to Ra-223 therapy. This is a subject of ongoing research as part of the REASSURE trial (NCT02141438) [22].

Radium-223 is not approved in the United States for treatment of bone metastases from other neoplasms such as breast cancer and osteosarcoma; this is the subject of ongoing research (e.g., NCT02258464, NCT01833520) [22].

30.6 Strontium-89 and Samarium-153

Like Ra-223, strontium-89 (Sr-89) is in an alkaline earth metal in Group II of the periodic table along with calcium. As such, it is directly incorporated into hydroxyapatite [30]. The FDA approved Sr-89 chloride (commercial name, Metastron) in 1993 for palliation of confirmed, painful skeletal metastases [2] with a recommended dose of 4 mCi or a body weight-based dose of 40–60 μCi/kg (Table 30.2). In this patient population, about 1/3 of administered Sr-89 is excreted in the feces, and 2/3 is excreted in the urine. Onset of pain relief takes approximately 7–20 days, with about 50–60% of patients showing benefit [31]. This is similar to the 56% response rate seen for patients with symptomatic skeletal metastases who were administered a single 50 kBq/kg does of Ra-223 [32]. Per the package insert [2], platelet counts decline about 30% from baseline with a nadir between 12 and 16 weeks after injection, though others with extensive experience with Sr-89 report a decrease of up to 47% with a nadir at about 9 weeks post administration [33]. It can take up to 6 months for recovery. The physical half-life of 50.5 days can complicate subsequent use of myelosuppressive therapy should the need arise. However, patients can have prolonged relief from bone pain for an average of 6 months [34]. Repeated therapy is possible, but this can have a cumulative suppressive effect on platelet counts [33].

Samarium-153-ethylenediaminetetramethylenephosphonic acid (Sm-153-EDTMP or Sm153 lexidronam) targets bone likely via the affinity of EDTMP for hydroxyapatite [11, 35]. The FDA approved Sm-153 lexidronam pentasodium (commercial name, Quadramet) in 1997 for pain relief of osteoblastic bone metastases that are visible on radionuclide bone scan, with a recommended dosage of 1.0 mCi/kg [3]. Pain relief occurs in an average of 70% of patients [31] and takes approximately one week with maximal effect occurring at about 3–4 weeks [3]. Platelet counts decline about 40–50% from baseline with a nadir between 3 and 5 weeks after injection. It can take up to eight weeks for recovery. Per the Quadramet package insert [3], the percentages of treated patients in clinical trials showing combined grade 3 and 4 toxicities (National Cancer Institute Criteria) were 13% for hemoglobin (vs. 8% placebo), 8% for leukocytes (vs. 0% placebo), and 6% for platelets (0% placebo). With a physical half-life of 1.9 days, the nadir and recovery are faster than for Sr-89.

Guidelines published by the Society of Nuclear Medicine and Molecular Imaging [36] recommend that blood counts be obtained no more than 7 days prior to therapy with Sr-89 or Sm-153, with levels being at least 60,000/μL for platelets, at least 2400–3000/μL for white blood cells (2000/μL for the absolute granulocyte count), and more than 10 g/dL for the hemoglobin level (Table 30.2). The package insert for Metastron states to use caution if the white blood cell count is below 2400 or if the platelet count is below 60,000 [2]. Leukocyte and platelet counts should be monitored beginning 2 weeks after the injection and continued every 1–3 weeks thereafter for a 12–16 week period [36]. Repeated therapy, if desired, should be given no earlier than 3 months after prior therapy and only if sufficient marrow recovery has occurred. Patients who have diffuse skeletal metastases and a "superscan" on scintigraphic bone imaging may not be appropriate candidates for therapy with Sr-89 and Sm-153 [18]. The package insert for Quadramet states that caution should be exercised if there is suspicion for disseminated intravascular coagulation [3]. Though not specifically stated in the package insert for Metastron, it is logical to extend this recommendation to Sr-89. Some consider disseminated intravascular coagulation to be an absolute contraindication to therapy with Sr-89 and Sm-153 [37]. Pathologic fractures and spinal cord compression should be treated by standard care (e.g., orthopedic fixation, external beam radiation therapy) before initiating therapy with Sr-89 or Sm-153. A negative pregnancy test is required prior to therapy for breast and other cancers in women with reproductive potential. There is no specific guidance on how to make dose adjustments for patients with renal dysfunction.

Decay energy from Sr-89 and Sm-153 is primarily released as beta particles with maximum tissue penetration of about 0.8 cm for Sr-89 and 0.3 cm for Sm-153 [2, 3, 11, 35, 38]. Sm-153 also releases enough gamma photons (29%) to allow for scintigraphic imaging at 103-keV max [31, 34, 39]. Direct contact with body fluids, including accidental ingestion, is the major potential source of beta particle exposure to caregivers. Thus, instructions are provided to wear gloves to clean up body fluids, to wash hands after contact, and to be particularly cognizant about urine (the primary route of Sr-89 and Sm-153 elimination). About 1/3 of Sr-89 is eliminated in feces, so this too deserves special attention. Caregivers should minimize time spent in close proximity to patients treated with Sm-153 (e.g., not to sleep in the same bed) in order to reduce exposure to gamma rays (29% abundance). Beta emitters also produce secondary bremsstrahlung x-rays.

Neither Sr-89 nor Sm-153 has been definitively shown to extend survival as monotherapy in prostate cancer. However, some interesting observations have been made. Sr-89 combined with doxorubicin as consolidation therapy showed improved survival (median 27.7 months; range 4.9–37.7) compared to doxorubicin alone (16.8 months; range 4.4–34.2) in patients who had undergone induction therapy with ketoconazole and doxorubicin alternating with vinblastine and estramustine [40]. In patients with hormone refractory prostate cancer metastatic to the skeleton, Collins et al. [41] noted in a nonrandomized trial that single-dose administration of 2.5 mCi (93 MBq)/kg of Sm-153 resulted in a median survival of 9 vs. 6 months in men who received 1.0 mCi (37 MBq)/kg. In another trial [42], breast cancer patients with painful bone metastases showed a trend toward increased survival when randomized to 1.0 vs. 0.5 mCi/kg Sm-153. A survival advantage was not seen for prostate cancer patients that were also assessed in this study.

The package insert for Quadramet recommends against concurrent myelosuppressive therapy unless benefits are judged to outweigh risks [3]. No specific comment about concurrent therapy is made in the package insert for Metastron, but extreme caution is warranted given the long half-life of Sr-89. It should be noted that Sr-89 and Sm-153 were approved before the introduction of docetaxel and cabazitaxel.

Conclusion

Ra-223, an alkaline earth metal in the same group as calcium, is approved for use in men with symptomatic skeletal metastases from castrate-resistant metastatic prostate cancer and no known visceral metastases. It relieves bone pain and extends survival. Sm-153 and Sr-89 are options for palliation of bone pain in individuals with documented painful skeletal metastases.

Ra-223 is advantageous because approximately 95% of its decay energy is released as alpha particles. Alpha particles are equivalent to helium nuclei and are composed of two protons and two neutrons. Due to size and mass, they deposit considerable energy over a span of only 2–10 cells and leave a localized trail of damage including difficult to repair (and thus lethal) double-stranded DNA breaks. In contrast, almost all decay energy from Sr-89, and the majority of decay energy from Sm-153, is released as beta particles (high-energy electrons). An electron is less than 1/1800 the mass of a single proton and can travel several millimeters through matter before hitting another atomic structure. Less energy is deposited at the site of tumor, and DNA damage often manifests repairable single-stranded breaks.

Radiation directly leaves the body in the excreta of patients treated with Ra-223, Sr-89, and Sm-153. Thus, instructions are given to reduce the potential exposure of others to the patient's body fluids, particularly feces and urine. Sm-153 decay generates a significant number of gamma photons (29% abundance). Thus, patients treated with this agent are given additional instructions for minimizing time in the presence of caregivers and bystanders.

All three agents, Ra-223, Sr-89, and Sm-153, have varying effects on bone marrow function. Monitoring required for Ra-223 (baseline and q-monthly just prior to next therapy) is less stringent than that for Sr-89 and Sm-153 (baseline, q 1–3 weeks for

12–16 weeks, and just prior to any subsequent therapy). Concurrent use of these agents with myelosuppressive chemotherapy is either currently not approved (Ra-223) or discouraged (Sr-89 and Sm-153).

References

1. Bayer. Xofigo prescribing information. 2016 [cited 2017 May 27]. Available from: http://labeling.bayerhealthcare.com/html/products/pi/Xofigo_PI.pdf.
2. GE. Metastron prescribing information. 2013 [cited 2017 May 27]. Available from: https://www.accessdata.fda.gov/scripts/cder/daf/index.cfm?event=overview.process&applno=020134.
3. Lantheus. Quadramet prescribing information. 2014. Available from: http://www.lantheus.com/products/overview/quadramet/.
4. USNRC. Code of Federal Regulations, Title 10, Part 35 (10 CFR Part 35) – Medical use of byproduct material. 2017 [cited 2017 Jun 04]. Available from: https://www.nrc.gov/reading-rm/doc-collections/cfr/part035/.
5. Larson RH, Henriksen G, Bruland ØS. Preparation and use of radium-223 to target calcified tissues for pain palliation, bone cancer therapy, and bone surface conditioning. 2003: United States patent US6635234 B1.
6. Henriksen G, et al. Targeting of osseous sites with alpha-emitting 223Ra: comparison with the beta-emitter 89Sr in mice. J Nucl Med. 2003;44(2):252–9.
7. Nilsson S, et al. First clinical experience with alpha-emitting radium-223 in the treatment of skeletal metastases. Clin Cancer Res. 2005;11(12):4451–9.
8. Carrasquillo JA, et al. Phase I pharmacokinetic and biodistribution study with escalating doses of (2)(2)(3)Ra-dichloride in men with castration-resistant metastatic prostate cancer. Eur J Nucl Med Mol Imaging. 2013;40(9):1384–93.
9. Abou DS, et al. Whole-body and microenvironmental localization of radium-223 in naive and mouse models of prostate cancer metastasis. J Natl Cancer Inst. 2016;108(5):djv380.
10. Frankenberg-Schwager M, Frankenberg D. Rejoining of radiation-induced DNA double-strand breaks in yeast. In: Obe G, editor. Advances in mutagenesis research. Berlin: Springer; 1991. p. 1–25.
11. Finlay IG, Mason MD, Shelley M. Radioisotopes for the palliation of metastatic bone cancer: a systematic review. Lancet Oncol. 2005;6(6):392–400.
12. Parker C, et al. Alpha emitter radium-223 and survival in metastatic prostate cancer. N Engl J Med. 2013;369(3):213–23.
13. Saad F, et al. Radium-223 and concomitant therapies in patients with metastatic castration-resistant prostate cancer: an international, early access, open-label, single-arm phase 3b trial. Lancet Oncol. 2016;17(9):1306–16.
14. Lowrance WT, et al. Castration-resistant prostate cancer: AUA guideline amendment 2015. J Urol. 2016;195(5):1444–52.
15. Shore ND. When to initiate treatment with radium-223 in patients with metastatic castration-resistant prostate cancer. Clin Adv Hematol Oncol. 2016;14(1):26–9.
16. Modi D, et al. Radium-223 in heavily pretreated metastatic castrate-resistant prostate cancer. Clin Genitourin Cancer. 2016;14(5):373. e2–380.e2.
17. Cornford P, et al. EAU-ESTRO-SIOG guidelines on prostate cancer. Part II: treatment of relapsing, metastatic, and castration-resistant prostate cancer. Eur Urol. 2017;71(4):630–42.
18. Baldari S, et al. Management of metastatic castration-resistant prostate cancer: A focus on radium-223: opinions and suggestions from an expert multidisciplinary panel. Crit Rev Oncol Hematol. 2017;113:43–51.
19. Umeweni N, Knight H, McVeigh G. NICE guidance on gadium-223 dichloride for hormone-relapsed prostate cancer with bone metastases. Lancet Oncol. 2016;17(3):275–6.
20. Crawford ED, et al. The role of therapeutic layering in optimizing treatment for patients with castration-resistant prostate cancer (prostate cancer radiographic assessments for detection of advanced recurrence II). Urology. 2017;104:150–9.
21. Bayer. Product Monograph Xofigo. Radium Ra 223 dichloride solution for injection. [Monograph] 2016 [cited 2017 Apr 02]. Available from: http://omr.bayer.ca/omr/online/xofigo-pm-en.pdf.
22. NLM, ClinicalTrials.gov. 2017.
23. Finkelstein S, et al. External beam radiation therapy (EBRT) use and safety with radium-223 dichloride (Ra-223) in patients with castration-resistant prostate cancer (CRPC) and symptomatic bone metastases (mets) from the ALSYMPCA trial. Int J Radiat Oncol Biol Phys. 2015;93(3):S20. [Abstract 1107].
24. USNRC. Revision to the National Institute of Standards and Technology standard for radium-223 and impact on dose calibration for the medical use of radium-223 dichloride. 2016 [cited 2017 Jun 18]. Available from: https://www.nrc.gov/docs/ML1526/ML15264B095.pdf.
25. Hague C, Logue JP. Clinical experience with radium-223 in the treatment of patients with advanced castrate-resistant prostate cancer and symptomatic bone metastases. Ther Adv Urol. 2016;8(3):175–80.
26. NCCN. NCCN Clinical Practice Guidelines in Oncology (NCCN Guidelines). Prostate Cancer. Version 2.2017 2017 [cited 2017 Apr 02]. Available from: https://www.nccn.org/professionals/physician_gls/pdf/prostate.pdf.
27. Dauer LT, et al. Radiation safety considerations for the use of (2)(2)(3)RaCl(2) DE in men with castration-resistant prostate cancer. Health Phys. 2014;106(4):494–504.

28. Sartor O, et al. An exploratory analysis of alkaline phosphatase, lactate dehydrogenase, and prostate-specific antigen dynamics in the phase 3 ALSYMPCA trial with radium-223. Ann Oncol. 2017;28(5):1090–7.
29. Benjegerdes KE, Brown SC, Housewright CD. Focal cutaneous squamous cell carcinoma following radium-223 extravasation. Proc (Bayl Univ Med Cent). 2017;30(1):78–9.
30. Brady D, Parker CC, O'Sullivan JM. Bone-targeting radiopharmaceuticals including radium-223. Cancer J. 2013;19(1):71–8.
31. Jong JM, et al. Radiopharmaceuticals for palliation of bone pain in patients with castration-resistant prostate cancer metastatic to bone: a systematic review. Eur Urol. 2016;70(3):416–26.
32. Nilsson S, et al. A randomized, dose-response, multicenter phase II study of radium-223 chloride for the palliation of painful bone metastases in patients with castration-resistant prostate cancer. Eur J Cancer. 2012;48(5):678–86.
33. Preston DF, Dusing RW. Therapy for painful skeletal metastases. In: Henkin RE, editor. Nuclear medicine. Philadelphia: Mosby Elsevier; 2006.
34. Pandit-Taskar N, Batraki M, Divgi CR. Radiopharmaceutical therapy for palliation of bone pain from osseous metastases. J Nucl Med. 2004; 45(8):1358–65.
35. Nilsson S. Radionuclide therapies in prostate cancer: integrating radium-223 in the treatment of patients with metastatic castration-resistant prostate cancer. Curr Oncol Rep. 2016;18(2):14.
36. Silberstein EB, et al. Society of Nuclear Medicine procedure guideline for palliative treatment of painful bone metastases. 2003 [cited 2017 May 27]. Available from: http://snmmi.files.cms-plus.com/docs/pg_ch25_0403.pdf.
37. Henkin RE, et al. ACR-ASTRO practice guideline for the performance of therapy with unsealed radiopharmaceutical sources. Clin Nucl Med. 2011;36(8):e72–80.
38. UCSD. Radionuclide Data Sheets. 2017 [cited 2017 Jun 04]. Available from: https://blink.ucsd.edu/safety/radiation/research/RUA/radionuclide.html.
39. Eary JF, et al. Samarium-153-EDTMP biodistribution and dosimetry estimation. J Nucl Med. 1993;34(7):1031–6.
40. Tu SM, et al. Bone-targeted therapy for advanced androgen-independent carcinoma of the prostate: a randomised phase II trial. Lancet. 2001;357(9253):336–41.
41. Collins C, et al. Samarium-153-EDTMP in bone metastases of hormone refractory prostate carcinoma: a phase I/II trial. J Nucl Med. 1993;34(11):1839–44.
42. Resche I, et al. A dose-controlled study of 153Sm-ethylenediaminetetramethylenephosphonate (EDTMP) in the treatment of patients with painful bone metastases. Eur J Cancer. 1997;33(10):1583–91.

Part V

Lymphomas

Radioimmunotherapy of Lymphomas

31

Stefano Luminari, Silvia Morbelli, Lucia Garaboldi, Mahila Esmeralda Ferrari, and Alberto Biggi

Abstract

Radioimmunotherapy (RIT) using radionuclide labeled anti-CD20 monoclonal antibodies allows for the delivery of the radionuclides directly to the surface of targeted B-cell non-Hodgkin's lymphoma (NHL) achieving additional cytotoxic effect.

Actually the only RIT agent is 90Y-ibritumomab tiuxetan registered and commercialized as Zevalin® in the USA since February 2002 and in European Union since 2004.

In the first part, the main characteristics of the radiopharmaceutical are described including the different steps of RIT, i.e., radiolabeling and quality control procedure, the preparation of the patients for the treatment, the preparation and administration of the individual dose, and the main contraindications, risks, and collateral effects. The entire procedure reported in this chapter follows the Annex I summary of product characteristics.

In the second part dedicated to radiation protection issue, the current modalities of the treatment are reported in order to obtain the best clinical results and at the same time to respect the radiation protection recommendations, considering the patients, their relatives, and the nuclear medicine staff.

In the third part on clinical experience with Zevalin®, the most important clinical results are discussed. These studies highlight the safety and efficacy of the treatment especially in relapsed/refractory low-grade follicular lymphoma but also in other CD20-positive lymphomas. Despite these evidences, 90Y-ibritumomab tiuxetan during the time missed its

S. Luminari
Haematology Department, Arcispedale Santa Maria Nuova, IRCCS and Univerità di Modena e Reggio Emilia, Reggio Emilia, Italy

S. Morbelli • L. Garaboldi
Nuclear Medicine Department, IRCCS San Martino – IST, Genova, Italy

M.E. Ferrari
Medical Physics Unit, European Institute of Oncology, Milano, Italy

A. Biggi (✉)
Nuclear Medicine Department, Santa Croce e Carle Hospital, Cuneo, Italy
e-mail: biggi.a@ospedale.cuneo.it

E. Bombardieri et al. (eds.), *Clinical Applications of Nuclear Medicine Targeted Therapy*,
https://doi.org/10.1007/978-3-319-63067-0_31

high initial interest for hematologists, and at present its use became limited for various reasons. These treatments in different countries require protected dedicated rooms not always available in all hospitals; the use of this radioisotope therapy includes several complex multidisciplinary steps, and some alternative nonradioactive options to 90Y-ibritumomab tiuxetan have demonstrated several comparable advantages in terms of feasibility and efficacy. However this targeted therapy still remains an important example of the successful therapeutic use of radiolabeled antibodies in the clinical routine of hematology.

31.1 Introduction

The treatment of B-cell non-Hodgkin's lymphoma (NHL) has undergone significant transformation since the approval of rituximab in November 26, 1997, by the US Food and Drug Administration (FDA). This chimeric monoclonal antibody is specifically targeted to the CD20 which is expressed on the surface of normal (except for pre-B cells and secretory B cells) and malignant B lymphocytes. Evidence suggests a role of CD20 in B-cell cycle progression as well as regulation of calcium influx necessary for B-cell activation. Rituximab exerts a cytotoxic effect via numerous different mechanisms including induction of apoptosis, antibody-dependent cell-mediated toxicity, and complement-mediated cytotoxicity; this cytotoxic response requires the physical association of the monoclonal antibody with the particular target cell [1]. Thus, a fractionated approach is necessary as evidenced by approved regimens for rituximab as sole therapy and in combination with chemotherapy.

It was recognized early that the addition of a radionuclide to a monoclonal antibodies would be a rational approach to achieving additional cytotoxic effects. This approach, termed radioimmunotherapy (RIT), allows for the delivery of the radionuclides directly to the surface of targeted tumor cells [2].

To date, two RIT agents have been approved by the FDA for the treatment of B-cell NHL: yttrium-90 (90Y)-ibritumomab tiuxetan (Zevalin®) (IDEC Pharmaceuticals, San Diego, CA) and iodine-131 (131I)-tositumomab (Bexxar®) (Corixa Corporation, South San Francisco, CA).

Ibritumomab is a murine monoclonal IgG1 kappa antibody directed against CD20 antigen, the parent from which the widely used chimeric monoclonal antibody rituximab (Mabthera®) was derived. The use of unlabeled ibritumomab together with 90Y-labeled tiuxetan was approved by the US Food and Drug Administration (FDA) in February 2002 as a radioimmunotherapeutic-based regimen for the treatment of adult patients with relapsed or refractory, low-grade, or follicular B-cell non-Hodgkin's lymphoma (NHL) and of previously untreated follicular NHL who achieve a partial or complete response to first-line chemotherapy. 90Y-ibritumomab tiuxetan was registered and commercialized as Zevalin® [3–5].

Tositumomab is a murine IgG2a lambda monoclonal antibody directed against CD20 antigen. The use of unlabeled tositumomab together with 131I-labeled tositumomab was approved by the US FDA on June 27, 2003, as a radioimmunotherapeutic-based regimen for the treatment of patients with CD20-positive relapsed or refractory, low-grade, follicular, or transformed non-Hodgkin's lymphoma who have progressed during or after rituximab therapy, including patients with rituximab-refractory non-Hodgkin's lymphoma. 131I-tositumomab was registered and commercialized as Bexxar® [6, 7].

Marketing approval Bexxar® was withdrawn in 2014 despite the high rate of response in 2014 due to marked decline in usage. Date of issue of marketing authorization valid throughout the European Union of Zevalin® was 16.01.2004 (agency product number: EMEA/H/C/000547).

31.2 The Radioimmunotherapy Agent Zevalin®

The entire procedure described in this chapter follows the *ANNEX I SUMMARY OF PRODUCT CHARACTERISTICS* (http://www.ema.europa.eu/ema/index).

31.2.1 What Is Zevalin®?

Zevalin® consists of ibritumomab and tiuxetan which is the MX-DTPA chelating agent for the radionuclide 90Y.

90Y is a pure β-emitter with physical characteristics suitable for therapy, i.e., $T_{1/2} = 2.67$ days, $E_{Max} = 2.27$ MeV, $E_{Mean} = 939$ keV, and an effective path length (R50) of 5.3 mm, meaning that 90% of its energy is absorbed within a sphere with 5.3 mm radius. This path length corresponds to 100–200 cell diameters, giving 90Y a broad cross-fire effect when it is conjugated to monoclonal antibody such as ibritumomab [8].

Pharmacokinetic studies have shown that almost the entire radioactivity of Zevalin® is retained within the body after injection. The median effective half-life for a standard dose of 15 MBq/kg of Zevalin® in blood is 28 h (range 14–44 h), provided that pretreatment with rituximab with a standard dose of 250 mg/m2 is performed. Urinary excretion is the primary clearance mechanism, and it accounts for the elimination of only 7.3 ± 3.2% of the administered activity over 7 days [9].

31.2.2 Radiolabeling

Zevalin® is supplied as a kit containing the non-radioactive components required for generating a single dose of 90Y-labeled ibritumomab tiuxetan. The kit must be stored at 2–8 °C and should not be frozen. The preparation of 90Y-Zevalin® is performed at room temperature. After radiolabeling 90Y-Zevalin® must be injected as soon as possible. Eventually the preparation may be stored at 2–8 °C (in a refrigerator) and protected from light for a maximum of 8 h.

The kit of Zevalin® contains:

- A bottle with piercable seal contains 3.2 mg (1.6 mg/mL) ibritumomab tiuxetan
- 2 mL sodium acetate solution in a bottle with piercable seal
- 10 mL formulated buffer solution in a bottle with piercable seal
- An empty 10 mL reaction vial

After radiolabeling the final formulation contains 2.08 mg ibritumomab tiuxetan in a total volume of 10 mL.

The radioactive component, 90Y (1.5 GBq), must be obtained separately upon order from the manufacturer. Sterile and pyrogen-free yttrium-90 chloride ($90YCl_3$), approved for radiolabeling of human drugs, should be used. The $90YCl_3$ activity must be in the range 1.67–3.34 GBq/mL, radiochemical purity range the radionuclidic purity ≤0.74 MBq 90Sr/37 GBq $90YCl_3$ activity must be in the range 1.67–3.34 GBq/mL, the radiochemical purity >95%, the radionuclidic purity ≤0.74 MBq 90Sr/37 GBq 90Y.

The labeling procedures must be carried out in a dedicated hot lab, using a hot cell made of a special material to shield both 90Y β-rays and bremsstrahlung spectrum. Protective shields for needles and containers and at least 1-cm-thick Perspex or lead-loaded Perspex shields during labeling must be used. Local regulations for procedures involving unsealed radioactive sources must be observed.

The labeling procedure follows the different steps described in Fig. 31.1:

Step 1: Transfer sodium acetate solution to the reaction vial.

A 10-mL 0.22-μm ventilated vial containing a volume of sodium acetate buffer equal to 1.2 $90YCl_3$ volume is used as reaction vial and placed inside a cylindrical polymethylmethacrylate (PMMA) shield.

Step 2: Transfer $90YCl_3$ to the reaction vial.

Generally the $90YCl_3$ vial is self-shielded with 8-mm plexiglass plus 4-mm lead containers; at the top of the plexiglass shielding, a small

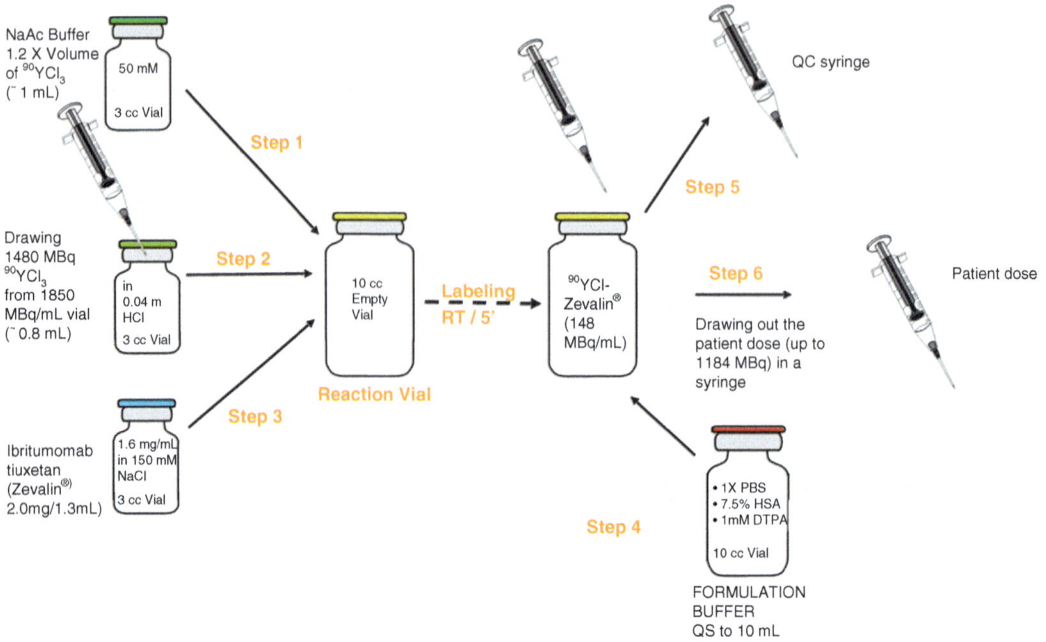

Fig. 31.1 Labeling procedure steps

hole allowed the insertion of the syringe needle and a second 0.22-μm ventilated needle. Whenever possible, activity concentration is kept constant at 1.85 GBq·mL⁻1. By means of a shielded syringe with a spinal needle reaching the V-shaped bottom, the correct 90YCl$_3$ activity (1.5 GBq) is drawn up and transferred into the reaction vial in a few seconds.

Step 3: Transfer ibritumomab tiuxetan solution to the reaction vial.

The corresponding amount of ibritumomab tiuxetan (1.3 mL) is added to the shielded reaction vial.

The reaction mixture is gently shaken and allowed to react for 5 min at room temperature. Labeling time longer than 6 min or shorter than 4 min will result in inadequate radioincorporation.

Step 4: Add the formulation buffer to the reaction vial.

Using a 10-mL syringe with a large bore needle (18–20 G), the formulation buffer was then added to the vented reaction vial up to 10 mL to block the reaction.

Step 5: Radiochemical purity (RCP) determination (see Sect. 31.2.3, Quality Control).

If the average radiochemical purity is less than 95%, the preparation must not be administered.

Step 6: Preparation of the patient dose (see Sect. 31.2.5, Preparation of the Patient Dose and Administration).

31.2.3 Quality Control

Radiochemical purity is performed by instant thin layer chromatography (ITLC) and must be carried out according to the following procedure.

The procedure requires materials not supplied in the Zevalin kit:

- Developing chamber for chromatography
- Mobile phase: sodium chloride 9 mg/mL (0.9%) solution, bacteriostatic-free
- ITLC strips (e.g., ITLC TEC-Control Chromatography Strips, Biodex, Shirley,

New York, USA, Art. Nr. 150–772 or equivalent, dimensions: approximately 0.5–1 × 6 cm)
- Scintillation vials
- Liquid scintillation cocktail (e.g., Ultima Gold, catalog No. 6013329, Packard Instruments, USA or equivalent)

Assay procedure:

- Add approximately 0.8-mL sodium chloride 9-mg/mL (0.9%) solution to developing chamber assuring the liquid will not touch the 1.4-cm origin mark on the ITLC strip.
- Using a 1-mL insulin syringe with a 25- to 26-G needle, place a hanging drop (7–10 μL) of [^{90}Y]-radiolabeled Zevalin onto the ITLC strip at its origin. Spot one strip at a time and run three ITLC strips. It may be necessary to perform a dilution (1:100) before application of the [^{90}Y]-radiolabeled Zevalin to the ITLC strips.
- Place ITLC strip in the developing chamber and allow the solvent front to migrate past the 5.4-cm mark.
- Remove ITLC strip and cut in half at the 3.5-cm cut line. Place each half into separate scintillation vials to which 5-mL LSC cocktail must be added (e.g., Ultima Gold, catalog No. 6013329, Packard Instruments, USA or equivalent). Count each vial in a beta counter or in an appropriate counter for 1 min (CPM), record net counts, corrected for background.
- Calculate the average radiochemical purity (RCP) as follows:

  Average % RCP = net CPM bottom half × 100/ net CPM top half + net CPM bottom half

  A labeling efficiency of 95% or more is required otherwise ^{90}Y-Zevalin® cannot be injected. The in vivo stability of ^{90}Y-Zevalin® is extremely high.

Alternately the radiochemical yield can be evaluated with different beta-counting systems for quantification, like autoradiography system (AS) and TLC scanner or dose calibrator (DC).

An example of AS is a high-resolution filmless autoradiography phosphor imager, employing a multisensitive and high-performance storage phosphor screen. The screen, protected from wet samples and radio contamination with a transparent film, was exposed to the radio-ITLC-SG strips, absorbed the energy emitted by the radioactivity, and later reemitted that energy as blue light (measured as a digital light unit, DLU) when excited by a red laser scanner device. The triplicate ITLCs can be analyzed at the same time by the storage phosphor screen, requiring no more than 10 s for exposure and 3 min for imaging and quantitation. All the triplicate values usually obtained in each labeling were self-consistent and had very high precision, with a maximum RCP deviation of 0.5%.

Using a TLC scanner, the triplicate radioactive strips can be scanned one at a time and their chromatograms acquired using a dedicated software and analyzed for radiolabeling yield calculation.

To calculate the radiolabeling yield, it is also possible to use a dose calibrator but only if the DC has been properly calibrated and if it is equipped with a specific and suitable sample holder for beta measurement. The isotope-specific calibration factors have to be determined employing a certified $^{90}YCl_3$ source, by comparing the theoretical ^{90}Y activity with the measured ^{90}Y activity, for each specific measurement condition (geometry, filling amount, and activity). The radioactive strips in triplicate have to be cut and separately counted by DC for calculation of radiolabeling yield. As expected, with ITLC silica gel in saline, ^{90}Y-Zevalin remain at the point of spotting (RF = 0.0), while ^{90}Y-DTPA moved toward the solvent front (RF = 0.8–1.0).

31.2.4 Preparation of the Patients (Pre-targeting with Unlabeled Mab)

Pre-targeting the patients with unlabeled rituximab (Mabthera®) is part of a treatment with Zevalin® necessary to obtain a more favorable biodistribution of the subsequently injected radiolabeled antibody by clearing peripheral B cells from the circulation. Not only does the unlabeled rituximab prevent the radiolabeled antibody to bind non-tumor sites (normal B cells, spleen), but

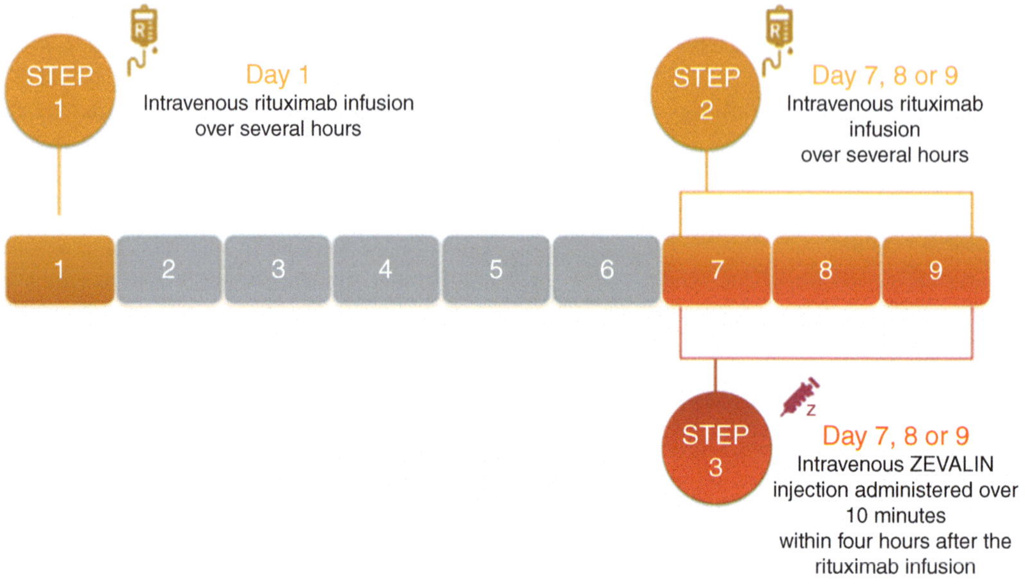

Fig. 31.2 Preparation of the patient for Y^{90}-Zevalin therapy

it is also said to facilitate deeper penetration into the tumor, translating into a more homogenous distribution. Furthermore, rituximab itself induces several mechanisms of tumor cell killing such as antibody-dependent cellular cytotoxicity (ADCC) and complement-dependent cytotoxicity (CDC), but also direct induction of apoptosis and possibly cell cycling blockade. In radioimmunotherapy the biological effects of the monoclonal antibody and of radiation are thought to be synergistic.

In Fig. 31.2 is reported the administration scheme of pre-targeting with rituximab. Briefly on day 1, intravenous infusion of 250-mg/m2 rituximab is administered to the patient. The volume of normal saline solution, which contains the rituximab stock solution, and the infusion must comply with the recommendations contained in the package insert of the preparation. The administration of rituximab at the same dosage is repeated on day 7, 8, and 9 and at these time points is followed by administration of 90Y-Zevalin® over 10 min.

31.2.5 Preparation of the Patient Dose and Administration

The therapeutic dose of Zevalin® is calculated in functions of the patient's weight and baseline platelet count. If the platelet count is normal (≥150,000 cells/mm3), the recommended dose is 15 MBq/kg (0.4 mCi/kg); if the platelet count is between 100 and 150,000 cells/mm3, the dose is 11 MBq/kg (0.3 mCi/kg). If the platelet count is below 100 cells/mm3, treatment cannot be performed. In any case, the administered dose should not exceed 1.18 GBq (32 mCi).

If administered after first-line chemotherapy, RIT with Zevalin® should be performed between 6 and 12 weeks after the last dose of first-line chemotherapy to allow the recovery of platelet counts to ≥150,000 cells/mm3.

The patient dose is drawn out with a shielded syringe, or alternatively, the slight excess of activity present in the shielded reaction vial is drawn out with a remotely controlled dispensing unit or manually, to leave the prescribed dose for the patient in the reaction vial, which was immediately measured. An infusion system in which the prescribed dose is administered through a shielded vial pushed out by gravimetric pressure with saline can be used.

The 90Y activity is measured by a dose calibrator set for the geometry in use. For β-emitters the precise measurement of injected activity depends significantly from the geometry of measurement. Thus the best approach consists in setting the dose calibrator for a standard geometry (i.e., a volume of 8-mL 90Y in a 10-mL syringe) [10].

Ideally Zevalin® should be administered within 4 h of completion of the rituximab dose as a slow intravenous push over approximately 10 min; Zevalin® should not be administered as an intravenous. When the drug is administered, the syringe shields made of materials such as acrylic are preferred; in addition to the 1 cm of plastic surrounding the syringe, lead or more plastic can be used for shielding the low-energy bremsstrahlung.

31.2.6 Contraindication

The main contraindication to treatment is previous hypersensitivity to ibritumomab tiuxetan, to rituximab, and to yttrium.

The presence of human anti-mouse antibodies (HAMA) should be tested before treatment in patients previously treated with rituximab or Zevalin.

To perform radioimmunotherapy, patients had to be not pregnant or lactating and following reliable birth control methods.

31.2.7 Risks and Collateral Effects

The most common adverse events reported during the trial are hematological. The hematological toxicity is related to a mielodepression that involves all the bone marrow population and implies thrombocytopenia, neutropenia, and anemia. Mielodepression usually starts 2–3 weeks after the treatment; the nadir for thrombocyte and granulocyte is reached after 4–8 weeks with a complete recovery after 12 weeks; mean recovery time are 27 days for granulocyte, 23 days for thrombocytes, and 15 days for hemoglobin. Usually a moderate toxicity is observed. However in 40–50% of the patients, a grade 3 or 4 thrombocytopenia is observed with a median time of recovery of 13 and 21 days, respectively, while in 30–40% of the patients, a grade 3 or 4 neutropenia is observed with a median time of recovery of 8 and 14 days, respectively [11, 12].

The most common nonhematologic adverse events reported during clinical trials of 90Y-ibritumomab tiuxetan included, but were not limited to, asthenia, nausea, infection, chills, fever, and abdominal pain [13].

Because of the potential for anaphylactic and other hypersensitivity reactions related to the administration of proteins to patients, medications for the treatment of such reactions, such as epinephrine, antihistamines, and corticosteroids, should be readily available during the administration of both rituximab and 90Y-ibritumomab tiuxetan. However the incidence of HAMA and of human anti-chimeric antibodies (HACA) in patients treated with Zevalin® and rituximab is low, around 2%, and anaphylactic, and other hypersensitivity reactions are observed in less than 1% of patients [14].

31.2.8 Radiation Protection Issue

Precautions taken for radiation protection purposes are aimed at three general objectives: (1) protecting the patient, (2) protecting the people close to the patient and household contacts of patients, and (3) protecting the nuclear medicine staff.

Even though the radiation exposure to medical workers and others is low, radiation precautions consistent with time, distance, and shielding principles should be followed to keep the exposure as low as reasonably achievable (ALARA).

31.2.9 Staff Safety

90Y, the therapeutic radionuclide in the Zevalin® regimen, is a pure β-emitter with physical characteristics suitable for therapy [8]; however, bremsstrahlung radiation is produced and is readily detectable externally.

During the different steps of therapy, hospital personnel may be exposed to intense radiation fields, and in particular major attention has to be paid to the preparation and administration of the radiopharmaceutical, due to the possible direct irradiation of the hands by an intense field of high-energy β-particles. As a general rule, plastic or acrylic is the preferred shielding for the beta emissions of 90Y, because lead or tungsten shielding leads to the production of bremsstrahlung [15].

The radiopharmaceutical labeling was identified as the procedures at higher risk [16]: the mean absorbed dose to fingertips during single-labeling procedures, with 1.5 GBq of Zevalin®, was 2.9 mGy (range 0.20–41.8 mGy), while the effective dose to the operator was negligible (<10 μSv/labeling), as expected. The doses measured by the "conventional" ring dosimeter provide only a rough estimation of the dose to the whole hand, but cannot reveal local "hot spots." Therefore, the regular monitoring of fingertip doses is strongly recommended.

During the patient administration, the standard universal precautions are suitable for shielding hospital workers, and the bremsstrahlung irradiation of the personnel during systemic administration and assistance of patients was very low (physician's hands <0.1 mGy/patient; nurse's and physician's thorax <5 μGy/patient).

31.2.10 Population Safety

Due to the physical and pharmacokinetics characteristics of Zevalin®, a low exposure to the people close to the patient and household contacts is expected. Patient hospitalization of less than 6 h after the injection guarantees the recommended limits of the Council Directive 97/43/Euratom. No people of the general population is expected to be exposed to a dose higher than 0.3 mSv/year, while no people of the family members is expected to be exposed to a dose higher than 3 mSv/year for those aged <60 years and of 10 mSv/year for those aged ≥60 years.

After the injection of 1036 MBq (28 mCi) of Zevalin® to a normal type patient, the intensity of the irradiation field around the patient is 15.7 μGy/h at a distance of 10 cm and 0.63 μGy/h at a distance of 50 cm.

A study was conducted to determine the radiation exposure to family members who had unrestricted contact with patients who had been treated with the ibritumomab tiuxetan regimen [15]: 13 family members wore personal dosimeters for the first 7 days after treatment, and no precautions were given aside from avoiding the patient's body wastes. The median deep dose equivalent radiation exposure to the family members was 3.5 μSv, which is within the range of normal background radiation.

Nevertheless, patients require some reassurance and instruction about intimacy and contact with family and friends. In general, patients are advised to avoid contamination of others with body fluids (saliva, blood, urine, seminal fluid, and stool), but instructions about distance and duration of contact are not considered necessary.

31.2.11 Patients Safety

Pre-therapeutic imaging with 111In-ibritumomab tiuxetan is mandatory in Switzerland and the USA. The imaging is performed not for dosimetric purposes but to confirm the expected biodistribution, as an additional safety measure before administering the Zevalin® therapy.

In the EU, EMEA has accepted that no dosimetry studies are required, because, probably due to methodological problems, the dosimetry performed during the registration trials showed a poor absorbed dose-response relationship, meaning that the pre-therapeutic dosimetry predicted neither therapeutic efficacy nor toxicity of the treatment [17].

In Zevalin® regimen, the injected activity is determined according to body weight and platelet counts. Dosimetry should be performed, however, when Zevalin® is used as an investigational treatment at higher activities [18] or for indications different from those defined in the registration trials in patients with indolent B-cell lymphomas [17].

Table 31.1 reports the dosimetry evaluations based on pre-therapeutic 111In imaging performed (1) during the registration trials [19] and (2) during a phase I–II trials based on high-dose 90Y-ibritumomab tiuxetan followed by autologous stem cell transplantation established by a more refined dosimetric approach performed [20].

Table 31.1 Organ radiation absorbed doses (median and range—mGy/MBq) for 90Y-ibritumomab tiuxetan

Organ	From Wiseman et al. [19]	From Cremonesi et al. [20]
Spleen	7.35 (0.37–29.7)	1.9 (0.8–5.0)
Liver	4.32 (0.85–17.5)	2.8 (1.8–10.6)
Lungs	2.05 (0.59–4.86)	1.7 (0.3–3.5)
Red marrow (blood derived)	0.59 (0.09–1.84)	0.8 (0.4–1.0)
Red marrow (sacrum derived)	0.97	
Kidneys	0.22 (0–0.95)	1.7 (0.6–3.8)
Bone surfaces	0.53 (0.09–1.31)	
Urinary bladder wall	0.89 (0.38–2.32)	
Other organs	0.41 (0.06–0.62)	0.4 (0.3–0.6)
Testes		2.8 (1.3–4.7)
Total body	0.54 (0.27–0.78)	0.5 (0.4–0.8)

The differences are due to different dosimetric approaches (in the first study, a whole-body-averaged attenuation correction factor was used instead of a transmission scan for attenuation correction, kidneys were not identified as major source organs, and the selection of curve fitting can further contribute to differences in the biokinetics of the liver and spleen, which typically show a prolonged uptake phase not easily interpretable by monoexponential) and to the quite diverse number of patients included in the studies (179 vs 22). In any case, a study shows that true altered bio distribution that disqualified patients from further treatment has been observed in only 6 (0.6%) of 953 patients [21].

31.3 Radioimmunotherapy in Lymphoma: Clinical Aspects

The potential clinical applications of RIT include relapsed/refractory (RR) indolent B-cell NHL (iNHL), diffuse large B-cell lymphoma (DLBCL), indolent lymphoma in the frontline setting, and mantle cell lymphoma (MCL).

The value of radioimmunotherapy (RIT) for the treatment of CD20-positive NHL has been first proved as monotherapy in patients with relapsed follicular lymphoma.

In a phase II study for RR iNHL, 59 patients were enrolled and treated with 131I-tositumomab, of whom 31 had transformed iNHL or aggressive NHL. The reported overall response (OR) rate and complete response (CR) rate were 71% and 34%, respectively, with higher activity for iNHL and transformed cases. The median progression-free survival (PFS) was around 1 year but it was greater than 20 months for those achieving a CR after RIT [22]. In a similar study of patients with RR or transformed iNHL, 47 patients were treated, with an OR rate of 57% and a CR rate of 32%, respectively [23].

On a phase III trial comparing 90Y-ibritumomab tiuxetan vs rituximab on 143 patients with RR, the higher activity of RIT was confirmed by the higher OR rate (80 vs 56%), CR rate (30 vs 16%), and median time to progression (24.7 vs 13.7 months) [5, 24]. Moreover patients with follicular lymphoma treated with RIT in first relapse experienced a higher CR than those treated later (51 vs 28%). In the same study, median PFS was also significantly better for those treated earlier (15.4 vs 9.2 months) [25].

In summary, RIT with either ^{131}I-tositumomab or ^{90}Y-ibritumomab tiuxetan has been shown to be an effective treatment option for patients with relapsed or refractory indolent B-cell NHL. OR rates range from approximately 60 to 80%, with nearly 40% of patients achieving a CR. Responses are seen both in patients who are rituximab refractory and in naïve subjects, and data evidence suggests higher activity when RIT is used early during the course of the disease.

The FIT trial first investigated the early use of RIT as consolidation therapy in patients with FL responding to initial chemotherapy [26]. The study enrolled 414 patients with follicular lymphoma; 90Y-ibritumomab tiuxetan consolidation significantly prolonged median PFS in all patients (36.5 vs 13.3 months in control arm). Median PFS with consolidation was prolonged in all Follicular Lymphoma International Prognostic Index (FLIPI) risk subgroups. The major criticism with the FIT study that was recently updated with confirmed results was that only approximately 14% of subjects received rituximab during the induction phase [27].

In the S0016 trial, consolidation with ^{131}I-tositumomab RIT after CHOP chemotherapy was compared in a randomized fashion with six cycles of standard R-CHOP chemotherapy [28]. A total of 526 patients were evaluated, and after 5 years of follow-up, no significant differences in OR rates, CR rates, or 2-year PFS or OS were observed. In addition, there were also no differences between the arms for toxicity (hematologic or nonhematologic) and for secondary malignancies, including secondary myelodysplastic syndrome (MDS).

More recently, based on the results of the PRIMA trial [29], 12 bimonthly doses of rituximab have been shown to improve PFS in patients responding to induction immunochemotherapy compared to observation. The question whether a single dose of 90Y-ibritumomab tiuxetan could be compared to standard maintenance treatment with rituximab has been recently addressed in the ZAR trial conducted by the Spanish intergroup PETHEMA/GELTAMO/GELCAB [30]. The study compared, in a randomized phase II trial, the use of consolidation with 90Y-RIT versus rituximab maintenance in 146 FL patients with high tumor burden, who had responded to R-CHOP. A total of 124 patients were randomized, and after a median follow-up of 37 months from randomization, PFS was of 64% in the 90Y-RIT and 86% in the rituximab maintenance arm.

Until now a "total treatment strategy" of immunochemotherapy, RIT, and maintenance has been investigated in FL only in a single phase II study by the MDACC groups [31]. A total of 46 valuable patients, high-risk stage III or IV FL, most of them with bone marrow involvement, were treated with four cycles of R-FND followed by 90Y-IT and rituximab maintenance (a single infusion every 2 months for 1 year) in the frontline setting. After R-FND, CR was 87% and following 90Y-RIT, it increased to 91%.

More interestingly the Fondazione Italiana Linfomi (FIL) is currently recruiting patients in two different randomized trials designed to compare RIT consolidation with ASCT in patients with RR FL responding to salvage immunochemotherapy (FLAZ trial) [32] and to try to overcome the bad prognostic features of patients with FL who have incomplete metabolic response to induction immunochemotherapy (FOLL12 study) [33]. If these two trials will be successful, novel indication to the use of RIT shall be identified in the next future.

The use RIT has also been investigated in DLBCL and MCL mostly with phase II trials but never with randomized studies.

In 104 patients with relapsed or primary refractory DLBCL treated with ^{90}Y-ibritumomab tiuxetan, CR rates ranged from 12 to 40%, with a discouraging median PFS ranging from 1.6 to 5.9 months was observed [34].

Similarly to FL RIT consolidation was also assessed in DLBCL patients following CHOP-based chemotherapy. Hamlin et al. reported results of a trial of 61 high-risk elderly patients. Patients received six cycles of R-CHOP, and then those with responding or stable disease received Zevalin 6–9 weeks later. Following R-CHOP treatment, 50 patients were eligible for Zevalin and 44 were ultimately treated. Zevalin was generally well tolerated, and 86% of patients experienced a complete response (CR) or unconfirmed complete response (CRu), while 2% experienced a partial response. Response improvement (from PR to CR or CRu to CR) occurred in 16% of patients. At 42 months, the overall survival for Zevalin-treated patients was 83.5%, and the progression-free survival was 74.5% [35].

More recently the 7-year update was provided of a multicenter phase II study in which 55 elderly high-risk untreated diffuse large B-cell lymphoma patients were treated with ^{90}Y-ibritumomab tiuxetan after a short course of R-CHOP. The overall response rate to the entire regimen was 80%, including 73% of CR. With a median follow-up of 7 years, the disease-free survival was 43.3%, and the progression-free survival was 36.1%. The overall survival at 7.9 years was 38.9% (27 deaths mainly because of lymphoma). Two patients developed secondary hematological malignancies, an acute myeloid leukemia and a myelodysplastic syndrome, at 4 and 3 years from RIT, respectively [36].

Data from RIT consolidation after R-CHOP in DLBCL confirm the feasibility, efficacy, and safety of this approach. A randomized trial is currently ongoing to try to address the question of the utility of a consolidation RIT in elderly patients responding to induction R-CHOP [37].

As far as mantle cell lymphoma (MCL) is concerned, activity of RIT in this lymphoma subtype has been first documented in a phase II study of 34 patients treated with single-agent ^{90}Y-ibritumomab tiuxetan for relapsed or refractory disease; they reported an OR rate of 31%, a CR rate of 15%, and a median event- free survival of 28 months for responders [38].

Two studies investigated the use of RIT in newly diagnosed MCL. In the first study, 25 MCL patients were treated with frontline 131I-tositumomab, before CHOP consolidation. The OR rate was 86%, the CR rate was 67%, and the OS rate at 2 years was 92% [39]. In the second study, 53 patients with newly diagnosed MCL were treated with four cycles of R-CHOP chemotherapy followed by planned 90Y-ibritumomab tiuxetan consolidation. The complete response rate (CR/CRu) improved from 19% after R-CHOP to 56% after consolidation; RIT consolidation also met the primary endpoint of 50% prolongation of time to treatment failure (TTF) over that expected for R-CHOP x 6 alone. While there was no apparent plateau in TTF, median overall survival (OS) has not been reached, with an estimated 5-year OS of 73% [40].

Key Points

- Radioimmunotherapy with ^{90}Y-Zevalin was approved by FDA as a radioimmunotherapeutic-based regimen for the treatment of adult patients with relapsed or refractory, low-grade, or follicular B-cell non-Hodgkin's lymphoma (NHL) and of previously untreated follicular NHL who achieve a partial or complete response to first-line chemotherapy.
- The use of consolidation with ^{90}Y-Zevalin versus rituximab maintenance in follicular lymphoma is under investigation.
- The potential clinical application includes diffuse large B-cell lymphoma, indolent lymphoma in the frontline setting, and mantle cell lymphoma.
- Treatment is usually safe, but hematological toxicity related to mielodepression and potential for anaphylactic and other hypersensitivity reactions should be taken into account.
- Even if radiation exposure to medical workers and others is low, radiation precautions consistent with time, distance, and shielding principles should be followed to keep the exposure as low as reasonably achievable (ALARA).

References

1. Seyfizadeh N, Seyfizadeh N, Hasenkamp J, Huerta-Yepez S. A molecular perspective on rituximab: a monoclonal antibody for B cell non Hodgkin lymphoma and other affections. Crit Rev Oncol Hematol. 2016;97:275–90. https://doi.org/10.1016/j.critrevonc.2015.09.001.
2. Alcindor T, Witzig TE. Radioimmunotherapy with yttrium-90 ibritumomab tiuxetan for patients with relapsed CD20+ B-cell non-Hodgkin's lymphoma. Curr Treat Options in Oncol. 2002;3(4):275–82.
3. Knox SJ, Goris ML, Trisler K, et al. Yttrium- 90-labeled anti-CD20 monoclonal antibody therapy of recurrent B-cell lymphoma. Clin Cancer Res. 1996;2:457–70.
4. Witzig TE, White CA, Wiseman GA, et al. Phase I/II trial of IDEC-Y2B8 radioimmunotherapy for treatment of relapsed or refractory CD20(+) B-cell non-Hodgkin's lymphoma. J Clin Oncol. 1999;17:3793–803.
5. Witzig TE, Gordon LI, Cabanillas F, et al. Randomized controlled trial of yttrium-90-labeled ibritumomab tiuxetan radioimmunotherapy versus rituximab immunotherapy for patients with relapsed or refractory low-grade, follicular, or transformed B-cell non-Hodgkin's lymphoma. J Clin Oncol. 2002;20:2453–63.
6. Kaminski MS, Zelenetz AD, Press OW, et al. Pivotal study of iodine I^{131} tositumomab for chemotherapy-refractory low-grade or transformed low-grade B-cell non-Hodgkin's lymphomas. J Clin Oncol. 2001;19:3918–28.
7. Kaminski MS, Tuck M, Estes J, et al. ^{131}I-tositumomab therapy as initial treatment for follicular lymphoma. N Engl J Med. 2005;352:441–9.
8. Delacroix D, Guerre JP, Leblanc P, Hickman C. Radionuclide and radiation protection data handbook 2002 (2nd edition). Radiat Prot Dosim. 2002;98:1–168.

9. Chinn PC, Leonard JE, Rosenberg J, Hanna N, Anderson DR. Preclinical evaluation of ^{90}Y-labeled anti-CD20 monoclonal antibody for treatment of non-Hodgkin's lymphoma. Int J Oncol. 1999;15:1017–25.
10. Siegel JA, Zimmerman BE, Kodimer K, Dell MA, Simon WE. A single dose calibrator dial setting accurately measures ^{90}Y-ibritumomab tiuxetan activity. J Nucl Med. 2003;44:317.
11. Borghaei H, Schilder RJ. Safety and efficacy of radio immunotherapy with Yttrium 90 ibritumomab tiuxetan (Zevalin). Semin Nucl Med. 2004;34:4–9.
12. Juweid ME. Radio immunotherapy of B-cell non-Hodgkin's lymphoma; from clinical trial to clinical practice. J Nucl Med. 2002;43:1507–29.
13. Bischof Delaloye A. The role of nuclear medicine in tre treatment of non-Hodgkin's lymphoma (NHL). Leuk Lymphoma. 2003;44(Supplement 4):S29–36.
14. Silverman DH, Delpassand ES, Torabi F, Goy A, McLaughlin P, Murray JL. Radiolabeled antibody therapy in non-Hodgkin lymphoma: radiation protection, isotope comparisons and quality of life issue. Cancer Treat Rev. 2004;30:165–72.
15. Wagner HN Jr, Wiseman GA, Marcus CS, Nabi HA, Nagle CE, Fink-Bennett DM, Lamonica DM, Conti PS. Administration guidelines for radio immunotherapy of non-Hodgkin's lymphoma with (90)Y-labeled anti-CD20 monoclonal antibody. J Nucl Med. 2002;43(2):267–72.
16. Cremonesi M, Ferrari M, Paganelli G, Rossi A, Chinol M, Bartolomei M, Prisco G, Tosi G. Radiation protection in radionuclide therapies with (90)Y-conjugates: risks and safety. Eur J Nucl Med Mol Imaging. 2006;33(11):1321–7.
17. Tennvall J, Fischer M, Delaloye AB, Bombardieri E, Bodei L, Giammarile F, Lassmann M, Oyen W, Brans B. EANM procedure guideline for radio-immunotherapy for B-cell lymphoma with ^{90}Y-radiolabelled ibritumomab tiuxetan (Zevalin). Eur J Nucl Med Mol Imaging. 2007;34:616–22.
18. Ferrucci PF, Vanazzi A, Grana CM, Cremonesi M, Bartolomei M, Chinol M, Ferrari M, Radice D, Papi S, Martinelli G, Paganelli G. High activity ^{90}Y-ibritumomab tiuxetan (Zevalin) with peripheral blood progenitor cells support in patients with refractory/resistant B-cell non-Hodgkin lymphomas. Br J Haematol. 2007;139(4):590–9.
19. Wiseman GA, Kornmehl E, Leigh B, Erwin WD, Podoloff DA, Spies S, Sparks RB, Stabin MG, Witzig T, White CA. Radiation dosimetry results and safety correlations from ^{90}Y-ibritumomab tiuxetan radioimmunotherapy for relapsed or refractory non-Hodgkin's lymphoma: combined data from 4 clinical trials. J Nucl Med. 2003;44(3):465–74.
20. Cremonesi M, Ferrari M, Grana CM, Vanazzi A, Stabin M, Bartolomei M, Papi S, Prisco G, Ferrucci PF, Martinelli G, Paganelli G. High-dose radioimmunotherapy with ^{90}Y-ibritumomab tiuxetan: comparative dosimetric study for tailored treatment. J Nucl Med. 2007;48(11):1871–9. Erratum in: J Nucl Med. 2007;48(12):2027
21. Meredith RF. Logistics of therapy with the ibritumomab tiuxetan regimen. Int J Radiat Oncol Biol Phys. 2006;66(2 Supplement):S35–8.
22. Kaminsky MS, Ester J, Zasadny KR, Francis IR, Ross CW, Tuck M, et al. Radioimmunotherapy with iodine 131 tositumomab for relapsed or refractory B-cell non-Hodgkin's lymphoma: update results and long term follow-up of the University of Michigan experience. Blood. 2000;96:1259–66.
23. Vose JM, Wahl RL, Saleh M, et al. Multicenter phase II study of iodine ^{131}I tositumomab for chemotherapy-relapsed/refractory low-grade and transformed low-grade B-cell non-Hodgkin's lymphomas. J Clin Oncol. 2000;18:1361–23.
24. Witzig TE, Flinn IW, Gordon LI, et al. Treatment with ibritumomab tiuxetan radioimmunotherapy in patients with rituximab-refractory follicular non-Hodgkin's lymphoma. J Clin Oncol. 2002;20:3262–9.
25. Emmanouilides C, Witzig TE, Gordon LI, et al. Treatment with Yttrium 90 ibritumomab tiuxetan at early relapse is safe and effective in patients with previously treated B-cell non-Hodgkin's lymphoma. Leuk Lymphoma. 2006;47(4):629–36.
26. Morschhauser F, Radford J, Van Hoof A, et al. Phase III trial of consolidation therapy with yttrium-90-ibritumomab tiuxetan compared with no additional therapy after first remission in advanced follicular lymphoma. J Clin Oncol. 2008;26:5156–64.
27. Morschhauser F, Radford J, Van Hoof A, Botto B, Rohatiner AZ, Salles G, Soubeyran P, Tilly H, Bischof-Delaloye A, van Putten WL, Kylstra JW, Hagenbeek A. ^{90}Yttrium-ibritumomab tiuxetan consolidation of first remission in advanced-stage follicular non-Hodgkin lymphoma: updated results after a median follow-up of 7.3 years from the international, randomized, phase III first-line indolent trial. J Clin Oncol. 2013;31:1977–83.
28. ClinicalTrials.gov. NCT00006721 S0016 - Combination chemotherapy with monoclonal antibody therapy in treating patients with newly diagnosed non-Hodgkin's lymphoma.
29. Salles G, Seymour JF, Offner F, López-Guillermo A, Belada D, Xerri L, Feugier P, Bouabdallah R, Catalano JV, Brice P, Caballero D, Haioun C, Pedersen LM, et al. Rituximab maintenance for 2 years in patients with high tumour burden follicular lymphoma responding to rituximab plus chemotherapy (PRIMA): a phase 3, randomised controlled trial. Lancet Oncol. 2011;377:42–51.
30. ClinicalTrial.gov. NCT00662948 Geltamo/Pethema Open study in Phase II to evaluate efficacy of initial R-CHOP combination in follicular lymphoma no treated previously. Consolidation with one dose of ^{90}Y ibritumomab Tiuxetan (Zevalin) versus maintenance treatment with Rituximab.
31. Fowler NH, Neelapu SS, Fanale MA, et al. Phase II study with R-FND followed by 90-Y ibritumomab

tiuxetan radioimmunotherapy and rituximab maintenance for untreated high-risk follicular lymphoma. Blood. 2011;118:99.
32. FIL-FLAZ12 trial EudraCT Number 2012-000251-14 A phase III multicenter, randomized study comparing consolidation with (90)Yttrium-labeled Ibritumomab Tiuxetan (Zevalin) radioimmunotherapy vs autologous stem cells transplantation (ASCT) in patients with relapsed/refractory follicular lymphoma (FL) aged 18–65 years.
33. FIL-FOLL12 trial EudractCT Number 2012-003170-60 Randomized, multicentre, phase III, response-adapted trial to define maintenance after standard treatment in advanced Follicular Lymphoma.
34. Morschhauser F, Illidge T, Huglo D, Martinelli G, Paganelli G, Zinzani PL, Rule S, Liberati AM, Milpied N, Hess G, Stein H, Kalmus J, Marcus R. Effiacy and safety of yttrium-90 ibritumomab tiuxetan in patients with relapsed or refractory diffuse large B-cell lymphoma not appropriate for autologous stem-cell transplantation. Blood. 2007;110:54–8.
35. Hamlin PA, Rodriguez MA, Noy A, et al. Final results of a phase II study of sequential R-CHOP and Yttrium-90 Ibritumomab Tiuxetan (RIT) for elderly high risk patients with untreated diffuse large B-cell lymphoma (DLBCL). Blood. 2010;116(21):1793.
36. Stefoni V, Casadei B, Bottelli C, et al. Short-course R-CHOP followed by ^{90}Y-Ibritumomab tiuxetan in previously untreated high-risk elderly diffuse large B-cell lymphoma patients: 7-year long-term results. Blood Cancer J. 2016;6(5):e425. https://doi.org/10.1038/bcj.2016.29.
37. ClinicalTrials.gov. NCT00322218 – Study comparing the Zevalin regimen with no further treatment in DLBC patients who are in complete remission after R-CHOP.
38. Wang M, Oki Y, Pro B, Romaguera JE, Rodriguez MA, Samaniego F, McLaughlin P, Hagemeister F, Neelapu S, Copeland A, Samuels BI, Loyer EM, Ji Y, Younes A. Phase II Study of Yttrium-90–ibritumomab tiuxetan in patients with relapsed or refractory mantle cell lymphoma. J Clin Oncol. 2009;27:5213–8.
39. Zelenetz AD, Noy A, Pandit-Taskar N, Scordo M, Rijo I, Zhou Y, O'Donoghue JA, Divgi C. Sequential radioimmunotherapy with tositumomab/iodine I^{131} tositumomab followed by CHOP for mantle cell lymphoma demonstrates RIT can induce molecular remissions. J Clin Oncol. 2006;24(18 suppl):7560.
40. Smith MR, Li H, Gordon L, Gascoyne RD, Paietta E, Forero-Torres A, Kahl BS, Advan R, Hong F, Horning SJ. Phase II study of rituximab plus cyclophosphamide, doxorubicin, vincristine, and prednisone immunochemotherapy followed by yttrium-90–ibritumomab tiuxetan in untreated mantle-cell lymphoma: Eastern Cooperative Oncology Group Study E1499. J Clin Oncol. 2012;30:3119–26.

32 Radioimmunotherapy in the Transplant Setting

Liliana Devizzi

Abstract

High-dose chemotherapy (HDC) conditioning regimens with autologous stem cell transplantation (ASCT) or reduced intensity conditioning (RIC) with allogeneic stem cell transplantation (allo-SCT) are consolidate approaches for patients with chemotherapy-sensitive, relapsed, aggressive, or indolent non-Hodgkin's lymphoma (NHL). These approaches have been shown to be the only curative option for the majority of patients. Despite results that can be achieved with SCT combined with HDC, there are some problems that may limit the utility of this approach for a broad patient population, for example, older age or comorbidities. Furthermore SCT has limited success in chemorefractory disease or in heavily pretreated patients; recurrent disease is the major cause of treatment failure and the majority of patients relapsed. Consequently, there is the need for other effective and well-tolerated modality that will eradicate disease thus improving outcomes for both unfit patients and younger with refractory disease. Because lymphomas are highly sensitive to radiation, radioimmunotherapy (RIT) has been used with great success in consolidation therapy, and there is great interest in exploring the use of RIT, either as a single agent or as part of a conditioning regimen for autologous SCT. RIT was also considered as part of RIC to reduce the toxic effects of HDC. The data so far suggest that the use of RIT in the autologous setting can improve clinical outcome with no added toxicity, whereas similar positive findings have been reported in studies of yttrium-90-ibritumomab tiuxetan combined with RIC and allograft SCT in high-risk patients.

32.1 Introduction

Although most patients with follicular lymphoma (FL) and diffuse large B-cell lymphoma (DLBCL) obtain a CR following primary rituximab

L. Devizzi
Hematology and BMT Unit, IRCCS Istituto Nazionale Tumori, Milan, Italy
e-mail: lilli.devizzi@istitutotumori.mi.it

E. Bombardieri et al. (eds.), *Clinical Applications of Nuclear Medicine Targeted Therapy*,
https://doi.org/10.1007/978-3-319-63067-0_32

implemented chemotherapy, 15–40% of patients with DLBCL are treated and almost all patients with FL will relapse and require salvage chemotherapies [1, 2]. Detection and thus elimination of minimal residual disease are the goal of a modern approach in non-Hodgkin's lymphoma and may be achieved either by using conditioning regimens followed by stem cell transplantation or with an immunological approach using stem cells from a matched donor (allo-SCT). Guidelines from the National Comprehensive Cancer Network [3] identify autologous stem cell transplantation the treatment of choice for relapsed follicular lymphoma. SCT has been in fact the only therapy able to achieve a potential of a cure for younger NHL patients who have relapsed or are resistant to chemotherapy [4–17]. Randomized trials have demonstrated that ASCT provide benefit to patients with either DLBCL or FL [8, 10, 15].

32.2 Rationale for Radioimmunotherapy

Radioimmunotherapy (RIT) for NHL targets cells expressing the CD20 antigen that is present exclusively on mature B cells and B-cell lymphomas [18].

In contrast to TBI, traditionally integrated into transplant regimens in the past for many NHL patients, RIT can be used in elderly patients with comorbidities as a conditioning regimen [19–21]. Moreover, RIT delivers targeted radiation, thus sparing the HDC-associated toxicity and increasing the therapeutic index and the treatment options for older and frailer patients. Phase I and II trial data show that ibritumomab tiuxetan may be safely added to HDC preparative regimens for high-risk B-cell NHL (Table 32.1) [22, 23, 26, 27, 31, 32, 36, 38, 42]. Currently, three approaches of RIT in the SCT setting are studied and approved. The first combines standard-dose, non-myeloablative RIT with HDC prior to ASCT [27–42], the second includes high-dose myeloablative RIT prior to ASCT using in vivo dosimetry to limit radiation exposure to critical organs [43–57], and the last approach with either conventional-dose chemotherapy (i.e., a reduced intensity regimen) in the allo-SCT setting [24, 58–61].

Table 32.1 Selected trial and results of non-myeloablative RIT chemotherapy before ASCT

Reference	No of Pts	Treatment	PFS (%)	OS (%)
Press et al. [54]	52	^{90}Y-IT-HD-CTX-VP16	67	83
Nademanee et al. [27]	31	^{90}Y-IT-CTX-VP16	74	93
Vose et al. [55]	40	^{131}I-T-BEAM	70	
Shimoni et al. [31]	23	^{90}Y-BEAM	52	67
Krishnan et al. [32]	46	^{90}Y-BEAM	NR	81
Siddiqui et al. [36]	36	^{90}Y-BEAM	64	79
Shimoni et al. [38]	22	^{90}Y-BEAM	59	91
Hertzberg et al. [39]	42	^{90}Y-BEAM	67	78
Briones et al. [40]	30	^{90}Y-BEAM	61	63
Wondergem et al. [42]	24	^{90}Y-BEAM	80	100
Winter et al. [51]	44	^{90}Y-BEAM	43	60

32.3 Standard-Dose Non-myeloablative RIT with HDC Prior to ASCT

Promising results from numerous trials suggest that incorporating RIT may significantly improve disease control with negligible added toxicity. Combining HDC regimens with 90Y-ibritumomab tiuxetan has produced impressive long-term OS rates of 81–93% in chemotherapy-sensitive patients in a variety of histologic lymphoma subtypes [26–28]. Reports investigating RIT in combination with HDC regimens in patients with chemotherapy-refractory disease have demonstrated high OS rates of 55% and 87% at 38 months [29]; Vose et al. reported an estimated 2-year OS rate of 67%, and another study investigating RIT and high-dose carmustine, etoposide, cytarabine, and melphalan (BEAM) chemotherapy with ASCT reported 2-year OS and PFS rates of 67% (95% CI, 46–87%) and 52% (95% CI, 31–72%), respectively [31]. Such improvements in OS rates demonstrate the benefit of adding RIT to ASCT for patients with chemotherapy-refractory NHL. Such improvement in OS rates suggested the benefit of adding RIT to ASCT in chemorefractory patients.

The use of standard-dose 90Y-ibritumomab tiuxetan (0.4 mCi/kg) plus HDC (BEAM) has been evaluated as a conditioning regimen prior to ASCT in patients with relapsed/refractory NHL. In one study, 90Y-ibritumomab tiuxetan at this dose was well tolerated and effective in 41 older patients (median age, 60 years) undergoing ASCT for poor-risk NHL [32]. With a median follow-up of 18.4 months (range, 5.5–53.3 months), the estimated 2-year OS and disease-free survival rates were 88.9% and 69.8%, respectively, and the rate and types of toxicities observed were similar to those with high-dose BEAM alone. Similar activity was reported in two other studies. In the GELA phase II trial, a conventional dose of 90Y-ibritumomab tiuxetan was combined with BEAM in 74 patients with low-grade B-cell lymphomas (68 with FL and 6 with marginal zone lymphoma (MZL)). At a minimum 1-year follow-up, the estimated 1-year EFS rate was 80% [22]. The second phase II trial, reporting data for the first ten patients treated with standard-dose 90Y-ibritumomab tiuxetan and high-dose BEAM conditioning chemotherapy followed by ASCT, demonstrated similar results [33]. A comparative trial of Z-BEAM and a TBI-based conditioning regimen (i.e., 1200 cGy plus etoposide and cyclophosphamide) in 92 DLBCL patients showed a trend toward improvement of 2-year PFS in the Z-BEAM group (60% vs. 42%, $P = 0.10$). Overall survival at 4 years was 81% for the Z-BEAM group and 53% for the TBI group [27]. Comparison of outcomes with RIT + ASCT in poor-risk, aggressive lymphoma, with historic controls, suggests that ibritumomab tiuxetan/CT may be more effective than conventional regimens (e.g., myeloablative doses of RIT ± CT or standard non-myeloablative doses of RIT combined with HDC) [36, 37]. In the study by Shimoni et al. [38], 43 patients with CD20 (+) aggressive lymphoma were randomized to a treatment arm (Z-BEAM, $n = 22$) or control arm (BEAM alone, $n = 21$). Engraftment kinetics and toxicity profile were similar between the two groups. Two-year progression-free survival (PFS) for all patients was 48% and 59% and 37% after Z-BEAM and BEAM, respectively ($P = 0.2$). Multivariate analysis identified advanced age ($P = 0.001$), high-risk disease ($P = 0.04$), and BEAM alone ($P = 0.03$) as poor prognostic factors. Two-year overall survival was 91% and 62% after Z-BEAM and BEAM, respectively ($P = 0.05$) (Fig. 32.1). Conclusion of this such impressive study is that standard-dose ibritumomab tiuxetan combined with BEAM is safe and possibly more effective than BEAM alone as a conditioning regimen for ASCT in the era of rituximab-containing chemotherapy regimens.

The impact of 90Y-ibritumomab tiuxetan was evaluated in a PET-driven prospective trial [39]. Patients with DLBCL received four cycles of R-CHOP-14, followed by a centrally reviewed PET. Median age of the 151 evaluable patients was 57 years, with 79% stages 3–4, 54% bulk, and 54% International Prognostic Index 3–5. Among the 143 patients undergoing interim PET, 101 (71%) were PET-negative (96 of whom completed R-CHOP) and 42 (29%) were PET-positive and underwent a treatment intensification with R-ICE (rituximab, ifosfamide, carboplatin, and etoposide) chemotherapy followed by 90Y-ibritumomab tiuxetan-BEAM (32 of whom completed R-ICE and 90Y-ibritumomab tiuxetan-BEAM). At a median follow-up of 35 months, the 2-year progression-free survival for PET-positive patients was 67%, a rate similar to that of PET-negative patients treated with R-CHOP-14 (74%, $P = 0.11$); overall survival was 78% and 88% ($P = 0.11$), respectively. These data encourage and suggest new prospective studies in refractory DLBCL. Thirty refractory patients, 18 primary refractory patients and 12 refractory to salvage immunochemotherapy at relapse, were enrolled in a study by Briones et al. [40]. All patients received 90Y-ibritumomab tiuxetan at a fixed dose of 0.4 mCi/kg (maximum dose 32 mCi) 14 days prior to the preparative CT regimen. Histologic examination showed that 22 patients had de novo DLBCL and 8 had transformed DLBCL. All patients had persistent disease at the time of transplantation, with 25 patients considered to be chemorefractory. The ORR at day +100 was 70% (95% CI, 53.6–86.4) with 60% (95% CI, 42.5–77.5) of patients obtaining a CR. After a median follow-up of 31 months, the estimated 3-year OS and PFS rates were 63% (95% CI, 48–82) and 61% (95% CI, 45–80), respectively. Krishnan et al. [41]

Fig. 32.1 PFS and OS according to conditioning regimen: standard-dose ibritumomab tiuxetan combined with high-dose BEAM (Z-BEAM) versus BEAM. Shimoni et al. [38]

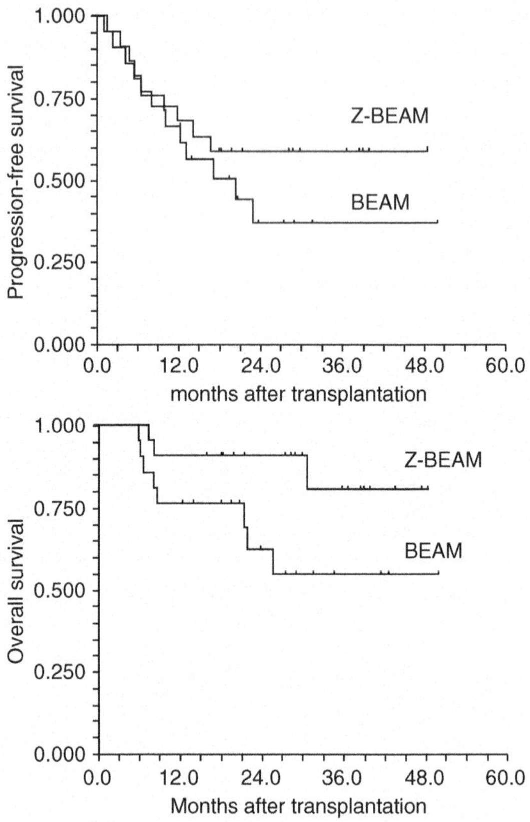

report the outcomes of a single-center, single-arm phase II trial of Z-BEAM conditioning in high-risk CD20+ non-Hodgkin's lymphoma: diffuse large B-cell (DLBCL), mantle cell, follicular, and transformed. Overall survival and notably low non-relapse mortality rates (0.9% at day +100 for the entire cohort), with few short- and long-term toxicities, confirm the safety and tolerability of the regimen. In addition, despite a high proportion of induction failure patients (46%), the promising response and progression-free survival (PFS) rates seen in DLBCL (3-year PFS, 71%; 95% confidence interval, 55–82%) support the premise that the Z-BEAM regimen is particularly effective in this histologic subtype. Transformation from indolent NHL to DLBCL is historically associated with a poor prognosis. The results of a multicenter retrospective trial that evaluated ASCT in patients with transformed lymphoma using the Z-BEAM conditioning regimen (ibritumomab tiuxetan plus with high-dose BEAM) in 63 patients were reported by Wondergem et al. [42]. Median patient age at ASCT was 59.5 years, median number of prior regimens was 2, and all patients were exposed to rituximab. Disease status at ASCT was first CR ($n = 30$), first PR ($n = 11$), first relapse ($n = 14$), and at least second CR ($n = 8$). The median time from diagnosis of histologic transformation to ASCT was 7.5 months. Two-year non-relapse mortality was 0%. Median follow-up for living patients was 28 months. Two-year PFS was 68% (95% CI, 58–75) and OS was 90% (95% CI, 80–95).

32.4 High-Dose Myeloablative RIT and ASCT

Data from studies of RIT plus HDC and ASCT are promising, but the use of HDC in this setting may still be too aggressive for many patients who may benefit from ASCT such as elderly and unfit patients. Therefore, high-dose, single-agent RIT prior to ASCT may be a promising new approach for patients with relapsed B-cell lymphoma. Because of the acceptable tolerability of RIT, a conditioning regimen that includes high-dose RIT but excludes HDC may be appropriate for a broader range of patients for whom myeloablative chemotherapy regimens are too toxic. In dose-finding studies, the maximum-tolerated dose and dose-limiting toxicities of RIT were defined. For high-dose 90Y-ibritumomab tiuxetan prior to ASCT, 1.2 mCi/kg (45 MBq/kg) was defined as the maximum recommended dose because the radiation absorbed by non-hematologic critical organs approached the protocol-defined upper safety limit. Table 32.2 summarize selected trial with myeloablative RIT before ASCT.

In phase I dose escalation studies of 131I-tositumomab, 27 Gy was determined to be the maximum-tolerated level of radiation that can be delivered to normal critical organs, with limited non-hematologic toxicity and maintained efficacy [44, 50]. These data established the optimal therapeutic dose as 2.5 mg/kg antibody labeled with 5–10 mCi 131I. However the use of high-dose 131I-tositumomab treatment can be complicated for both healthcare professionals and patients, because therapeutic doses may have a long total-body residence time and patients may require radiation isolation in specialist hospital for many days. In contrast, following treatment with 90Y-ibritumomab tiuxetan, patients are readily discharged with minor advices. Furthermore, unlike treatment with 131I-tositumomab, patients are not required to minimize contact with others [52, 53].

Table 32.2 Selected trial and results of myeloablative RIT alone before ASCT

Reference	No of Pts	Treatment	PFS (%)	OS (%)
Vanazzi et al. [45]	24	^{90}Y-IT	NR	NR
Devizzi et al. [48]	30	^{90}Y-IT	69	87
Gopal et al. [43]	24	^{131}I-T-IT	51	59
Liu et al. [44]	29	^{131}I-T-IT	42	68
Swinnen et al. [46]	24	^{90}Y-IT	NR	NR

In our phase II study [47], 30 patients with relapsed/refractory (n = 25) or de novo high-risk (n = 5) NHL received ibritumomab tiuxetan 0.8 mCi/kg, and 17 patients received 1.2 mCi/kg followed by tandem autologous stem cell transplantation after a cytoreductive phase with rituximab implemented sequential intermediate high-dose chemotherapy (ZHDS) (Fig. 32.2). At 1.2 mCi/kg, the radiation absorbed by critical non-hematologic organs approached the protocol-defined upper safety limit, defining this as the recommended dose for subsequent study. Hematologic toxicity was mild to moderate and of short duration. Infections occurred in 27% of patients (0 had a severity grade >3). At a median follow-up of 30 months, the OS rate was 87%, and the PFS rate was 69%. We found that high-dose ibritumomab tiuxetan to be an innovative myeloablative regimen with wide clinical applicability. A 5-year update in a larger series of 60 patients with poor-risk CD20+ NHL who were not eligible for BEAM was published in 2013 [48]. Fifty-four patients (90%) experienced a CR, and one patient a PR, for an ORR of 92%. At a median follow-up of 5.9 years, 44 patients were alive and 38 in continuous CR: 5-year PFS and OS are 62.7% and 72.9%, respectively (Fig. 32.3). The 5-year cumulative incidence of relapse was 32.5%, and non-relapse mortality was only 1.7%. The antitumor activity of the program was noteworthy, and the tolerability of myeloablative RIT was remarkable for patients otherwise ineligible for CT-based autotransplant regimens. In this study, an 8-year cumulative incidence of sMDS of 9.4% was observed, suggesting an increased risk compared with younger patients receiving high-dose therapy and autograft. However, when the occurrence of sMDS was analyzed in the pair-matched group of patients treated with a conventional myeloablative regimen, a comparable 8-year cumulative incidence of sMDS of 10.3% was observed (Fig. 32.4). These results confirm the benefit of myeloablative RIT in the transplant setting for patients who experience relapse after rituximab-containing regimens. The long-term toxicity profile of ibritumomab tiuxetan in

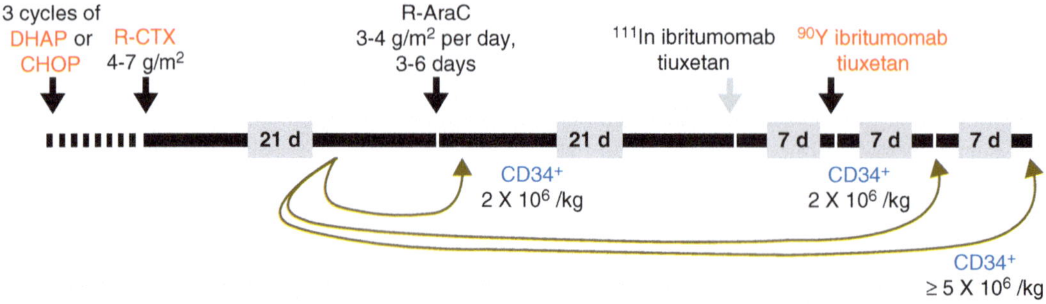

Fig. 32.2 Treatment plan of patients receiving myeloablative 90Y-ibritumomab tiuxetan (Z-HDS)

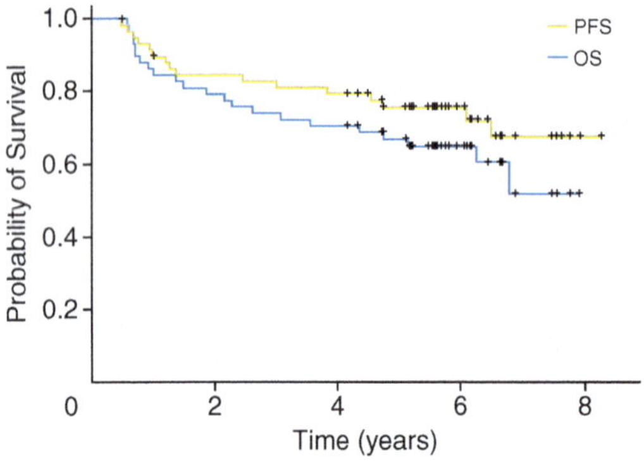

Fig. 32.3 Kaplan-Meyer estimate of OS and PFS probabilities for patients who received high-dose sequential chemotherapy followed by myeloablative 90Y-ibritumomab tiuxetan (Z-HDS). Devizzi et al.: JCO [48]

this trial was comparable to other, more toxic, high-dose myeloablative regimens. Its high efficacy in this population of frail patients otherwise ineligible for HDC should encourage additional, large-scale trials particularly in patients with unfavourable histologies such as transformed DLBCL and MCL to confirm these favorable findings. Superimposable results with excellent similar safety profile have been previously published by Nademanee and coworkers with high-dose 90Y-ibritumomab tiuxetan plus high dose etoposide and cyclophosphamide before ASCL in poor risk NHL [29].

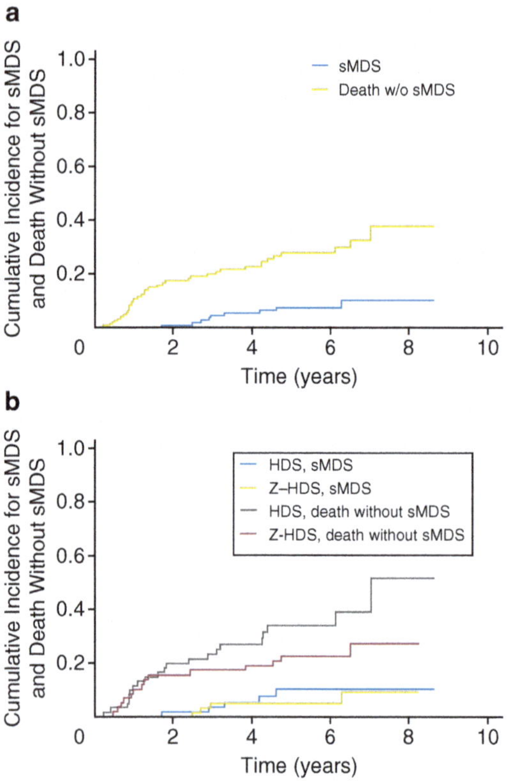

Fig. 32.4 Cumulative incidence of secondary myelodysplastic syndrome (sMDS) and mortality stratified by treatment regimens. (**a**) Cumulative incidence of sMDS or death for patients who received high-dose sequential chemotherapy (HDS) followed by myeloablative 90Y-ibritumomab tiuxetan (Z-HDS). (**b**) Cumulative incidence of sMDS or death for patients receiving Z-HDS or HDS. Devizzi et al.: JCO [48]

32.5 Standard-Dose Non-myeloablative RIT with Conventional-Dose Chemotherapy (RIC) and Allo-SCT

Reduced intensity conditioning (RIC) regimens have been developed to permit elderly patients or patients with comorbidities, contraindicated for myeloablative HDC, to undergo allogeneic stem cell transplant (SCT). To increase the efficacy of the allogeneic graft, ibritumomab tiuxetan was added to the RIC conditioning regimen in different subpopulation of patients including those with CT-resistant or bulky disease or with aggressive histology (Table 32.3). In a study of 12 patients with CT-refractory NHL, Shimoni et al. [59] evaluated ibritumomab tiuxetan 0.4 mCi/kg given on day −14 and fludarabine combined with busulfan (BU) ($n = 6$) or melphalan ($n = 6$) starting on day −6. Graft-versus-host disease (GVHD) prevention was tapered 3 months after allogeneic SCT to augment the graft-versus-lymphoma effect. All patients engrafted at a median of 14 days after SCT. Eighty-three percent achieved either a CR or PR. With a median follow-up of 21 months, 2-year PFS was 33%. Only three patients relapsed; non-relapse mortality was high 42%, predominantly due to acute GVHD. The authors concluded that ibritumomab tiuxetan-RIC was feasible with consistent engraftment but with a high rate of acute GVHD. The low incidence of relapse showed an augmented anti-lymphoma effect in this study, and investigators suggested that better results may be achieved in patients earlier in the course of disease and with a longer duration of immunosuppression. Forty patients with low-grade advanced NHL were enrolled in the phase II study, combining RIT using a standard dose of ibritumomab tiuxetan with RIC using fludarabine and 2 Gy TBI followed by ASCT [60]. The combination of RIT with RIC did not increase toxicity, in comparison with previous experience in patients conditioned with fludarabine/2 Gy TBI alone even in elderly and heavily pretreated patients. Similar data were previously reported in a study by Gopal et al. [24] where the combined use of RIT with RIC (fludarabine and 2 Gy TBR) for a non-myeloablative ASCT was examined. Forty patients were enrolled, 18 with indolent lymphoma, 14 with DLBCL, and 8 with MCL. At a median follow-up of 30 months, the estimated 2-year OS and PFS were 54% and 31%, respectively. Combined RIT/RIC was safe and feasible in this study and was able to induce objective remissions in the majority of the high-risk patients enrolled (i.e., those not previously considered candidates for either standard myeloablative or non-myeloablative transplants). Very recently the GELTAMO group [61] designed a phase II clinical trial including 90Y-ibritumomab tiuxetan as part of RIC-allo-SCT in patients with high-risk relapsed/refractory aggressive lymphoma. At the time of transplantation, responses were complete remission (CR) ($n = 7$, 39%), partial remission ($n = 6$, 33%), or refractory disease ($n = 4$, 28%). 90Y-Ibritumomab infusions were well tolerated, with no adverse reactions. Non-relapse mortality at 1 year was 28%. Median follow-up was 46 (range, 39–55) months. Estimated 1-year progression-free survival (PFS) was 50%, and 4-year OS and PFS were both 44.4%. CR at the moment of allo-SCT had significant impact on PFS (71% versus 27%, $P = 0.046$) and OS (71% versus 27%, $P = 0.047$). The authors concluded that 90Y-ibritumomab tiuxetan as a component of RIC for allo-SCT is feasible in patients with high-risk B-cell lymphoma and that the need for phase III clinical trials to better clarify the contribution of radioimmunotherapy to RIC-allo-SCT is recommended.

Table 32.3 Selected trial and results of non-myeloablative RIT and RIC

Reference	No of Pts	Treatment	PFS (%)	OS (%)
Shimoni et al. [59]	12	^{90}Y-Flu-2GyTBI	33%	42%
Gopal et al. [24]	40	^{90}Y-Flu-2GyTBI	31	54
Bouabdallah et al. [60]	31	^{90}Y-Flu-2GyTBI	80	60.8
Cabrero et al. [61]	18	^{90}Y-IT	44.4	44.4

Feasibility and activity of 90Y-ibritumomab tiuxetan after intensive chemotherapy including myeloablative ASCT were also reported: At least three studies published interesting results with limited toxicity suggesting a potential role of RIT improving long-term remissions in patients with different subtypes of NHL, relapsed or with minimal residual disease after myeloablative regimes [55, 57, 58].

Conclusion

Although HDC with ASCT is one curative option for eligible patients with chemotherapy-sensitive, relapsed, aggressive NHL leading to prolonged PFS, some patients who undergo this therapeutic option will eventually relapse. Additionally, it has limited success in chemotherapy-refractory disease or in heavily pretreated, multiple-relapsed patients and, because of its highly toxic nature, is unsuitable for elderly or frail patients. Allo-SCT is another curative option that may also be appropriate for elderly, but relapse rates are high in active disease. Consequently, there is much interest in evaluating new treatment regimens that can be used to improve the outcome with SCT in NHL without increasing the toxicity level of the existing regimens. In this chapter, the data supporting the safety and efficacy of RIT with 90Y-ibritumomab tiuxetan and 131I-tositumomab as part of the conditioning regimen before SCT were reported. Three approaches have been explored relating to the use of RIT as a conditioning agent for ASCT: standard-dose, non-myeloablative RIT with HDC, high-dose myeloablative RIT with or without chemotherapy, and non-myeloablative RIC allotransplantation. The data show that all these approaches appear to provide promising outcomes and disease control without greater toxicity. Interestingly, in both chemotherapy-sensitive and chemotherapy-refractory disease, adding RIT to HDC prior to ASCT appears to provide better clinical outcomes than with historical data for pure HDC pretransplant conditioning regimens. Data from phase I–III trials clearly show that RIT may be safely used as a single agent or added to either a high dose or standard dose to HDC preparative regimens for high-risk B-cell NHL histotypes (DLBCL, FL, MCL, and MZL). Published data also suggest that RIT in combination with RIC in allo-SCT may improve outcome, by better disease eradication and prevention of recurrence, while maintaining the low toxicity of RIC.

Based on these data, application of high-dose RIT in aggressive lymphoma subtypes with poor prognosis such transformed DLBCL or MCL, particularly in patients not suitable to standard/high-dose ASCT, is expected in the next future.

References

1. Feugier P, Van Hoof A, Sebban C, et al. Long-term results of the R-CHOP study in the treatment of elderly patients with diffuse large B-cell lymphoma: a study by the Groupe d'Etude des Lymphomes de l'Adulte. J Clin Oncol. 2005;23:4117–26.
2. Armitage JO. Treatment of non-Hodgkin's lymphoma. N Engl J Med. 1993;328:1023–30.
3. National Comprehensive Cancer Network. NCCN clinical practice guidelines in oncology: Non-Hodgkin's lymphomas.
4. Baron F, Maris MB, Sandmaier BM, et al. Graft-versus-tumor effects after allogeneic hematopoietic cell transplantation with nonmyeloablative conditioning. J Clin Oncol. 2005;23:1993–2003.
5. Deconinck E, Foussard C, Milpied N, et al. High-dose therapy followed by autologous purged stem-cell transplantation and doxorubicin-based chemotherapy in patients with advanced follicular lymphoma: a randomized multicenter study by GOELAMS. Blood. 2005;105:3817–23.
6. Lenz G, Dreyling M, Schiegnitz E, et al. Myeloablative radiochemotherapy followed by autologous stem cell transplantation in first remission prolongs progression-free survival in follicular lymphoma: results of a prospective, randomized trial of the German Low-Grade Lymphoma Study Group. Blood. 2004;104:2667–74.
7. Sebban C, Mounier N, Brousse N, et al. Standard chemotherapy with interferon compared with CHOP followed by high-dose therapy with autologous stem cell transplantation in untreated patients with advanced follicular lymphoma: the GELF-94 randomized study from the Groupe d'Etude des Lymphomes de l'Adulte (GELA). Blood. 2006;108:2540–4.
8. Philip T, Guglielmi C, Hagenbeek A, et al. Autologous bone marrow transplantation as compared with salvage chemotherapy in relapses of chemotherapy-sensitive non-Hodgkin's lymphoma. N Engl J Med. 1995;333:1540–5.

9. Bertz H, Zeiser R, Lange W, et al. Long-term follow-up after high-dose chemotherapy and autologous stem-cell transplantation for high-grade B-cell lymphoma suggests an improved outcome for high-risk patients with respect to the age-adjusted International Prognostic Index. Ann Oncol. 2004;15:1419–24.
10. Schouten HC, Kvaloy S, Sydes M, et al. The CUP trial: a randomized study analyzing the efficacy of high dose therapy and purging in low-grade non-Hodgkin's lymphoma (NHL). Ann Oncol. 2000;11(Suppl 1):91–4.
11. Schouten HC, Qian W, Kvaloy S, et al. High-dose therapy improves progression-free survival and survival in relapsed follicular non-Hodgkin's lymphoma: results from the randomized European CUP trial. J Clin Oncol. 2003;21:3918–27.
12. Rohatiner AZS, Nadler L, Davies AJ, et al. Myeloablative therapy with autologous bone marrow transplantation for follicular lymphoma at the time of second or subsequent remission: long-term follow-up. J Clin Oncol. 2007;25:2554–9.
13. Gianni AM, Berinstein NL, Evans PA, et al. Stem-cell transplantation in non-Hodgkin's lymphoma: improving outcome. Anti-Cancer Drugs. 2002;13(Suppl 2):S35–42.
14. Gribben JG, Freedman AS, Neuberg D, et al. Immunologic purging of marrow assessed by PCR before autologous bone marrow transplantation for B-cell lymphoma. N Engl J Med. 1991;325:1525–33.
15. Tomblyn MR, Ewell M, Bredeson C, et al. Autologous versus reduced-intensity allogeneic hematopoietic cell transplantation for patients with chemosensitive follicular non-Hodgkin lymphoma beyond first complete response or first partial response. Biol Blood Marrow Transplant. 2011;17(7):1051–7.
16. Weaver CH, Petersen FB, Appelbaum FR, et al. High-dose fractionated total-body irradiation, etoposide, and cyclophosphamide followed by autologous stem-cell support in patients with malignant lymphoma. J Clin Oncol. 1994;12:2559–66.
17. Gisselbrecht C, Mounier N. Rituximab: enhancing outcome of autologous stem cell transplantation in non-Hodgkin's lymphoma. Semin Oncol. 2003;30(Suppl 2):28–33.
18. Stashenko P, Nadler LM, Hardy R, et al. Characterization of a human B lymphocyte-specific antigen. J Immunol. 1980;125:1678–85.
19. Gregory SA, Hohloch K, Gisselbrecht C, et al. Harnessing the energy: development of radioimmunotherapy for patients with non-Hodgkin's lymphoma. Oncologist. 2009;14(Suppl 2):4–16.
20. Montoto S, Canals C, Rohatiner AZS, et al. Long-term follow-up of high-dose treatment with autologous haematopoietic progenitor cell support in 693 patients with follicular lymphoma: an EBMT registry study. Leukemia. 2007;21:2324–31.
21. Morschhauser F, Illidge T, Huglo D, et al. Efficacy and safety of yttrium-90 ibritumomab tiuxetan in patients with relapsed or refractory diffuse large B-cell lymphoma not appropriate for autologous stem-cell transplantation. Blood. 2007;110:54–8.
22. Gisselbrecht C. Completing the picture: results of the GELA-Z-BEAM trial in follicular lymphoma. Presented at the EBMT 2008; Month dd,-dd 7777; location. Painting a brighter future: improving clinical outcomes in transplant patients with NHL and CLL. Google Scholar.
23. Gisselbrecht C, Bethge W, Duarte RF, et al. Current status and future perspectives for yttrium-90 (90Y)-ibritumomab tiuxetan in stem cell transplantation for non-Hodgkin's lymphoma. Bone Marrow Transplant. 2007;40:1007–17.
24. Gopal AK, Pagel JM, Rajendran JG, et al. Improving the efficacy of reduced intensity allogeneic transplantation for lymphoma using radioimmunotherapy. Biol Blood Marrow Transplant. 2006;12:697–702.
25. Shimoni A, Nagler A. Radioimmunotherapy and stem-cell transplantation in the treatment of aggressive B-cell lymphoma. Leuk Lymphoma. 2007;48:2110–20.
26. Khouri IF, Saliba RM, Hosing C, et al. Efficacy and safety of yttrium 90 (90Y) ibritumomab tiuxetan in autologous and nonmyeloablative stem cell transplantation (NST) for relapsed non-Hodgkin's lymphoma (NHL). Blood. 2006;108. Abstract 315.
27. Nademanee A, Forman S, Molina A, et al. A phase 1/2 trial of high-dose yttrium-90-ibritumomab tiuxetan in combination with high-dose etoposide and cyclophosphamide followed by autologous stem cell transplantation in patients with poor-risk or relapsed non-Hodgkin lymphoma. Blood. 2005;106:2896–902.
28. Nademanee A, Raubitschek A, Molina A, et al. Updated results of high-dose yttrium 90 (90Y) ibritumomab tiuxetan with high-dose etoposide (VP-16) and cyclophosphamide (CY) followed by autologous hematopoietic cell transplant (AHSCT) for poor-risk or refractory B-cell non-Hodgkin's lymphoma. Blood. 2007;110. Abstract 1891.
29. Vose JM, Bierman PJ, Enke C, et al. Phase I trial of iodine-131 tositumomab with high-dose chemotherapy and autologous stem-cell transplantation for relapsed non-Hodgkin's lymphoma. J Clin Oncol. 2005;23:461–7.
30. Krishnan A, Palmer JM, Tsai NC, et al. Matched-cohort analysis of autologous hematopoietic cell transplantation with radioimmunotherapy versus total body irradiation-based conditioning for poor-risk diffuse large cell lymphoma. Biol Blood Marrow Transplant. 2012;18:441–50.
31. Shimoni A, Zwas ST, Oksman Y, et al. Yttrium-90-ibritumomab tiuxetan (Zevalin) combined with high-dose BEAM chemotherapy and autologous stem cell transplantation for chemo-refractory aggressive non-Hodgkin's lymphoma. Exp Hematol. 2007;35:534–40.
32. Krishnan A, Nademanee A, Fung HC, et al. Phase II trial of a transplantation regimen of yttrium-90 ibritumomab tiuxetan and high-dose chemotherapy

in patients with non-Hodgkin's lymphoma. J Clin Oncol. 2008;26:90–5.
33. Shimabukuro-Vornhagen A, Josting A, Hübel K, et al. Yttrium-90 ibritumomab tiuxetan combined with high-dose BEAM chemotherapy and autologous stem cell transplantation for relapsed/refractory B-cell non-Hodgkin's lymphoma. J Clin Oncol. 2008;26(15 Suppl). Abstract 8615.
34. Vose J, Bierman P, Bociek G, et al. Radioimmunotherapy with 131-I tositumomab enhanced survival in good prognosis relapsed and high-risk diffuse large B-cell lymphoma (DLBCL) patients receiving high-dose chemotherapy and autologous stem cell transplantation. J Clin Oncol. 2007;25(18 Suppl). Abstract 8013.
35. Voegeli M, Rondeau S. Berardi Vilei S, et al. Y90-Ibritumomab tiuxetan (Y90 -IT) and high-dose melphalan as conditioning regimen before autologous stem cell transplantation for elderly patients with lymphoma in relapse or resistant to chemotherapy: a feasibility trial (SAKK 37/05). Hematol Oncol. 2016 Sep 28. https://doi.org/10.1002/hon.2348.
36. Siddiqi T, Tsai NC, Palmer JM, Forman SJ, et al. Effect of radioimmunotherapy-based poor-risk molecular profiling in diffuse large B-cell lymphoma. 2012 Annual meeting of the American Society of Clinical Oncology. 2012.
37. Witzig TE, Hong F, Micallef IN, et al. A phase II trial of RCHOP followed by radioimmunotherapy for early stage (stages I/II) diffuse large B-cell non-Hodgkin lymphoma. Br J Haematol. 2015;170:679–86.
38. Shimoni A, Avivi I, Rowe JM, et al. A randomized study comparing yttrium-90 ibritumomab tiuxetan (Zevalin) and high-dose BEAM chemotherapy versus BEAM alone as the conditioning regimen before autologous stem cell transplantation in patients with aggressive lymphoma. Cancer. 2012;118(19):4706–14.
39. Hertzberg M, Gandhi MK, Trotman J, Australasian Leukaemia Lymphoma Group (ALLG), et al. Early treatment intensification with R-ICE and 90Y-ibritumomab tiuxetan (Zevalin)-BEAM stem cell transplantation in patients with high-risk diffuse large B-cell lymphoma patients and positive interim PET after 4 cycles of R-CHOP-14. Haematologica. 2017;102(2):356–63.
40. Briones J, Novelli S, García-Marco JA, et al. Grupo Español de Linfomas y Trasplante Autologo de Médula Ósea (GELTAMO). Haematologica. 2014;99(7):e126.
41. Krishnan AY, Palmer J, Nademanee A, et al. Phase II study of yttrium-90 ibritumomab tiuxetan plus high-dose BCNU, etoposide, cytarabine, and melphalan for non-hodgkin lymphoma: the role of histology. Biol Blood Marrow Transplant. 2017;23(6):922–9.
42. Wondergem MJ, Palmer JM, Shimoni A, et al. Autologous transplantation for transformed non-Hodgkin lymphoma using an yttrium-90 ibritumomab tiuxetan conditioning regimen. Biol Blood Marrow Transplant. 2014;20(12):2072–5.
43. Gopal AK, Rajendran JG, Gooley TA, et al. High-dose 131I tositumomab (anti-CD20) radioimmunotherapy and autologous hematopoietic stem-cell transplantation for adults ≥60 years old with relapsed or refractory B-cell lymphoma. J Clin Oncol. 2007;25:1396–402.
44. Liu SY, Eary JF, Petersdorf SH, et al. Follow-up of relapsed B-cell lymphoma patients treated with iodine-131-labeled anti-CD20 antibody and autologous stem-cell rescue. J Clin Oncol. 1998;16:3270–8.
45. Vanazzi A, Ferrucci P, Grana C, et al. High dose 90yttrium ibritumomab tiuxetan with PBSC support in refractory-resistant NHL patients [abstract 1890]. Presented at the 2008 American Society for Hematology Annual Meeting; December 6–9, 2008; San Francisco.
46. Swinnen LJ, Flinn IW, Kahl B, et al. Phase I trial of yttrium 90 ibritumomab tiuxetan 90Y-RIT with autologous stem cell transplantation (ASCT) in patients with relapsed or refractory B-cell non-Hodgkin's lymphoma (NHL). J Clin Oncol. 2008;26(15 Suppl). Abstract 8565.
47. Devizzi L, Seregni E, Guidetti A, et al. High-dose yttrium-90-ibritumomab tiuxetan with tandem stem-cell reinfusion: an outpatient preparative regimen for autologous hematopoietic cell transplantation. J Clin Oncol. 2008;26(32):5175–82.
48. Devizzi L, Guidetti A, Seregni E, et al. Long-term results of autologous hematopoietic stem-cell transplantation after high-dose 90Y-ibritumomab tiuxetan for patients with poor-risk non-Hodgkin lymphoma not eligible for high-dose BEAM. J Clin Oncol. 2013;31(23):2974–6.
49. Press OW, Eary JF, Appelbaum FR, et al. Phase II trial of 131I-B1 (anti-CD20) antibody therapy with autologous stem cell transplantation for relapsed B cell lymphomas. Lancet. 1995;346:336–40.
50. Press OW, Eary JF, Appelbaum FR, et al. Radiolabeled-antibody therapy of B-cell lymphoma with autologous bone marrow support. N Engl J Med. 1993;329:1219–24.
51. Winter JN, Inwards DJ, Spies S, et al. Yttrium-90 ibritumomab tiuxetan doses calculated to deliver up to 15 Gy to critical organs may be safely combined with high-dose BEAM and autologous transplantation in relapsed or refractory B-cell non-Hodgkin's lymphoma. J Clin Oncol. 2009;27:1653–9.
52. Wagner HN Jr, Wiseman GA, Marcus CS, et al. Administration guidelines for radioimmunotherapy of non-Hodgkin's lymphoma with 90Y-labeled anti-CD20 monoclonal antibody. J Nucl Med. 2002;43:267–72.
53. Meredith RF. Logistics of therapy with the ibritumomab tiuxetan regimen. Int J Radiat Oncol Biol Phys. 2006;66(2 suppl):S35–8.
54. Press OW, Eary JF, Gooley T, et al. A phase I/II trial of iodine-131-tositumomab (anti-CD20), etoposide, cyclophosphamide, and autologous stem cell transplantation for relapsed B-cell lymphomas. Blood. 2000;96:2934–42.

55. Vose JM, Bierman PJ, Loberiza FR Jr, et al. Phase I trial of 90Y-ibritumomab tiuxetan in patients with relapsed B-cell non-Hodgkin's lymphoma following high-dose chemotherapy and autologous stem cell transplantation. Leuk Lymphoma. 2007;48:683–90.
56. Kaminski MS, Estes J, Zasadny KR, et al. Radioimmunotherapy with iodine 131I tositumomab for relapsed or refractory B-cell non-Hodgkin lymphoma: updated results and long-term follow-up of the University of Michigan experience. Blood. 2000;96:1259–66.
57. Jacobs SA, Vidnovic N, Joyce J, et al. Full-dose 90Y ibritumomab tiuxetan therapy is safe in patients with prior myeloablative chemotherapy. Clin Cancer Res. 2005;11(19 Suppl):7146s–50s.
58. Mondello P, Steiner N, Willenbacher W, et al. 90Y-ibritumomab-tiuxetan consolidation therapy for advanced-stage mantle cell lymphoma after first-line autologous stem cell transplantation: is it time for a step forward? Clin Lymphoma Myeloma Leuk. 2016;16(2):82–8.
59. Shimoni A, Zwas ST, Oksman Y, et al. Ibritumomab tiuxetan (Zevalin) combined with reduced intensity conditioning and allogeneic stem-cell transplantation (SCT) in patients with chemorefractory non-Hodgkin's lymphoma. Bone Marrow Transplant. 2008;41:355–61.
60. Bouabdallah K, Furst S, Asselineau J, Chevalier P, et al. 90Y-ibritumomab tiuxetan, fludarabine, busulfan and antithymocyte globulin reduced-intensity allogeneic transplant conditioning for patients with advanced and high-risk B-cell lymphomas. Ann Oncol. 2015;26(1):193–8.
61. Cabrero M, Martin A, Briones J, et al. Phase II study of yttrium-90-ibritumomab tiuxetan as part of reduced-intensity conditioning (with melphalan, fludarabine ± thiotepa) for allogeneic transplantation in relapsed or refractory aggressive B cell lymphoma: a GELTAMO trial. Biol Blood Marrow Transplant. 2017;23(1):53–9.

33 Guidelines on Radioisotope Treatment of Lymphomas

Mariapaola Cucinotta and Laura Evangelista

33.1 Introduction

The present chapter has the aim to provide the current position of radioimmunotherapy for the treatment of lymphoma, in the main national and international clinical guidelines. In Table 33.1, a summary of clinical indications is reported.

33.2 Comments and Suggestions

For lymphomas RIT, nuclear physicians usually refer to current guidelines formulated by the Therapy, Oncology and Dosimetry Committees of EANM, published in 2007 [2]. The purpose of these guidelines is to support nuclear physicians in the management of patients undergoing ^{90}Y-ibritumomab tiuxetan treatment, covering the main practical aspects of this radionuclide therapy. They provide information about the chemical and physical characteristics of the radiopharmaceutical, about its kinetics and mechanism of action, also dealing with the procedural issues concerning personnel and facility, patient's preparation and instruction, radiopharmaceutical labeling and administration, possible treatment's side effects, and dosimetric features. Moreover, these guidelines have been endorsed by the SNMMI in 2012. Due to their "procedural" nature and considering the date of redaction (2006), the only indication to therapy they report is treatment of adult patients affected by follicular B-cell non-Hodgkin's lymphoma (NHL), CD20+, and relapsed or refractory after rituximab that is the indication for which ^{90}Y-ibritumomab tiuxetan or Zevalin® (the only radiopharmaceutical approved and commercialized in Europe for lymphomas RIT) has been initially approved by the European Agency for the Evaluation of Medicinal Products (EMEA) in 2004. However, the authors conclude the discussion with a very brief list of issues requiring further clarification, such as the use of Zevalin® in a wider spectrum of indications, including bone marrow suppression, and the possibility of retreatment (it can be administered only once in the clinical history of patients so far).

The NHMRC Australian guidelines of 2005 already suggested the use of RIT in case of low-grade lymphoma as a preferable alternative to rituximab, especially in case of bone infiltration <25% [1].

On the contrary, London cancer guidelines (2014) do not recommend RIT in lymphoma patients [3].

M. Cucinotta (✉)
Department of Medical-Surgical Sciences and Translational Medicine, "Sapienza" University, Rome, Italy
e-mail: mariapaola.cucinotta@gmail.com

L. Evangelista
Nuclear Medicine and Molecular Imaging Unit, Veneto Institute of Oncology IOV – IRCCS, Padua, Italy

E. Bombardieri et al. (eds.), *Clinical Applications of Nuclear Medicine Targeted Therapy*,
https://doi.org/10.1007/978-3-319-63067-0_33

Table 33.1 A schematic information about the available guidelines on radioisotope treatment of lymphoma

	Name of guidelines	Year of pub.	Useful link	Clinical indications	Level of evidence/ grade of recommendation[a]
1	National Health and Medical Research Council (NHMRC) Australian guidelines for the diagnosis and management of lymphoma [1]	2005	https://www.nhmrc.gov.au/guidelines-pubblications/cp107	For patients with low-grade lymphoma who fulfill specific criteria (specifically <25% bone marrow infiltration), the use of RIT is associated with a higher rate of disease control and should be considered in preference to single-agent rituximab	II/NA
2	European Association of Nuclear Medicine (EANM) procedure guideline of radioimmunotherapy for B-cell non-Hodgkin's lymphoma with ^{90}Y-radiolabeled ibritumomab tiuxetan (Zevalin®) [2]	2007	http://eanm.org/publications/guidelines/gl_radio_ther_radioimmun.pdf	Adult patients with rituximab relapsed or refractory CD20+ follicular B-cell NHL	NA
3	American Society of Nuclear Medicine and Molecular Imaging (SNMMI) procedure standard = EANM procedure guideline of radioimmunotherapy for B-cell lymphoma with ^{90}Y-radiolabeled ibritumomab tiuxetan (Zevalin®) [2] endorsed by SNNMI	2012	http://snmmi.files.cms-plus.com/docs/EANM_Guideline_for_Radioimmunotherapy_(Zevalin).pdf	Adult patients with rituximab relapsed or refractory CD20+ follicular B-cell NHL	NA
4	London cancer for the management of lymphoma [3]	2014	https://londoncancer.org	No data are available about the use of RIT in patients with lymphoma	NA
5	European Association of Medical Oncology (ESMO) Clinical Practice Guidelines for diagnosis, treatment, and follow-up of newly diagnosed and relapsed *mantle cell* lymphoma [4]	2014	http://www.esmo.org/Guidelines/Haematological-Malignancies/Newly-Diagnosed-and-Relapsed-Mantle-Cell-Lymphoma	• As consolidation after CHT in front-line treatment of elderly patients with advanced MCL, because RIT prolongs PFS after CHT, but its benefit seems to be inferior in comparison to rituximab maintenance	II/B
				• In relapsed MCL patients, because RIT seems to result in extended remission durations, especially in elderly patients with comorbidities not eligible for dose intensification	IV/B

Table 33.1 (continued)

	Name of guidelines	Year of pub.	Useful link	Clinical indications	Level of evidence/ grade of recommendation[a]
6	*Diffuse large B-cell* lymphoma (DLBCL): ESMO Clinical Practice Guidelines for diagnosis, treatment, and follow-up [5]	2015	http://www.esmo.org/Guidelines/Haematological-Malignancies/Diffuse-Large-B-Cell-Lymphoma	No mention about the use of RIT for patients with DLBCL lymphoma	NA
7	ESMO Clinical Practice Guidelines for diagnosis, treatment, and follow-up: newly diagnosed and relapsed *follicular* lymphoma [6]	2016	http://www.esmo.org/Guidelines/Haematological-Malignancies/Newly-Diagnosed-and-Relapsed-Follicular-Lymphoma	• As single agent in front-line treatment of advanced FL patients with low risk or not eligible for conventional CHT	III/B
				• As consolidation after CHT in front-line treatment of advanced FL patients with high tumor burden, because it prolongs PFS after CHT, but its benefit seems to be inferior in comparison with rituximab maintenance for 2 years	II/B
				• Treatment of recurrent advanced FL and high tumor burden in elderly patients with comorbidities not appropriate for CHT	IV/B
8	*Associazione Italiana di Oncologia Medica* (AIOM) guidelines (on DLBCL, FL, and HL) [7]	2016	http://www.aiom.it/professionisti/documenti-scientifici/linee-guida/1,413,1,#TopList	• Patients with FL:	
				- Front-line treatment of advanced FL as consolidation after CHT, because RIT improves PFS and conversion rate from partial to complete response in comparison with simple observation after	1++ (B)/weakly positive
				- CHT	++ (B)/weakly positive
				- Treatment of recurrent FL as monotherapy or consolidation after CHT, because RIT improves rates and duration of response in comparison with rituximab	1
				- As part of conditioning regimens before stem cell transplantation only in clinical trials	NA
				• Patients with DLBCL:	
				- As part of conditioning regimens before stem cell transplantation only in clinical trials	NA

(continued)

Table 33.1 (continued)

	Name of guidelines	Year of pub.	Useful link	Clinical indications	Level of evidence/grade of recommendation[a]
9	National Cancer Comprehensive Network (NCCN) Guidelines for B-cell lymphoma [8]	2017	http://www.nccn.org	• First-line therapy for elderly or infirm patients of FL (grades 1–2)	2B
				• Consolidation or extended dosing of FL (grades 1–4)	
				• Histological transformation to DLBCL	
				• Partial responder or non-responder patients with histological transformation to DLBCL	
				• Relapsed patients with generalized DLBCL (skin only), T3	

RIT radioimmunotherapy, *NA* not available, *NHL* non-Hodgkin's lymphoma, *FL* follicular lymphoma, *CHT* chemotherapy, *PFS* progression-free survival, *DLBCL* diffuse large B-cell lymphoma, *HL* Hodgkin's lymphoma

[a]*Level of evidence*: for NHMRC Australian guidelines, II (at least one properly designed randomized control trial); for ESMO guidelines (classification adapted from the "Infectious Diseases Society of America-United States Public Health Service Grading System"), II (small randomized trials or large randomized trials with a suspicion of bias—lower methodological quality—or meta-analyses of such trials or of trials with demonstrated heterogeneity), III (prospective cohort studies), IV (low evidence by retrospective or case-control studies); for AIOM guidelines (criteria of the "Scottish Intercollegiate Guidelines Network," SIGN), 1++ (B) (very low risk of bias). *Grade of recommendation*: for ESMO guidelines (classification adapted from the "Infectious Diseases Society of America-United States Public Health Service Grading System"), B (strong or moderate evidence for efficacy but with a limited clinical benefit, generally recommended); for NCCN guidelines, 2B (based upon lower level of evidence; alternative approaches may be better for some patients under some circumstances)

The ESMO guidelines take in consideration RIT for two different histological types of lymphoma, respectively, for mantle cell lymphoma (MCL) and FL. In the first disease, RIT is recommended in elderly patients not able to tolerate heavier therapeutic schemes, because it prolongs the PFS and thus extend the remission [4]. However, the level of evidence ranges between II and IV indicating the need for randomized controlled trials (RCT) in this subtype of lymphoma. In FL, the ESMO guidelines recommend RIT if CHT cannot be performed or is inappropriate, with evidence again ranging between II and IV. The strongest evidence is related to the consolidation treatment after CHT, but maintenance with rituximab seems to have more efficacy [6]. Studies about efficacy and safety in larger patient population comparing RIT with actual standard therapies are missing, also in FL. ESMO guidelines do not mention the use of RIT for treatment of DLBCL [5].

The Italian guidelines have an optimistic vision about the quality of evidence concerning the use of RIT in advanced FL, as consolidation therapy after CHT in front-line treatment as well as in case of relapsed/refractory FL, attributing a high level of evidence (1++/B) [7]. However, the editors underline the limits of the available studies regarding their control arm not representing actual standard therapy anymore. They consider RIT for DLBCL, but only as conditioning therapy prior to autologous stem cell transplantation (ASCT) and only in the context of clinical trials (as for FL), because high level of evidence is missing.

The NCCN guidelines are more specific than the others, because it indicates the role of RIT as first-line therapy in elderly FL patients, in relapsed FL patients after other treatment regimens, and in case of histological transformation [8]. However, 2B level of recommendation is considered weak and therefore cannot be definitive.

From the careful analysis of all the abovementioned guidelines, two main points appear:

1. In FL, RIT can be useful in elderly patients, because it has demonstrated significant advantages in terms of PFS.
2. The loss of RCT represents the major limitation of the RIT against rituximab, and therefore its utility in clinical practice is limited.

A simplifying flowchart has been drawn (Fig. 33.1), only for the FL treatment (more scientific evidences).

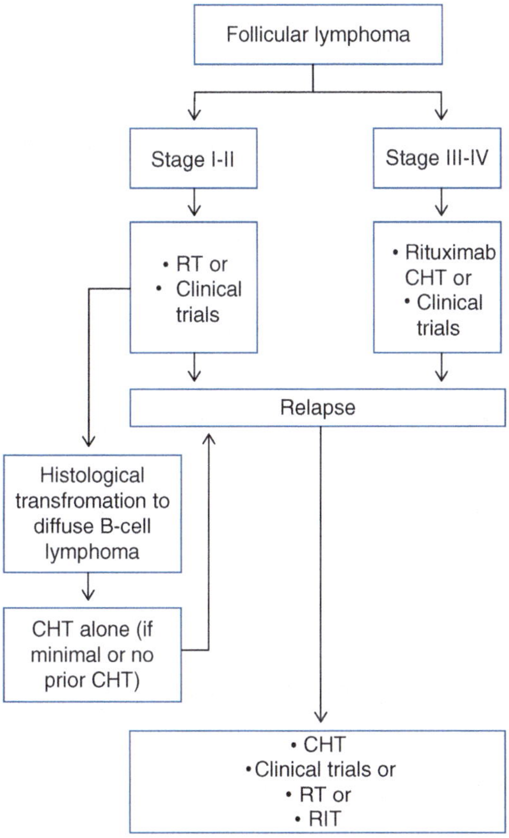

Fig. 33.1 A simplifying flowchart for the treatment of follicular lymphoma. *RT* radiotherapy, *CHT* chemotherapy, *RIT* radioimmunotherapy

References

1. Australian Cancer Network Diagnosis and Management of Lymphoma Guidelines Working Party. Guidelines for the diagnosis and management of lymphoma. The Cancer Council Australia and Australian Cancer Network, Sydney. 2005.
2. Tennvall J, Fischer M, Delaloye AB, Bombardieri E, Bodei L, Giammarile F, Lassmann M, Oyen W, Brans B, Therapy Committee EANM, Oncology Committee EANM, Dosimetry Committee EANM. EANM procedure guideline for radio-immunotherapy for B-cell lymphoma with ^{90}Y-radiolabelled ibritumomabtiuxetan (Zevalin®). Eur J Nucl Med Mol Imaging. 2007;34(4):616–22.
3. London cancer north and east. London cancer guidelines for the management of lymphoma. June 2014; available from the link: https://londoncancer.org.
4. Dreyling M, Geisler C, Hermine O, Kluin-Nelemans HC, LeGouill S, Rule S, Shpilberg O, Walewski J, Ladetto M, on behalf of the ESMO Guidelines Working Group. Newly diagnosed and relapsed mantle cell lymphoma: ESMO Clinical Practice Guidelines for diagnosis, treatment and follow-up. Ann Oncol. 2014;25(3):83–92.
5. Tilly H, Gomes da Silva M, Vitolo U, Jack A, Meignan M, Lopez-Guillermo A, Walewski J, André M, Johnson PW, Pfreundschuh M, Ladetto M, on behalf of the ESMO Guidelines Committee. Diffuse large B-cell lymphoma (DLBCL): ESMO Clinical Practice Guidelines for diagnosis, treatment and follow-up. Ann Oncol. 2015;26(5):116–25.
6. Dreyling M, Ghielmini M, Rule S, Salles G, Vitolo U, Ladetto M, on behalf of the ESMO Guidelines Committee. Newly diagnosed and relapsed follicular lymphoma: ESMO Clinical Practice Guidelines for diagnosis, treatment and follow-up. Ann Oncol. 2016;27(5):63–90.
7. Balzarotti M, Carbone A, Castagna L, Pinotti G, Ricardi U, Spina M, Tedeschi L, AIOM Linee Guida Linfomi. 2016; available from the link: http://www.aiom.it/professionisti/documenti-scientifici/linee-guida/1,413,1,#TopList.
8. NCCN guidelines version 3.2017; available from the link: http://www.nccn.org.

Part VI

New Approaches of Radiometabolic Therapy

PSMA-Based Therapy of Metastasized Castrate-Resistant Prostate Cancer

34

Sarah Marie Schwarzenböck, Jens Kurth, Sascha Nitsch, and Bernd Joachim Krause

Abstract

Despite clinically established therapeutic regimens, mCRPC patients have a poor prognosis indicating the need for more effective therapies. In recent years, therapeutic radiolabelled PSMA-ligands have shown promising results in therapy of mCRPC patients with favourable safety and efficacy. A positive response to therapy in terms of PSA decline occurs in about 70% of patients; PSA reduction ≥50% is observed in up to 50% of patients. Pain release and improvement of quality of life are observed in a major proportion of symptomatic patients. Preliminary data show that decline of PSA values is accompanied by morphological and/or metabolic changes which can be assessed by CT, bone scintigraphy and/or ^{68}Ga-PSMA PET/CT. The most common side effects of RLT are mild fatigue as well as mild and in most cases transient xerostomia. In the majority of studies, no acute or long-term side effects and high-grade haematological or renal toxicity were observed. Even though currently therapeutic PSMA-ligands have not yet been approved, ^{177}Lu-PSMA RLT is a promising treatment option to be potentially offered following approved therapies in patients with mCRPC. In the future the use of PSMA-ligands labelled with alpha emitters such as ^{225}Ac could be beneficial in patients with compromised bone marrow. Additionally, other novel theranostic agents addressing the gastrin-releasing peptide receptor (GRPR) might be promising treatment options in the future.

34.1 Introduction

The prostate-specific membrane antigen (PSMA) is a transmembrane protein also named folate hydrolase 1 which is located on the short arm of chromosome 11. PSMA is expressed on the surface of prostate cancer (PC) cells and therefore makes it a highly attractive target structure for

S.M. Schwarzenböck (✉) • J. Kurth • S. Nitsch
B.J. Krause
Department of Nuclear Medicine, Rostock University Medical Centre, Rostock, Germany
e-mail: sarah.schwarzenboeck@med.uni-rostock.de

E. Bombardieri et al. (eds.), *Clinical Applications of Nuclear Medicine Targeted Therapy*,
https://doi.org/10.1007/978-3-319-63067-0_34

molecular imaging and therapy. PSMA expression on PC cell surface is 100- to 1000-fold higher than in normal cells [1]. The most widely used PSMA-ligands for PET imaging are ^{68}Ga-PSMA-11 (^{68}Ga-PSMA HBED-CC) [2] and the theranostic agents ^{68}Ga-PSMA-617 and ^{68}Ga-PSMA-I&T [3, 4]; besides ^{18}F-DCFBC and ^{18}F-DCFPyL [5–7], ^{18}F-PSMA-1007 has recently been introduced as another ^{18}F-labelled agent for PSMA PET/CT imaging [8].

Molecular imaging of PC with PSMA-ligands has become an increasingly used imaging procedure for the assessment of recurrent disease as well as primary staging of high-risk PC. Recently, Perera et al. published a meta-analysis on sensitivity and specificity of PSMA-ligand PET/CT in PC. Based on a systematic review, 16 articles with a total of 1309 patients were further analysed. For detection of recurrent disease and for primary staging, the percentage of PSMA-positive PET was 76% (95% confidence interval (CI) 66–85%) and 40% (95% confidence interval (CI) 19–64%), respectively. For PSA values of 0.2–1, 1–2 and > 2 ng/ml, detection rates were 58%, 76% and 95% in recurrent PC [9]. Besides the use of PSMA-ligand PET/CT for restaging of patients with biochemical recurrence and primary staging of high-risk PC, therapeutic stratification and treatment monitoring of advanced metastasized castration-refractory PC (mCRPC) might become future indications of PSMA-ligand PET/CT.

After salvage treatment options, patients with metastatic PC are usually treated with androgen deprivation therapy (ADT). However, after 2–8 years of ADT, PSA rises despite ADT indicating the onset of mCRPC. Chemotherapies such as cytotoxic taxane-based agents are frequently administered in mCRPC patients [10]. Additionally, agents targeting the androgen receptor signalling axis, such as abiraterone and enzalutamide, have shown to improve survival in clinical trials [11, 12]. For bone metastases the bone-seeking α-emitter ^{223}Ra has also demonstrated to improve overall survival and quality of life [13]. Despite the use of those therapeutic regimens, mCRPC patients have a poor prognosis with an expected survival of ≤19 months [14]. Therefore, effective therapies for mCRPC patients are urgently needed. In recent years, therapeutic PSMA-ligands have shown promising results in therapy of mCRPC patients.

The first therapeutic PSMA-ligand developed by the 'Heidelberg group' was ^{131}I-MIP-1095 showing high tumour uptake, considerable symptom relief and a decline of PSA level [15]. As ^{177}Lu has certain advantages over ^{131}I with respect to synthesis and radiotoxicity [16], studies increasingly focused on the use of ^{177}Lu for PSMA-based radioligand therapies, mainly using ^{177}Lu-PSMA-617 and ^{177}Lu-PSMA-I&T.

This article gives an overview on procedural aspects, dosimetry and current literature on ^{177}Lu-PSMA radioligand therapy (RLT).

34.2 Therapy Procedure and Practical Aspects

An expert panel constituted by the German Association of Nuclear Medicine published a consensus document with recommendations of a German consortium of nuclear medicine therapy centres for indication, baseline tests, therapy protocol, concomitant therapy, dosimetry as well as follow-up of ^{177}Lu-PSMA RLT [17].

For patients with mCRPC – after having received first- and second (third)-line therapies according to guidelines and current clinical practice – ^{177}Lu-PSMA RLT can be offered in specialized nuclear medicine therapy units. As most of the PSMA RLTs have been carried out with ^{177}Lu-PSMA-617 at the present time, the consensus recommendation summarizes the expert view on the current procedure of therapy with ^{177}Lu-PSMA-617 [17].

^{177}Lu-PSMA-617 RLT should be considered in mCRPC patients after first- and second (third)-line therapies according to guidelines and current clinical practice; sufficient organ function and increased PSMA expression are crucial prerequisites for RLT. As ^{177}Lu-PSMA-617 RLT is not a routine indication in current clinical practice, indication should be discussed in an interdisciplinary tumour board on an individual basis [17].

^{177}Lu-PSMA-617 RLT is administered in multiple cycles similar to the therapy of neuroendocrine neoplasias/neuroendocrine carcinomas with ^{177}Lu-labelled peptides. The following specifications with respect to the therapy regimen have been consented: (1) Two ^{177}Lu-PSMA-617 RLTs are planned 8 weeks apart. (2) Four to seven weeks after the two therapy cycles, restaging takes place; provided that ^{177}Lu-PSMA-617 RLT is sufficiently tolerated and tumour manifestations show PSMA expression, further cycles can be considered. (3) 6 GBq is considered as standard activity. (4) A cumulative activity of 18 GBq is considered to be the upper limit [17].

Patient preparation should – among other clinically relevant parameters – comprise an evaluation of the renal function, as well as sufficient hydration before, during and after the therapy. Pretherapeutic renal function test including renal scintigraphy with ^{99m}Tc-MAG3 and salivary gland scintigraphy with ^{99m}Tc-pertechnetate can be considered. ^{177}Lu-PSMA-617 is administered intravenously. The activity administration should be given as a slow bolus (>30 s). During therapy the following procedures and co-medication might be considered: forced diuresis, ice packs for the salivary glands, anti-emetic medication as well as steroid therapy [17]. The influence of continued ADT-based therapy during RLT is still under debate [18–20].

Dosimetric measurements following ^{177}Lu-PSMA-617 RLT are recommended as discussed below. The follow-up examination should comprise (but has not to be limited to) patient history, physical examination, imaging as well as laboratory measurements. For more details on the recommendations for ^{177}Lu-PSMA-617 RLT, see Fendler et al. [17].

34.3 Dosimetry

^{177}Lu has a physical half-life of about 6.7 days, emits β-particles (E_{max} = 497 keV, E_{mean} = 149 keV) and has a penetration range in tissue of R_{max} = 2 mm, which is lower compared to ^{90}Y, for instance, and hence reduces the cross-fire effect. However, this might be partially compensated by a higher percentage of the radiation energy absorbed in small volumes. ^{177}Lu also emits γ-particles with low energy (E_γ, 113 kev, 208 keV) and with a relatively low transition probability of 6% and 11%, respectively, but enabling imaging of the biodistribution of ^{177}Lu-labelled compounds in vivo by a gamma camera. This allows for determination of patient-specific biokinetics and to perform patient-specific dosimetry before and during treatment offering the opportunity to improve safety and efficacy of targeted radionuclide therapies as the dose to tumour lesions can be optimized and the dose to organs at risk can be used as an early predictor of organ toxicity [21].

34.3.1 Imaging

To perform calculations for post-therapeutic dosimetry, patients need to be imaged at multiple time points during treatment. From these images the time-activity curve (TAC) for each organ and lesion of interest can be extracted individually. According to the EANM guideline, at least three measurements in every kinetic phase are necessary [22]. ^{177}Lu-PSMA-ligands exhibit two kinetic phases; therefore at least six measurements are required. The more time points are acquired, the more accurate the dose calculation will be. However, in clinical practice, it is also mandatory to match the requirements of a reliable dosimetry with patient comfort. Patients with mCRPC who are referred for PSMA-targeted therapy are often in poor general condition not able to tolerate many or long-lasting imaging sessions. Considering this limitation and the kinetics of ^{177}Lu-PSMA compounds, the German consensus guideline recommends a standardized imaging protocol for dosimetry purposes of PSMA-ligands (4 time points at 2, 24, 48 and 72 h post-injection) [23].

The spatially and temporally varying distribution of the therapeutic radiopharmaceutical within the patient can be extracted from planar images or SPECT series. Due to the fact that for dosimetry purposes absolute activity estimate is needed, a proper calibration of the gamma camera is mandatory, both for planar and SPECT imaging. Quantitative imaging also demands an appropriate post-processing of the images. For planar imaging correction for attenuation, scatter and source depth should be included [24–26].

SPECT images should be reconstructed using iterative algorithms (ML-EM, OSEM) including corrections for scattered and attenuated photons, dead time and distant-dependent detector blurring. A recently published review by Ljungberg et al. and the current EANM guideline give an excellent overview on the prerequisites for imaging in radionuclide therapies [21, 27].

Ideally, on every time point, quantitative SPECT/CT should be performed. However, in the clinical routine, imaging is always a trade-off between the requirements of treatment on one side and the compliance and the comfort of the patient on the other side. In principle, calculations of the absorbed dose can be made from planar 2D images, but some limitations do exist, for example, the structure overlap, e.g. of the upper pole of the right kidney and the lower liver segments, and overestimation of calculated dose to organs by tumour lesions [28]. In contrast, using SPECT/CT facilitates a high level of trust in quantitative data, which is very important in the case of dosimetric applications. However, in some situations multiple SPECT/CT imaging is not possible, and/or the axial field of view (FOV) obtained from whole body (WB) imaging is desired. In these cases a combination of WB imaging and SPECT/CT can be applied which is a frequently used approach (so-called 2.5D imaging). WB imaging is performed on all time points. Time-activity data obtained from WB images for each organ of interest are used to determine TAC. On one time point, a quantitative SPECT/CT study is acquired. The amplitude of WB curve is then renormalized making the curve pass through the organ activity as determined from quantitative SPECT/CT data being more accurate than the planar-derived ones. A study by He et al. showed the significant improvement in quantitative accuracy by this approach compared to 2D imaging [29]. For an example of WB and SPECT/CT imaging, see Fig. 34.1.

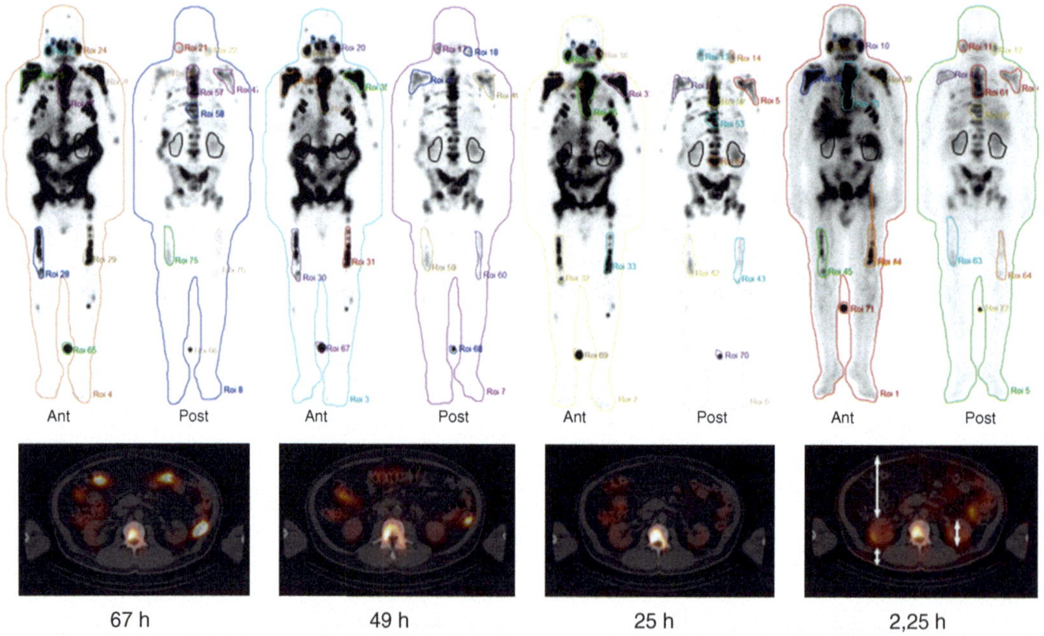

Fig. 34.1 Whole body images (anterior and posterior view) and slices of the corresponding SPECT series of a patient with mCRPC at four time points after the administration of ^{177}Lu-PSMA-617. To minimize radiation exposure, an actual SPECT/CT was only acquired 1d p.i.. At the other time points, only SPECT series were acquired, and subsequently a retrograde fusion of SPECT and CT was performed. Besides the high uptake in the tumour lesions (e.g. femoral bone, both scapulars, ribs, spine, lymph nodes), also the uptake in the kidneys and the salivary and the lacrimal glands can be seen. The interference of the ROI of the kidneys with colon shows the organ overlap as one of the main disadvantages of WB imaging for dosimetry

34.3.2 Dose Calculation

The integral of the activity over time until infinity (calculated from the fitted TAC) is equal to the number of decays that occur in the specific organ and describes the cumulated activity from which the absorbed dose can be calculated. Estimations of the doses to organs and target lesions are generally performed using the MIRD scheme [30]. Cumulative activity in organs and tumour lesions of interest are determined by numeric or compartmental models [25]. Calculations of the absorbed doses are performed using special software tools, e.g. OLINDA/EXM or NUKDOSE [31, 32]. These tools use diverse phantoms and kinetic models and therefore provide reference parameters for patients of different age, weight, size and sex. The adaptation of the standard models to patient-specific parameters (e.g. the mass of the organs) is also possible.

Different approaches such as blood-based and imaging-based methods are used to calculate the red marrow dose (for details, see [33]).

34.3.3 Dosimetry Studies

Estimations of biokinetic parameters and dosimetric calculations are part of the protocols of ^{177}Lu-PSMA-targeted therapies [23, 34, 35]. The reported results confirm a rapid blood clearance and activity elimination from the body mainly through the kidneys. Besides uptake in prostate cancer lesions, physiological uptake of therapeutic PSMA-ligands can also be seen in the lacrimal, parotid and submandibular glands, liver and spleen. Additionally, the kidneys and the bladder wall are exposed to an increased irradiation due to the excretion via the urogenital system. Table 34.1 summarizes the results of currently published studies [34–41].

Despite the fact that two different PSMA-ligands were used (PSMA-617 and PSMA-I&T), the survey does not show clear differences in the calculated doses. It can be summarized that the accumulated doses for the most sensitive organs (lacrimal and salivary glands, kidney, red bone marrow) are remarkably lower compared to those of malignant lesions. It is likely that absorbed doses of ^{177}Lu-PSMA-617 therapy are not critical for the kidneys and red bone marrow. Kidney-absorbed dose related to ^{177}Lu-PSMA RLT has been reported to be well below the 23 Gy dose-limiting threshold, which is regarded as critical. Delker et al. reported an absorbed kidney dose of 2.2 Gy in a quantitative SPECT/CT study of five patients after the administration of 3.6 GBq (range 3.4–3.9 GBq) ^{177}Lu-PSMA-617 per cycle [36]. The study by Baum et al. on 56 mCRPC patients found comparable results with an average kidney dose of 0.8 Gy/GBq based on WB data [35]. The administered activity of ^{177}Lu-PSMA per cycle was 5.76 GBq (range 3.6–8.7 GBq). Both groups reported that parotid glands received higher doses than the kidneys, with an average parotid-absorbed dose per cycle of 5.1 Gy and 7.5 Gy (calculated from the reported median activity), respectively. The role of the lacrimal and the salivary glands as dose-limiting organs is under debate [37].

All the studies present a high variability of intra-patient and intra-lesion tumour uptake. However, the wide range of tumour doses is mostly related to localization and biological and pathological factors (heterogeneity in binding affinity, receptor density, differences in tumour volume, viability and many more).

The study by Okamoto et al. on ^{177}Lu-PSMA-I&T therapy also evaluated the changes of tumour doses from cycle to cycle [39]. They showed that absorbed doses to organs of risk were relatively constant across four different cycles. The doses to tumour lesions decreased slightly, with 3.5 Gy/GBq for the first, 3.3 Gy/GBq for the second, 2.7 Gy/GBq for the third and 2.4 Gy/GBq for the fourth cycle. Additionally, the authors reported a moderate correlation of the SUV of pretherapeutic ^{68}Ga-PSMA PET with the absorbed dose and with the change of SUV during therapy.

Kabasakal et al. [41] evaluated the usefulness of pretherapeutic dosimetry to estimate the absorbed dose of ^{177}Lu-PSMA-617 in different organs. Seven patients with mCRPC were analysed after a single diagnostic dose (mean activity of 192.6 MBq). These pretherapeutically calculated absorbed doses are comparable to intrath-

Table 34.1 Dosimetric results for organs at risk and tumours

Study	Absorbed doses per unit administered activity (Gy/GBq)[a]					
	Kidneys	Parotid (salivary) glands	Lacrimal glands	Liver	Red bone marrow	Tumour
Baum et al. [35][c]	0.80 ± 0.40	1.3 ± 2.3	n. r.	n. r.	0.025 ± 0.01	3.0 ± 10.0 (bone lesions) 4.0 ± 20.0 (lymph nodes)
Delker et al. [36][b]	0.60 ± 0.18	1.41 ± 0.53	n. r.	0.11 ± 0.06	0.01 ± 0.01	5.3 ± 3.7 (bone lesions) 4.2 ± 5.3 (lymph nodes) 2.1 ± 0.8 (soft tissue)
Hohberg et al. [37]	0.53	0.72	2.82			
Yadav et al. [38][b]	0.99 ± 0.31	1.24 ± 0.26	n. r.	0.36 ± 0.10	0.048 ± 0.05	n. r.
Okamoto et al. [39][c]	0.72 ± 0.21	0.55 ± 0.14 (parotid) 0.64 ± 0.40 (submandibular)	3.8 ± 1.4	0.12 ± 0.06	n. r.	3.2 ± 2.6
Scarba et al. [40][b]	0.60 ± 0.36	0.56 ± 0.25 (parotid) 0.50 ± 0.15 (submandibular)	1.01 ± 0.69		0.04 ± 0.03	3.4 ± 1.9 (bone lesions) 2.6 ± 0.4 (lymph nodes) 2.4 ± 0.8 (liver)
Fendler et al. [34][b]	0.55 ± 0.20	1.00 ± 0.60	n. r.	0.1 ± 0.1	0.002 ± 0.005	6.10 ± 4.90
Kabasakal et al. [41][b] (pretherapeutic)	0.88 ± 0.40				0.03 ± 0.01	

[a]Results are given as mean value ± 1SD
[b]^{177}Lu-PSMA-617
[c]^{177}Lu-PSMA-I&T
n. r. not reported

erapeutic dosimetric results reported by other groups (see Table 34.1) demonstrating that a pretherapeutic dose estimation is thus possible and reliable.

Regarding renal dose limits, it has to be considered that the value of 23 Gy which is associated with a 5 % probability of developing severe kidney damages within 5 years [42, 43] is derived from external beam radiation therapy (EBRT). It is under debate if it is possible to directly transfer this value from EBRT to peptide receptor radionuclide therapy (PRRT) and ^{177}Lu-PSMA-targeted therapy. Important factors, like the dose rate, the radiation type and the heterogeneity of dose delivery (e.g. micro-biodistribution within the organs), are completely different from EBRT. For instance, the radiation dose rate is much higher in EBRT (1–3 Gy/min) compared to PRRT (<3 mGy/min) and more variable, with a continuous exponential decrease related to effective half-life [44]. It is well known that the dose rate is an important radiobiological factor influencing the recovery from radiation damage. This issue results in a higher tissue tolerance in terms of PRRT [44]. Also the concept of biologically effective dose (BED) is applied to measure biological effects resulting from different dose patterns [44]. Based on the BED concept, recent studies proposed higher kidney toxicity thresholds of 28 and 40 Gy (depending on the presence of additional risk factors) for PRRT [45, 46]. Of course, these considerations also apply to the other organs at risk.

34.4 Summary

Due to substantial individual variance, dosimetry is mandatory for a patient-specific approach in ^{177}Lu-PSMA-targeted therapy – the maximally tolerable dose to organs of risk calculated by an individualized method may be higher in a considerable number of patients allowing for administration of a higher cumulative dose to the tumour. Therefore, higher activities and/or shorter treatment intervals might be tested in the future. Newest dosimetric concepts, like the calculation and generation of 3D dose maps by S-voxel-kernel convolution, will help to further optimize PSMA-targeted therapies.

34.5 Review of the Current Literature on PSMA-Ligand RLT

34.5.1 Current RLT Studies: Biochemical and Clinical Response

In a study by Baum et al., 56 mCRPC patients underwent PSMA RLT with ^{177}Lu-PSMA-I&T. A decline in PSA levels was found in 80.4% of patients (PSA decline was ≥80% in 23.2% and ≥50% in 58.9% of patients). The severity of pain was significantly reduced in 2 of 6 patients (33.3%). Karnofsky performance status score improved in several patients; worsening was not observed [35].

The same group reported on their experience in 119 mCRPC patients (between 2013 and 2016) who underwent 300 cycles of PRLT using different ^{177}Lu-PSMA radioligands (1–7 treatments per patient, median activity of 6.0 GBq/cycle). In PSA assessment of 80 patients after at least 1 therapy cycle, PSA reduction was shown in 76.3% of patients (>50% of reduction in 57.5% of patients and >80% in 27.5% of patients). Pain release and improvement of quality of life were significant in symptomatic patients [47].

Similar results with respect to PSA decline were demonstrated by Ahmadzadehfar et al. reporting on early side effects and response rate of ^{177}Lu-PSMA-617 (mean administered activity of 5.6 GBq) in ten patients suffering from hormone- and/or chemo-refractory prostate cancer in a two-centre study. Seven (70%) patients experienced a PSA decline (with five patients >50%) [48].

These results were confirmed by a subsequent study of the same group in which side effects and the response rate of 24 hormone- and/or chemo-refractory metastasized PC patients were retrospectively analysed according to the PSA level. Patients were treated with 46 cycles of RLT with ^{177}Lu-PSMA-617 (22 patients received 2 cycles). Decline in PSA was observed in 79.1% and in 68.2% of patients 8 weeks after the first and second cycle of RLT, respectively [49].

Kratochwil et al. retrospectively reported on 30 treatment-resistant mCRPC patients treated with ^{177}Lu-PSMA-617-targeted radionuclide therapy. Twenty-one of 30 patients showed a PSA response; in 13 of 30 patients, PSA decreased more than 50%. After 3 cycles, 8 of 11 patients achieved a sustained PSA response (>50%) for over 24 weeks, which was also correlated with radiologic response (decrease in lesion number and size) [50].

Rahbar et al. reported on 50 therapies using ^{177}Lu-PSMA-617 performed in 28 consecutive patients with mCRPC (after conventional therapies) (mean activity of 5.9 ± 0.44 GBq and 5.9 ± 0.7 GBq at the first and second therapy, respectively). In this cohort, any PSA decline occurred in 59% and 75% of patients after 1 and 2 therapies, respectively. PSA decline was ≥ 50% (representing relevant response according to Prostate Cancer Working Group (PCWG) 2 criteria) in 32% and 50% of the patients, respectively [51].

Subsequently, the same group performed a multicentre retrospective analysis on response and tolerability of a single dose of

^{177}Lu-PSMA-617 (mean applied activity of 5.9 ± 0.5 GBq) in 74 patients with mCRPC. Sixty-four percent of patients showed a PSA decline, 31% showed a decline of more than 50%, 47% of patients had stable disease (defined by change of PSA ranging from a decrease of <50% to an increase of >25%) and only 23% of patients showed progressive disease (with a PSA increase of more than 25%) during therapy [52].

Heck et al. reported on 22 patients with mCRPC and treatment failure after chemotherapy and novel androgen receptor-targeted therapy who were treated for 8 weeks with up to 4 cycles of ^{177}Lu-PSMA-I&T. The administered activity was 3.7 GBq in the first cycle of the first 3 patients; due to a favourable safety profile, the activity was increased to 7.4 GBq in 19 subsequent patients who completed a total of 40 cycles.

A maximum PSA decrease of ≥30%, ≥50% and ≥90% was achieved in 56%, 33% and 11% of patients, respectively. ECOG performance status improved or was stable in 74% of patients. Of men with bone pain, 56% achieved complete resolution or reduced pain [53].

Yadav et al. found a reduction of mean serum PSA (baseline, 275 ng/mL; after the first cycle of therapy, 141.75 ng/mL) in 31 mCRPC patients treated with ^{177}Lu-PSMA-617 (mean applied activity of 5.07 ± 1.85 GBq ranging from 1 to 4 cycles). Based on biochemical response criteria, 2/31, 20/31, 3/31 and 6/31 of patients had complete response (CR), partial response (PR), stable disease (SD) and progressive disease (PD), respectively. With respect to clinical response assessment, the mean visual analogue score (VAS_{max}) decreased from 7.5 to 3; the mean analgesic score decreased from 2.5 to 1.8 after therapy. The mean Karnofsky performance score improved from 50.32 to 65.42; the mean ECOG performance status improved from 2.54 to 1.78 after therapy [54].

These results on biochemical and clinical response were confirmed by Fendler et al. including 15 patients who received 2 cycles of 3.7 GBq or 6 GBq of ^{177}Lu-PSMA-617. Any PSA decline was observed in 12/15 (80%) patients; a PSA decline of ≥50% was observed in 9/15 (60%) patients. Significant pain relief was described in 7/10 (70%) symptomatic patients, and quality of life improved in 9/15 (60%) patients [34].

A recently published retrospective German multicentre study investigated ^{177}Lu-PSMA-617 therapy in mCRPC patients. Two hundred forty eight therapy cycles were performed in 145 patients (1–4 therapy cycles) in 12 therapy centres. An average activity of 5.9 GBq of ^{177}Lu-PSMA-617 was administered (range 2–8 GBq).

The overall biochemical response rate (defined as a decrease of PSA ≥50% from baseline to at least 2 weeks after the start of RLT) was 45% after all therapy cycles. Forty percent of the patients already showed biochemical response after a single cycle. In a multivariate analysis, alkaline phosphatase, number of therapy cycles and the presence of visceral metastases were significant predictors associated with the rate of biochemical response. The results of the German multicentre study are indicative of a favourable safety and efficacy of ^{177}Lu-PSMA-617 therapy in patients with mCRPC [55].

In summary, a positive response to therapy in terms of decline in PSA occurs in about 70% of patients; a PSA reduction ≥50% is observed in up to 50% of patients. Pain release and improvement of quality of life were significant in symptomatic patients. Karnofsky and ECOG performance status score improved or remained stable in the majority of patients.

34.5.2 Current RLT Studies: Imaged-Based Therapy Response Assessment

Baum et al. evaluated metabolic response revealing partial remission in 14, stable disease in 2 and progressive disease in 9 patients out of 25 patients monitored for at least 6 months after 2 or more PSMA RLT cycles by ^{68}Ga-PSMA PET/CT (EORTC criteria). Contrast-enhanced CT revealed partial remission in 5, stable disease in 13 and progressive disease in 7 patients (according to RECIST 1.1). Morphologic response was better in lymph nodes compared to bone metastases possibly due to better delineation of lymph nodes on CT compared to osseous metastases

[35]. This finding is in line with the results by Ahmadzadehfar et al. showing that ^{68}Ga-PSMA PET/CT might outperform CT due to its superiority regarding response assessment of bone metastases. Nevertheless, therapy response assessed by CT (according to RECIST criteria) was also significantly correlated with the change of PSA values. The authors showed partial response, stable disease and progressive disease in 40%, 55% and 5% of patients using RECIST CT criteria as well as in 80%, 0% and 20% using PSMA PET for therapy response assessment [49].

Yadav et al. showed similar results – sustained PSA response for over 24 weeks in 8/11 patients after 3 therapy cycles was correlated with radiologic response (decrease in lesion number and size). Metabolic response assessed using ^{68}Ga-PSMA PET/CT revealed complete response in 2/6 patients, partial response in 3/6 and stable disease in 1/6 patients [54].

In the study by Kratochwil et al., imaging-based restaging revealed a positive response in 10 of the 11 patients; surprisingly, a positive imaging response was even found in 1 of the 2 patients with rising PSA. Of six patients who were restaged with ^{68}Ga-PSMA PET/CT, all presented with a decrease of more than 50% (average of index lesions) in SUV_{max} [50].

Heck et al. who showed complete remission in 5% of patients, stable disease in 63% and progressive disease in 32% in combined assessment of bone and soft tissue metastases (CT/RECIST criteria for soft tissue lesions and ^{68}Ga-PSMA PET/CT/PCWG2 criteria for bone lesions) [53].

According to those results, in the recent study by Fendler et al., 27% of patients showed partial response, 40% stable disease and 33% progressive disease according to RECIST 1.1. In ^{68}Ga-PSMA PET/CT, 73% of patients showed partial response, 20% stable disease and 7% progressive disease according to PERCIST 1.0. [34].

In summary, preliminary data show that decline of PSA values is accompanied by morphological and/or metabolic changes assessed by CT (RECIST criteria) and/or ^{68}Ga-PSMA PET/CT (PCWG2 criteria or PERCIST criteria); for a patient example of therapy response assessed by ^{68}Ga-PSMA PET/CT, see Fig. 34.2. For an overview on the results of treatment efficacy of PSMA-ligand therapy, see Table 34.2.

34.5.3 Current RLT Studies: Side Effects

The majority of studies observed no acute or long-term side effects and high-grade haematological or renal toxicity [34, 35, 48–54]. Kratochwil et al. found diffuse bone marrow involvement to be a risk factor for higher-grade myelosuppression which however could be identified by ^{68}Ga-PSMA PSMA PET/CT imaging in advance [50]. In accordance with this observation, Kulkarni et al. described grade 3 or 4 haematological toxicity in only 3.4% of patients who were heavily pretreated with chemotherapy or ^{223}Ra therapy [47]. The most common side effects were mild fatigue (during a few days after therapy) and mild and in most cases transient xerostomia [47]. These results were confirmed by other studies [35, 48, 50, 53].

In the German multicentre study in none of the therapy centres, a therapy-related death was documented. During the follow-up (median 16 weeks, range 2–30), 19 patients died. Data for laboratory-based toxicity were available for 121 patients. Grade 3–4 haematological toxicity was observed in 18 patients. Of all patients 105 presented with anaemia, 4% with thrombocytopenia and 3% with leukopenia. Xerostomia occurred in 8% of the treated patients. For further details on toxicity of PSMA-ligand therapy, see [56].

The role of potential kidney protection has to be evaluated in further studies; however according to the available data, kidney protection procedures might not be obligatorily necessary in patients with normal kidney function. Uptake of salivary glands could be reduced by cooling procedure before and after therapy administration minimizing dryness of the mouth.

34.5.4 Current RLT Studies: Survival

In their patient cohort treated with RLT, Baum et al. reported a median progression-free sur-

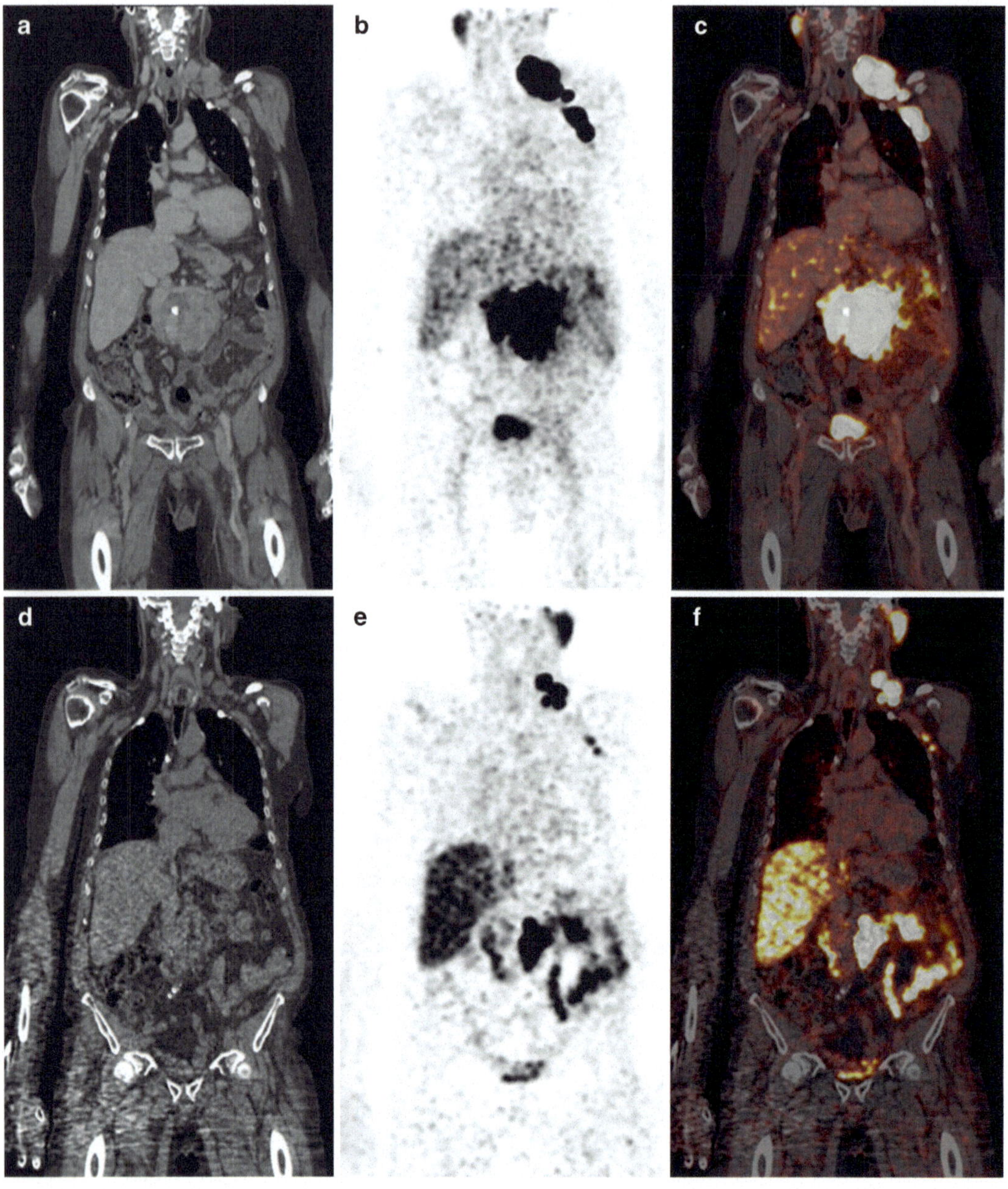

Fig. 34.2 Image example of a 77-year-old patient with metastasized castration-refractory prostate cancer (initially cT3a cN1 cM0 G2b, Gleason score of 7). Patient received hormone ablation therapy, local radiation treatment and numerous systemic therapies (Zytiga®, Taxotere® and Xtandi®). Due to progressive disease, patient was referred for three cycles of ^{177}Lu PSMA therapy. Baseline ^{68}Ga-PSMA PET/CT showed PSMA-positive nodal metastases (coronal (**a**) CT, (**b**) PET, (**c**) fused PET/CT). Therapy response assessment using ^{68}Ga-PSMA PET/CT after three cycles of ^{177}Lu-PSMA therapy showed reduced tumour load (coronal (**d**) CT, (**e**) PET, (**f**) fused PET/CT), and PSA significantly decreased

vival of 13.7 months; the median overall survival was not reached during follow-up for 28 months [35]. These results are in line with those by Kulkarni et al. analysing survival in 104 patients. Over a follow-up period of 34 months, 25% of patients died. Progression-free survival was estimated to be 10.7 months (potentially underestimated due to already-com-

Table 34.2 Overview of previously published studies

Study	Therapy response (% of patients)					
	Any PSA reduction	PSA reduction ≥50%	PSA-PD	CT (RECIST)	PSMA PET (EORCT, PERCIST)	Clinical response
Ahmadzadehfar et al. [48]	70	50	30	–	–	–
Ahmadzadehfar et al. [49]	79/68[a]	42/60[a]	21/32[a]	PR 40	PR 80	–
				SD 55	SD 0	
				PD 5	PD 20	
Kratochwil et al. [50]	70	43	27	–	–	–
Baum et al. [35]	80	59	11	PR 20	PR 56	Decrease of severity in pain (33), improvement of KPS in several patients
				SD 52	SD 8	
				PD 28	PD 36	
Rahbar et al. [51]	59/75[a]	32/50[a]	17	–	–	–
Rahbar et al. [52]	64	31	23	–	–	–
Kulkarni et al. [47]	76	58	–	–	CR 9	Significant pain release and improvement in QoL
					PR 21	
Heck et al. [53]		33	32	PR 11	CR 5[b]	Stable/improved ECOG (74), complete/partial bone pain resolution (56)
				SD 56	SD 63[b]	
				PD 33	PD 32[b]	
Yadav et al. [54]	–	–	19	–	CR 33	CR 23
					PR 50	PR 45
					SD 17	
Fendler et al. [34]	80	60	20	PR 27	PR 73	Significant pain relief (70) and improvement in QoL (60)
				SD 40	SD 20	
				PD 33	PD 7	

CR complete response, *PR* partial response, *SD* stable disease, *PD* progressive disease, *ECOG* Eastern Cooperative Oncology Groups, *KPS* Karnofsky performance status, *QoL* quality of life

[a]After the first/second therapy cycle

[b]Combined therapy response assessment (CT and PSMA PET)

promised bone marrow function); median overall survival had not yet been reached [47].

Rahbar et al. compared survival in a RLT group and a historical group of best supportive care. The estimated median survival of the RLT group was significantly longer compared to the best supportive care group; however, improved overall survival has to be shown within a controlled randomized trial due to the retrospective character of this study. The authors concluded that RLT with ^{177}Lu-PSMA-617 might increase overall survival compared to conventional therapy approaches [51]. Heck et al. showed a median progression-free survival of 175 days (95% CI 35–315) [53]. In the study by Yadav et al., median progression-free and overall survival was 12 and 15 months, respectively [54].

Conclusion

Even though currently therapeutic PSMA-ligands have not yet been approved, ^{177}Lu-PSMA RLT is a promising safe and effective treatment option to be offered in patients with mCRPC after all approved therapies.

In patients with bulky disease, ^{90}Y as a high-energy beta emitter may represent an alternative to ^{177}Lu given the fact that the range of beta particles emitted by ^{90}Y is higher compared to ^{177}Lu being advantageous in such patients.

The use of PSMA-ligands labelled with alpha emitters such as ^{225}Ac (which is currently only available in Heidelberg, Germany) could in the future be beneficial in patients with compromised bone marrow (due to heavily myelosuppressive pretreatment) [57, 58]. Additionally, other novel theranostic agents addressing the gastrin-releasing peptide receptor (GRPR) also being overexpressed in prostate cancer, such as the GRPR antagonist ^{68}Ga/^{177}Lu-RM2, might be promising treatment options in the future [59–61].

Conflict of Interest The authors declare that they have no conflict of interest.

References

1. Evans MJ, Smith-Jones PM, Wongvipat J, Navarro V, Kim S, Bander NH, et al. Noninvasive measurement of androgen receptor signaling with a positron-emitting radiopharmaceutical that targets prostate-specific membrane antigen. Proc Natl Acad Sci U S A. 2011;108(23):9578–82.
2. Eder M, Neels O, Muller M, Bauder-Wust U, Remde Y, Schafer M, et al. Novel preclinical and radiopharmaceutical aspects of [68Ga]Ga-PSMA-HBED-CC: a new PET tracer for imaging of prostate cancer. Pharmaceuticals (Basel). 2014;7(7):779–96.
3. Afshar-Oromieh A, Hetzheim H, Kratochwil C, Benesova M, Eder M, Neels OC, et al. The theranostic PSMA ligand PSMA-617 in the diagnosis of prostate cancer by PET/CT: biodistribution in humans, radiation dosimetry, and first evaluation of tumor lesions. J Nucl Med. 2015;56(11):1697–705.
4. Weineisen M, Schottelius M, Simecek J, Baum RP, Yildiz A, Beykan S, et al. 68Ga- and 177Lu-labeled PSMA I&T: optimization of a PSMA-targeted theranostic concept and first proof-of-concept human studies. J Nucl Med. 2015;56(8):1169–76.
5. Cho SY, Gage KL, Mease RC, Senthamizhchelvan S, Holt DP, Jeffrey-Kwanisai A, et al. Biodistribution, tumor detection, and radiation dosimetry of 18F-DCFBC, a low-molecular-weight inhibitor of prostate-specific membrane antigen, in patients with metastatic prostate cancer. J Nucl Med. 2012;53(12):1883–91.
6. Rowe SP, Macura KJ, Ciarallo A, Mena E, Blackford A, Nadal R, et al. Comparison of prostate-specific membrane antigen-based 18F-DCFBC PET/CT to conventional imaging modalities for detection of hormone-naive and castration-resistant metastatic prostate cancer. J Nucl Med. 2016;57(1):46–53.
7. Szabo Z, Mena E, Rowe SP, Plyku D, Nidal R, Eisenberger MA, et al. Initial evaluation of [(18)F] DCFPyL for prostate-specific membrane antigen (PSMA)-targeted PET imaging of prostate cancer. Mol Imaging Biol. 2015;17(4):565–74.
8. Giesel FL, Hadaschik B, Cardinale J, Radtke J, Vinsensia M, Lehnert W, et al. F-18 labelled PSMA-1007: biodistribution, radiation dosimetry and histopathological validation of tumor lesions in prostate cancer patients. Eur J Nucl Med Mol Imaging. 2017;44(4):678–88.
9. Perera M, Papa N, Christidis D, Wetherell D, Hofman MS, Murphy DG, et al. Sensitivity, specificity, and predictors of positive 68Ga-prostate-specific membrane antigen positron emission tomography in advanced prostate cancer: a systematic review and meta-analysis. Eur Urol. 2016;70(6):926–37.
10. Seruga B, Tannock IF. Chemotherapy-based treatment for castration-resistant prostate cancer. J Clin Oncol. 2011;29(27):3686–94.
11. de Bono JS, Logothetis CJ, Molina A, Fizazi K, North S, Chu L, et al. Abiraterone and increased survival in metastatic prostate cancer. N Engl J Med. 2011;364(21):1995–2005.
12. Scher HI, Beer TM, Higano CS, Anand A, Taplin ME, Efstathiou E, et al. Antitumour activity of MDV3100 in castration-resistant prostate cancer: a phase 1-2 study. Lancet. 2010;375(9724):1437–46.
13. Parker C, Nilsson S, Heinrich D, Helle SI, O'Sullivan JM, Fossa SD, et al. Alpha emitter radium-223 and survival in metastatic prostate cancer. N Engl J Med. 2013;369(3):213–23.
14. Heidenreich A, Bastian PJ, Bellmunt J, Bolla M, Joniau S, van der Kwast T, et al. EAU guidelines on prostate cancer. part 1: screening, diagnosis, and local treatment with curative intent-update 2013. Eur Urol. 2014;65(1):124–37.
15. Zechmann CM, Afshar-Oromieh A, Armor T, Stubbs JB, Mier W, Hadaschik B, et al. Radiation dosimetry and first therapy results with a (124)I/(131)I-labeled small molecule (MIP-1095) targeting PSMA for prostate cancer therapy. Eur J Nucl Med Mol Imaging. 2014;41(7):1280–92.
16. Kassis AI. Therapeutic radionuclides: biophysical and radiobiologic principles. Semin Nucl Med. 2008;38(5):358–66.
17. Fendler WP, Eiber M, Beheshti M, Bomanji J, Ceci F, Cho S, et al. 68Ga-PSMA PET/CT: joint EANM and SNMMI procedure guideline for prostate cancer imaging: version 1.0. Eur J Nucl Med Mol Imaging. 2017;44(6):1014–24.
18. Liu T, LY W, Fulton MD, Johnson JM, Berkman CE. Prolonged androgen deprivation leads to downregulation of androgen receptor and prostate-specific membrane antigen in prostate cancer cells. Int J Oncol. 2012;41(6):2087–92.
19. Meller B, Bremmer F, Sahlmann CO, Hijazi S, Bouter C, Trojan L, et al. Alterations in androgen deprivation enhanced prostate-specific membrane antigen (PSMA) expression in prostate cancer cells as a target for diagnostics and therapy. EJNMMI Res. 2015;5(1):66.
20. Wright GL Jr, Grob BM, Haley C, Grossman K, Newhall K, Petrylak D, et al. Upregulation of prostate-specific membrane antigen after androgen-deprivation therapy. Urology. 1996;48(2):326–34.

21. Ljungberg M, Celler A, Konijnenberg MW, Eckerman KF, Dewaraja YK, Sjogreen-Gleisner K, et al. MIRD pamphlet No. 26: joint EANM/MIRD guidelines for quantitative 177Lu SPECT applied for dosimetry of radiopharmaceutical therapy. J Nucl Med. 2016;57(1):151–62.
22. Lassmann M, Chiesa C, Flux G, Bardies M, Committee EDEANM. Dosimetry Committee guidance document: good practice of clinical dosimetry reporting. Eur J Nucl Med Mol Imaging. 2011;38(1):192–200.
23. Fendler WP, Kratochwil C, Ahmadzadehfar H, Rahbar K, Baum RP, Schmidt M, et al. 177Lu-PSMA-617 therapy, dosimetry and follow-up in patients with metastatic castration-resistant prostate cancer. Nuklearmedizin. 2016;55(3):123–8.
24. Fleming JS. A technique for the absolute measurement of activity using a gamma camera and computer. Phys Med Biol. 1979;24(1):176–80.
25. Siegel JA, Thomas SR, Stubbs JB, Stabin MG, Hays MT, Koral KF, et al. MIRD pamphlet no. 16: techniques for quantitative radiopharmaceutical biodistribution data acquisition and analysis for use in human radiation dose estimates. J Nucl Med. 1999;40(2):37S–61S.
26. Ogawa K, Harata Y, Ichihara T, Kubo A, Hashimoto S. A practical method for position-dependent Compton-scatter correction in single photon emission CT. IEEE Trans Med Imaging. 1991;10(3):408–12.
27. Ljungberg M, Gleisner KS. Hybrid imaging for patient-specific dosimetry in radionuclide therapy. Diagnostics (Basel). 2015;5(3):296–317.
28. Sandstrom M, Garske U, Granberg D, Sundin A, Lundqvist H. Individualized dosimetry in patients undergoing therapy with (177)Lu-DOTA-D-Phe (1)-Tyr (3)-octreotate. Eur J Nucl Med Mol Imaging. 2010;37(2):212–25.
29. He B, Wahl RL, Du Y, Sgouros G, Jacene H, Flinn I, et al. Comparison of residence time estimation methods for radioimmunotherapy dosimetry and treatment planning – Monte Carlo simulation studies. IEEE Trans Med Imaging. 2008;27(4):521–30.
30. Bolch WE, Eckerman KF, Sgouros G, Thomas SR. MIRD pamphlet No. 21: a generalized schema for radiopharmaceutical dosimetry – standardization of nomenclature. J Nucl Med. 2009;50(3):477–84.
31. Stabin MG, Sparks RB, Crowe E. OLINDA/EXM: the second-generation personal computer software for internal dose assessment in nuclear medicine. J Nucl Med. 2005;46(6):1023–7.
32. Kletting P, Schimmel S, Hanscheid H, Luster M, Fernandez M, Nosske D, et al. The NUKDOS software for treatment planning in molecular radiotherapy. Z Med Phys. 2015;25(3):264–74.
33. Hindorf C, Glatting G, Chiesa C, Linden O, Flux G, Committee EDEANM. Dosimetry Committee guidelines for bone marrow and whole-body dosimetry. Eur J Nucl Med Mol Imaging. 2010;37(6):1238–50.
34. Fendler WP, Reinhardt S, Ilhan H, Delker A, Boning G, Gildehaus FJ, et al. Preliminary experience with dosimetry, response and patient reported outcome after 177Lu-PSMA-617 therapy for metastatic castration-resistant prostate cancer. Oncotarget. 2017;8(2):3581–90.
35. Baum RP, Kulkarni HR, Schuchardt C, Singh A, Wirtz M, Wiessalla S, et al. 177Lu-labeled prostate-specific membrane antigen radioligand therapy of metastatic castration-resistant prostate cancer: safety and efficacy. J Nucl Med. 2016;57(7):1006–13.
36. Delker A, Fendler WP, Kratochwil C, Brunegraf A, Gosewisch A, Gildehaus FJ, et al. Dosimetry for (177)Lu-DKFZ-PSMA-617: a new radiopharmaceutical for the treatment of metastatic prostate cancer. Eur J Nucl Med Mol Imaging. 2016;43(1):42–51.
37. Hohberg M, Eschner W, Schmidt M, Dietlein M, Kobe C, Fischer T, et al. Lacrimal glands may represent organs at risk for radionuclide therapy of prostate cancer with [(177)Lu]DKFZ-PSMA-617. Mol Imaging Biol. 2016;18(3):437–45.
38. Yadav MP, Ballal S, Tripathi M, Damle NA, Sahoo RK, Seth A, et al. Post-therapeutic dosimetry of 177Lu-DKFZ-PSMA-617 in the treatment of patients with metastatic castration-resistant prostate cancer. Nucl Med Commun. 2017;38(1):91–8.
39. Okamoto S, Thieme A, Allmann J, D'Alessandria C, Maurer T, Retz M, et al. Radiation dosimetry for 177Lu-PSMA I&T in metastatic castration-resistant prostate cancer: absorbed dose in normal organs and tumor lesions. J Nucl Med. 2017;58(3):445–50.
40. Scarpa L, Buxbaum S, Kendler D, Fink K, Bektic J, Gruber L, et al. The 68Ga/177Lu theragnostic concept in PSMA targeting of castration-resistant prostate cancer: correlation of SUVmax values and absorbed dose estimates. Eur J Nucl Med Mol Imaging. 2017;44(5):788–800.
41. Kabasakal L, AbuQbeitah M, Aygun A, Yeyin N, Ocak M, Demirci E, et al. Pre-therapeutic dosimetry of normal organs and tissues of (177)Lu-PSMA-617 prostate-specific membrane antigen (PSMA) inhibitor in patients with castration-resistant prostate cancer. Eur J Nucl Med Mol Imaging. 2015;42(13):1976–83.
42. Cassady JR. Clinical radiation nephropathy. Int J Radiat Oncol Biol Phys. 1995;31(5):1249–56.
43. Dale R. Use of the linear-quadratic radiobiological model for quantifying kidney response in targeted radiotherapy. Cancer Biother Radiopharm. 2004;19(3):363–70.
44. Cremonesi M, Ferrari M, Bodei L, Tosi G, Paganelli G. Dosimetry in peptide radionuclide receptor therapy: a review. J Nucl Med. 2006;47(9):1467–75.
45. Sundlov A, Sjogreen-Gleisner K, Svensson J, Ljungberg M, Olsson T, Bernhardt P, et al. Individualised 177Lu-DOTATATE treatment of neuroendocrine tumours based on kidney dosimetry. Eur J Nucl Med Mol Imaging. 2017;44(9):1480–9.
46. Bodei L, Cremonesi M, Ferrari M, Pacifici M, Grana CM, Bartolomei M, et al. Long-term evaluation of renal toxicity after peptide receptor radionuclide therapy with 90Y-DOTATOC and 177Lu-DOTATATE:

the role of associated risk factors. Eur J Nucl Med Mol Imaging. 2008;35(10):1847–56.
47. Kulkarni HR, Singh A, Schuchardt C, Niepsch K, Sayeg M, Leshch Y, et al. PSMA-based radioligand therapy for metastatic castration-resistant prostate cancer: the Bad Berka experience since 2013. J Nucl Med. 2016;57(Suppl 3):97S–104S.
48. Ahmadzadehfar H, Rahbar K, Kurpig S, Bogemann M, Claesener M, Eppard E, et al. Early side effects and first results of radioligand therapy with (177) Lu-DKFZ-617 PSMA of castrate-resistant metastatic prostate cancer: a two-centre study. EJNMMI Res. 2015;5(1):114.
49. Ahmadzadehfar H, Eppard E, Kurpig S, Fimmers R, Yordanova A, Schlenkhoff CD, et al. Therapeutic response and side effects of repeated radioligand therapy with 177Lu-PSMA-DKFZ-617 of castrate-resistant metastatic prostate cancer. Oncotarget. 2016;7(11):12477–88.
50. Kratochwil C, Giesel FL, Stefanova M, Benesova M, Bronzel M, Afshar-Oromieh A, et al. PSMA-targeted radionuclide therapy of metastatic castration-resistant prostate cancer with 177Lu-labeled PSMA-617. J Nucl Med. 2016;57(8):1170–6.
51. Rahbar K, Bode A, Weckesser M, Avramovic N, Claesener M, Stegger L, et al. Radioligand therapy with 177Lu-PSMA-617 as a novel therapeutic option in patients with metastatic castration resistant prostate cancer. Clin Nucl Med. 2016;41(7):522–8.
52. Rahbar K, Schmidt M, Heinzel A, Eppard E, Bode A, Yordanova A, et al. Response and tolerability of a single dose of 177Lu-PSMA-617 in patients with metastatic castration-resistant prostate cancer: a multicenter retrospective analysis. J Nucl Med. 2016;57(9):1334–8.
53. Heck MM, Retz M, D'Alessandria C, Rauscher I, Scheidhauer K, Maurer T, et al. Systemic radioligand therapy with (177)Lu labeled prostate specific membrane antigen ligand for imaging and therapy in patients with metastatic castration resistant prostate cancer. J Urol. 2016;196(2):382–91.
54. Yadav MP, Ballal S, Tripathi M, Damle NA, Sahoo RK, Seth A, et al. 177Lu-DKFZ-PSMA-617 therapy in metastatic castration resistant prostate cancer: safety, efficacy, and quality of life assessment. Eur J Nucl Med Mol Imaging. 2017;44(1):81–91.
55. Rahbar K, Ahmadzadehfar H, Kratochwil C, Haberkorn U, Schafers M, Essler M, et al. German multicenter study investigating 177Lu-PSMA-617 radioligand therapy in advanced prostate cancer patients. J Nucl Med. 2017;58(1):85–90.
56. Emmett L, Willowson K, Violet J, Shin J, Blanksby A, Lee J. Lutetium 177 PSMA radionuclide therapy for men with prostate cancer: a review of the current literature and discussion of practical aspects of therapy. J Med Radiat Sci. 2017;64(1):52–60.
57. Kratochwil C, Bruchertseifer F, Giesel FL, Weis M, Verburg FA, Mottaghy F, et al. 225Ac-PSMA-617 for PSMA-targeted alpha-radiation therapy of metastatic castration-resistant prostate cancer. J Nucl Med. 2016;57(12):1941–4.
58. Zhu C, Bandekar A, Sempkowski M, Banerjee SR, Pomper MG, Bruchertseifer F, et al. Nanoconjugation of PSMA-targeting ligands enhances perinuclear localization and improves efficacy of delivered alpha-particle emitters against tumor endothelial analogues. Mol Cancer Ther. 2016;15(1):106–13.
59. Kahkonen E, Jambor I, Kemppainen J, Lehtio K, Gronroos TJ, Kuisma A, et al. In vivo imaging of prostate cancer using [68Ga]-labeled bombesin analog BAY86-7548. Clin Cancer Res. 2013;19(19):5434–43.
60. Minamimoto R, Hancock S, Schneider B, Chin FT, Jamali M, Loening A, et al. Pilot comparison of (6)(8)Ga-RM2 PET and (6)(8)Ga-PSMA-11 PET in patients with biochemically recurrent prostate cancer. J Nucl Med. 2016;57(4):557–62.
61. Roivainen A, Kahkonen E, Luoto P, Borkowski S, Hofmann B, Jambor I, et al. Plasma pharmacokinetics, whole-body distribution, metabolism, and radiation dosimetry of 68Ga bombesin antagonist BAY 86-7548 in healthy men. J Nucl Med. 2013;54(6):867–72.

35 Locoregional Treatment of Brain Tumors

Jolanta Kunikowska, Alfred Morgenstern, Frank Bruchertseifer, and Leszek Krolicki

Abstract

Glioblastoma multiforme (GBM), primary brain tumor, is the most common and most malignant of the glia tumors. It is characterized by the worst prognosis with a median overall survival time of only 9–15 months. The infiltrating character of the tumor, its molecular heterogeneity, as well as the protective effects of the blood-brain barrier are the main causes for the insufficiency of established frontline treatments (surgery, radiotherapy, and chemotherapy).

The best treatment strategy for patients with recurrent GBM is unclear and controversial. Even with established state-of-the-art treatment in almost 90% of patients, the recurrence of disease is observed and median survival after recurrence is less than 6 months.

An alternative method of treatment is to apply the drug locally. It has been shown that GBM overexpresses the of NK-1 receptor and substance P (SP) can be used as a ligand. Alpha emitters, with shorter range and higher energy than beta emitters, offer the new potential for selective irradiation of tumors, with minimizing damage to adjacent tissue.

This chapter describes the use of radiolabeled SP for intratumoral treatment of the glia tumors.

Glioblastoma multiforme (GBM) is the most common and most malignant of the glia tumors. It has a dismal prognosis with 12–15-month median survival despite the use of aggressive standard treatment which includes surgery, radiotherapy, and chemotherapy [1–3].

Therefore, there is urgent need for the development and testing of new therapy strategies.

A variety of chemotherapy agents have been tried in this setting, with response rates in the range of 0–20% [4, 5]. The external radiotherapy has limitations (dose 60 Gy in 2-Gy fractions,

J. Kunikowska (✉) • L. Krolicki
Department of Nuclear Medicine, Medical University of Warsaw, Warsaw, Poland
e-mail: jolanta.kunikowska@wum.edu.pl

A. Morgenstern • F. Bruchertseifer
European Commission, Joint Research Centre, Directorate for Nuclear Safety and Security, Karlsruhe, Germany

E. Bombardieri et al. (eds.), *Clinical Applications of Nuclear Medicine Targeted Therapy*, https://doi.org/10.1007/978-3-319-63067-0_35

recommended by the radiation therapy oncology group—RTOG), because higher doses affect the normal tissue. For this reason, the combination of radiotherapy and chemotherapy was examined. Combining temozolomide (TMZ) with radiation improves median survival by 2.5 months compared with radiation therapy alone and results in median survival of 14.6 months [2].

Treatment options are especially limited at recurrence. Even with optimal treatment in almost 90% of patients, recurrence of disease is observed and median survival after recurrence is less than 6 months. The documented benefit from second operation is described only in patients of younger age (70 years or younger), with smaller tumor volume (<50 cm^3) and preoperative Karnofsky performance score greater than 80% [6, 7].

An alternative method of treatment is to apply the drug locally. It was proposed by Riva et al. in 1995 [8] and subsequently by Merlo et al. [9]. This method allows for a higher concentration of drug in the tumor and omits the blood-brain barrier. For this approach surgical implementation of a special port-path into the tumor or the post-resection cavity is required. Furthermore a ligand-receptor system is needed to address the drug selectively to tumor cells.

Firstly, anti-tenascin antibodies were proposed as targeting molecule; tenascin is a biologically active peptide that plays an important role in angiogenesis in glioblastoma [10, 11]. Merlo et al. described the effect of radiolabeled somatostatin analogs; overexpression of SSTR-2 receptor system is observed in about 80% of GBM tumors, especially in grades II and III, less common in grade IV [9]. Inconsistent expression of SSTR2 limited application in glioblastoma. Similar results were presented by Schumacher et al. [12].

Kneifel et al. applied substance P (SP) as a major ligand of neurokinin type 1 (NK-1) receptor [13]. The low molecular weight of SP, allowing for rapid diffusion in the brain, and the high incidence of increased expression of NK-1 in GBM cells, regardless of the degree of malignancy, render radiolabeled SP analogs very promising candidates for local treatment of glia tumors.

The therapeutic effect of nuclear medicine procedures also depends on the type of radiation emitted: its energy and range. Each of these properties plays a critical role in the radiobiological processes that lead to cell damage. Two types of radioisotopes are typically used: beta (^{131}I, ^{90}Y, ^{177}Lu) and alpha emitters (^{225}Ac, ^{213}Bi). Alpha emitters seem particularly promising for targeted brain tumor treatment.

35.1 Radiopharmaceutical

Alpha-emitting radionuclides have distinct advantages for use in targeted therapy. The short range (<100 μm) and high linear energy transfer (LET $\approx$ 100 keV/μm) of alpha particles in human tissue allow to deliver a highly cytotoxic dose to targeted cells while minimizing damage to surrounding healthy tissue. Cell death induced by alpha radiation is predominantly due to DNA double-strand breaks occurring along the densely ionizing particle trajectory and is largely independent of cell cycle phase and cell oxygenation status [14–17]. As alpha radiation is able to overcome resistance to chemotherapeutic drugs and beta and gamma radiation [18], targeted alpha therapy can offer an alternative therapy option for patients refractory to standard therapies. It must be stressed that the effect of radiation is not dependent on MGMT promoter methylation status—the most important predictor factor in treatment of temozolomide.

Among the few alpha emitters suitable for application in cancer therapy, the generator-derived radionuclide pair ^{225}Ac and ^{213}Bi has emerged as particularly promising.

^{225}Ac is a pure alpha emitter with a half-life of 9.9 days. It decays via a cascade of six relatively short-lived radionuclide daughters to long-lived ^{209}Bi ($T_{1/2} = 1.9 \times 10^{19}$ *y*). The predominant decay path of ^{225}Ac yields four net alpha particles with a large cumulative energy of 28 MeV and two beta disintegrations of 1.6 and 0.6 MeV maximum energy. Gamma emissions with limited use for in vivo imaging are generated in the ^{225}Ac decay path from disintegration of ^{221}Fr (218 keV, 11.6% emission probability) and ^{213}Bi (440 keV, 26.1% emission probability). Its relatively long half-life of 9.9 days and the multiple alpha particles generated in the rapid decay chain render ^{225}Ac a particularly cytotoxic radionuclide.

Its short-lived daughter nuclide ^{213}Bi is a mixed alpha/beta emitter with a half-life of 46 min. It mainly decays via beta emission to the ultrashort-lived, pure alpha emitter ^{213}Po ($T_{1/2}$ = 4.2 μs, E = 8.4 MeV) with a branching ratio of 97.8%. The remaining 2.2% of ^{213}Bi decays lead to ^{209}Tl via alpha particle emission (E = 5.5 MeV, 0.16%, E = 5.9 MeV, 2.01%). Both ^{213}Po and ^{209}Tl finally decay via ^{209}Pb ($T_{1/2}$ = 3.25 h, beta-) into long-lived ^{209}Bi. The 8.4 MeV alpha particle emitted by ^{213}Po has a path length of 85 μm in human tissue. It is contributing more than 98% of the alpha particle energy emitted per disintegration of ^{213}Bi and can therefore be considered as mainly responsible for its cytotoxic effects. With 92.7% the majority of the total particle energy emitted per disintegration of ^{213}Bi originates from alpha decay, while only 7.3% of decay energy is contributed by beta particle emission, including the decay of ^{209}Pb [14]. As mentioned above, the decay of ^{213}Bi is accompanied by the emission of a 440 keV photon (emission probability of 26.1%) that allows to monitor ^{213}Bi biodistribution and to conduct pharmacokinetic and dosimetric studies using gamma cameras equipped with commercially available high-energy collimators.

The favorable chemical properties of the trivalent metal ions Ac(III) and Bi(III) allow the stable linking to biomolecules using the established chelate molecules DOTA (1,4,7,10-tetraazacyclo dodecane-1,4,7,10-tetraacetic acid).

Substance P (SP) belongs to a group of neurokinins (NKs), small peptides that are broadly distributed in the central nervous system and peripheral nervous system. The biological effects of substance P in the central nervous system are mediated by its binding to the transmembrane neurokinin type 1 (NK-1) receptor. Autoradiography disclosed overexpression of neurokinin type 1 receptor in 55 of 58 gliomas of WHO grade II. NK1-receptors have also been detected on tumor cells infiltrating the intratumoral and peritumoral vasculature [19]. SP, the natural ligand for NK-1 receptor, is an undecapeptide composed of the amino acid chain Arg-Pro-Lys-Pro-Gln-Gln-Phe-Phe-Gly-Leu-Met, with an amidation at the C-terminus. Conjugation of SP with DOTA or DOTAGA allows for stable radiolabeling of SP with a variety of radionuclides, including ^{225}Ac and ^{213}Bi. The radiolabeled pharmaceutical has a preserved affinity for the NK-1 receptor in the low nanomolar range. The vector has a low molecular weight of only 1.8 kDa, which is a prerequisite for sufficient and rapid intratumoral distribution following local injection.

35.2 Clinical Experience of Local Treatment With Radiolabeled Substance P

The principal indications for TAT in glia tumors are:

- Recurrent primary brain tumor
- Critically located primary brain tumor
- Recurrent secondary brain tumor

35.2.1 Implantation of Catheter and Preparation for Local Injection

For local administration of radiolabeled drugs, catheter systems are implanted intratumorally or into the post-resection cavity typically 2–4 weeks before treatment. For confirmation of catheter positions, functioning, and an exclusion of connection with ventricular system, MRI is performed after injection of gadolinium contrast agent to the cath-path reservoir. Before administration of ^{213}Bi-DOTA-SP or ^{225}Ac-DOTAGA-SP, corticosteroids and antiepileptic drugs are recommended. Injection of the radiopharmaceutical is performed via implanted catheter/catheters (port-a-cath system) with low speed of injections (1 mL/2 min) (Fig. 35.1).

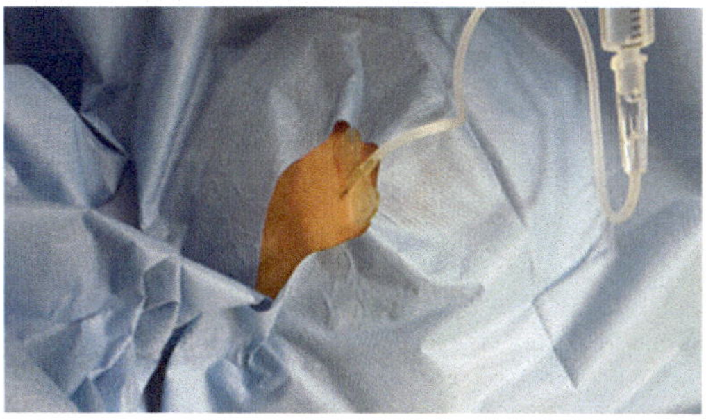

Fig. 35.1 Treatment procedure ^{213}Bi-DOTA-SP injection by catheters to the postsurgical cavity

35.2.2 Inclusion Criteria and Critical Point of Therapy

The criteria for inclusion to TAT are:

- Histologically confirmed glia tumor
- One focal tumor diameter not more than 10 cm
- No evidence for obstruction of CSF circulation or decompensating intracranial pressure
- Karnofsky performance score >40
- No pregnancy or lactation
- Age older than 18 years, absence of psychological, familiar, sociological conditions potentially hampering compliance with the study protocol

A critical point for successful therapy is the adequate positioning and functioning of catheters. For these reasons, MRI controls of catheters should be performed few weeks after implantation of cath-cap system to control the position of catheter. In addition, MRI control is performed 1 week before each administration to control function and patency.

Another important aspect is to control the distribution of injected doses of ^{213}Bi-DOTA-SP or ^{225}Ac-DOTAGA-SP. In a previous study with ^{213}Bi-DOTA-SP, biodistribution was monitored by SPECT/CT, using the 440 keV gamma emission of ^{213}Bi [20]. However, the acquisition took about 30 min and yielded images of limited resolution.

In the Medical University of Warsaw, Poland, control with ^{68}Ga-DOTA-SP PET/CT was implemented. ^{68}Ga-DOTA-SP is co-injected with therapeutic doses of ^{213}Bi-DOTA-SP or ^{225}Ac-DOTAGA-SP, allowing to monitor distribution in the brain and in the whole body with PET/CT with acquisition times of 5 min (brain) and 10 min (whole body), respectively. (Figs. 35.2 and 35.3). Potential problems with catheter systems (obstruction, enlargement) are illustrated in Figs. 35.4 and 35.5.

35.2.3 Results of Clinical Experience With TAT

A pilot study in 20 patients with gliomas of WHO grades II–IV provided proof of principle that, following local intratumoral injection of radiolabeled SP, there is sufficient and specific intratumoral distribution of the radiopharmaceutical. Most patients (15/20) were treated with SP labeled with the long-range beta emitter ^{90}Y. To reduce the "cross-fire effect," the low-energy beta emitter ^{177}Lu (3/20) and the alpha emitter ^{213}Bi (2/20) were used in a subset of patients with critically located tumors.

The short-term and long-term toxicity observed in the patients with 14 WHO IV and the six patients with WHO II-III was limited; the only relevant toxicity was a symptomatic radiogenic edema in one patient. Disease stabilization

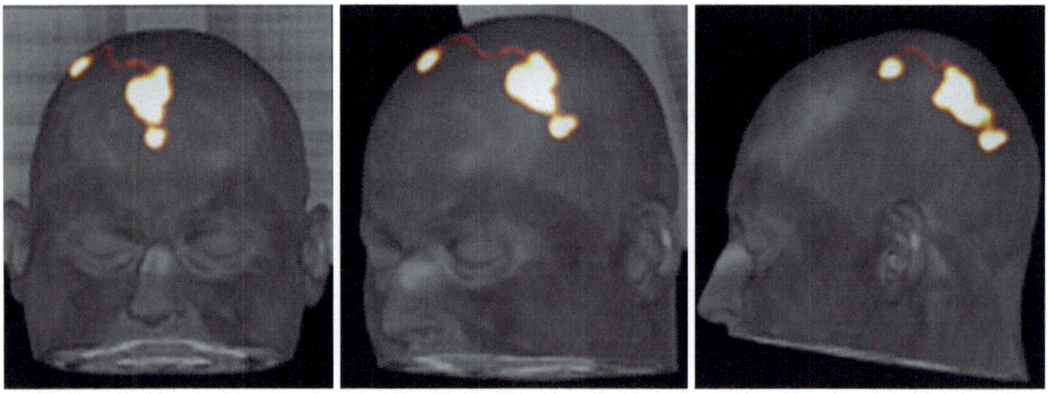

Fig. 35.2 ^{68}Ga-DOTA-SP PET/CT of local co-injection with therapeutic dose of ^{213}Bi-DOTA-SP to cavity of glia tumor. The picture shows small activity in capsule and catheter and major activity in cavity

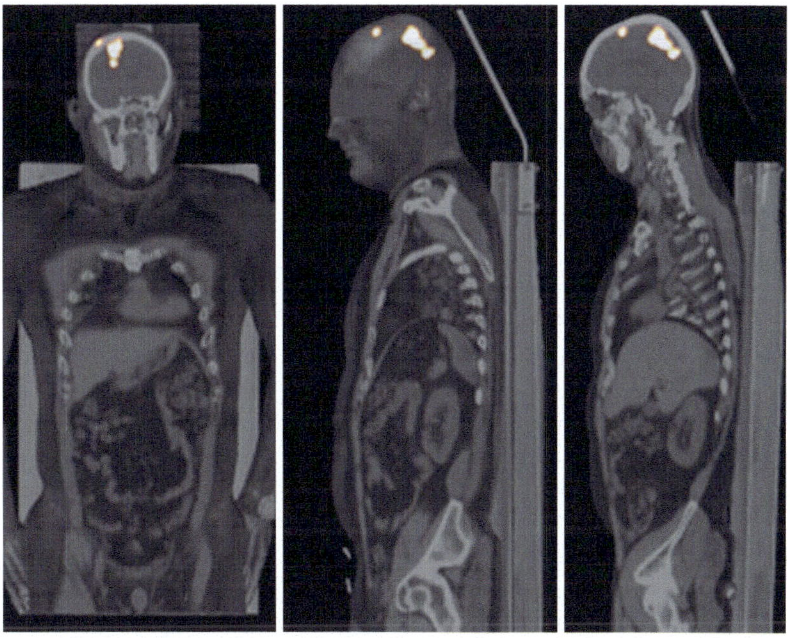

Fig. 35.3 Whole body PET/CT biodistribution 30 min after intracavital injection of 10 MBq ^{68}Ga-DOTA-SP

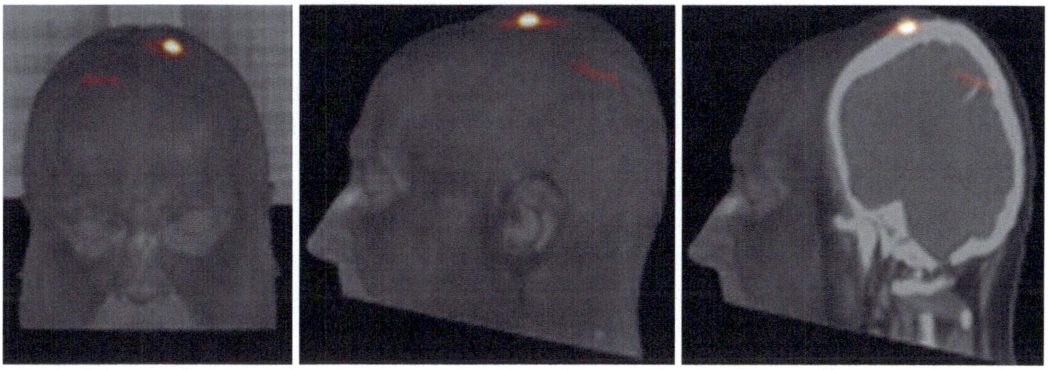

Fig. 35.4 Problems with catheter. ^{68}Ga-DOTA-SP PET/CT after intracavital injection of 10 MBq ^{68}Ga-DOTA-SP. The picture shows obstruction of catheter

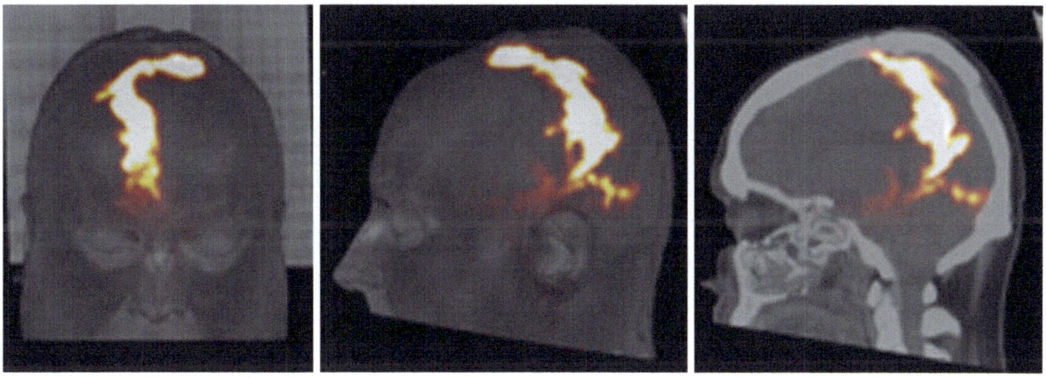

Fig. 35.5 Problems with catheter. ^{68}Ga-DOTA-SP PET/CT after intracavital injection of 10 MBq ^{68}Ga-DOTA-SP. The picture shows enlarged catheter

or improved neurologic status was observed in 13 of the 20 patients. Secondary resection disclosed widespread radiation necrosis with improved demarcation of the tumor [13].

^{90}Y-DOTAGA-SP as a neoadjuvant treatment was studied in 17 patients with GBM. After one to four intratumoral injections of ^{90}Y-DOTAGA-SP, patients underwent surgical resection. It was found that neoadjuvant injection ^{90}Y-DOTAGA-SP was feasible without decompensation of intracranial pressure. Fifteen of seventeen patients had stabilization or improved their functional status. The mean extent of resection in subsequent surgery was 96%. Neoadjuvant therapy of GBM using locally injected radiolabeled DOTAGA-substance P was feasible and of low toxicity and furthermore helpful to achieve a prognostically relevant high extent of resection [21].

The pilot study of local injections of ^{213}Bi-DOTA-[Thi8,Met(O2)11]-substance P (^{213}Bi-DOTA-SP) included five patients with critically located gliomas [20]. Application of the radiopeptide was straightforward and well tolerated by all patients. No additional neurologic deficit was observed. Repeated MRI was suggestive of radiation-induced necrosis and demarcation of the tumors, and this finding was validated by subsequent resection. Therefore, the study concluded that targeted local radiotherapy with ^{213}Bi-DOTA-SP may represent an innovative and effective treatment strategy for critically located malignant gliomas, because primarily nonoperable gliomas may become resectable over the course of treatment.

The study with ^{213}Bi-DOTA-SP has been continued and further developed at the Medical University of Warsaw, Poland, including patients with glioma II–IV.

The first interim analysis in a group of 18 patients with primary GBM (glioma grade IV) treated with ^{213}Bi-DOTA-SP showed from start of radioisotope treatment, the PFS was 3.7 months and overall survival (OS-t) 8.5 months. The median overall survival from the start of primary diagnosis (OS-d) was 21.5 months, and the median survival from the diagnosis of the recurrence (OS-r) was 9 months [22].

In a group of seven patients with secondary GBM (transmission from grade II/III to grade IV) treated with ^{213}Bi-DOTA-SP, median PFS was 13.6 months and OS-t was 16.4 months. Median overall survival from the first diagnosis (OS-d) was 46.8 months [23].

Longer survival was observed in patients who received multiple ^{213}Bi-SP doses which may be due to higher administered doses and/or better clinical status in the beginning of therapy. Examples of therapeutic effects are shown in Figs. 35.6, 35.7, and 35.8.

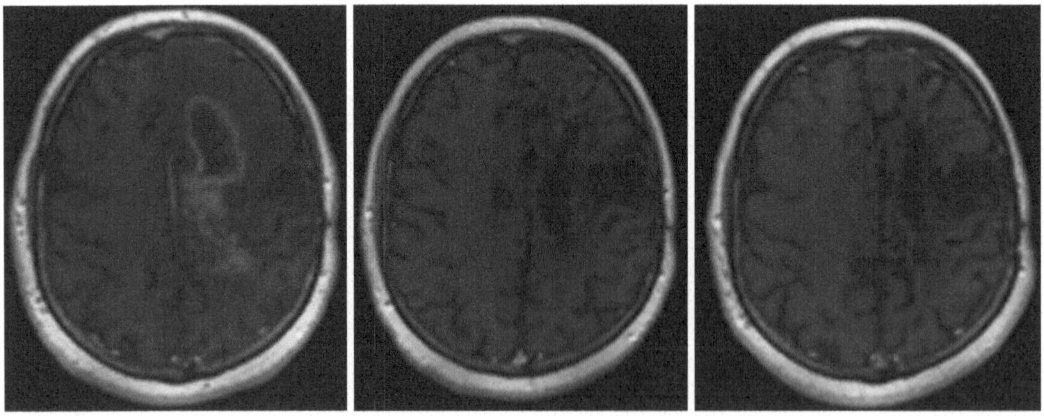

Fig. 35.6 Example of ^{213}Bi-DOTA-SP therapy effect. A 27-year-old man, with recurrence of glioma grade III (1 year after standard treatment-surgery, radiotherapy) treated with eight cycles, up to total doses of 14.1 GBq ^{213}Bi-DOTA-SP. The following MRI (T1-weighted contrast-enhanced) examinations revealed shrinkage of the tumor

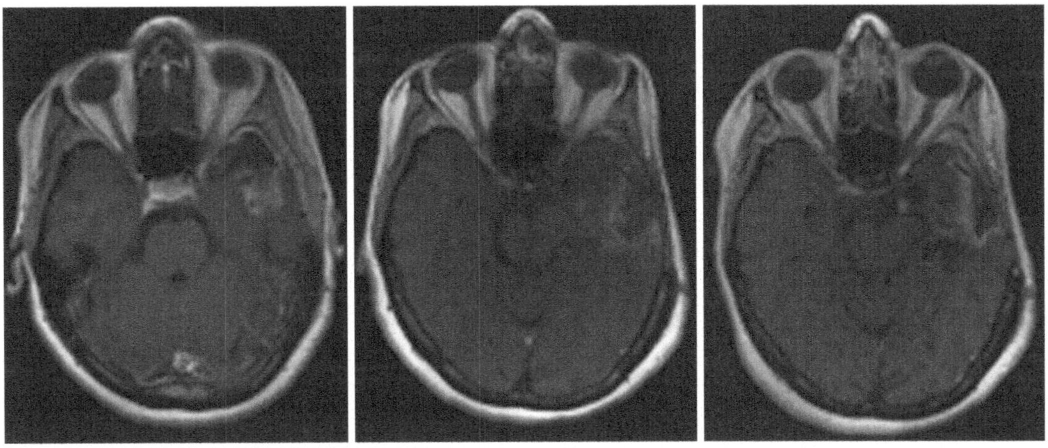

Fig. 35.7 Example of ^{213}Bi-DOTA-SP therapy effect. A 41-year-old woman, with recurrence of astrocytoma grade III (6 years after standard treatment-surgery, radiotherapy) treated with three cycles, up to total doses of 5.1 GBq ^{213}Bi-DOTA-SP. The following MRI (T1-weighted contrast-enhanced) examinations revealed shrinkage of the tumor

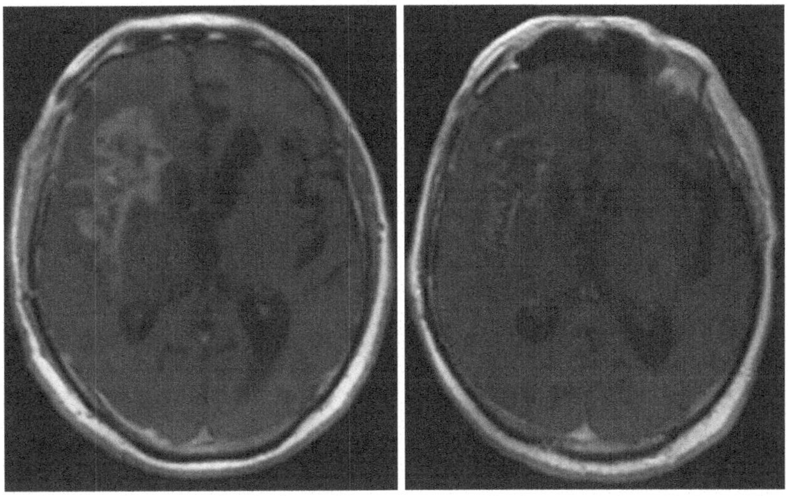

Fig. 35.8 Example of ^{213}Bi-DOTA-SP therapy effect. A 68-year-old man, with recurrence of glioblastoma multiforme grade IV (4 months after standard treatment-surgery, radiotherapy) treated only with one cycle, of 1.9 GBq ^{213}Bi-DOTA-SP. The MRI (T1-weighted contrast-enhanced) examinations performed 6 weeks after injection revealed shrinkage of the tumor with central necrosis and decrease in contrast-enhanced volume

Due the short half-life of ^{213}Bi of 46 min, diffusion of the radiolabeled drug into the infiltration zone might be limited. This might be overcome using SP labeled with longer-lived ^{225}Ac. We have recently initiated clinical testing to investigate the safety, tolerability, and therapeutic efficacy of ^{225}Ac-DOTAGA-SP in GBM patients, and patient follow-up is ongoing.

35.2.4 Side Effects and Toxicity

Intratumorally injected ^{213}Bi-DOTA-SP and ^{225}Ac-DOTAGA-SP are well tolerated by patients; no relevant acute local or systemic toxicity could be found according to the National Cancer Institute (NCI) Common Toxicity Criteria (CTC) scale (version 2.0).

Only in two patients, during ^{213}Bi-DOTA-SP infusion, flashed face was observed, as a systemic SP effect when small amount of tracer was absorbed in the blood. In one patient transient (5 days) worsening of paresis was observed. No other severe adverse events occurred.

Follow-up of therapeutic responses and toxicity is continued and patient recruitment is ongoing.

Conclusion

Targeted therapy of gliomas (WHO grades II–IV) with locally injected ^{213}Bi-DOTA-SP and ^{225}Ac-DOTAGA-SP is safe and well tolerated without relevant toxicity.

TAT may evolve as a promising novel option for treatment of recurrent GBM.

Acknowledgments The authors are indebted for use of parts of the ^{225}Ac/^{213}Bi to the US Department of Energy, Office of Nuclear Physics, Isotope Development and Production for Research and Applications Program.

References

1. Yung WK, Albright RE, Olson J, Fredericks R, Fink K, Prados MD, et al. A phase II study of temozolomide vs. procarbazine in patients with glioblastoma multiforme at first relapse. Br J Cancer. 2000;83:588–93.
2. Stupp R, Mason WP, van den Bent MJ, Weller M, Fisher B, Taphoorn MJ, European Organisation for Research and Treatment of Cancer Brain Tumor and Radiotherapy Groups, National Cancer Institute of Canada Clinical Trials Group, et al. Radiotherapy plus concomitant and adjuvant temozolomide for glioblastoma. N Engl J Med. 2005;10:987–96.
3. Lamborn KR, Yung WK, Chang SM, Wen PY, Cloughesy TF, DeAngelis LM, North American Brain Tumor Consortium, et al. Progression-free survival: an important end point in evaluating therapy for recurrent high-grade gliomas. Neuro-Oncology. 2008;10:162–70.
4. Tatter SB. Recurrent malignant glioma in adults. Curr Treat Options in Oncol. 2002;3:509–24.
5. Chang SM, Theodosopoulos P, Lamborn K, Malec M, Rabbitt J, Page M, Prados MD. Temozolomide in the treatment of recurrent malignant glioma. Cancer. 2004;100:605–11.
6. Barbagallo GM, Jenkinson MD, Brodbelt AR. 'Recurrent' glioblastoma multiforme, when should we reoperate? Br J Neurosurg. 2008;22:452–5.
7. Park JK, Hodges T, Arko L, Shen M, Dello Iacono D, McNabb A, et al. Scale to predict survival after surgery for recurrent glioblastoma multiforme. J Clin Oncol. 2010;28:3838–43.
8. Riva P, Arista A, Franceschi G, Frattarelli M, Sturiale C, Riva N, et al. Local treatment of malignant gliomas by direct infusion of specific monoclonal antibodies labeled with 131I: comparison of the results obtained in recurrent and newly diagnosed tumors. Cancer Res. 1995;55:5952s–6s.
9. Merlo A, Hausmann O, Wasner M, Steiner P, Otte A, Jermann E. Locoregional regulatory peptide receptor targeting with the diffusible somatostatin analogue 90Y-labeled DOTA0-D-Phe1-Tyr3-octreotide (DOTATOC): a pilot study in human gliomas. Clin Cancer Res. 1999;5:1025–33.
10. Bigner DD, Brown MT, Friedman AH, Coleman RE, Akabani G, Friedman HS, et al. Iodine-131-labeled antitenascin monoclonal antibody 81C6 treatment of patients with recurrent malignant gliomas: phase I trial results. J Clin Oncol. 1998;16:2202–12.
11. Zalutsky MR. Targeted radiotherapy of brain tumours. Br J Cancer. 2004;90:1469–73.
12. Schumacher T, Hofer S, Eichhorn K, Wasner M, Zimmerer S, Freitag P, et al. Local injection of the 90Y-labelled peptidic vector DOTATOC to control gliomas of WHO grades II and III: an extended pilot study. Eur J Nucl Med Mol Imaging. 2002;29: 486–93.
13. Kneifel S, Cordier D, Good S, Ionescu MC, Ghaffari A, Hofer S, et al. Local targeting of malignant gliomas by the diffusible peptidic vector 1,4,7,10-tetraaz acyclododecane-1-glutaric acid-4,7,10-triacetic acid-substance p. Clin Cancer Res. 2006;12:3843–50.
14. Sgouros G, Roeske JC, McDevitt MR, Palm S, Allen BJ, Fisher DR, et al. MIRD Pamphlet No. 22 (abridged): radiobiology and dosimetry of alpha-particle emitters for targeted radionuclide therapy. J Nucl Med. 2010;51(2):311–28.
15. Barendsen GW. Modification of radiation damage by fractionation of dose anoxia + chemical protectors in relation to LET. Ann N Y Acad Sci. 1964;114(1):96–114.
16. Barendsen GW, Koot CJ, van Kerson GR, Bewley DK, Field SB, Parnell CJ. The effect of oxygen on the impairment of the proliferative capacity of human cells in culture by ionizing radiations of different LET. Int J Radiat Biol. 1966;10:317–27.
17. Wulbrand C, Seidl C, Gaertner FC, Bruchertseifer F, Morgenstern A, Essler M, Senekowitsch-Schmidtke R. Alpha-particle emitting (213)Bi-anti-EGFR immunoconjugates eradicate tumor cells independent of oxygenation. PLoS One. 2013;8(5):e64730.
18. Friesen C, Glatting G, Koop B, Schwarz K, Morgenstern A, Apostolidis C, et al. Breaking chemoresis- tance and radioresistance with [213Bi]anti-CD45 antibodies in leu- kemia cells. Cancer Res. 2007;67(5):1950–8.
19. Hennig IM, Laissue JA, Horisberger U, Reubi JC. Substance-P receptors in human primary neoplasms: tumoral and vascular localization. Int J Cancer. 1995;61:786–92.

20. Cordier D, Forrer F, Bruchertseifer F, Morgenstern A, Apostolidis C, Good S, et al. Targeted alpha-radionuclide therapy of functionally critically located gliomas with 213Bi-DOTA-[Thi8,Met(O2)11]-substance P: a pilot trial. Eur J Nucl Med Mol Imaging. 2010;37:1335–44.
21. Cordier D, Forrer F, Kneifel S, Sailer M, Mariani L, et al. Neoadjuvant targeting of glioblastoma multiforme with radiolabeled DOTAGA-substance P: results from a phase I study. J Neuro-Oncol. 2010;100:129–36.
22. Krolicki L, Morgenstern A, Kunikowska J, Koziara H, Królicki B, Jakuciński M, et al. Recurrent glioblastoma multiforme - local alpha emiters targeted therapy with 213Bi-DOTA-substance P. Eur J Nucl Med Mol Imaging. 2015;42:S84–5.
23. Krolicki L, Morgenstern A, Kunikowska J, Koziara H, Królicki B, Jakuciński M, et al. Secondary glioblastoma multiforme - local alpha emiters targeted therapy with Bi-213-DOTA-substance P. Eur J Nucl Med Mol Imaging. 2016;43:S158.

36 CXCR4-Directed Endoradiotherapy as New Treatment Option in Advanced Multiple Myeloma

Constantin Lapa, K. Martin Kortüm, and Ken Herrmann

Abstract

Multiple myeloma (MM) accounts for approximately 1% of all cancers and around 10% of hematological malignancies. Although various novel drugs and treatment options including proteasome inhibitors, immunomodulators, antibodies, or the implementation of autologous and allogeneic stem cell transplantation have improved overall survival over the last decades, MM essentially remains an incurable disease. In relapsed/refractory disease, even the most intense treatment regimens frequently fail to efficiently reduce the tumor burden, and patients eventually succumb to their disease.

Given the paramount importance of C-X-C chemokine receptor CXCR4 for both multiple myeloma and bone marrow microenvironment, development of radiolabeled receptor ligands for both CXCR4-directed imaging and therapy has opened new exciting opportunities in the field of radionuclide therapies. Endoradiotherapy can be safely performed as part of the conditioning regimen prior to autologous or allogeneic stem cell transplantation. First experience has hinted at high tumor cell kill in even very advanced MM including extramedullary disease. Further prospective studies to evaluate the efficacy in earlier disease stages are about to be initiated and will also provide further evidence on synergistic multimodality treatment.

C. Lapa
Department of Nuclear Medicine, Universitätsklinikum Würzburg, Würzburg, Germany

K. Martin Kortüm
Department of Internal Medicine II, Universitätsklinikum Würzburg, Würzburg, Germany

K. Herrmann (✉)
Department of Nuclear Medicine, Universitätsklinikum Essen, Essen, Germany
e-mail: Ken.Herrmann@uk-essen.de

36.1 Multiple Myeloma

Multiple myeloma (MM) is a malignant plasma cell dyscrasia that accounts for approximately 1% of all cancers and around 10% of hematological malignancies. The clinical picture is characterized by a remarkably variable course, but most patients suffer from infection, bone marrow

E. Bombardieri et al. (eds.), *Clinical Applications of Nuclear Medicine Targeted Therapy*, https://doi.org/10.1007/978-3-319-63067-0_36

insufficiency, osteo-destruction, and kidney failure. Treatment options were highly limited for decades; however the introduction of the so-called novel agents more than 10 years ago dramatically improved the outlook for MM patients. Since then significant improvements in progression-free and overall survival could be achieved. Today various treatment regimens are available for MM patients including conventional (mainly alkylating) chemotherapy agents, proteasome inhibitors (PIs), and immunomodulators (IMiDs). Just recently a number of monoclonal antibodies were added to the therapeutic armament. In medically fit MM patients, current treatment strategies combine high-dose chemotherapy with autologous stem cell transplantation (ASCT) after a novel agent-based tumor-debulking induction therapy, followed by a long-term remission-maintaining therapy. This leads to prolonged disease-free survival in most patients and high-quality remissions, including complete responses (CR), in the majority of patients. Still, literally all patients relapse after variable time frames; develop drug resistance, extramedullary disease, or plasma cell leukemia; and finally succumb to their disease. Most recently the detection of minimal residual disease (MRD) by flow cytometry or next-generation sequencing demonstrated significant impact on the survival of CR patients, and the "sustained MRD-negative CR" has been added as the highest grade of remission to the response criteria of the International Myeloma Working Group [1].

To date, no MRD assessment has been implemented to standard diagnostics in MM, and the debate how to best achieve this ultimate aim of therapy is topic of ongoing clinical trials. However, it is clear that additional therapeutic approaches are needed, of which CXCR4-targeted endoradiotherapy (ERT) might be a promising option. CXCR4 has paramount importance for both multiple myeloma cells and bone marrow microenvironment. In patients with upregulated CXCR4 expression, radiolabeled receptor ligands with high binding affinity represent a new therapy option opening a new therapy option in MM patients.

36.1.1 Treatment Approaches to Multiple Myeloma

Modern anti-MM strategies combine two or three drug combinations, in which steroids, proteasome inhibitors, and/or immunomodulators are the main backbone partners. To date we have a substantial number of compounds available for the treatment of MM, all of them with significant anti-MM single-agent activity. This includes three generations of IMiDs (thalidomide, lenalidomide, and pomalidomide) and three PIs (bortezomib, carfilzomib, and ixazomib) as well as growing number of targeted immunotherapies, of which panobinostat, elotuzumab, and daratumumab were recently added to the list of approved anti-MM therapies and other promising agents are currently being tested in early-phase clinical trials. The role of radiotherapy in MM generally declined the recent years despite known MM radiosensitivity, and its use is mainly limited for symptomatic treatment or in extramedullary disease.

36.2 The CXCR4/CXCL12 Axis

Chemokine receptors form a large family of proteins that mediate chemotaxis of cells toward a gradient of chemokines. C-X-C motif chemokine receptor 4 (CXCR4) is a G-protein-coupled receptor, encoded on chromosome 2 [2]. The receptor has a seven-transmembrane structure with seven helical regions connected by six extramembrane loops. CXCR4 exerts its biological effects by binding its ligand CXCL12 activating the downstream signaling pathway, leading to alteration of gene expression, actin polymerization, cell skeleton rearrangement, and cell migration [3, 4].

CXCR4 expression plays a key role during embryonic development as CXCR4 is expressed on progenitor cells, allowing the targeted migration from the respective place of origin to the destination where the progenitor cells will differentiate into organs and tissues. CXCR4-/CXCL12-deficient mice show a lethal phenotype, confirming the critical importance of CXCR4/CXCL12 in embryonic development [5].

The CXCR4 pathway is also important in immunity and infections. Innate immune cells such as neutrophils and macrophages express CXCR4 allowing them to migrate along a gradient of CXCL12 present at the site of inflammation [6]. In the late 1990s, CXCR4 expressed on CD4+ T cells was discovered to serve as a co-entry receptor for human immunodeficiency virus (HIV-1) [7]. The role of CXCR4 has been elucidated in numerous physiological and pathological circumstances like systemic lupus erythematosus, rheumatoid arthritis, and multiple sclerosis [4].

CXCR4 and CXCL12 play a decisive role in tumorigenesis including enhancement of cell proliferation migration and invasion and in cancer cell-tumor microenvironment interaction, angiogenesis, and metastasis. Overexpression of CXCR4 has been demonstrated for more than 20 different tumor entities and linked to unfavorable prognosis, including MM [8, 9]. Tumor-associated stromal cells constitutively express CXCL12. This paracrine signaling stimulates the proliferation and survival of CXCR4-positive tumor cells. Moreover, CXCR4-expressing tumor cells migrate along the CXCL12 gradient to distant organs showing peak levels of CXCL12 expression, eventually leading to metastases [10]. Tumor cells utilize CXCR4 to access the CXCL12-rich bone marrow microenvironment that favors their growth and survival. Furthermore, high expression of CXCL12 by tumor cells and tumor-associated stromal cells forms a local gradient of the chemokine in the tumor region. CXCR4-expressing bone marrow-derived progenitor cells are then recruited to the tumor, where they contribute to the process of vasculogenesis by supporting newly formed blood vessels and by releasing other pro-angiogenic factors [11]. In MM, the CXCR4/CXCL12 axis is critically for the homing of MM cells to the protective bone marrow (BM) niche [12]; it induces the proliferation of MM cells and protects them from drug-induced apoptosis [13, 14]. CXCL12 is secreted by BM stromal cells and bone endothelium as well as from MM cell lines and primary myeloma cells [15].

36.3 CXCR4 Receptor Imaging in MM

Given the paramount importance of the CXCL12/CXCR4 axis in a multitude of tumors, the chemokine receptor represents a very promising target for imaging and therapy. Recently, noninvasive molecular imaging of CXCR4 expression has become feasible by the introduction of radiolabeled receptor ligands that allow for whole-body single photon emission computed tomography (SPECT) or positron emission tomography (PET) [16–18]. Among these tracers, the development of [^{68}Ga]Pentixafor can be regarded as milestone for clinical PET imaging of CXCR4 expression. Proof-of-concept visualization with this tracer could be demonstrated for several different hematologic and other neoplasms including leukemia, lymphoma, MM, adrenocortical carcinoma, or small-cell lung cancer, as well as in other solid tumors and disease conditions, such as stroke, atherosclerosis, and myocardial infarction [19–25].

Most experience with CXCR4-directed PET imaging has been gained in MM in which around two thirds of patients could be demonstrated to overexpress the receptor on the myeloma cell surface (Fig. 36.1, [24]). As for many tumor entities, CXCR4 positivity represented a negative prognostic factor. Interestingly, patients can present with striking inter- and intraindividual receptor expression heterogeneity which has to be investigated regarding the underlying mechanisms and implication by future studies [26]. Additionally receptor expression seems to be a dynamic process which can be severely influenced by preceding or concomitant chemotherapy [unpublished data]. Current investigations try to identify underlying biological implication and potential targets to exploit synergistic combinations of different treatment modalities, e.g., combinations of CXCR4 upregulating agents prior to scheduled [^{68}Ga]Pentixafor-PET (to improve sensitivity) or chemokine-directed therapy.

To date—whereas [^{68}Ga]Pentixafor-PET proves a higher sensitivity in myeloma detection as compared to [^{18}F]FDG in a relevant percentage of patients [24, 25]—the main value of

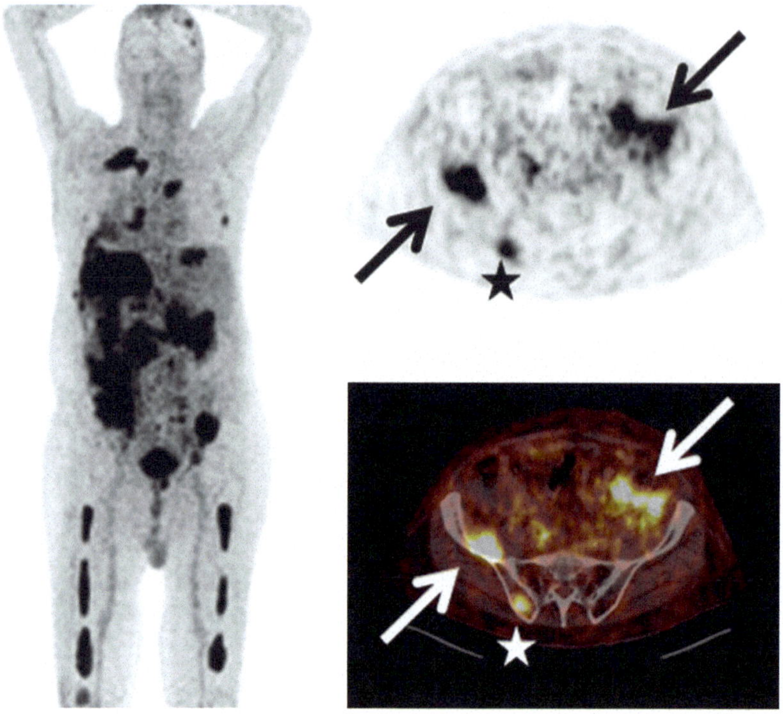

Fig. 36.1 Display of a patient with MM Ig A λ and rising free serum light chains. [^{68}Ga]Pentixafor-PET depicts intense tracer uptake in multiple intramedullary (stars) as well as extramedullary (arrows) lesions. Taken with friendly permission from [24]

CXCR4 imaging in MM is not staging of disease but identification of suitable candidates for chemokine receptor-targeted treatment, in particular CXCR4-directed ERT.

36.4 CXCR4-Directed Radionuclide Therapy

As a main achievement of the so-called theranostic approach for individualized therapy, a peptide CXCR4 ligand which can be labeled with α- and/or β-emitters (Pentixather) was recently developed representing a therapeutic counterpart to the diagnostic PET/SPECT agents [27].

Before CXCR4-directed ERT can be considered, confirmation of sufficient target expression by means of [^{68}Ga]Pentixafor-PET/CT is mandatory. Given the high intraindividual heterogeneity of CXCR4 expression by the various myeloma lesions, a comparison to [^{18}F]FDG should be performed. Until now ERT is preceded in every patient by a pre-therapeutic dosimetry study with a low activity of [^{177}Lu]Pentixather to exclude relevant retention in critical organs, to allow safely administrable activities, and to estimate the achievable tumor doses. Assessment of estimated radiation doses to the kidneys, liver, spleen, bone marrow, and—if applicable—tumorous lesions is performed by SPECT/CT and planar scintigraphy. Planar whole-body scans are taken over several days, and regions of interest are drawn for the organs of interest and corresponding background regions. The resulting count statistics are fitted by bi-exponential decay functions in order to approximate the activity kinetics in the organs. The fit functions are integrated and normalized to activity concentrations measured quantitatively by SPECT/CT. Generally, the kidneys represent the dose-limiting organs with an according to the Food and Drug Administration (FDA) tolerable maximum estimated dose of 23 Gy. Based on individual dosimetry, patients are treated by intravenous injection of ^{177}Lu- or ^{90}Y-labeled Pentixather approximately 3–7 days after pre-therapy dosimetry. The radionuclide to be administered for ERT is chosen depending on tumor burden, biological half-life of the radiopharmaceutical, and the associated time interval to stem cell transplantation (SCT).

To prevent renal toxicity, 2 L of a solution containing arginine and lysine (25 g/L each) is co-infused in analogy to the joint IAEA, EANM, and SNMMI practical guidance on peptide receptor radionuclide therapy [28]. The therapy itself is very well-tolerated without any acute adverse effects. However, given the high tumor cell kill, tumor lysis syndrome has been observed in a single patient with very high tumor burden and high proliferation. Therefore, prophylaxis should be initiated in selected cases [29].

First encouraging results could be obtained from small pilot studies in end-stage MM patients, in whom CXCR4-directed ERT was well-tolerated and resulted in high initial response rates (Fig. 36.2, [27, 29]). Experience and promising data have also been gained for other hematologic malignancies beyond MM like (relapsed/refractory) AML and diffuse large B-cell lymphoma on single case basis which could also be effectively targeted by radionuclide therapy (unpublished data). In all cases, ERT was added to standard high-dose chemotherapy as part of the conditioning regimen prior to SCT in order to augment tumor cell kill. In addition, stem cell rescue mediates bone marrow ablation that is also an effect of CXCR4-directed therapy due to receptor expression on tumor but also physiological bone marrow progenitor cells. In general, myeloablation can be expected at approximately 2 weeks after ERT. Therefore, ERT is especially suitable in hematologic disease in which tumor bone marrow ablation is highly desirable and stem cell rescue not a concern. Of note, the use of the shorter-lived ^{90}Y has proven advantageous over ^{177}Lu due to exact interval of 14 days between ERT and SCT in comparison to the more variable outcomes of ^{177}Lu. Given the risk of infectious complications during a prolonged phase of aplasia, most of current ERT are performed with [^{90}Y] Pentixather notwithstanding the disadvantage of insufficient post-therapeutic dosimetry due to pure beta-emission of this radionuclide.

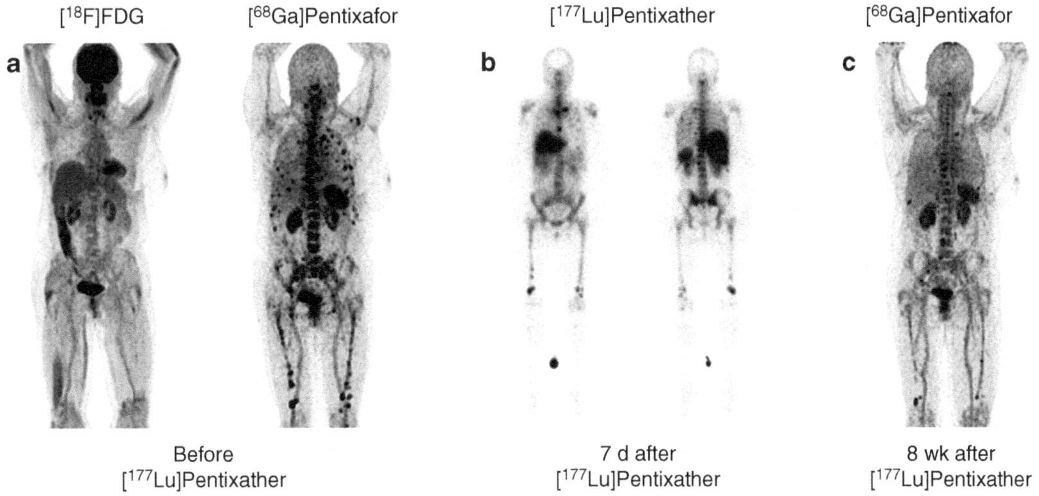

Fig. 36.2 Example of partial response to CXCR4-directed treatment with [177Lu]Pentixather. (**a**) Maximum intensity projections (MIP) of [^{68}Ga]Pentixafor- and [^{18}F] FDG-PET/CT prior to Pentixather therapy indicating high CXCR4 expression in multiple intramedullary [^{18}F]FDG-negative myeloma lesions. (**b**) Scintigraphic images 7 days after administration of [^{177}Lu]Pentixather confirming the long-lasting binding to the CXCR4 target after treatment. The patient is seen from ventral (left) and dorsal (right). (**c**) MIP of [^{68}Ga]Pentixafor-PET/CT 8 weeks after [^{177}Lu]Pentixather therapy displaying partial response with disappearance of most of the myeloma manifestations. In concordance, serological response was assessed as stable disease. Taken with friendly permission from [29]

Whereas side effects on the bone marrow have prevented the use of radionuclide therapy in solid cancers so far, ERT could be considered an option in malignancies like adrenocortical cancer or small-cell lung cancer, given the intense receptor expression in relapsed stages with otherwise dismal prognosis. Additionally, future trials will investigate the benefit of ERT in patients with MM or lymphoma at earlier disease stages (COLPRIT trial, EudraCT 2015-001817-28). Additionally, the use of alpha-emitters like ^{225}Ac of ^{213}Bi, which have been successfully implemented in the care of prostate cancer patients, might prove beneficial in homogenously CXCR4 expression malignancies like diffuse large B-cell lymphoma or SCLC [30, 31]. Future research will also focus on combinations of ERT and "conventional" therapies which could lead to synergistic effects. Both preclinical studies in myeloma cell lines and clinical observations in patients with various diseases (myeloma, diffuse large B-cell lymphoma, AML) have suggested the possibility to up- and/or downregulate CXCR4 on the cell surface.

References

1. Kumar S, Paiva B, Anderson KC, Durie B, Landgren O, Moreau P, et al. International myeloma working group consensus criteria for response and minimal residual disease assessment in multiple myeloma. Lancet Oncol. 2016;17:e328–46.
2. Caruz A, Samsom M, Alonso JM, Alcami J, Baleux F, Virelizier JL, et al. Genomic organization and promoter characterization of human CXCR4 gene. FEBS Lett. 1998;426:271–8.
3. Burger JA, Kipps TJ. CXCR4: a key receptor in the crosstalk between tumor cells and their microenvironment. Blood. 2006;107:1761–7.
4. Domanska UM, Kruizinga RC, Nagengast WB, Timmer-Bosscha H, Huls G, de Vries EG, et al. A review on CXCR4/CXCL12 axis in oncology: no place to hide. Eur J Cancer. 2013;49:219–30.
5. Nagasawa T, Hirota S, Tachibana K, Takakura N, Nishikawa S, Kitamura Y, et al. Defects of B-cell lymphopoiesis and bone-marrow myelopoiesis in mice lacking the CXC chemokine PBSF/SDF-1. Nature. 1996;382:635–8.
6. Loetscher P, Moser B, Baggiolini M. Chemokines and their receptors in lymphocyte traffic and HIV infection. Adv Immunol. 2000;74:127–80.
7. Feng Y, Broder CC, Kennedy PE, Berger EA. HIV-1 entry cofactor: functional cDNA cloning of a seven-transmembrane, G protein-coupled receptor. Science. 1996;272:872–7.
8. Zhao H, Guo L, Zhao H, Zhao J, Weng H, Zhao B. CXCR4 over-expression and survival in cancer: a system review and meta-analysis. Oncotarget. 2015;6:5022–40.
9. Vande Broek I, Leleu X, Schots R, Facon T, Vanderkerken K, Van Camp B, et al. Clinical significance of chemokine receptor (CCR1, CCR2 and CXCR4) expression in human myeloma cells: the association with disease activity and survival. Haematologica. 2006;91:200–6.
10. Muller A, Homey B, Soto H, Ge N, Catron D, Buchanan ME, et al. Involvement of chemokine receptors in breast cancer metastasis. Nature. 2001;410:50–6.
11. Guo F, Wang Y, Liu J, Mok SC, Xue F, Zhang W. CXCL12/CXCR4: a symbiotic bridge linking cancer cells and their stromal neighbors in oncogenic communication networks. Oncogene. 2016;35:816–26.
12. Alsayed Y, Ngo H, Runnels J, Leleu X, Singha UK, Pitsillides CM, et al. Mechanisms of regulation of CXCR4/SDF-1 (CXCL12)-dependent migration and homing in multiple myeloma. Blood. 2007;109:2708–17.
13. Azab AK, Runnels JM, Pitsillides C, Moreau AS, Azab F, Leleu X, et al. CXCR4 inhibitor AMD3100 disrupts the interaction of multiple myeloma cells with the bone marrow microenvironment and enhances their sensitivity to therapy. Blood. 2009;113:4341–51.
14. Hideshima T, Chauhan D, Hayashi T, Podar K, Akiyama M, Gupta D, et al. The biological sequelae of stromal cell-derived factor-1alpha in multiple myeloma. Mol Cancer Ther. 2002;1:539–44.
15. Beider K, Bitner H, Leiba M, Gutwein O, Koren-Michowitz M, Ostrovsky O, et al. Multiple myeloma cells recruit tumor-supportive macrophages through the CXCR4/CXCL12 axis and promote their polarization toward the M2 phenotype. Oncotarget. 2014;5:11283–96.
16. Demmer O, Gourni E, Schumacher U, Kessler H, Wester HJ. PET imaging of CXCR4 receptors in cancer by a new optimized ligand. ChemMedChem. 2011;6:1789–91.
17. Gourni E, Demmer O, Schottelius M, D'Alessandria C, Schulz S, Dijkgraaf I, et al. PET of CXCR4 expression by a (68)Ga-labeled highly specific targeted contrast agent. J Nucl Med. 2011;52:1803–10.
18. Hartimath SV, Domanska UM, Walenkamp AM, Rudi AJOD, de Vries EF. [(9)(9)mTc]O(2)-AMD3100 as a SPECT tracer for CXCR4 receptor imaging. Nucl Med Biol. 2013;40:507–17.
19. Herhaus P, Habringer S, Philipp-Abbrederis K, Vag T, Gerngross C, Schottelius M, et al. Targeted positron emission tomography imaging of CXCR4 expression in patients with acute myeloid leukemia. Haematologica. 2016;101:932–40.

20. Vag T, Gerngross C, Herhaus P, Eiber M, Philipp-Abbrederis K, Graner FP, et al. First experience with chemokine receptor CXCR4-targeted PET imaging of patients with solid cancers. J Nucl Med. 2016;57:741–6.
21. Bluemel C, Krebs M, Polat B, Linke F, Eiber M, Samnick S, et al. 68Ga-PSMA-PET/CT in patients with biochemical prostate cancer recurrence and negative 18F-choline-PET/CT. Clin Nucl Med. 2016;41:515.
22. Lapa C, Luckerath K, Rudelius M, Schmid JS, Schoene A, Schirbel A, et al. [68Ga]Pentixafor-PET/CT for imaging of chemokine receptor 4 expression in small cell lung cancer - initial experience. Oncotarget. 2016;7:9288.
23. Lapa C, Reiter T, Werner RA, Ertl G, Wester HJ, Buck AK, et al. [(68)Ga]Pentixafor-PET/CT for imaging of chemokine receptor 4 expression after myocardial infarction. JACC Cardiovasc Imaging. 2015;8:1466–8.
24. Lapa C, Schreder M, Schirbel A, Samnick S, Kortum KM, Herrmann K, et al. [68Ga]Pentixafor-PET/CT for imaging of chemokine receptor CXCR4 expression in multiple myeloma - comparison to [18F]FDG and laboratory values. Theranostics. 2017;7:205–12.
25. Philipp-Abbrederis K, Herrmann K, Knop S, Schottelius M, Eiber M, Luckerath K, et al. In vivo molecular imaging of chemokine receptor CXCR4 expression in patients with advanced multiple myeloma. EMBO Mol Med. 2015;7:477–87.
26. Lapa C, Schirbel A, Samnick S, Luckerath K, Kortum KM, Knop S, et al. The gross picture: intraindividual tumour heterogeneity in a patient with nonsecretory multiple myeloma. Eur J Nucl Med Mol Imaging. 2017;44:1097–8.
27. Herrmann K, Schottelius M, Lapa C, Osl T, Poschenrieder A, Hanscheid H, et al. First-in-human experience of CXCR4-directed endoradiotherapy with 177Lu- and 90Y-labeled pentixather in advanced-stage multiple myeloma with extensive intra- and extramedullary disease. J Nucl Med. 2016;57:248–51.
28. Bodei L, Mueller-Brand J, Baum RP, Pavel ME, Horsch D, O'Dorisio MS, et al. The joint IAEA, EANM, and SNMMI practical guidance on peptide receptor radionuclide therapy (PRRNT) in neuroendocrine tumours. Eur J Nucl Med Mol Imaging. 2013;40:800–16.
29. Lapa C, Herrmann K, Schirbel A, Hänscheid H, Lückerath K, Schottelius M, et al. CXCR4-directed endoradiotherapy induces high response rates in extramedullary relapsed multiple myeloma. Theranostics. 2017;7:1589.
30. Kratochwil C, Bruchertseifer F, Giesel FL, Weis M, Verburg FA, Mottaghy F, et al. 225Ac-PSMA-617 for PSMA-targeted alpha-radiation therapy of metastatic castration-resistant prostate cancer. J Nucl Med. 2016;57:1941–4.
31. Sathekge M, Knoesen O, Meckel M, Modiselle M, Vorster M, Marx S. 213Bi-PSMA-617 targeted alpha-radionuclide therapy in metastatic castration-resistant prostate cancer. Eur J Nucl Med Mol Imaging. 2017;44:1099–100.

37 Radiolabeled Somatostatin Analogues in the Treatment of Non-GEP-NET Tumors

Annibale Versari, Angelina Filice, Massimiliano Casali, Martina Sollini, and Andrea Frasoldati

Abstract

In the last two decades Peptide Receptor Radionuclide Therapy (PRRT) has acquired great importance as an alternative or complementary tool in the treatment of neuroendocrine tumors (NETs) and other somatostatin receptor (SSTR) positive tumors. Many experiences of PRRT using different radiopharmaceuticals, mainly beta-emitters 90Yttrium (90Y) and 177Lutetium (177Lu) labeled peptides, are reported in the literature with encouraging results in terms of tumor regression, self-assessed quality of life, and overall survival. SSTRs are mainly expressed in Gastro-Entero-Pancreatic neuroendocrine tumors (GEP-NETs) but in many other neoplasms (NETs and non-NETs) it is possible to find a high SSTR expression. Some of these are pheochromocytoma/paraganglioma, bronchial NET, thymic NET, meningioma, thyroid cancer (differentiated and medullary) and Merkel cell carcinoma.

Theranostics (therapy and diagnosis) using radiolabeled somatostatin analogues has proved to be a valuable tool in the management of SSTR-expressing tumors. Many studies are available for PRRT in GEP-NETs demonstrating very interesting results. Other neoplasms with SSTR expression can be evaluated and treated according to the same rationale: the experience is limited but sometimes promising. Further studies are necessary to confirm these interesting results.

A. Versari (✉) • A. Filice • M. Casali
Nuclear Medicine Unit, Arcispedale Santa Maria Nuova-IRCCS, Reggio Emilia, Italy
e-mail: annibale.versari@ausl.re.it

M. Sollini
Department of Biomedical Sciences, Humanitas University, Milan, Italy

A. Frasoldati
Endocrinology Unit, Arcispcdale Santa Maria Nuova-IRCCS, Reggio Emilia, Italy

37.1 Introduction

Differently from other therapies, the first requirement for radiolabeled somatostatin analogue (SSTA) treatment is that the target should be clearly visualized by specific molecular imaging. The "in vivo" use of molecular imaging is useful to circumvent screen target expression by using

E. Bombardieri et al. (eds.), *Clinical Applications of Nuclear Medicine Targeted Therapy*,
https://doi.org/10.1007/978-3-319-63067-0_37

immunohistochemistry or serum assays [1]. Moreover, the use of a diagnostic radiopharmaceutical with pharmacokinetic characteristics similar to the therapeutic compound may offer some additional advantages as compared to the radiometabolic treatment planning based on target expression identification alone [1]. Firstly, the diagnostic scans may serve as support for dose estimation and rationalization of treatments based on dose-effect relationships; secondly, they are helpful to monitor response to therapy in follow-up studies and can be repeated in order to detect any change of target expression which may possibly occur during target therapy or cancer progression [1].

In this regard, radiolabeled SSTA imaging studies demonstrating the expression of somatostatin receptors (SSTR) may be used to guide PRRT. Radiolabeled SSTA imaging has proven useful in diagnosing SSTR positive tumors [1]. Both radiolabeled SSTA scintigraphy (preferentially with SPECT or SPECT/CT acquisition) and PET/CT may be used to demonstrate SSTR expression. Scintigraphy has some limitations in detecting small lesions (due to suboptimal isotopes physical resolution [2, 3]) and in organs characterized by a high physiological tracer uptake (e.g., liver) [4]. PET/CT imaging with SSTA radiolabeled with 68Gallium (^{68}Ga) offers higher spatial resolution and a better pharmacokinetic profile as compared to radiolabeled SST analogues scintigraphy [5–7]. Different PET tracers such as [^{68}Ga-DOTA0-Tyr3]octreotide (^{68}Ga-DOTATOC, ^{68}Ga-edotreotide), [^{68}Ga-DOTA0-1NaI3]octreotide (^{68}Ga-DOTANOC), [^{68}Ga-DOTA0-Tyr3]octreotate (^{68}Ga-DOTATATE), and ^{68}Ga-DOTA-Lanreotide (^{68}Ga-DOTALAN) may alternatively be used. All these PET tracers bind SSTR subtype 2 and they have different affinity profiles for the other SSTR subtypes [8–12]. Although neuroendocrine tumors (NETs) especially gastro-entero-pancreatic ones (GEP-NETs) are the main indication for radiolabeled SSTA imaging, other neoplasms as well as a variety of inflammatory granulomatous and autoimmune conditions may also be accurately imaged by radiolabeled STTA [4]. Neoplasms that arise from adrenal medulla, pituitary, parathyroid, and thyroid glands or from endocrine islets in the thyroid, the pancreas, or the respiratory and gastrointestinal tract often express a high density of SSTR [4]. These heterogeneous group of neoplasms (i.e., other than GEP-NETs) may thus be imaged using radiolabeled SSTA although this imaging modality is not to be considered the first-choice, having its major role in the determination of SSTR status [4]. In tumors other than GEP-NETs, ^{68}Ga-labeled SSTA PET/CT has been reported mainly in case reports or in small series of patients and in a variety of clinical settings, including diagnosis, staging, restaging, follow-up, treatment selection and response assessment.

37.2 ^{68}Ga-DOTA-Peptide PET/CT: Clinical Application in Non-GEP NET Tumors

Radiolabeled somatostatin analogues imaging, particularly ^{68}Ga-labeled SSTA PET/CT, is the main procedure to select patients for PRRT (Tables 37.1, 37.2, 37.3, 37.4, and 37.5).

^{68}Ga-DOTA peptide PET/CT may provide additional diagnostic information in patients with sympathoadrenal system tumors (e.g., primary tumor site localization, metastases diagnosis). Therefore, in case of negative ^{123}I-MIBG scan in patients with a high pretest probability of pheochromocytomas or paragangliomas, ^{68}Ga-labeled SSTA PET/CT should be considered as the next investigation. Additionally, ^{68}Ga-labeled SSTA PET/CT should be considered in the staging of patients in whom metastatic spread is suspected (Table 37.1).

^{68}Ga-SSTA PET/CT has been evaluated in all types of lung cancer including typical and atypical carcinoids, large cell neuroendocrine tumor, small cell neuroendocrine carcinoma, non-small cell lung cancer and small cell lung cancer. The comparison of uptake patterns on [^{18}F]FDG and ^{68}Ga-SSTA PET/CT may be helpful in differentiating between typical and atypical carcinoids. Additionally, ^{68}Ga-SSTA PET/CT may be useful to stage lung NETs and to select patients candidate to PRRT [4]. Among thoracic neoplasms, thymic malignancies have also been evaluated with ^{68}Ga-labeled SSTA PET/CT (Table 37.2).

Table 37.1 Studies reporting 68Ga-SSTA imaging related to PRRT in pheochromocytoma and paraganglioma

References	Tumor type(s)	Tracer	Clinical purpose	Results
Haug et al. [17]	Paraganglioma (*n* = 1); lung NET (*n* = 4)	^{68}Ga-DOTATATE	Outcome prediction	Decreased ^{68}Ga-DOTATATE uptake in tumors after the first cycle of PRRT predicted time to progression and correlated with an improvement in clinical symptoms
Kroiss et al. [18]	Pheochromocytoma (*n* = 6); neuroblastoma (*n* = 5)	^{68}Ga-DOTATOC	PRRT selection	Sensitivity: = 92% for pheochromocytoma; = 97% for neuroblastoma
Kroiss et al. [19]	Paraganglioma (*n* = 20)	^{68}Ga-DOTATOC	PRRT selection	Lesions detection rate = 100%
Mittal et al. [20]	Paraganglioma (*n* = 3); pheochromocytoma (*n* = 2); neuroblastoma (*n* = 8); DTC (*n* = 5); thymic carcinoid (*n* = 1); mesenchymal tumor (*n* = 8)	^{68}Ga-DOTATATE	Staging/restaging/ treatment response assessment	Positive in 20/27 cases[a]
Gupta et al. [21]	Paraganglioma (*n* = 1)	^{68}Ga-DOTANOC	PRRT selection	Positive
Puranik et al. [22]	Paraganglioma (*n* = 9)	^{68}Ga-DOTATOC	PRRT selection/ treatment response assessment	All positive

PRRT peptide radioreceptor therapy,
[a]Overall results (no specific results for each tumor type)

Table 37.2 Studies reporting ^{68}Ga-SSTA imaging related to PRRT in thoracic neoplasms

References	Tumor type(s)	Tracer	Clinical purpose	Results
Vasamiliette et al. [23]	Thymoma (*n* = 1)	^{68}Ga-DOTATOC[a]	PRRT selection	Positive only in primary tumor
Haug et al. [17]	Paraganglioma (*n* = 1); lung NET (*n* = 4)	^{68}Ga-DOTATATE	Outcome prediction	Decreased ^{68}Ga-DOTATATE uptake in tumors after the first cycle of PRRT predicted time to progression and correlated with an improvement in clinical symptoms
Mittal et al. [20]	Paraganglioma (*n* = 3); pheochromocytoma (*n* = 2); neuroblastoma (*n* = 8); DTC (*n* = 5); thymic carcinoid (*n* = 1); mesenchymal tumor (*n* = 8)	^{68}Ga-DOTATATE	Staging/restaging/ treatment response assessment	Positive in 20/27 cases
Sollini et al. [24]	SCLC (*n* = 24)	^{68}Ga-DOTATOC/ DOTATATE	PRRT selection	Positive in 20/24 cases
Lapa et al. [25]	SCLC (*n* = 21)	^{68}Ga-DOTATATE	PRRT selection	Positive in 10/21 cases
Parghane et al. [26]	Lung NET (*n* = 22)	^{68}Ga-DOTATATE	PRRT selection/ treatment response assessment	Positive in 21/22

SCLC small cell lung cancer, *PRRT* peptide radioreceptor therapy, *NET* neuroendocrine tumor
[a]Only PET images without CT components

Table 37.3 Studies reporting ^{68}Ga-SSTA imaging related to PRRT in primary brain tumors

References	Tumor type(s)	Tracer	Clinical purpose	Results
Gehler et al. [27]	Meningioma (*n* = 26)	^{68}Ga-DOTATOC	EBRT planning	Change in clinical target volume = 54%
Heute et al. [28]	Glioblastoma (*n* = 3)	^{68}Ga-DOTATOC[a]	PRRT selection	All positive
Nyuyki et al. [29]	Meningioma (*n* = 42)	^{68}Ga-DOTATOC	EBRT planning	Change in gross tumor volume = 93%
Gains et al. [30]	Neuroblastoma (*n* = 8)	^{68}Ga-DOTATATE	PRRT selection	Positive in 6/8 cases
Kroiss et al. [18]	Pheochromocytoma (*n* = 6); neuroblastoma (*n* = 5)	^{68}Ga-DOTATOC	PRRT selection	Sensitivity: = 92% for pheochromocytoma; = 97% for neuroblastoma
Waitz et al. [31]	Meningioma (*n* = 22); glioma (*n* = 33); medulloblastoma (*n* = 2); anaplastic astrocytoma (*n* = 1); glioblastoma (*n* = 13)	^{68}Ga-DOTATOC[a]	PRRT selection	Positive in 39/41 cases
Graf et al. [32]	Meningioma (*n* = 16)	^{68}Ga-DOTATOC	EBRT planning	All positive
Hänscheid et al. [33]	Meningioma (*n* = 11)	^{68}Ga-DOTATOC/^{68}Ga-DOTATATE[a]	Prediction PRRT radionuclide retention	Significant correlations between: SUVmax and the therapeutic uptake; SUVmax and the maximum voxel dose from PRRT
Graf et al. [34]	Meningioma (*n* = 48)	^{68}Ga-DOTATOC	EBRT planning	Change in gross tumor volume = 67%
Combs et al. [35]	Meningioma (*n* = 70)	^{68}Ga-DOTATOC[a]	EBRT planning	Reduction in target volume = 40%
Golemi et al. [36]	Anaplastic meningioma (*n* = 1)	^{68}Ga-DOTANOC	PRRT selection	Positive
Mittal et al. [20]	Paraganglioma (*n* = 3); pheochromocytoma (*n* = 2); neuroblastoma (*n* = 8); TC (*n* = 5); thymic carcinoid (*n* = 1); mesenchymal tumor (*n* = 8)	^{68}Ga-DOTATATE	Staging/restaging/treatment response assessment	Positive in 20/27 cases
Collamati et al. [37]	Meningioma (*n* = 11); high-grade glioma (*n* = 12)	^{68}Ga-DOTATOC	PRRT selection	All positive
Madani et al. [38]	Meningioma (*n* = 5)	^{68}Ga-DOTATATE	EBRT planning	All positive
Seystahl et al. [39]	Meningioma (*n* = 20)	^{68}Ga-DOTATOC/^{68}Ga-DOTATATE	Treatment response prediction	Higher baseline tracer uptake in stable lesion

EBRT external beam radiotherapy, *PRRT* peptide radioreceptor therapy, *TC* thyroid cancer, *NET* neuroendocrine tumor
[a]Only PET images without CT components

The overexpressions of SSTR have been reported in brain tumors including meningioma, neuroblastoma, and glioma, which may therefore be an interesting target for PRRT. Particularly, in meningiomas ^{68}Ga-labeled SSTA imaging may provide additional information in patients with uncertain or equivocal results on MRI and could help to confirm a diagnosis based on MRI find-

Table 37.4 Studies reporting ^{68}Ga-SSTA imaging related to PRRT in thyroid cancer

References	Tumor type(s)	Tracer	Clinical purpose	Results
Gabriel et al. [40]	TC (*n* = 6)	^{68}Ga-DOTALAN/^{68}Ga-DOTATOC[a]	PRRT selection	NA
Damle et al. [41]	MTC (*n* = 15)	^{68}Ga-DOTATOC	PRRT selection	All positive
Mittal et al. [20]	Paraganglioma (*n* = 3); pheochromocytoma (*n* = 2); neuroblastoma (*n* = 8); DTC (*n* = 5); thymic carcinoid (*n* = 1); mesenchymal tumor (*n* = 8)	^{68}Ga-DOTATATE	Staging/restaging/treatment response assessment	Positive in 20/27 cases
Versari et al. [42]	TC (*n* = 41)	^{68}Ga-DOTATOC	PRRT selection/treatment response assessment	Positive in 24/41 cases
Traub-Weidinger et al. [43]	TC (*n* = 23); MTC (*n* = 8)	^{68}Ga-DOTATOC and ^{8}Ga-DOTALAN	PRRT selection	Positive in – 18/31 cases for ^{8}Ga-DOTALAN – 12/28 cases for ^{8}Ga-DOTATOC
Basu et al. [44]	TC (*n* = 1)	^{68}Ga-DOTATATE	Treatment response assessment	Positive
Elboğa et al. [45]	TC (*n* = 1)	^{68}Ga-DOTATATE	PRRT selection	Positive

MTC medullary thyroid cancer, *TC* thyroid cancer, *PRRT* peptide radioreceptor therapy
[a]Only PET images without CT components

Table 37.5 Studies reporting ^{68}Ga-SSTA imaging related to PRRT in Merkel cell carcinoma

References	Tumor type(s)	Tracer(s)	Clinical purpose	Results
Salavati et al. [46]	Merkel cell carcinoma (*n* = 1)	^{68}Ga-DOTATOC	PRRT selection	Positive
Schmidt et al. [47]	Merkel cell carcinoma (*n* = 2)	^{68}Ga-DOTATATE	PRRT selection	All positive
Epstude et al. [48]	Merkel cell carcinoma (*n* = 1)	^{68}Ga-DOTATATE	PRRT selection	Positive

PRRT peptide radioreceptor therapy

ings in case not accessible to biopsy or with non-diagnostic biopsy results. Finally, ^{68}Ga-labeled SSTA imaging may be useful to delineate the target volume for external beam radiotherapy and to select patients for PRRT [4] (Table 37.3).

The usefulness of ^{68}Ga-STTA PET/CT has been demonstrated to identify recurrent disease in thyroid cancer especially in case of iodine refractory tumors; in recurrent medullary thyroid carcinoma, the diagnostic role of ^{68}Ga-SSTA appears controversial since these tumors show a variable and often low SSTR subtype cell expression although a high ^{68}Ga-SSTA uptake could be used to accurately define the tumor biology "map" and therefore may be potentially helpful in selecting the most appropriate therapeutic option [4] (Table 37.4).

^{68}Ga-labeled SSTA PET/CT has also been used in Merkel cell carcinoma. Merkel cell tumors are aggressive neoplasms that often metastasize and, despite therapy, disease-related death is high. Ultrastructurally and immunocytochemically, the majority of these tumors have neuroendocrine characteristics. Establishing the extent of the disease may ensure an optimal choice of treatment for these rare tumors [4] (Table 37.5).

In addition to these neoplasms, ^{68}Ga-labeled SSTA PET and PET/CT has been used also in other type of cancers (e.g., prostate cancer, breast cancer, lymphoma) [4].

Preliminary promising results in tumors non GEP-NETs have also been obtained using [^{18}F]-SSTA PET/CT [4] and ^{68}GA-SSTA PET/MRI [13–16].

In the following paragraphs, the results of PRRT in different types of non-GEP-NET tumors will be concisely described.

37.3 Peptide Receptor Radionuclide Therapy (PRRT) in Non-GEP NET Tumors

37.3.1 Pheochromocytoma and Paraganglioma

Pheochromocytomas (PCC) and paragangliomas (PGL) are rare neuroendocrine tumors (NETs) arising from adrenal (80%) or extra-adrenal (20%) chromaffin tissue, respectively. Whilst most PCC/PGLs are benign, with surgical excision frequently curative, malignant progression occurs in 10–20% of patients, either due to metastatic spread at the time of diagnosis or recurrence after radical treatment. Radionuclide therapy with [131I]-meta-iodo-benzyl-guanidine ([131I]-MIBG) for mPGL has been in use since 1980s, producing radiologic responses in a third of patients and disease stabilization in 43% [49], with median survival time of 4.7 years [50]. However, significant adverse events including hypertension, hypothyroidism, gastrointestinal and hematological toxicity limit the utility of this treatment. Novel PRRT using radiolabeled somatostatin analogues, such as 177Lu-DOTATATE, has been shown to be well tolerated and highly effective in these NETs, with an overall disease control rate of 82% and durable responses confirmed by a median time to radiologic progression of 36 months [51]. Pinato et al., in their retrospective study, reviewed treatment records of all patients with neuroendocrine malignancies treated with PRRT at Imperial College London between 2008 and 2014, and identified five consecutive patients with histologically confirmed mPGL. Treatment cycles were repeated with a 12-week interval, with patients being given a maximum of 4 courses. Patients received 177Lu-DOTATATE PRRT at between 6.600 and 7.600 MBq per session. Response to treatment, assessed by surveillance imaging with CT and PET following each cycle, included: one partial response (20%), with imaging following each treatment showing good uptake within target lesions and a significant reduction in size of the large retroperitoneal mass; disease stabilization in three patients (60%), and progression disease through the treatment in one patient (20%). Patient population was exclusively composed of succinate dehydrogenase B (SDH-B) mutation carriers, a highly prevalent genetic trait indicative of aggressive malignant progression of PCC/PGL. Mean OS was 53 months (SD 22.7 months) and mean PFS was 36.4 months (SD 27.4 months). Van Essen et al. reported 12 PGLs treated with PRRT with cumulative doses ranging between 14.800 and 29.600 MBq. The median time to progression was not reached, following a median follow-up of 13 months, whilst radiologic restaging after treatment showed one partial response, disease stabilization in six patients, and disease progression in another three [52]. However, in this report, 25% of patients had non-metastatic PGL, and only 33% displayed documented evidence of progressive disease prior to PRRT; this may have affected estimates of response and survival outcomes due to the favorable prognostic outlook of such patients. Ameya et al. described PRRT in head and neck paragangliomas (HNPGLs), considering nine patients affected by a critical head and neck location of the tumor or recurrent/metastatic disease. Currently, the main treatment options for HNPGL are surgery and radiotherapy, external beam (EBRT) or stereotactic (STR). In the majority of patients, the disease is confined to the local site in the head and neck region. Multicentricity is seen in some patients, especially those with certain genetic mutations, and distant metastases are extremely rare. Patients received 90Y/177Lu, by slow intravenous infusion over 20 min, and 1500 ml of amino acid infusion (Lysine HCl 5%, Larginine HCl 10%, NaCl) over 4 h, with 20 mg Furosemide for assisted diuresis nephroprotection. Patients received up to four courses of PRRT (3–6 months between therapies) using 90Y/177Lu-labeled DOTATOC/DOTATATE between June 2006 and June 2014. The decision regarding the number of courses of PRRT to be administered was primarily based on four factors: size of the tumor, severity of symptoms (primarily related to cranial nerve involvement), presence or absence of synchronous sites or distant metastases, and renal and hematological parameters at baseline and during subsequent courses of PRRT. The patients received 2–4 PRRT cycles (90Y-DOTA peptide: 1.500–5.700 MBq; 177Lu-DOTA peptide: 5.400–7.500 MBq). Response to PRRT was documented on the basis of metabolic and morphological parameters, defined by European Organization for Research and Treatment of Cancer (EORTC) criteria and Response Evaluation Criteria In Solid Tumors version 1.1 (RECIST 1.1), respectively, as assessed on 68Ga-DOTATOC PET/CT images. Four patients showed molecular PR, while the remaining five patients showed molecular SD [8, 22]. In another study by Zovato et al. [9, 53], four patients with inoperable hereditary HNPGL (multifocal) were treated with 177Lu-DOTATATE (three to five courses) and SD or PR was documented on SSTR imaging. The authors therefore concluded that PRRT with 177Lu-DOTATATE is an active and well-tolerated treatment, with limited and predictable side effects, and can be proposed as a viable alternative for the treatment of PGL when no other options are available. 177Lu-DOTATATE has also been tried in a case with multiple spinal canal and cranial PGLs with a mean tumor volume reduction of 70% [54]. Recently, Makis et al. suggested that in patients with paragangliomas, 177Lu-DOTATATE should be administered over 2 h at least (preferably over 4 h), and not over 15–30 min as previously described, in order to prevent adverse reactions or reduce their severity [55]. In conclusion, PRRT seems a promising therapy for PGLs; nevertheless, further investigations in larger patient cohorts are needed (Fig. 37.1).

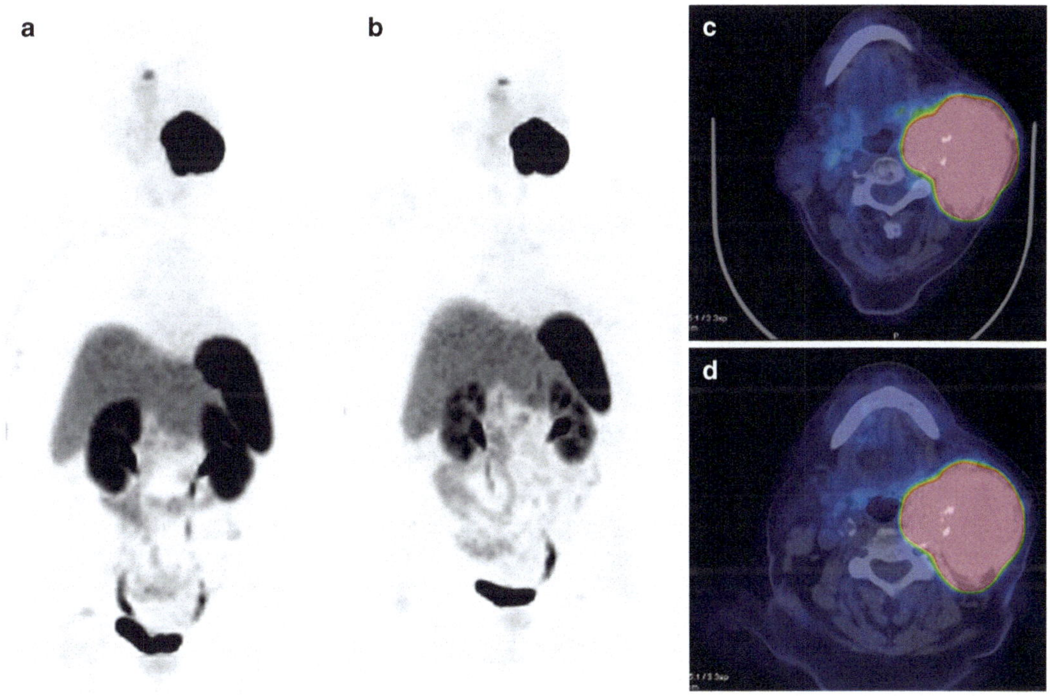

Fig. 37.1 Left latero-cervical paraganglioma. ^{68}Ga-DOTATOC PET/CT before (**a**, **c**) and after (**b**, **d**) PRRT (2 cycles of ^{177}Lu-DOTATOC +2 cycles of ^{90}Y-DOTATOC): lesion slightly reduced in extension but unchanged in terms of uptake intensity. Final response: stable disease

37.4 Thoracic Neoplasms

37.4.1 Neuroendocrine Bronchial Tumors

Neuroendocrine bronchial tumors are a relatively rare entity, accounting for up to 5% of all lung cancers. Possible treatment options for patients suffering from these particular neoplasms are as follows: surgery (for localized tumors), somatostatin analogues, as first-line therapy in metastatic cancers with high expression of somatostatin-receptors, chemotherapy (for the most aggressive forms of neuroendocrine cancer), target therapies (not yet well-established role), and, finally, PRRT. Most of the studies and, consequently, of the PRRT results were obtained in gastro-entero-pancreatic neuroendocrine tumors (GEP-NETs), while at the moment there are no ongoing clinical phase 3 trials specific for patients with neuroendocrine bronchial tumors (B-NETs). Available PRRT on B-NETs related data are therefore few, and extrapolated from more general studies. In a review of 11 publications, Lo Russo et al. in 2016 investigated the role of PRRT in B-NETs and found that PRRT with both Lu177- and Y90-labeled SSAs has been shown to provide ORR ranging from 20 to 35%. In terms of OS and PFS, PRRT results seem to be favorable also compared with the other available therapies (median PFS of more than 30 months and median OS of 40–72 months from diagnosis). Moreover, PRRT is able to produce a decrease in biomarker levels with an improvement in symptom control and patients reported QOL. The AA concluded that, despite the paucity of data, PRRT is certainly an evaluable strategy also in patients with B-NETs, especially if progressive after multiple treatment lines [56]. In 2001 Waldherr et al. reported results of 39 patients with NETs (7 of them with B-NETs) treated by PRRT at the dose of 6000 MBq/m^2 every 6 weeks. Treatments were well tolerated and, after PRRT, patients with B-NETs showed one CR, one PR, and five SD [57]. The next year the same authors published a new paper on 39 patients with NETs (3 of them with B-NETs), treated with PRRT: all B-NETs showed SD after treatment [58]. Bodei et al. in 2003 and 2004 published results of two studies (phase I–II) on NETs patients treated with PRRT. In the first study 141 NET patients in total were treated with a cumulative activity of 7.4–26.4 GBq of Y90-octreotide [59]. 8/11 patients affected by B-NETs after therapy showed SD, and one PR; while in the second paper [60] one patient showed SD and the other PR. In another phase II study, Bodei et al. (2011) treated 51 advanced SSTR2-positive NET tumors with escalating activities of Lu177-octreotate. The radiopeptide was well tolerated up to 29 GBq cumulative activity (up to 7.4 GBq/cycle). Five B-NETs were included and showed two PR, two minor responses, and one SD [61]. In the phase II single-center open-label trial by Imhof et al., the authors reported 84 B-NETs treated with Y90-octreotide with 28.6% achieving objective response [62]. Van Essen et al. described 131 patients with advanced GEP-NETs treated with an intended cumulative dose of Lu177-octreotate of 22.2–29.6 GBq. In patients with B-NETs, the authors reported a median TTP of 31 months with five PR, one minor response, two SD, and one PD. These results were comparable to those obtained in the total group of GEP-NETs [63]. In one study of 34 patients with progressive B-NETs, treatment with 177Lu-DOTATATE was associated with an ORR of 15% and SD of 47%. The median PFS and OS were 19 and 49 months, respectively [64]. Mariniello et al. analyzed 114 patients with advanced B-NETs treated with three different PRRT protocols (Y90-octreotide versus Lu177-octreotate versus Y90-octreotide +Lu177-octreotate). Median PFS and median OS were 28.0 and 58.8 months, respectively. Lu177-octreotate protocol showed the highest 5-year OS (61.4%), and was associated with longer OS and PFS, with a morphological RR (PR + minor responses) of 26.5%. Finally, Khan et al. evaluated quality of life (QOL) and symptom control after PRRT with Lu177-octreotate in 265 patients with GEP or B-NETs. Patients completed the QOL questionnaire of the European Organization for the Research and Treatment of Cancer before and after therapy. Results indicated that Lu177-octreotate therapy clearly improved the patients' self-assessed QOL [65]. In summary, reported studies demonstrate efficacy of PRRT in patients suffering from B-NETs comparable to those reported for GEP-NETs [66]. However, some limitations have to be taken into account: (1) the lack of perspective phase III trials, (2) the relative low number of publications about PRRT in

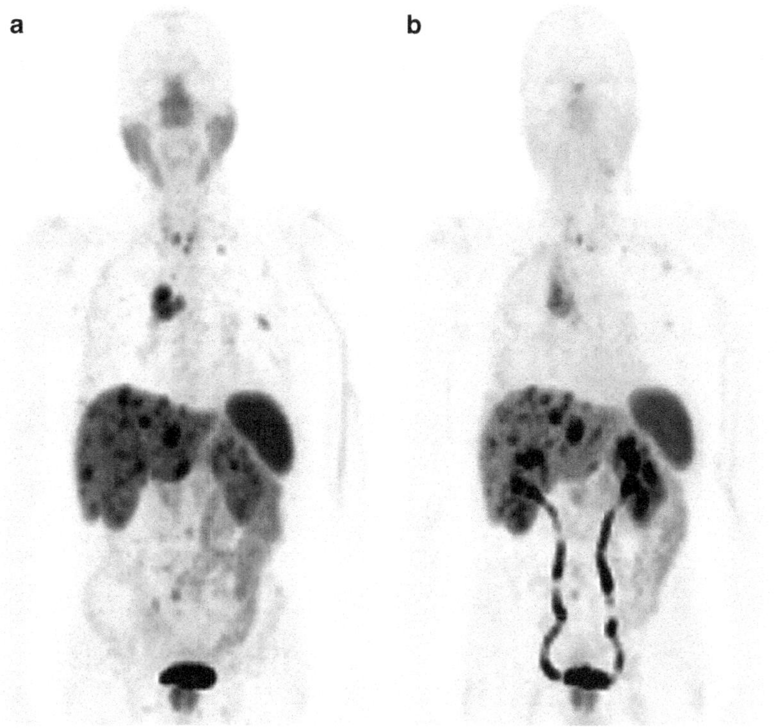

Fig. 37.2 Neuroendocrine lung tumor (G2) with lymph nodes, liver, bone metastases. 68Ga-DOTATOC PET/CT before (**a**) and after (**b**) PRRT (5 cycles of 177Lu-DOTATOC): improvement after treatment. Final response: partial response

B-NETs; (3) often authors do not report the specific outcome of B-NETs compared to the global study population; (4) not all B-NETs overexpress SSRs (e.g., atypical carcinoid tumors), and consequently a percentage of neuroendocrine lung tumors result not eligible for PRRT [67] (Fig. 37.2).

37.4.2 Thymic Malignancies

Thymic tumors are uncommon, corresponding to 0.2–1.5% of all malignancies with an incidence of 0.15 per 100,000 population. They are generally regarded as indolent tumors. Whilst this is often true for thymomas, thymic adenocarcinoma and thymic neuroendocrine tumors can be quite aggressive, with a poor prognosis. Understanding the biology of these tumors is important for prognosis and management. NETs of thymus are a heterogeneous group of neoplasms with a variety of morphological features and different levels of clinical aggressiveness. The current classification of thymus NETs follows the WHO criteria published in 2015 that identifies low-grade NETs (corresponding to the typical carcinoids—TC), intermediate-grade tumors (corresponding to atypical carcinoids—AC), high-grade NE carcinoma (large cell—LCNEC) or small cell carcinoma (SCC). Most thymic NENs belong to the category of intermediate AC while the forms of LCNECs are exceedingly rare. Carcinoid syndrome in patients with thymic carcinoid occurs very rarely (less than 1%), whereas ectopic Cushing's syndrome occurs in up to 17%. Furthermore thymic carcinoids can occur sporadically as part of MEN-1 syndrome and more frequently in male than in female patients [68]. Few data are available about the role of 68Ga-SST-analogues PET in thymic malignancies [69–71]. When there is a high expression of somatostatin receptors, anti-tumor benefit has been reported in patients treated with PRRT. This has become an established therapy in management of gastro-entero-pancreatic neuroendocrine tumors but, at the moment, the PRRT in all thoracic neuroendocrine tumors is used when the disease is in progression, at an advanced stage and there are no therapeutic alternatives. This clearly reduces the chances of complete response which, according to the data available in literature, varies between 0 and 10%. The partial response range is 9–40%, the stabilization of disease range is 27–61%, and progression varies between 9 and 20%. There are no significant differences in survival between patients with com-

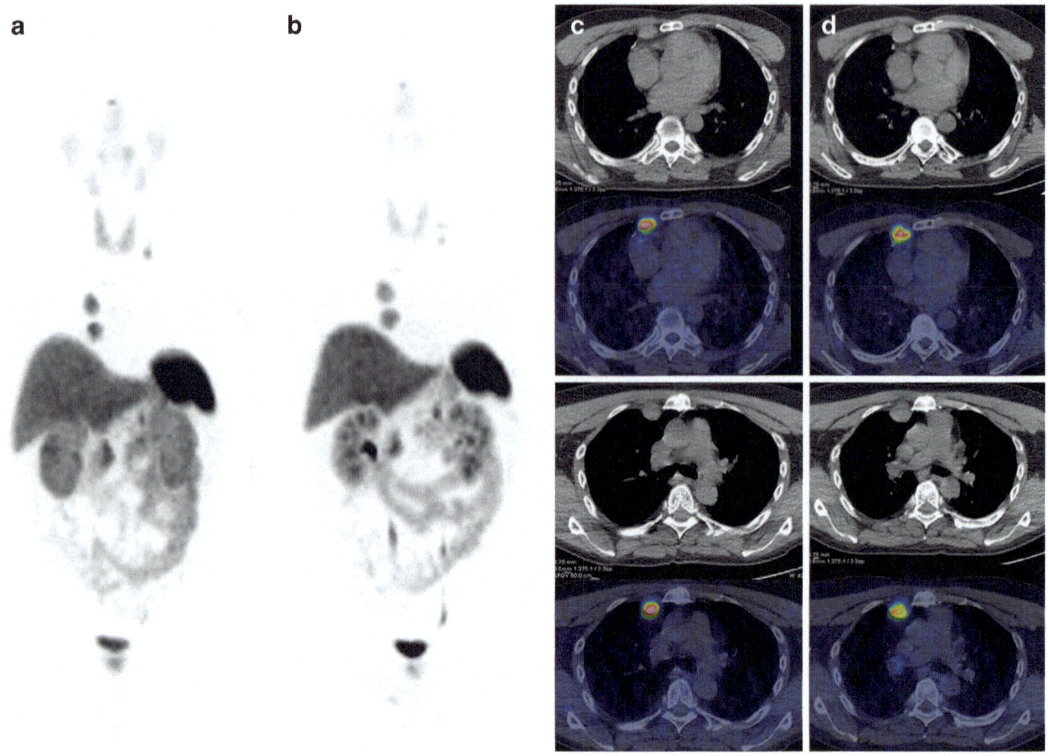

Fig. 37.3 Neuroendocrine tumor of the thymus. 68Ga-DOTATOC PET/CT at baseline (**a**, **c**) demonstrated multiple sites of pathological uptake in lymph nodes. The patient underwent five cycles of 177Lu/90Y-DOTATOC (total activity: 23.8 GBq). 68Ga-DOTATOC PET/CT after treatment (**b**, **d**) revealed a slight uptake reduction. Final response: stable disease

plete or partial response and patients with stable disease [68, 72]. It also reported a significant impact on quality of life [73]. Unfortunately many published results are related to experiences of mixed neuroendocrine tumors mainly gastro-entero-pancreatic, lung, and unknown where it is not always possible to extrapolate the data of thymic tumors. Some authors present the effects of PRRT in a subgroup of patients with foregut carcinoids of bronchial, gastric, or thymic origin. Nine patients with bronchial, five with gastric, and two with thymic carcinoids were treated. All patients had metastasized disease. The intended cumulative dose of 177Lu-octreotate was 22.2–29.6 GBq. In patients with bronchial carcinoids they obtained partial remission (PR) in five patients, one patient had minor response (MR, tumor size reduction: $\geq$25%, <50%), two had stable disease (SD) and one had progressive disease (PD). In patients with gastric carcinoids one had complete remission, one had MR and two had SD, including one with PD at baseline. One patient developed PD. In thymic carcinoids, one patient had SD. In the other patient, disease remained progressive, in all patients overall remission rate was 50%, including MR. The authors concluded that 177Lu-octreotate treatment can be effective in patients with bronchial and gastric carcinoids but its role in thymic carcinoids cannot be determined yet because of the limited number of patients. However the overall remission rate of 50% in patients with the studied foregut carcinoids is comparable to that in the total group of GEP NETs [69]. The use of PRRT in an advanced stage of the disease is certainly limitative for the clinical condition of the patient, frequently deteriorated, which does not allow the use of adequate doses. Moreover, the long response time of PRRT often is not suitable for patients in advanced stage. The PRRT is definitely very promising, but for a complete validation is necessary to wait for confirmation from experimental studies in progress. It is also desirable in the future the opportunity to experience the PRRT at an earlier stage of the disease and/or in combination with other treatments (Fig. 37.3).

37.5 Meningioma

Meningiomas are the most common primary intracranial tumors classified, according to WHO classification, as grade I (80–90%), grade II (5–15%), or grade III (1–3%) lesions on the basis of local invasiveness and cellular features of atypia [74]. Depending on age, tumor size, and treatment, 5-year survival is 70% for benign and 55% for malignant meningiomas [75]. The vast majority of patients can be cured by surgery alone, particularly patients with WHO grade I tumors in favorable locations (e.g., convexity and/or easily accessible skull-base meningiomas). Beyond surgery, various radiotherapy approaches are often used to increase local control, especially if surgery alone seems insufficient. By contrast, pharmacotherapy has a minor role in the management of meningiomas. A subgroup exhibits a diffuse en plaque growth pattern, and attachment of tumor segments to critical neural or vascular structures does not allow complete resection. Attempts to resect meningiomas involving these critical structures may cause devastating vascular injury or disabling cranial neuropathies. Tumor remnants are treated radiotherapeutically, which leads to 5-year progression-free survival rates in 89% of benign and 48% of malignant cases [76]. However, fractionated external-beam radiotherapy may also cause serious neurologic complications and secondary tumors [77]. Stereotactic radiotherapy represents an option for selected cases, leading to 5-year tumor control rates of 93% [78].

Meningiomas have been uniformly found to be positive for SSTR, the receptor density reaching even more than 400 fmol/mg protein [79]. Moreover, a prominent expression of subtype 2 sstr has also been reported in endothelial cells of peritumoral blood vessels [80] suggesting that PPRT may exert its action also through an antiangiogenic effect, and a correlation between sstr2A expression and the entity of neo-angiogenesis [81] has been demonstrated in meningiomas. Few data are available about the use of radiolabeled somatostatin analogues to treat meningiomas.

Sabet et al. reported the case of a 62-year-old female affected by intracranial anaplastic meningioma with pulmonary metastases presenting with progressive facial pain and treated with PRRT (three cycles of 177Lu-DOTATATE, cumulative activity: 691 mCi): the patient had no serious side effects and experienced a dramatic reduction of facial pain together with a significant improvement in quality of life; at 3 month follow-up she was considered in SD [82].

Van Essen et al. described 177Lu-DOTATATE therapy in five patients (cumulative activity up to 29.6 GBq) with high-grade cranial or cervical meningiomas (two patients had extremely large, exophytic, cranial tumors—one of them also had cervical metastases—one patient had a large, exophytic, cervical meningioma with rapid progression; two patients had a cavernous sinus meningioma) reporting PD in three patients and SD in 2. They proposed 177Lu-DOTATATE therapy in cases in which the disease is slowly progressive and other options are absent or not considered effective. Moreover, they stated that if 177Lu-DOTATATE is given earlier in the course of the disease or in combination with other therapies, results could possibly be better [83].

Bartolomei et al. reported about 29 patients with inoperable (n = 3) or recurrent (n = 26) meningiomas (14 grade I, 9 grade II, and 6 grade III) treated with 90Y-DOTATOC (cumulative activity up to 15 GBq); 20 patients had a single lesion whereas nine patients had multifocal meningiomas. The authors reported SD in 19/29 patients (66%) and PD in 10/29 (34%), 3 months after PRRT. Better results were achieved in patients with grade I meningioma than in patients with grade II or III; namely, median time to progression (i.e., from PRRT) was 61 months in patients with grade I meningioma and 13 months in patients with grade 2 or 3 meningioma [84].

Moreover, the combination of EBRT and PRRT has been used in advanced cases, which is feasible and well-tolerated. Namely, Kreissl et al. described ten patients with inoperable or recurrent meningioma who have been treated with either 177Lu-DOTATATE (four patients) or 177Lu-DOTATOC (six patients) and external beam radiotherapy. EBRT dose was 42–60 Gy whereas the median tumor dose at each PRRT was 7.2 Gy (specific dose: 30–3890 mGy/GBq). CR occurred in one patient, SD in eight patients,

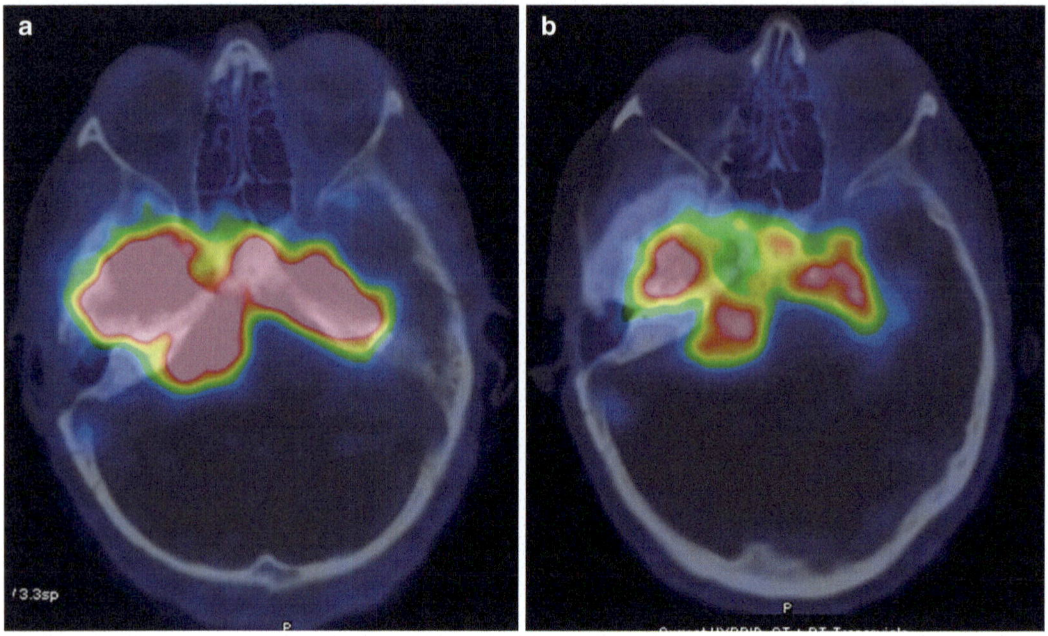

Fig. 37.4 Right parietal meningioma with invasion of the anterior cranial fossa, both cavernous sinuses, middle cranial fossa floor, right ponto-cerebellar angle and both ear canals. 68Ga-DOTATATE PET/CT before (**a**) and after (**b**) PRRT (11,063 MBq of 177Lu-DOTATATE and 8140 MBq of 90Y-DOTATATE): Improvement after treatment. Final response: partial response

and PD in one patient. Moreover, the authors reported that lesion volume after therapy, as estimated by PET/CT imaging, became 81–21% of the baseline volume; mean time to progression was 13.4 months [85].

According to Minutoli et al., the higher specific activity of 111In-Pentetreotide as compared to that reached by 90Y- or 177Lu-labeled DOTA-peptides and a lower injected mass of peptide may be additional favorable features. In fact, increasing the mass dose of ligand or radioligand (i.e., the injected mass of peptide) will eventually result in a saturation of the receptors, since, in vivo, high affinity SSTRs may be expressed at low capacity. As a consequence, less of the administered radioactivity will bind to receptors and become internalized by receptor-expressing tissues and tumors. Actually, the uptake expressed as percentage of the administered dose is a bell-shaped function of the injected mass. This finding might be the result of two opposing effects, (1) a positive effect of increasing ligand concentrations on the rate of internalization by ligand-induced receptor clustering and (2) a negative effect due to saturation of the receptor at increasing ligand concentrations. This retrospective analysis shows that PRRT with 111In-Pentetreotide is safe, well tolerated, and effective on disease control in patients with meningiomas. Moreover, the results are better than that obtained in the majority of the reported series by using hydroxyurea, IFN, somatostatin, or bevacizumab [86] (Fig. 37.4).

37.6 Thyroid Cancer

37.6.1 Differentiated Thyroid Cancer (DTC)

Differentiated non-medullary (follicular and papillary) thyroid cancer is the most common endocrine malignancy (approximately 95% of incident diagnosed cases) and usually has a good long-term prognosis with a 10-year survival rate of 85% to 99% [87, 88]. However, tumor recurrences occur in about 20% of patients, sometimes decades after initial therapy. Radioactive iodine is used for the detection (^{123}I, ^{131}I) and treatment (^{131}I) of recurrent DTC, but 20–30% of recurrent tumors does not uptake radioiodine [89, 90]. The prognosis of patients with DTC is usually favorable when metastatic 131I-avid disease is present. For this reason, 131I is considered the gold standard in the treatment of metastatic disease. Despite the good prognosis, sometimes the conventional therapy may fail. Some DTC patients with advanced disease do not respond or become refractory to 131I, with some of these patients dying within 3–5 years, but there are also long-term survivors with very slow progressive disease. When a patient with DTC is classified as refractory to 131I, there is no indication for further radioiodine treatment and therapy options are limited.

Several studies demonstrated the involvement of SSTRs in the regulation of normal and tumoral thyroid cell proliferation and there is a tendency for less differentiated carcinomas to express a greater variety of SSTR subtypes and thyroid tumor cell lines have been shown to be SSTR positive [91]. Somatostatin receptor subtypes are frequently expressed in pathologically altered thyrocytes in contrast to normal thyroid follicular epithelium. These findings support the concept that PRRT could be a therapeutic tool [92] in patients with advanced thyroid cancer [93–96]. A preliminary experience with 90Y-DOTA-TOC in PPRT in patients with iodine-refractory thyroid cancer provided encouraging results [97]. Different radiolabeled somatostatin analogues have been suggested for therapeutic and diagnostic purposes in the management of non-radioiodine-avid DTC. 68Ga-DOTA-peptides in PET/CT have been suggested as an alternative imaging modality [98, 99]. The therapeutic efficacy of 111In-octreotide, 90Y-DOTATOC, 90Y-DOTA-lanreotide, and 177Lu-DOTATATE has also been studied in some series [100, 101].

In a retrospective analysis, Czepczyński et al. evaluated safety and efficacy of PRRT in patients with advanced, non-iodine avid DTC. Eleven patients, with a history of multiple cycles of radioiodine therapy, increasing thyroglobulin (Tg) and negative whole body scan, were enrolled. After confirming receptor expression by somatostatin receptor scintigraphy, PRRT with 90Y-STT analogues was performed. The patients had lung metastases (nine patients), bone metastases (three patients), local or lymph node recurrences (four patients). Of 11 patients, five deceased before completing the treatment. In the remaining six patients, morphological response, evaluated 3 months after the last course using RECIST criteria showed 1 PR, 2 SD, and 3 PD. Biochemical response based on Tg measurements before and after PRRT showed 1 PR, 4 SD, and 1 PD. Median survival was 21 months from the first course of PRRT. Only minor and transient hematological toxicity was observed in some patients. The AA concluded that PRRT is generally well-tolerated and may be a valuable option for some patients with radioiodine-refractory DTC [102].

Versari et al. presented the results of ^{90}Y-DOTATOC PRRT in a series of patients with progressive radioiodine-negative DTC. ^{68}Ga-DOTATOC-PET/CT was performed to select patients with progressive DTC for PRRT. Forty-one patients with progressive radioiodine-negative DTC were enrolled. 68Ga-DOTATOC PET/CT was positive in 24/41 of radioiodine-negative DTC patients. Based on the high expression of SSTR detected by 68Ga-DOTATOC PET/CT, 13 patients were suitable for PRRT. Two out of 13 patients were not treated due to the lack of fulfillment of other study inclusion criteria. PRRT induced disease control in 7/11 patients (2 PR; 5 SD) with a duration of response of 3.5–11.5 months. Objective response was associated with symptom relief. Functional volume (FV) over time obtained by PET/CT was the only parameter demonstrating a significant difference between lesions responding and non-responding to PRRT ($p = 0.001$). Main PRRT adverse events were nausea, asthenia, and transient hematologic toxicity. One patient experienced permanent renal toxicity. The authors conclude that SSTR imaging provided positive results in more than half of the cases with radioiodine-negative DTC, and about one third of patients were eligible for PRRT.

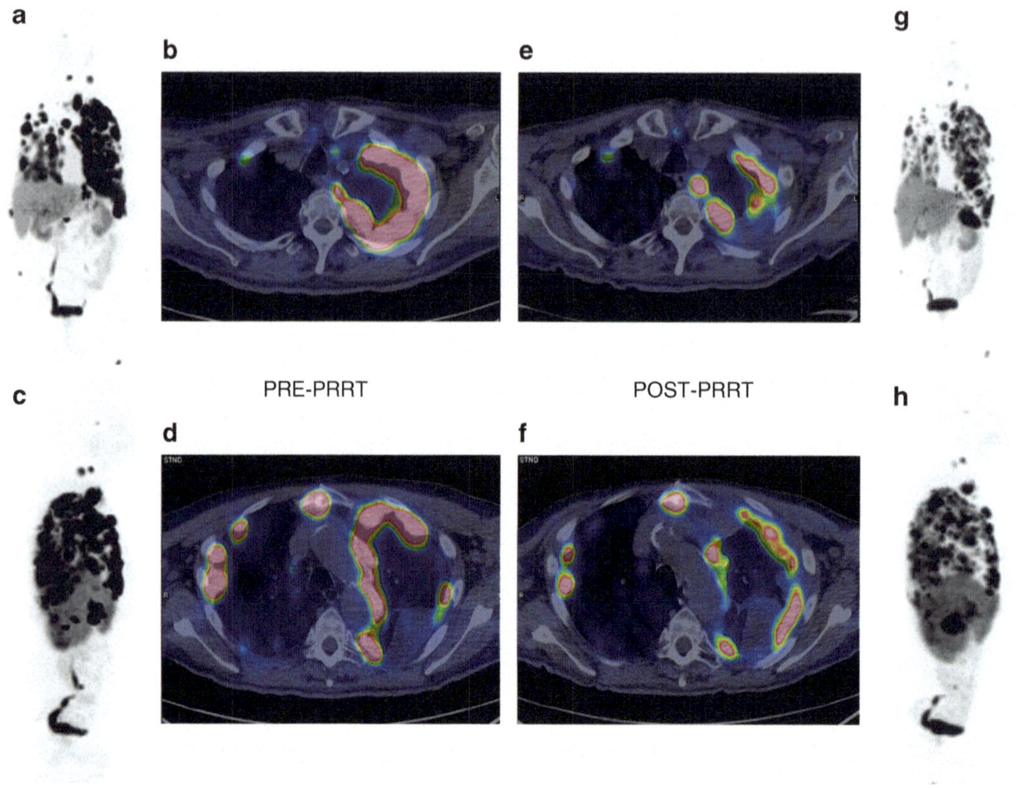

Fig. 37.5 Patient with a thyroid Hurthle cell carcinoma. 68Ga-DOTATOC PET/CT at baseline (**a**–**d**) shows multiple sites of disease in the thyroid bed, lymph nodes, lungs, and bone. The patient underwent six cycles of 90Y-DOTATOC (total activity: 11.7 GBq). At 68Ga-DOTATOC PET/CT after treatment (**e**–**h**), the radiopharmaceutical accumulation persisted but clearly decreased in intensity. The response after treatment was Partial Response and was associated with symptom relief

68Ga-DOTATOC PET/CT seems a reliable tool both for patient selection and evaluation of treatment response. FV determination over time seems to represent a reliable parameter to determine tumor response to PRRT [47] (Fig. 37.5).

37.6.2 Medullary Thyroid Cancer (MTC)

Medullary thyroid cancer is a rare malignancy arising from parafollicular or C cells of the thyroid gland which belongs to the diffuse neuroendocrine system that produces calcitonin (CT) and accounts for about 5% of thyroid malignancies. MTC occurs for 70–80% in sporadic form while 20–30% is hereditary familiar or associated with multiple endocrine neoplasia type MEN 2A and MEN 2B. Usually occurs in older than 40 years, with a slight prevalence in women. This cancer can spread across the lymphatic system, but also by blood to the skeletal, liver, and lung.

MTC has a 10-year survival ranging from 50% to 80% with a worse prognosis than the differentiated carcinoma.

The definitive treatment of this tumor is represented by total thyroidectomy associated with lymphadenectomy central neck lymph node compartment. Although primary surgery is curative in the vast majority of patients treated at an early stage, disease can persist or recur with deleterious effects on quality of life. Local and distant metastases can occur and are the major causes of mortality. Reoperation, embolization, and radiotherapy can improve the outcome for some patients who are not cured by primary surgery, but there is a need for new treatments. Single agent or combination cytotoxic chemotherapeutic regimens administered to patients with MTC are characterized by low response rates (15%–20%) of short duration, although they may be indicated in selected patients. Survival rate for MTC is not as good as for differentiated thyroid cancer. Distant metastases are present in 13% of patients at initial diagnosis and suggest a poor prognosis, with a 10-year survival rate of only 40%. This cancer usually behaves in a relatively indolent manner for most patients. However, approximately 20% of patients have a more aggressive course that requires effective management. In locally advanced unresectable disease with distant metastases or progression, systemic therapies are indicated. Available diagnostic and therapeutic options for this group of patients are limited and various alternative approaches have been investigated. Some authors have shown that metastatic MTC can express somatostatin receptors on ^{68}Ga-DOTA-somatostatin analogue PET-CT imaging. PRRT in metastatic thyroid tumors can be an opportunity after traditional treatment failure but are still under evaluation. In particular in patients with MTC the experience of PRRT is very limited.

Iten et al. in a retrospective analysis of 21 patients treated with ^{90}Y-PRRT DOTATOC at doses of 7.5-19.2GBq in 2–8 cycles, recorded 2 CR, 12 SD, and 7 PD. Patients with small lesions and high uptake had better response [103].

The same author, in a phase II study evaluated PRRT with ^{90}Y-DOTATOC, in 31 patients with MTC [103]. Only 30% of patients were classified as responders, based on the reduction of the levels of CT and showed an improvement in PFS compared to non-responders (PFS 74 months vs 11 months, respectively).

Salavati et al. evaluated response, survival, and long-term safety of systemic [^{90}Y-DOTA]-TOC in a phase II clinical trial with patients with advanced MTC, increasing serum CT levels, and tumor uptake on ^{111}In-octreoscan scintigraphy [104]. Out of 31 patients, 18 (58.1%) had a post-therapeutic prolongation of the serum CT doubling time by at least 100%. Only 9 (29%) of the 31 patients, however, experienced reduction of serum CT levels and were considered responders. The responders had a significantly longer median survival from the time of treatment compared to non-responders (74.5 months—range, 15.7–107 months versus 10.8 months—range, 1.4–85 months; $p = 0.02$). Thirteen percent of patients developed hematologic toxicities, and 23% developed renal toxicities. The degree of ^{111}In-octreoscan tumor uptake was not associated with treatment response or improvement in survival.

As therapeutic options in advanced medullary thyroid cancer are limited and associated with significant toxicity, PRRT using ^{177}Lu-labeled or ^{90}Y-labeled somatostatin analogues may have a significant role in the management of MTC in those patients where PET/CT with ^{68}Ga-labeled somatostatin analogues demonstrates significant SSTR expression. Further investigations are needed to better define the role of PRRT in thyroid cancer (Fig. 37.6).

37.7 Merkel Cell Carcinoma (MCC)

Merkel cell carcinoma is a rare, aggressive malignant neuroendocrine tumor of the skin, often diagnosed with lymph node and distant metastases. 18F-FDG and 68Ga DOTA peptide PET/CT can be used in the evaluation of the disease extent. In advanced patient, non-responders to conventional treatment and with DOTA-peptide PET/CT positivity, sporadic experiences with PRRT (90Y/177Lu DOTATOC/DOTATATE) are reported.

Schmidt MC et al. described two patients with the histopathological diagnosis of Merkel cell carcinoma suffering from extensive lymph node metastases, progressive after sunitinib followed by four chemotherapy cycles of cisplatin and etoposide. The patients underwent PRRT with 90Y-DotaTATE/177Lu-DotaTATE in combination with capecitabine and additional external

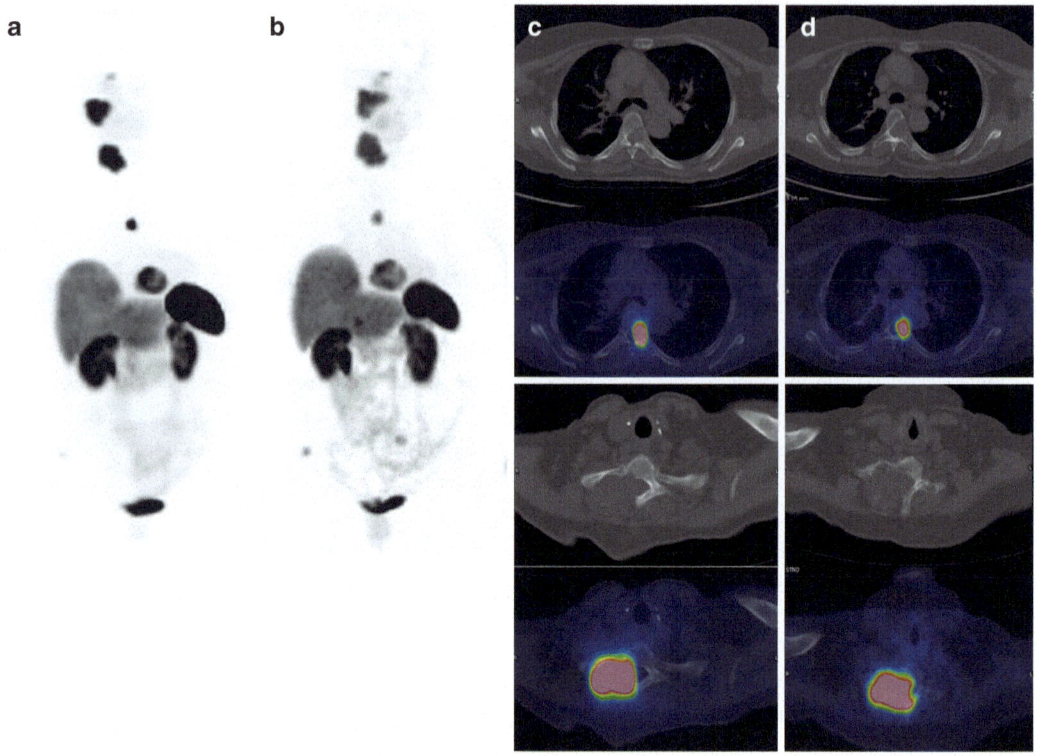

Fig. 37.6 Patient with medullary thyroid carcinoma. 68Ga-DOTATOC PET/CT at baseline (**a**, **c**) demonstrated multiple sites of pathological uptake in lymph nodes and bone. The patient underwent six cycles of 90Y-DOTATOC (total activity: 12.2 GBq). At 68Ga-DOTATOC PET/CT after treatment (**b**, **d**) pathological accumulations persist with a slight reduction in intensity of uptake. Final response to PRRT: stable disease

beam radiotherapy of the cervical and inguinal lymph nodes. Temporary partial response in both patients was achieved [47]. Salavati A et al. obtained an impressive improvement of the clinical symptoms with synchronous use of PRRT (1 cycle of 177Lu-DOTATATE) and radiosensitizing chemotherapy. However, follow-up PET/CT studies showed a mixed pattern of response [46]. Basu et al. reported an excellent partial response of Merkel cell carcinoma with multiple bilobar hepatic metastases to a single cycle of PRRT [105].

Conclusions

Theranostics (therapy and diagnosis) using radiolabeled somatostatin analogues has proven to be a valuable tool in the management of SSTR-expressing tumors. Many studies are available for PRRT in GEP-NETs demonstrating very interesting results. Other neoplasms with SSTR expression can be evaluated and treated according to the same rationale: the experience is limited but promising. Further studies are necessary to confirm these interesting results.

Acknowledgement The authors thank Chiara Coruzzi for the contribution in reference research and proof correction.

References

1. Sollini M, Boni R, Traino AC, Lazzeri E, Pasqualetti F, Modeo L, Mariani G, Petrini M, Erba PA. New approaches for imaging and therapy of solid cancer. Q J Nucl Med Mol Imaging. 2015;59:168–83.
2. Kowalski J, Henze M, Schuhmacher J, Maecke HR, Hofmann M, Haberkorn U. Evaluation of positron emission tomography imaging using [68Ga]-DOTA-D-Phe1-Tyr3-octreotide in comparison to [111In]-DTPAOC SPECT. First results in patients

with neuroendocrine tumors. Mol Imaging Biol. 2003;5:42–8.
3. Buchmann I, Henze M, Engelbrecht S, Eisenhut M, Runz A, Schäfer M, et al. Comparison of 68Ga-DOTATOC PET and 111In-DTPAOC (Octreoscan) SPECT in patients with neuroendocrine tumours. Eur J Nucl Med Mol Imaging. 2007;34(10):1617–26.
4. Sollini M, Erba PA, Fraternali A, Casali M, Di Paolo ML, Froio A, Frasoldati A, Versari A. PET and PET/CT with 68gallium-labeled somatostatin analogues in non GEP-NETs tumors. Sci World J. 2014;2014:194123. https://doi.org/10.1155/2014/194123.
5. Hofmann M, Maecke H, Börner R, Weckesser E, Schöffski P, Oei L, et al. Biokinetics and imaging with the somatostatin receptor PET radioligand (68) Ga-DOTATOC: preliminary data. Eur J Nucl Med. 2001;28(12):1751–7.
6. Wild D, Schmitt JS, Ginj M, Mäcke HR, Bernard BF, Krenning E, et al. DOTA-NOC, a high-affinity ligand of somatostatin receptor subtypes 2, 3 and 5 for labelling with various radiometals. Eur J Nucl Med Mol Imaging. 2003;30(10):1338–47.
7. Ambrosini V, Campana D, Bodei L, Nanni C, Castellucci P, Allegri V, et al. 68Ga-DOTANOC PET/CT clinical impact in patients with neuroendocrine tumors. J Nucl Med. 2010;51(5):669–73.
8. Antunes P, Ginj M, Zhang H, Waser B, Baum RP, Reubi JC, et al. Are radiogallium-labelled DOTA-conjugated somatostatin analogues superior to those labelled with other radiometals? Eur J Nucl Med Mol Imaging. 2007;34(7):982–93.
9. Ambrosini V, Campana D, Tomassetti P, Grassetto G, Rubello D, Fanti S. PET/CT with 68Gallium-DOTA-peptides in NET: an overview. Eur J Radiol. 2011;80:e116–9.
10. Smith-Jones PM, Bischof C, Leimer M, Gludovacz D, Angelberger P, Pangerl T, et al. DOTA-lanreotide: a novel somatostatin analog for tumor diagnosis and therapy. Endocrinology. 1999;140:5136–48.
11. Virgolini I, Szilvasi I, Kurtaran A, Angelberger P, Raderer M, Havlik E, Vorbeck F, Bischof C, Leimer M, Dorner G, Kletter K, Niederle B, Scheithauer W. Smith-Jones P.111In-DOTA-lanreotide: biodistribution, safety and radiation absorbed dose in tumor patients. J Nucl Med. 1998;39:1928–36.
12. Reubi JC, Schär JC, Waser B, Wenger S, Heppeler A, Schmitt JS, Mäcke HR. Affinity profiles for human somatostatin receptor subtypes SST1-SSt5 of somatostatinradiotracer selected for scintigraphic and radiothaerpeutic and radio therapeutic use. Eur J Nucl Med. 2000;27:273–82.
13. Vrachimis A, Stegger L, Wenning C, Noto B, Burg MC, Konnert JR, Allkemper T, Heindel W, Riemann B, Schäfers M. Weckesser M.[(68)Ga]DOTATATE PET/MRI and [(18)F]FDG PET/CT are complementary and superior to diffusion-weighted MR imaging for radioactive-iodine-refractory differentiated thyroid cancer. Eur J Nucl Med Mol Imaging. 2016;43(10):1765–72. https://doi.org/10.1007/s00259-016-3378-5.
14. Afshar-Oromieh A, Wolf MB, Kratochwil C, Giesel FL, Combs SE, Dimitrakopoulou-Strauss A, Gnirs R, Roethke MC, Schlemmer HP, Haberkorn U. Comparison of 68Ga-DOTATOC-PET/CT and PET/MRI hybrid systems in patients with cranial meningioma: initial results. Neuro-Oncology. 2015;17(2):312–9. https://doi.org/10.1093/neuonc/nou131.
15. Boss A, Bisdas S, Kolb A, Hofmann M, Ernemann U, Claussen CD, Pfannenberg C, Pichler BJ, Reimold M, Stegger L. Hybrid PET/MRI of intracranial masses: initial experiences and comparison to PET/CT. J Nucl Med. 2010;51(8):1198–205. https://doi.org/10.2967/jnumed.110.074773.
16. Thorwarth D, Müller AC, Pfannenberg C, Beyer T. Combined PET/MR imaging using (68) Ga-DOTATOC for radiotherapy treatment planning in meningioma patients. Recent Results Cancer Res. 2013;194:425–39.
17. Haug AR, Auernhammer CJ, Wängler B, Schmidt GP, Uebleis C, Göke B, Cumming P, Bartenstein P, Tiling R, Hacker M. ^{68}Ga-DOTATATE PET/CT for the early prediction of response to somatostatin receptor-mediated radionuclide therapy in patients with well-differentiated neuroendocrine tumors. J Nucl Med. 2010;51:1349–56.
18. Kroiss A, Putzer D, Uprimny C, Decristoforo C, Gabriel M, Santner W, Kranewitter C, Warwitz B, Waitz D, Kendler D, Virgolini IJ. Functional imaging in phaeochromocytoma and neuroblastoma with ^{68}Ga-DOTA-Tyr 3-octreotide positron emission tomography and 123I-metaiodobenzylguanidine. Eur J Nucl Med Mol Imaging. 2011;38:865–73.
19. Kroiss A, Putzer D, Frech A, Decristoforo C, Uprimny C, Gasser RW, Shulkin BL, Url C, Widmann G, Prommegger R, Sprinzl GM, Fraedrich G, Virgolini IJ. A retrospective comparison between 68Ga-DOTA-TOC PET/CT and 18F-DOPA PET/CT in patients with extra-adrenal paraganglioma. Eur J Nucl Med Mol Imaging. 2013;40(12):1800–8. https://doi.org/10.1007/s00259-013-2548-y.
20. Mittal BR, Agrawal K, Shukla J, Bhattacharya A, Singh B, Sood A, Bhansali A. Ga-68 DOTATATE PET/CT in neuroendocrine tumors: initial experience. J Postgrad Med Edu Res. 2013; 47:1–6.
21. Gupta SK, Singla S, Karunanithi S, Damle N, Bal C. Peptide receptor radionuclide therapy with (177) Lu DOTATATE in a case of recurrent carotid body paraganglioma with spinal metastases. Clin Nucl Med. 2014;39(5):440–1. https://doi.org/10.1097/RLU.0000000000000273.
22. Puranik AD, Kulkarni HR, Singh A, Baum RP. Peptide receptor radionuclide therapy with (90) Y/ (177)Lu-labelled peptides for inoperable head and neck paragangliomas (glomus tumours). Eur J Nucl Med Mol Imaging. 2015;42(8):1223–30. https://doi.org/10.1007/s00259-015-3029-2.

23. Vasamiliette J, Hohenberger P, Schoenberg S, Diehl S, Dinter DJ, Marx A, Stroebel P, Strauss LG, Dimitrakopoulou-Strauss A. Treatment monitoring with ^{18}F-FDG PET in metastatic thymoma after ^{90}Y-Dotatoc and selective internal radiation treatment (SIRT). Hell J Nucl Med. 2009;12:271–3.
24. Sollini M, Farioli D, Froio A, Chella A, Asti M, Boni R, Grassi E, Roncali M, Versari A, Erba PA. Brief report on the use of radiolabeled somatostatin analogs for the diagnosis and treatment of metastatic small-cell lung cancer patients. J Thorac Oncol. 2013;8:1095–101.
25. Lapa C, Hänscheid H, Wild V, Pelzer T, Schirbel A, Werner RA, Droll S, Herrmann K, Buck AK, Lückerath K. Somatostatin receptor expression in small cell lung cancer as a prognostic marker and a target for peptide receptor radionuclide therapy. Oncotarget. 2016;7(15):20033–40. 10.18632/oncotarget.7706.
26. Parghane RV, Talole S, Prabhash K, Basu S. Clinical response profile of metastatic/advanced pulmonary neuroendocrine tumors to peptide receptor radionuclide therapy with 177Lu-DOTATATE. Clin Nucl Med. 2017;42(6):428–35. https://doi.org/10.1097/RLU.0000000000001639.
27. Gehler B, Paulsen F, Oksüz MO, Hauser TK, Eschmann SM, Bares R, Pfannenberg C, Bamberg M, Bartenstein P, Belka C, Ganswindt U. [^{68}Ga]-DOTATOC-PET/CT for meningioma IMRT treatment planning. Radiat Oncol. 2009;4:56.
28. Heute D, Kostron H, von Guggenberg E, Ingorokva S, Gabriel M, Dobrozemsky G, Stockhammer G, Virgolini IJ. Response of recurrent high-grade glioma to treatment with (90)Y-DOTATOC. J Nucl Med. 2010;51:397–400.
29. Nyuyki F, Plotkin M, Graf R, Michel R, Steffen I, Denecke T, Geworski L, Fahdt D, Brenner W, Wurm R. Potential impact of (68)Ga-DOTATOC PET/CT on stereotactic radiotherapy planning of meningiomas. Eur J Nucl Med Mol Imaging. 2010;37: 310–8.
30. Gains JE, Bomanji JB, Fersht NL, Sullivan T, D'Souza D, Sullivan KP, Aldridge M, Waddington W, Gaze MN. ^{177}Lu-DOTATATE molecular radiotherapy for childhood neuroblastoma. J Nucl Med. 2011;52:1041–7.
31. Waitz D, Putzer D, Kostron H, Virgolini IJ. Treatment of high-grade glioma with radiolabeled peptides. Methods. 2011;55:223–9.
32. Graf R, Plotkin M, Steffen IG, Wurm R, Wust P, Brenner W, Budach V, Badakhshi H. Magnetic resonance imaging, computed tomography, and ^{68}Ga-DOTATOC positron emission tomography for imaging skull base meningiomas with infracranial extension treated with stereotactic radiotherapy--a case series. Head Face Med. 2012;8:1.
33. Hänscheid H, Sweeney RA, Flentje M, Buck AK, Löhr M, Samnick S, Kreissl M, Verburg FA. PET SUV correlates with radionuclide uptake in peptide receptor therapy in meningioma. Eur J Nucl Med Mol Imaging. 2012;39:1284–8.
34. Graf R, Nyuyki F, Steffen IG, Michel R, Fahdt D, Wust P, Brenner W, Budach V, Wurm R, Plotkin M. Contribution of 68Ga-DOTATOC PET/CT to target volume delineation of skull base meningiomas treated with stereotactic radiation therapy. Int J Radiat Oncol Biol Phys. 2013;85(1):68–73. https://doi.org/10.1016/j.ijrobp.2012.03.021.
35. Combs SE, Welzel T, Habermehl D, Rieken S, Dittmar JO, Kessel K, Jäkel O, Haberkorn U, Debus J. Prospective evaluation of early treatment outcome in patients with meningiomas treated with particle therapy based on target volume definition with MRI and 68Ga-DOTATOC-PET. Acta Oncol. 2013;52(3):514–20. https://doi.org/10.3109/0284186X.2013.762996.
36. Golemi A, Ambrosini A, Cecchi P, Ruiu A, Chondrogiannis S, Farsad M, Rubello D. (68) Ga-DOTANOC PET/CT detection of multiple extracranial localizations in a patient with anaplastic meningioma. Rev Esp Med Nucl Imagen Mol. 2015;34(4):258–60. https://doi.org/10.1016/j.remn.2015.03.003.
37. Collamati F, Pepe A, Bellini F, Bocci V, Chiodi G, Cremonesi M, De Lucia E, Ferrari ME, Frallicciardi PM, Grana CM, Marafini M, Mattei I, Morganti S, Patera V, Piersanti L, Recchia L, Russomando A, Sarti A, Sciubba A, Senzacqua M, Solfaroli Camillocci E, Voena C, Pinci D, Faccini R. Toward radioguided surgery with β-decays: uptake of a somatostatin analogue, DOTATOC, in meningioma and high-grade glioma. J Nucl Med. 2015;56(1):3–8. https://doi.org/10.2967/jnumed.114.145995.
38. Madani I, Lomax AJ, Albertini F, Trnková P, Weber DC. Dose-painting intensity-modulated proton therapy for intermediate- and high-risk meningioma. Radiat Oncol. 2015;10:72. https://doi.org/10.1186/s13014-015-0384-x.
39. Seystahl K, Stoecklein V, Schüller U, Rushing E, Nicolas G, Schäfer N, Ilhan H, Pangalu A, Weller M, Tonn JC, Sommerauer M, Albert NL. Somatostatin receptor-targeted radionuclide therapy for progressive meningioma: benefit linked to 68Ga-DOTATATE/−TOC uptake. Neuro-Oncology. 2016;18(11):1538–47.
40. Gabriel M, Andergassen U, Putzer D, Kroiss A, Waitz D, Von Guggenberg E, Kendler D, Virgolini IJ. Individualized peptide-related-radionuclide-therapy concept using different radiolabelled somatostatin analogs in advanced cancer patients. Q J Nucl Med Mol Imaging. 2010;54:92–9.
41. Damle NA, Bal C, Gupta S, Singhal A. Discordance in 68Ga-DOTANOC and 177Lu-DOTATATE uptake in diagnostic and post-therapy scans in patients with medullary thyroid cancer-likely reasons. J Cancer Res Ther. 2013;9(4):754–5.
42. Versari A, Sollini M, Frasoldati A, Fraternali A, Filice A, Froio A, Asti M, Fioroni F, Cremonini

N, Putzer D, Erba PA. Differentiated thyroid cancer: a new perspective with radiolabeled somatostatin analogues for imaging and treatment of patients. Thyroid. 2014;24(4):715–26. https://doi.org/10.1089/thy.2013.0225.
43. Traub-Weidinger T, Putzer D, von Guggenberg E, Dobrozemsky G, Nilica B, Kendler D, Bale R, Virgolini IJ. Multiparametric PET imaging in thyroid malignancy characterizing tumour heterogeneity: somatostatin receptors and glucose metabolism. Eur J Nucl Med Mol Imaging. 2015;42(13):1995–2001. https://doi.org/10.1007/s00259-015-3114-6.
44. Basu S, Joshi A. ^{68}Ga DOTATATE PET/CT in differentiated thyroid carcinoma with fibular metastasis and mixed response to sorafenib. Clin Nucl Med. 2016;41(10):772–3.
45. Elboğa U, Özkaya M, Sayiner ZA, Çelen YZ. Lu-177 labelled peptide treatment for radioiodine refractory differentiated thyroid carcinoma. BMJ Case Rep. 2016;8:2016.
46. Salavati A, Prasad V, Schneider CP, Herbst R, Baum RP. Peptide receptor radionuclide therapy of Merkel cell carcinoma using (177)lutetium-labeled somatostatin analogs in combination with radiosensitizing chemotherapy: a potential novel treatment based on molecular pathology. Ann Nucl Med. 2012;26(4):365–9. 1.
47. Schmidt MC, Uhrhan K, Markiefka B, et al. $^{(68)}$Ga-DotaTATE PET-CT followed by Peptide Receptor Radiotherapy in combination with capecitabine in two patients with Merkel Cell Carcinoma. Int J Clin Exp Med. 2012;5(4):363–6.
48. Epstude M, Tornquist K, Riklin C, di Lenardo F, Winterhalder R, Hug U, Strobel K. Comparison of (18)F-FDG PET/CT and $^{(68)}$Ga-DOTATATE PET/CT imaging in metastasized merkel cell carcinoma. Clin Nucl Med. 2013;38:283–4.
49. Chrisoulidou A, Kaltsas G, Ilias I, Grossman AB. The diagnosis and management of malignant phaeochromocytoma and paraganglioma. Endocr Relat Cancer. 2007;14:569–85.
50. Safford SD, Coleman RE, Gockerman JP, Moore J, Feldman JM, Leight GS Jr, Tyler DS, Olson JA Jr. Iodine −131 metaiodobenzylguanidine is an effective treatment for malignant pheochromocytoma and paraganglioma. Surgery. 2003;134:956–62. discussion 962–953
51. Kwekkeboom DJ, Teunissen JJ, Bakker WH, Kooij PP, de Herder WW, Feelders RA, van Eijck CH, Esser JP, Kam BL, Krenning EP. Radiolabeled somatostatin analog [177Lu-DOTA0, Tyr3]octreotate in patients with endocrine gastroenteropancreatic tumors. J Clin Oncol. 2005;23:2754–62.
52. Van Essen M, Krenning EP, Kooij PP, Bakker WH, Feelders RA, de Herder WW, Wolbers JG, Kwekkeboom DJ. Effects of therapy with [177Lu-DOTA0, Tyr3]octreotate in patients with paraganglioma, meningioma, small cell lung carcinoma, and melanoma. J Nucl Med. 2006;47:1599–606.
53. Zovato S, Kumanova A, Demattè S, Sansovini M, Bodei L, Di Sarra D, Casagranda E, Severi S, Ambrosetti A, Schiavi F, Opocher G, Paganelli G. Peptide receptor radionuclide therapy (PRRT) with 177LuDOTATATE in individuals with neck or mediastinal paraganglioma (PGL). Horm Metab Res. 2012;44:411–4.
54. Cecchin D, Schiavi F, Fanti S, Favero M, Manara R, Fassina A, Briani C, Allegri V, Sansovini M, Bui F, Paganelli G, Opocher G. Peptide receptor radionuclide therapy in a case of multiple spinal canal and cranial paragangliomas. J Clin Oncol. 2011;29:171–4.
55. Makis W, McCann K, McEwan AJB. The challenges of treating paraganglioma patients with 177Lu-DOTATATE PRRT: catecholamine crises, tumor lysis syndrome and the need for modification of treatment protocols. Nucl Med Mol Imaging. 2015;49:223–30. https://doi.org/10.1007/s13139-015-0332-6.
56. Lo Russo G, Pusceddu S, Prinzi N, Imbimbo M, Proto C, Signorelli D, Vitali M, Ganzinelli M, Maccauro M, Buzzoni R, Seregni E, de Braud F, Garassino MC. Peptide receptor radionuclide therapy: focus on bronchial neuroendocrine tumors. Tumor Biol. 2016;37:12991–3003. https://doi.org/10.1007/s13277-016-5258-9.
57. Waldherr C, Pless M, Maecke HR, Haldemann A, Mueller-Brand J. The clinical value of [90Y-DOTA]-D-Phe1-Tyr3-octreotide (90Y-DOTATOC) in the treatment of neuroendocrine tumours: a clinical phase II study. Ann Oncol. 2001;12:941–5.
58. Waldherr C, Pless M, Maecke HR, Schumacher T, Crazzolara A, Nitzsche EU, Haldemann A, Mueller-Brand J. Tumor response and clinical benefit in neuroendocrine tumors after 7.4 GBq (90) YDOTATOC. J Nucl Med. 2002;43:610–6.
59. Bodei L, Cremonesi M, Zoboli S, Grana C, Bartolomei M, Rocca P, Caracciolo M, Mäcke HR, Chinol M, Paganelli G. Receptor mediated radionuclide therapy with 90Y-DOTATOC in association with amino acid infusion: a phase I study. Eur J Nucl Med Mol Imaging. 2003;30:207–16.
60. Bodei L, Cremonesi M, Grana C, Rocca P, Bartolomei M, Chinol M, Paganelli G. Receptor radionuclide therapy with 90Y-[DOTA]0-Tyr3-octreotide (90Y-DOTATOC) in neuroendocrine tumours. Eur J Nucl Med Mol Imaging. 2004;31:1038–46.
61. Bodei L, Cremonesi M, Grana CM, Fazio N, Iodice S, Baio SM, Bartolomei M, Lombardo D, Ferrari ME, Sansovini M, Chinol M, Paganelli G. Peptide receptor radionuclide therapy with 177Lu-DOTATATE: the IEO phase I–II study. Eur J Nucl Med Mol Imaging. 2011;38:2125–35.
62. Imhof A, Brunner P, Marincek N, Briel M, Schindler C, Rasch H, Mäcke HR, Rochlitz C, Müller-Brand J, Walter MA. Response, survival, and long-term

toxicity after therapy with the radiolabeled somatostatin analogue [90YDOTA]-TOC in metastasized neuroendocrine cancers. J Clin Oncol. 2011;29:2416–23.
63. Van Essen M, Krenning EP, Bakker WH, de Herder WW, van Aken MO, Kwekkeboom DJ. Peptide receptor radionuclide therapy with 177Lu-octreotate in patients with foregut carcinoid tumours of bronchial, gastric and thymic origin. Eur J Nucl Med Mol Imaging. 2007;34:1219–27.
64. Ianniello A, Sansovini M, Severi S, Nicolini S, Grana CM, Massri K, Bongiovanni A, Antonuzzo L, Di Iorio V, Sarnelli A, Caroli P, Monti M, Scarpi E, Paganelli G. Peptide receptor radionuclide therapy with (177)Lu-DOTATATE in advanced bronchial carcinoids: prognostic role of thyroid transcription factor 1 and (18)F-FDG PET. Eur J Nucl Med Mol Imaging. 2016;43(6):1040–6.
65. Khan S, Krenning EP, van Essen M, Kam BL, Teunissen JJ, Kwekkeboom DJ. Quality of life in 265 patients with gastroenteropancreatic or bronchial neuroendocrine tumors treated with [177Lu-DOTA0,Tyr3]octreotate. J Nucl Med. 2011;52:1361–8.
66. Diakatou E, Alexandraki KI, Tsolakis AV, Kontogeorgos G, Chatzellis E, Leonti A, Kaltsas GA. Somatostatin and dopamine receptor expression in neuroendocrine neoplasms: correlation of immunohistochemical findings with somatostatin receptor scintigraphy visual scores. Clin Endocrinol. 2015;83(3):420–8.
67. Cives M, Strosberg J. Radionuclide therapy for neuroendocrine tumors. Curr Oncol Rep. 2017;19:9. https://doi.org/10.1007/s11912-017-0567-8.
68. Soga J, Yakuwa Y, Osaka M. Evaluation of 342 cases of mediastinal/thymic carcinoids collected from literature: a comparative study between typical carcinoids and atypical varieties. Ann Thorac Cardiovasc Surg. 1999;5:285–92.
69. Koukouraki S, Strauss LG, Georgoulias V, Eisenhut M, Haberkorn U, Dimitrakopoulou-Strauss A. Comparison of the pharmacokinetics of 68Ga-DOTATOC and [18F]FDG in patients with metastatic neuroendocrine tumours scheduled for 90Y-DOTATOC therapy. Eur J Nucl Med Mol Imaging. 2006;33(10):1115–22.
70. Ambrosini V, Nanni C, Zompatori M, Campana D, Tomassetti P, Castellucci P, Allegri V, Rubello D, Montini G, Franchi R, Fanti S. 68Ga-DOTA-NOC PET/CT in comparison with CT for the detection of bone metastasis in patients with neuroendocrine tumours. Eur J Nucl Med Mol Imaging. 2010;37(4):722–7.
71. Miederer M, Seidl S, Buck A, Scheidhauer K, Wester HJ, Schwaiger M, Perren A. Correlation of immunohistopathological expression of somatostatin receptor 2 with standardised uptake values in 68Ga-DOTATOC PET/CT. Eur J Nucl Med Mol Imaging. 2009;36(1):48–52.
72. Kwekkeboom DJ, de Herder WW, Kam BL, van Eijck CH, van Essen M, Kooij PP, Feelders RA, van Aken MO, Krenning EP. Treatment with the radiolabeled somatostatin analog [177 Lu-DOTA 0,Tyr3] octreotate: toxicity, efficacy, and survival. J Clin Oncol. 2008;26:2124–30.
73. Teunissen JJ, Kwekkeboom DJ, Krenning EP. Quality of life in patients with gastroenteropancreatic tumors treated with [177Lu-DOTA0,Tyr3] octreotate. J Clin Oncol. 2004;22:2724–9.
74. Louis DN, Ohgaki H, Wiestler OD, Cavenee WK, Burger PC, Jouvet A, Scheithauer BW, Kleihues P. The 2007 WHO classification of tumours of the central nervous system. Acta Neuropathol. 2007;114:97–109.
75. Gerster-Gilliéron K, Forrer F, Maecke H, Mueller-Brand J, Merlo A, Cordier D. 90Y-DOTATOC as a therapeutic option for complex recurrent or progressive meningiomas. J Nucl Med. 2015;56(11):1748–51. https://doi.org/10.2967/jnumed.115.155853.
76. Goldsmith BJ, Wara WM, Wilson CB, Larson DA. Postoperative irradiation for subtotally resected meningiomas: a retrospective analysis of 140 patients treated from 1967 to 1990. J Neurosurg. 1994;80:195–2015.
77. Nishio S, Morioka T, Inamura T, Takeshita I, Fukui M, Sasaki M, Nakamura K, Wakisaka S. Radiation-induced brain tumours: potential late complications of radiation therapy for brain tumours. Acta Neurochir. 1998;140:763–70.
78. Milker-Zabel S, Zabel A, Schulz-Ertner D, Schlegel W, Wannenmacher M, Debus J. Fractionated stereotactic radiotherapy in patients with benign or atypica intracranial meningioma: long-term experience and prognostic factors. Int J Radiat Oncol Biol Phys. 2005;61:809–16.
79. Reubi JC, Maurer R, Lamberts SW. Somatostatin binding sites in human leptomeninx. Neurosci Lett. 1986;70:183.
80. Dutour A, Kumar U, Panetta R, Ouafik L, Fina F, Sasi R, Patel YC. Expression of somatostatin receptor subtypes in human brain tumors. Int J Cancer. 1998;76:620.
81. Barresi V, Alafaci C, Salpietro F, Tuccari G. Sstr2A immunohistochemical expression in human meningiomas: is there a correlation with the histological grade, proliferation or microvessel density? Oncol Rep. 2008;20:485.
82. Sabet A, Ahmadzadehfar H, Herrlinger U, Wilinek W, Biersack HJ, Ezziddin S. Successful radiopeptide targeting of metastatic anaplastic meningioma: case report. Radiat Oncol. 2011;6:94.
83. Green S, Weiss GR. Southwest oncology group standard response criteria, endpoint definitions and toxicity criteria. Investig New Drugs. 1992;10:239.
84. Bartolomei M, Bodei L, De Cicco C, Grana CM, Cremonesi M, Botteri E, Baio SM, Aricò D, Sansovini M, Paganelli G. Peptide receptor radionuclide therapy with 90Y_DOTATOC in recur-

rent meningioma. Eur J Nucl Med Mol Imaging. 2009;36:1407.

85. Kreissl MC, Hänscheid H, Löhr M, Verburg FA, Schiller M, Lassmann M, Reiners C, Samnick SS, Buck AK, Flentje M, Sweeney RA. Combination of peptide receptor radionuclide therapy with fractionated external beam radiotherapy for treatment of advanced symptomatic meningioma. Radiat Oncol. 2012;7:99.
86. Minutoli F, Amato E, Sindoni A, Cardile D, Conti A, Herberg A, Baldari S. Peptide receptor radionuclide therapy in patients with inoperable meningiomas: our experience and review of the literature. Cancer Biother Radiopharm. 2014;29(5):193–9. https://doi.org/10.1089/cbr.2013.1599.
87. Eustatia-Rutten CF, Corssmit EP, Biermasz NR, Pereira AM, Romijn JA, Smit JW. Survival and death causes in differentiated thyroid carcinoma. J Clin Endocrinol Metab. 2006;91:313–9.
88. Sherman SI. Thyroid carcinoma. Lancet. 2003;361:501–11.
89. Durante C, Haddy N, Baudin E, Leboulleux S, Hartl D, Travagli JP, Caillou B, Ricard M, Lumbroso JD, De Vathaire F, Schlumberger M. Long-term outcome of 444 patients with distant metastases from papillary and follicular thyroid carcinoma: bene ts and limits of radio-iodine therapy. J Clin Endocrinol Metab. 2006;91:2892–9.
90. Rouxel A, Hejblum G, Bernier MO, Boëlle PY, Ménégaux F, Mansour G, Hoang C, Aurengo A, Leenhardt L. Prognostic factors associated with the survival of patients developing loco-regional recurrences of differentiated thyroid carcinomas. J Clin Endocrinol Metab. 2004;89(11):5362–8.
91. Forssell-Aronsson EB, Nilsson O, Bejegard SA, Kolby L, Bernhardt P, Molne J, Hashemi SH, Wangberg B, Tisell LE, Ahlman H. 111InDTPA-D-Phe1-octreotide binding and somatostatin receptor subtypes in thyroid tumors. J Nucl Med. 2000;41:636–42.
92. Pisarek H, Stepien T, Kubiak R, Borkowska E, Pawlikowski M. Expression of somatostatin receptor subtypes in human thyroid tumors: the immunohistochemical and molecular biology (RT-PCR) investigation. Thyroid Res. 2009;2:1.
93. De Jong M, Bernard BF, De Bruin E, Van Gameren A, Bakker WH, Visser TJ, Ma¨cke HR, Krenning EP. Internalization of radiolabeled [DTPA0] octreotide and [DOTA0,Tyr3]octreotide: peptides for somatostatin receptor-targeted scintigraphy and radionuclide therapy. Nucl Med Commun. 1998;19:283–8.
94. Eberle AN, Mild G. Receptor-mediated tumor targeting with radiopeptides. Part 1. General principles and methods. J Recept Signal Transduct Res. 2009;29:1–37.
95. Waldherr C, Schumacher T, Pless M, Crazzolara A, Maecke HR, Nitzsche EU, Haldemann A, Mueller-Brand J. Radiopeptide transmitted internal irradiation of noniodophil thyroid cancer and conventionally untreatable medullary thyroid cancer using. Nucl Med Commun. 2001;22:673–8.
96. Gorges R, Kahaly G, Müller-Brand J, Mäcke H, Roser HW, Bockisch A. Radionuclide-labeled somatostatin analogues for diagnostic and therapeutic purposes in nonmedullary thyroid cancer. Thyroid. 2011;11:647–59.
97. Iten F, Muller B, Schindler C, Rasch H, Rochlitz C, Oertli D, Maecke HR, Muller-Brand J. Walter MA. [(90)YttriumDOTA]-TOC response is associated with survival benefit in iodine-refractory thyroid cancer: long-term results of a phase 2 clinical trial. Cancer. 2009;115:2052–62.
98. Carreras C, Kulkarni HR, Baum RP. Rare metastases detected by (68)Ga-somatostatin receptor PET/CT in patients with neuroendocrine tumors. Recent Results Cancer Res. 2013;194:379–84.
99. Baum RP, Kulkarni HR, Carreras C. Peptides and receptors in image-guided therapy: theranostics for neuroendocrine neoplasms. Semin Nucl Med. 2012;42:190–207.
100. Baudin E, Schlumberger M. New therapeutic approaches for metastatic thyroid carcinoma. Lancet Oncol. 2007;8:148–56.
101. Bertagna F, Giubbini R, Savelli G, Pizzocaro C, Rodella C, Biasiotto G, Lucchini S, Maroldi R, Rosenbaum J, Alavi A. A patient with medullary thyroid carcinoma and right ventricular cardiac metastasis treated by (90)Y-Dotatoc. Hell J Nucl Med. 2009;12:161–4.
102. Czepczyński R, Matysiak-Grześ M, Gryczyńska M, Bączyk M, Wyszomirska A, Stajgis M, Ruchała M. Peptide receptor radionuclide therapy of differentiated thyroid cancer: efficacy and toxicity. Arch Immunol Ther Exp. 2015;63(2):147–54.
103. Iten F, Muller B, Schindler C, Rochlitz C, Oertli D, Macke HR, Muller-Brand J. Walter MA response to [90Yttrium-DOTA]-TOC treatment is associated with long-term survival benefit in metastasized medullary thyroid cancer: a phase II clinical trial. Clin Cancer Res. 2007;13(22 Pt 1):6696–702.
104. Salavati A, Puranik A, Kulkarni HR, Budiawan H, Baum RP. Peptide receptor radionuclide therapy (PRRT) of medullary and nonmedullary thyroid cancer using radiolabeled somatostatin analogues. Semin Nucl Med. 2016;46(3):215–24.
105. Basu S, Ranade R. Favorable response of metastatic merkel cell carcinoma to targeted 177Lu-DOTATATE therapy: will PRRT evolve to become an important approach in receptor-positive cases? J Nucl Med Technol. 2016;44(2):85–7. https://doi.org/10.2967/jnmt.115.163527. Review

The manufacturer's authorised representative in the EU is Springer Nature Customer Service Centre GmbH, Europaplatz 3, 69115 Heidelberg, Germany. If you have any concerns regarding our products, please contact ProductSafety@springernature.com

Printed and bound by CPI Group (UK) Ltd, Croydon, CR0 4YY

30/09/2026

02225231-0005